Ultrasound and Endoscopic Surgery in Obstetrics and Gynaecology

Springer-Verlag London Ltd.

Dirk Timmerman, Jan Deprest and Tom Bourne

Ultrasound and Endoscopic Surgery in Obstetrics and Gynaecology

A Combined Approach to Diagnosis and Treatment

With 150 Figures
including 73 Colour Plates

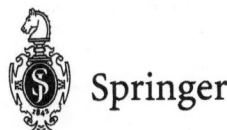

Springer

Dirk Timmerman, MD, PhD
Jan Deprest, MD, PhD
Department of Obstetrics and Gynaecology, U. Z. Gasthuisberg,
University Hospitals K.U. Leuven, Herestraat 49, B-3000 Leuven, Belgium

Tom Bourne, MBBS, MRCOG, PhD
Department of Obstetrics and Gynaecology, St George's Hospital Medical School,
Cranmer Terrace, London SW17 0RE, UK

British Library Cataloguing in Publication Data
Ultrasound and endoscopic surgery in obstetrics and
    gynaecology: a combined approach to diagnosis and
    treatment
    1. Ultrasonics in obstetrics 2. Generative organs, Female –
    Ultrasonic imaging 3. Generative organs, Female – Endoscopic
    surgery 4. Obstetrics – Surgery 5. Endoscopic surgery
    I. Timmerman, Dirk II. Deprest, Jan. A. III. Bourne, Tom
    618′.047543

Library of Congress Cataloging-in-Publication Data
Ultrasound and endoscopic surgery in obstetrics and gynaecology: a combined approach
to diagnosis and treatment / Dirk Timmerman, Jan Deprest, and Tom Bourne, (eds.).
    p. ; cm.
    Includes bibliographical references and index.

    1. Generative organs, Female – Ultrasonic imaging. 2. Ultrasonics in obstetrics. 3.
    Generative organs, Female – Endoscopic surgery. I. Timmerman, Dirk, 1964– II. Deprest,
    J. A. III. Bourne, Tom H., 1959–
    [DNLM: 1. Genital Diseases, Female – ultrasonography. 2. Pregnancy
    Complications – ultrasonography. 3. Endoscopy. 4. Gynecologic Surgical Procedures. 5.
    Obstetric Surgical Procedures. WP 141 U455 2002]
RG107.5.U4 U48 2002
618.2′07543–dc21   2002070752

Springer-Verlag London Berlin Heidelberg
a member of BertelsmannSpringer Science+Business Media GmbH
http://www.springer.co.uk

ISBN 978-1-4471-1170-2   ISBN 978-1-4471-0655-5 (eBook)
DOI 10.1007/978-1-4471-0655-5

Typeset by EXPO Holdings, Malaysia

28/3830-543210 Printed on acid-free paper SPIN 10637516

Foreword

This is a unique book in that it brings together the two key investigative techniques in Gynaecology and Obstetrics, namely ultrasound and endoscopy. So often in the past they were regarded by their exponents as rival techniques but it is now recognised that they are complementary to each other. Consequently future trainees in endoscopy should become efficient in transvaginal sonography and vice versa.

Ultrasound can be used to study the morphology of the pelvic organs such as the endometrium, myometrium and ovaries, and being non-invasive, safe and convenient can be repeated as often as is deemed necessary to monitor changes over time; for example in the investigation of the infertile woman the development of the dominant follicle, the maturation of the endometrium and the formation of the corpus luteum can be documented throughout the menstrual cycle while growth of ovarian cysts can be precisely measured to determine the need for surgery. A seldom-mentioned strength of the ultrasound examination is its interactive quality, for example by performing abdominal palpation during the scan, the mobility of the uterus and ovaries can be assessed. Also the images as they appear can be shown to the patient to aid understanding. Ultrasound can also determine function and the use of Doppler has been used for example to access endometrial receptivity, follicular maturity and the likelihood of malignancy in the endometrium or ovary.

Endoscopy is used to examine internal and external surfaces of organs under magnification and is superior to ultrasound for example in determining small lesions of the endometrium, peritoneal endometriosis or adhesions. However being invasive, anaesthesia usually has to be used and there is a limit to the number of times it can be repeated. Furthermore the technique does not assess function in the same way as ultrasound. Both techniques allow biopsy; ultrasound guided needle biopsy is mainly used in gynaecology to aspirate follicles in assisted conception treatment and in obstetrics the placenta and amniotic fluid are sampled for prenatal diagnosis. Tissue biopsy is usually performed by laparoscopy or hysteroscopy so that larger samples can be obtained.

With the advent of outpatient hysteroscopy under minimal or no sedation it was accepted that this was the optimal method of assessing the endometrium. However with the development of saline contrast sonohysterography (hydrosonography) and 3D ultrasound many of the advantages of hysteroscopy and indeed laparoscopy are being challenged. For example study of the endometrium for polyps and small fibroids and even early carcinoma may be equally effectively performed using hydrosonography while evaluation of the uterus for congenital malformations or assessment of fallopian tube patency with 3D ultrasound may become established as alternatives to laparoscopic investigations.

Probably the greatest advantage of endoscopy is that it is now used extensively to perform a large number of operative procedures and it is now possible to move seamlessly from investigative endoscopy to a definitive surgical procedure if it is required either through the laporoscope or hysteroscope. This book encompasses all aspects of ultrasonic and endoscopic diagnosis in gynaecology and also in early pregnancy complications and prenatal diagnosis. In addition all endoscopic surgical procedures are also described and discussed in impressive detail. The book is unashamedly postgraduate, to be read by the trainee who has already grasped the essentials of both techniques. An unusual aspect is that the techniques are described in relation to patient symptomatology such as menorrhagia, amenorrhoea, infertility, miscarriage etc. which gives the reader a strong clinical perspective to the relative strengths of these methods. Each chapter is equivalent to a high quality contemporary review by acknowledged masters in the field. For the trainee in gynaecological ultrasound and laparoscopic surgery it is essential reading and a book to return to again and again.

Professor Stuart Campbell, DSc, FRCP Ed, FACOG, FRCOG
Create Health Clinic
London
UK

Foreword

When performing surgery, a good view of the anatomy and pathology concerned is a basic requirement. The history of gynaecological surgery has evolved from the open abdominal and vaginal routes. Laparoscopy represents the most significant surgical advance in our specialty in recent times. Its development has led to a less aggressive approach to the organs being treated and their surrounding tissues. This in turn has led to a change in culture where conservative management strategies have become normal, and patients now expect less invasive approaches to their treatment. Surgeons now concentrate on preserving normal anatomy and physiology.

Laparoscopy is also remarkable for the quality of the images it obtains. It magnifies the view by a factor of 12 to 15 and gives a clearer, closer view of the surgical field. Greater details of the relationships between organs may be obtained. There is also the practical advantage that everyone in the operating theatre can see the images live, and can share in the surgical experience.

Originally when our team started its work in this field thirty years ago laparoscopy was largely perceived as a diagnostic procedure. It was always our aim to extend the role of laparoscopy to one of intervention. Today patients can have their disease diagnosed, assessed and treated under one anaesthetic without any delay.

In parallel to laparoscopy tremendous progress has been made in imaging techniques and in particular with ultrasonography. Today it is unusual for surgery to take place without an awareness of the pathology to be expected and a likely diagnosis. In this way surgical intervention can be more appropriately planned. Patients can also be given better information before the procedure.

Laparoscopy thus has a crucial role in surgical management and in my view is now a discipline in its own right within the great field of surgery. The trend today is to review all the classic surgical protocols that have been handed down to us, and to interpret them from an endoscopic point of view. Laparoscopy is now truly operative, and is having an expanding role in fields previously closed to it such as cancer and prolapse. For cancer the technique may facilitate more extensive treatment than has been previously possible. The information made available by laparoscopy has given a new view of the pathophysiology of the pelvic floor and ranks with the seminal radiological work of Bethoux and Huguier and the development of urodynamics.

I am convinced that the inspiration behind this book and its approach of integrating the use of ultrasonography and endoscopy are second to none, and that it will become essential reading for those working in the specialty. I am very pleased to contribute both to the introduction – together with our friend and colleague, Stuart Campbell – and with my colleagues to various chapters in the book.

M.A. Bruhat
Dean
Faculté de Médecine
Clermont-Ferrand
France

Preface

Since the introduction of ultrasonography by Donald and his first Lancet paper in 1958, the use of ultrasound in gynaecology has evolved rapidly. The introduction of the linear array real time scanner in the mid-seventies revolutionised the technique and turned it into a readily available and usable tool. The development of the transvaginal ultrasound probe went unnoticed by many gynaecologists, but has since had a major impact on many areas of gynaecological practice. The vaginal route has become standard for invasive ultrasound guided procedures, and colour Doppler has led to a greater understanding of how vessel growth is involved in reproductive pathophysiology. The more recent introduction of 3D ultrasonography will no doubt lead to further advances.

Advances seen in gynaecological ultrasonography have been paralleled by the rapid developments that have taken place in the technical aspects and practical applications of endoscopy. Both laparoscopy and hysteroscopy have evolved from being diagnostic tools to the present day when almost any gynaecological procedure can be performed with minimal access surgery.

However, as with many new techniques the advancement of both endoscopic surgery and ultrasonography has been driven by enthusiasts for one technique or the other, but rarely by practitioners who can do both. This was the experience that led to the development of this book. We feel that the modern gynaecologist should be conversant with both endoscopy and ultrasonography, and so we hope to move away from what might be termed "technique-driven" books and meetings.

The concept of an accurate ultrasound based diagnosis and minimal access treatment is an attractive one. The two techniques dovetail with each other. A good quality scan will often demonstrate that surgery is not necessary, whilst it is possible to select those cases that are suitable for a laparoscopic or hysteroscopic approach. When performing an operation on an ovarian cyst, the surgeon should already know the likely pathology on the basis of the preoperative scan and have planned accordingly.

For both techniques training is a major issue and varies greatly from country to country. There is no uniform agreement over the levels of training required. What is important, however, is that practitioners be made aware of what information can be available from an ultrasound scan and what procedures may be safely performed endoscopically. Conversely they must know the limitations of their own practice. In a small way we feel this book makes a contribution to this educational process. By bringing together many of the foremost authorities in ultrasonography and endoscopy we have aimed to get the best of both worlds. Whether we have succeeded in marrying these two special interests will be judged by the reader. However we hope the book will encourage a dialogue between experts in these fields, and persuade practitioners to learn both these techniques and use them to their maximum potential.

Dirk Timmerman
Jan Deprest
Tom Bourne
Leuven
June 2002

Contents

Part I Menorrhagia

Part II The Postmenopausal Endometrium

Part III Endometrial Malignancy

Part IV Urogynaecology

Part V Ovarian Masses

Part VI Endometriosis

Part VII Disorders of Ovarian Function and Subfertility

Part VIII Early Pregnancy Complications

Part IX Early Prenatal Diagnosis and Obstetric Endoscopy

List of Contributors

Wim M. Ankum
Department of Obstetrics and Gynaecology
Academic Medical Centre
University of Amsterdam
PO Box 22700
1100 DE Amsterdam
The Netherlands

Marie-Claude Anton
Department of Obstetrics, Gynaecology and Reproductive Medicine
CHU 13 Boulevard Charles de Gaulle
63033 Clermont-Ferrand
France

Amar Bhide
Department of Obstetrics and Gynaecology
St George's Hospital Medical School
Cranmer Terrace
London SW17 ORE
UK

Revaz Botchorishvili
Department of Obstetrics, Gynaecology and Reproductive Medicine
CHU 13 Boulevard Charles de Gaulle
63033 Clermont-Ferrand
France

Tom Bourne
Department of Obstetrics and Gynaecology
St George's Hospital Medical School
Cranmer Terrace
London SW17 ORE
UK

Hans Brölmann
Department of Obstetrics and Gynaecology
Maximà Medisch Centrum
De Run 4600
5504 DB Veldhoven
The Netherlands

Jonathan-David Broome
Department of Endo-Gynaecology
Royal Hospital for Women
Barker Street
Randwick NSW 2031
Australia

Ivo Brosens
Leuven Institute for Fertility and Embryology
Tiensevest 168
3000 Leuven
Belgium

Maurice-Antoine Bruhat
Faculté de Médecine
28 Place Henry Dunant
63000 Clermont-Ferrand
France

The-Hung Bui
Department of Molecular Medicine
Clinical Genetics Unit L08-02
Karolinska Hospital
17176 Stockholm
Sweden

Stuart Campbell
Create Health Clinic
21J Devonshire Place
London W1G 6HZ
UK

Rudi Campo
Leuven Institute for Fertility and Embryology
Tiensevest 168
3000 Leuven
Belgium

Michel Canis
Department of Obstetrics, Gynaecology and Reproductive Medicine
CHU Boulevard Leon Malfreyt
63058 Clermont-Ferrand
France

Charles Chapron
Department of Obstetrics and Gynaecology
Groupe Hospitalier Cochin
Saint-Vincent-de-Paul La Roche-Guyon
Pavillon Baudelocque
123 Boulevard Port-Royal
75079 Paris Cedex 14
France

Stephen Chew
Department of Obstetrics and Gynaecology
Polyclinique de l'Hôtel Dieu
Université de Clermont-Ferrand
65 Boulevard Gergovia
63003 Clermont-Ferrand
France

George Condous
Department of Obstetrics and Gynaecology
St George's Hospital Medical School
Cranmer Terrace
London SW17 ORE
UK

Michel R. Cosson
Department of Obstetrics and Gynaecology
Pôle de chirurgie gynécologique
Hôpital Jeanne de Flandres
CHRU Lille
59000 Lille
France

Gilles Crépin
Department of Obstetrics and Gynaecology
Pôle de chirurgie gynécologique
Hôpital Jeanne de Flandres
CHRU Lille
59000 Lille
France

Pino G. Cusumano
Department of Obstetrics, Gynaecology and Senology
Centre Hospitalier St-Joseph-Espérance
75 Rue de Hesbaye
4000 Liège
Belgium

Sjoerd de Blok
Department of Obstetrics and Gynaecology
Onze Lieve Vrouwe Gasthuis
PO Box 95500
1090 HM Amsterdam
The Netherlands

Filip De Bruyne
Department of Microsurgery and Gynaecological Endoscopy
Frauenklinik
Heinrich-Heine University Düsseldorf
Moorenstrasse 5
40225 Düsseldorf
Germany

Jan Decloedt
Department of Obstetrics and Gynaecology
St Blasius Hospitaal
Kroonveldlaan 50
9200 Dendermonde
Belgium

Michel Degueldre
Department of Obstetrics and Gynaecology
University Hospital St-Pierre
Hoogstraat 322
1000 Brussel
Belgium

Jan Deprest
Department of Obstetrics and Gynaecology
University Hospitals KULeuven
UZ Gasthuisberg
Herestraat 49
3000 Leuven
Belgium

Dirk De Ridder
Department of Urology
University Hospitals KU Leuven
UZ Gasthuisberg
Herestraat 49
3000 Leuven
Belgium

Jacques Donnez
Department of Gynaecology
Université Catholique de Louvain
Cliniques Universitaires St-Luc
10 Avenue Hippocrate
1200 Brussels
Belgium

Jean-Bernard Dubuisson1
Department of Obstetrics and Gynaecology
Groupe Hospitalier Cochin
Saint-Vincent-de-Paul La Roche-Guyon
Pavillon Baudelocque
123 Boulevard Port-Royal
75079 Paris Cedex 14
France

Erling Ekerhovd
Department of Obstetrics and Gynaecology
University of Göteborg
41345 Göteborg
Sweden

Marie Ellström
Scandinavian Center for Gynaecological Endoscopy
Department of Obstetrics and Gynaecology
Sahlgrenska University Hospital
University of Göteborg
41345 Göteborg
Sweden

Arnaud Fauconnier
Department of Obstetrics and Gynaecology
Groupe Hospitalier Cochin
Saint-Vincent-de-Paul La Roche-Guyon
Pavillon Baudelocque
123 Boulevard Port-Royal
75079 Paris Cedex 14
France

Hervé Fernandez
Department of Obstetrics and Gynaecology
Antoine Beclere Hospital
157 Rue de la Porte de Trivaux
92141 Clamart Cedex
France

Enrico Ferrazzi
Department of Obstetrics and Gynaecology
San Paolo Biomedical Sciences Institute
Università Degli Studi di Milano
Via di Rudini 8
20142 Milano
Italy

Reinaldo Goldchmit
Department of Obstetrics and Gynaecology
Polyclinique de l'Hôtel Dieu
Université de Clermont-Ferrand
65 Boulevard Gergovia
63003 Clermont-Ferrand
France

Steven R. Goldstein
New York University School of Medicine
530 First Avenue
Suite 10N
New York NY 10016
USA

Stephan Gordts
Leuven Institute for Fertility and Embryology
Tiensevest 168
3000 Leuven
Belgium

Seth Granberg
Ultrasound and Reproductive Medicine Unit
Department of Obstetrics and Gynaecology
Karolinska Hospital
PO Box 140
17176 Stockholm
Sweden

Eduard Gratacós
Department of Obstetrics and Gynaecology
Fetal Medicine Unit
University Hospitals Vall d'Hebron
Pg. Vall d'Hebron 129-139
08035 Barcelona
Spain

Beatrice Gulbis
Academic Department of Clinical Chemistry
Academic Hospital Erasme
Université Libre de Bruxelles
Lenniksebaan 808
1070 Brussels
Belgium

Petra J. Hajenius
Centre for Reproductive Medicine
Academic Medical Centre
University of Amsterdam
PO Box 22700
1100 DE Amsterdam
The Netherlands

Olav Istre
Department of Obstetrics and Gynaecology
Ullevaal Hospital
University of Oslo
Kirkev 166
0407 Oslo
Norway

Pascale Jadoul
Department of Gynaecology
Université Catholique de Louvain
Cliniques Universitaires St-Luc
10 Avenue Hippocrate
1200 Brussels
Belgium

Eric Jauniaux
Academic Departments of Obstetrics and Gynaecology
Royal Free and University College London Medical School
86-96 Chenies Mews
London WC1E 6HX
UK

Karen Jermy
Department of Obstetrics and Gynaecology
St George's Hospital Medical School
Cranmer Terrace
London SW17 ORE
UK

Davor Jurkovic
Department of Obstetrics and Gynaecology
King's College School of Medicine and Dentistry
University of London
Denmark Hill
London SE5 8RX
UK

Asma Khalid
Department of Obstetrics and Gynaecology
St George's Hospital Medical School
Cranmer Terrace
London SW17 ORE
UK

Philippe R. Koninckx
Department of Obstetrics and Gynaecology
Centre for Surgical Technologies
University Hospitals KU Leuven
UZ Gasthuisberg
Herestraat 49
3000 Leuven
Belgium

Ted T.M. Lee
Centre for Women's Care and Reproductive Surgery
1140 Hammond Drive
Building F
Suite 6230
Atlanta
Georgia GA 30328
USA

David T.Y. Liu
Department of Obstetrics and Gynaecology
City Hospital
Hucknall Road
Nottingham NG5 1PB
UK

Thomas L. Lyons
Centre for Women's Care and Reproductive Surgery
1140 Hammond Drive
Building F
Suite 6230
Atlanta
Georgia GA 30328
USA

Gérard Mage
Department of Obstetrics and Gynaecology
Polyclinique de l'Hôtel Dieu
Université de Clermont-Ferrand
65 Boulevard Gergovia
63003 Clermont-Ferrand
France

Hubert Manhes
Polyclinique 'La Pergola'
Allee des Ailes
03200 Vichy
France

Patrice Mille
Department of Obstetrics, Gynaecology and Reproductive Medicine
CHU 13 Boulevard Charles de Gaulle
63033 Clermont-Ferrand
France

Ben-Willem J. Mol
Department of Clinical Epidemiology and Biostatistics
Academic Medical Centre
University of Amsterdam
PO Box 22700
1100 DE Amsterdam
The Netherlands

Patrick Neven
Department of Gynaecological Oncology
University Hospitals KU Leuven
UZ Gasthuisberg
Herestraat 49
3000 Leuven
Belgium

Michelle Nisolle
Department of Gynaecology
Université Catholique de Louvain
Cliniques Universitaires St-Luc
10 Avenue Hippocrate
1200 Brussels
Belgium

Emeka Okaro
Department of Obstetrics and Gynaecology
St George's Hospital Medical School
Cranmer Terrace
London SW17 ORE
UK

Umberto Omodei
Department of Obstetrics and Gynaecology
San Paolo Biomedical Sciences Institute
Università Degli Studi di Milano
Via di Rudini 8
20142 Milano
Italy

Guiseppe Perugino
Department of Obstetrics and Gynaecology
San Paolo Biomedical Sciences Institute
Università Degli Studi di Milano
Via di Rudini 8
20142 Milano
Italy

Jean-Luc Pouly
Department of Obstetrics and Gynaecology
Polyclinique de l'Hôtel Dieu
Université de Clermont-Ferrand
65 Boulevard Gergovia
63003 Clermont-Ferrand
France

Federico Prefumo
Department of Obstetrics and Gynaecology
St George's Hospital Medical School
Cranmer Terrace
London SW17 ORE
UK

Denis Querleu
Department of Obstetrics and Gynaecology
Pôle de chirurgie gynécologique
Hôpital Jeanne de Flandres
CHRU Lille
59000 Lille
France

Rechad Rajabally
Department of Obstetrics and Gynaecology
Pavillon Maternité Paul Gellé 91
91 Avenue J Lagache
59056 Roubaix Cedex 1
France

Cristina Ruggeri
Department of Obstetrics and Gynaecology
San Paolo Biomedical Sciences Institute
Università Degli Studi di Milano
Via di Rudini 8
20142 Milano
Italy

Rehan Salim
Department of Obstetrics and Gynaecology
King's College School of Medicine and Dentistry
University of London
Denmark Hill
London SE5 8RX
UK

Jean Squifflet
Department of Gynaecology
Université Catholique de Louvain
Cliniques Universitaires St-Luc
10 Avenue Hippocrate
1200 Brussels
Belgium

Abdul H. Sultan
Department of Obstetrics and Gynaecology
Mayday University Hospital
Mayday Road
Thornton Heath
Croydon CR7 7YE
UK

Karin Sundberg
Department of Obstetrics and Gynaecology
State University Hospital
Rigshospitalet
Blegdamsvej 9
2100 Copenhagen
Denmark

Anil Tailor
Northern Gynaecological Oncology Centre
Queen Elizabeth Hospital
Sheriff Hill
Gateshead NE9 65X
UK

Basky Thilaganathan
Department of Obstetrics and Gynaecology
St George's Hospital Medical School
Cranmer Terrace
London SW17 ORE
UK

Dirk Timmerman
Department of Obstetrics and Gynaecology
University Hospitals KU Leuven
UZ Gasthuisberg
Herestraat 49
3000 Leuven
Belgium

Lil Valentin
Department of Obstetrics and Gynaecology
University Hospital Malmö
Lund University
20502 Malmö
Sweden

Yves Van Belle
St Jans ziekenhuis
Broekstraat 104
1000 Brussels
Belgium

Thierry G. Vancaillie
Department of Endo-Gynaecology
Royal Hospital for Women
Barker Street
Randwick NSW 2031
Australia

Thierry Van den Bosch
Department of Obstetrics and Gynaecology
AZ Heilig Hart
Kliniekstraat 45
3300 Tienen
Belgium

Axel Vandendael
Department of Obstetrics and Gynaecology
University of Stellenbosch and Tygerberg Hospital
Tygerberg 7505
South Africa

Fulco Van der Veen
Centre for Reproductive Medicine
Academic Medical Centre
University of Amsterdam
PO Box 22700
1100 DE Amsterdam
The Netherlands

Jean Vandromme
Department of Obstetrics and Gynaecology
University Hospital St-Pierre
Hoogstraat 322
1000 Brussels
Belgium

Ignace Vergote
Department of Gynaecological Oncology
University Hospitals KU Leuven
UZ Gasthuisberg
Herestraat 49
3000 Leuven
Belgium

Yves Ville
Department of Obstetrics and Gynaecology
CH de Poissy St-Germain
10 Rue du Champ Gaillard
78300 Poissy
France

Peter von Theobald
Centre Hospitalier Universitaire de Caen
Avenue George Clémenceau
14033 Caen Cedex
France

Arnaud Wattiez
Department of Obstetrics and Gynaecology
Polyclinique de l'Hôtel Dieu
Université de Clermont-Ferrand
65 Boulevard Gergovia
63003 Clermont-Ferrand
France

Wendy K. Winer
Centre for Women's Care and Reproductive Surgery
1140 Hammond Drive
Building F
Suite 6230
Atlanta
Georgia GA 30328
USA

Gerardo Zanetta
Department of Obstetrics and Gynaecology
San Gerardo Hospital
University of Milano Bicocca
Via Solferino 16
20052 Monza
Italy

Part I

Menorrhagia

Contents

Summary

Menorrhagia contributes a significant proportion of the workload for any gynaecologist. This section compares the use of ultrasound and hysteroscopy to evaluate the endometrial cavity. For many women, an ultrasound scan to exclude pathology and subsequent treatment with oral contraceptives, progestogens, tranexamic acid or a Mirena intrauterine system (IUS) is all that will be required. Others will need surgery. Hysteroscopic treatment is possible for many women and both the results that may be obtained and the possible complications of this surgery are discussed. For some women, a hysterectomy is required. The optimal approach for hysterectomy is not known; however, the arguments for and against total laparoscopic, subtotal laparoscopic and vaginal hysterectomy are outlined in detail. In our view, the logical approach to the management of menorrhagia is to exclude pathology on the basis of an ultrasound scan and outpatient biopsy. For women with a normal endometrial cavity, a Mirena IUS would be appropriate, while other patients can be selected for operative hysteroscopy. Hysterectomy or myomectomy will still be required in a proportion of cases.

Key points

- Patients with menorrhagia should be assessed in a "one stop" clinic
- The clinic can use ultrasonography as the primary investigation and to select women for hysteroscopy
- The diagnostic performance of ultrasound can be improved by introducing saline into the endometrial cavity to act as a negative contrast agent (hydrosonography)
- Office hysteroscopy is indicated if the ultrasound scan is inconclusive. The rapid development of smaller hysteroscopes means that hysteroscopy may become the primary investigation in some cases
- Focal endometrial pathology can be dealt with by hysteroscopic resection. Fibroids should be considered for resection only if they are less than 5.0 cm and when a significant proportion lies within the endometrial cavity
- Laparoscopic myomectomy is best suited to small numbers of subserosal and mural fibroids of less than 8.0 cm in diameter
- The precise role of laparoscopic approaches to hysterectomy has not been defined. The relative merits of preserving the cervix at the time of hysterectomy are controversial. If a subtotal hysterectomy is considered, the laparoscopic approach is logical
- Mastering the technique of vaginal hysterectomy will enable 80% of hysterectomies to be performed via this route. The final role of laparoscopy may be in assisting vaginal hysterectomy in difficult cases

Chapter 1

Ultrasound and Menorrhagia

Karen Jermy and Tom Bourne

1.1 Introduction

The diagnosis and management of women with abnormal vaginal bleeding comprises a large proportion of the gynaecologist's workload. Up to a third of women referred to a general gynaecology outpatient clinic will have abnormal uterine bleeding, and it remains the most common indication for surgical intervention in gynaecology.

Up to 60% of abnormal uterine bleeding can be described as "dysfunctional" in nature, indicating that there is no underlying organic pathology. The aim of any group of investigations within this area of gynaecology should be to diagnose accurately the absence of pathology, thus facilitating reassurance and early treatment plans if required, without recourse to operative intervention unless indicated. The reverse is also true. As an increasing number of different strategies have been introduced in the management of menorrhagia, so has the need to diagnose accurately possible underlying pathology. A balance therefore needs to be established in order to provide accurate, early diagnosis and thus treatment, with the minimum of investigations.

The assessment of women with menstrual disorders has been taken out of the constraints of the general gynaecology clinic and operating theatre by the incorporation of transvaginal ultrasonography (TVS), along with outpatient endometrial sampling techniques, as part of a "one-stop" approach to diagnosis and management. When compared with outpatient hysteroscopy in the evaluation of endometrial pathology, TVS, with or without the addition of saline as a negative contrast agent, compares favourably.[1-3] It has been shown to be a well-tolerated part of the examination, providing not only an assessment of the uterine cavity and myometrium, but also of the adnexa at the same time.

In this chapter we will summarise the role of ultrasound in the diagnosis and management of the woman presenting with menorrhagia.

1.2 Aetiology of Abnormal Vaginal Bleeding

The differential diagnoses of women presenting with abnormal vaginal bleeding can be divided into genital tract disease, systemic disease and iatrogenic causes; these are summarised in Table 1.1. When all these have been excluded, a diagnosis of dysfunctional uterine bleeding can be made. Pregnancy should be excluded in all premenopausal women with abnormal vaginal bleeding. There needs to be a heightened suspicion of underlying systemic disease in younger patients presenting with heavy vaginal bleeding, as up to 20%[4] may have a coagulopathy. Screening for a coagulopathy is also advisable in women with anovulatory dysfunctional bleeding who fail to respond to medical or surgical therapy.

1.3 Investigations

The investigation of abnormal uterine bleeding will centre on an assessment of the endometrium. Undirected endometrial sampling alone has no role in the evaluation of abnormal uterine bleeding, as it will miss focal lesions, such as polyps and fibroids. Dilatation and curettage has a false-negative rate of up to 6% for diagnosing endometrial carcinoma and hyperplasia.[5,6] In one study[6] where dilatation and curettage was performed prior to hysterectomy, in 60% of patients less than half of the endometrial cavity was sampled. Hysteroscopy and directed biopsy remains the "gold standard" in the evaluation of intrauterine abnormalities, and it is against this that other techniques are still compared. Transvaginal ultrasound is highly sensitive in the diagnosis of intracavity pathology, but lacks specificity in many cases.[7,8] The sensitivity and specificity is improved

Table 1.1. Causes of abnormal vaginal bleeding

Genital tract disease	
Benign conditions	Cervical polyps and erosions
	Uterine leiomyomas
	Endometrial polyps
	Adenomyosis
	Endometriosis
Malignant tumours	Endometrial
	Cervical
	Vaginal
	Vulvar
	Fallopian tube
	Granulosa theca cell ovarian
Infection	Endometritis
	Salpingitis
Systemic disease	
Coagulopathy	Von Willebrand's disease
	Leukaemia
	Thrombocytopenia
	Chronic renal failure
Thyroid disorders	
Liver disease	Acute and chronic
Sarcoidosis	
Iatrogenic causes	
Anticoagulants	
Intrauterine contraceptive devices	
Phenytoin	
Sex steroids	
Dysfunctional uterine bleeding	Ovulatory
	Anovulatory

by hydrosonography (HS), to equal and in some studies[9] surpass, that of outpatient hysteroscopy. When patient preference is considered, TVS with HS is preferred to outpatient hysteroscopy,[9] making TVS an ideal first-line investigation for menstrual disorders (Figure 1.1).

1.3.1 Hydrosonography

This technique involves the introduction of a sonographic negative contrast agent into the uterine cavity, to enhance routine TVS in the identification of uterine cavity pathology (Figure 1.2).

A conventional transvaginal scan is performed to assess the uterus and adnexa in the coronal and sagittal planes. The examination should ideally be performed in the proliferative phase of the menstrual cycle, once menstruation has ceased. This not only enhances views of the uterine cavity, but also reduces the risk of disturbing an early intrauterine pregnancy. The ultrasound probe is removed and a bivalve Cuscoe's speculum inserted. The cervix is identified and cleaned with an antiseptic solution. The procedure should be postponed and an infection screen performed with appropriate antibiotic therapy if there are any signs of pelvic infection. The patient should be warned prior to the procedure that she may experience a dull ache like a period pain. Covering antibiotics may be given for potentially fertile women.

After the cervix has been cleaned, a fine-bore catheter (with or without a balloon), which has already been primed with sterile saline solution, is passed through the os using sponge holding forceps until the uterine fundus is reached. A volsellum may be needed to apply counter-traction to the cervix. The speculum is removed, taking care not to dislodge the catheter, and a 20 ml syringe of sterile saline is reattached to the catheter. The ultrasound probe is reintroduced and the saline is slowly infused, causing uterine distension. The uterine cavity is reassessed in both the sagittal and coronal planes for focal and global endometrial defects.

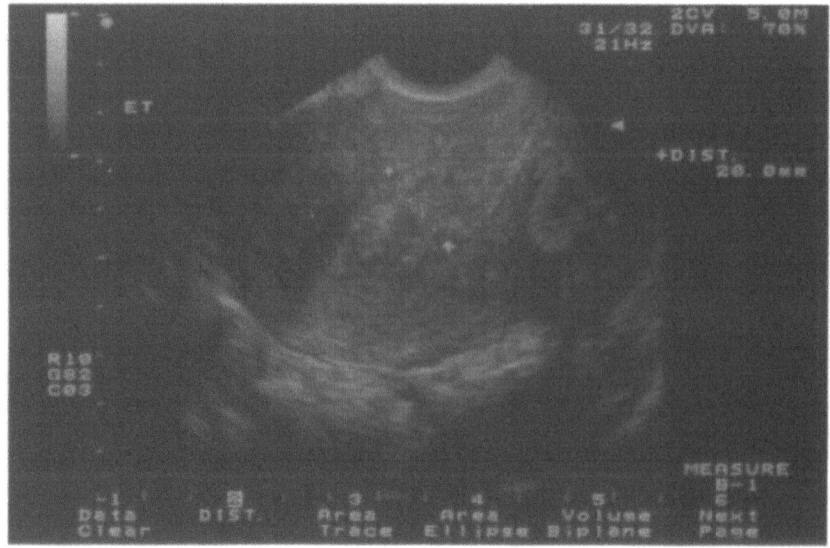

Figure 1.1 Sagittal view of an anteverted uterus. The endometrium is thickened and of mixed echoes.

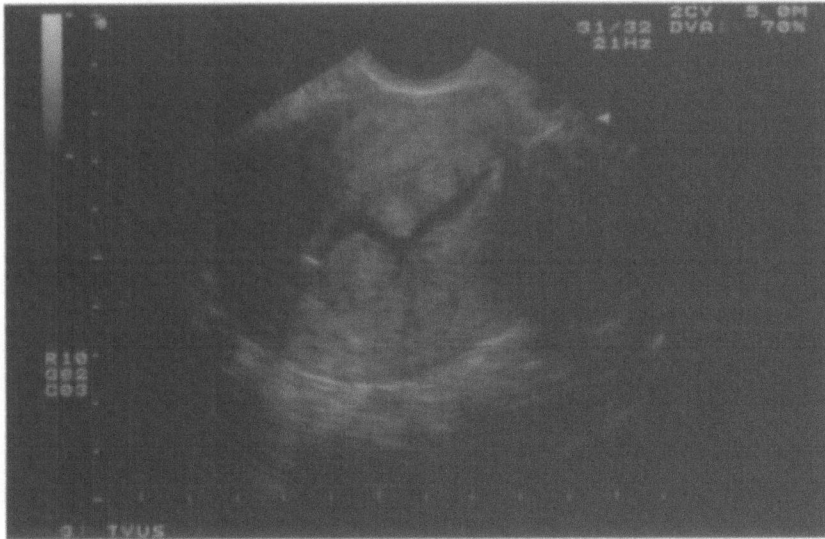

Figure 1.2 The same view as in Figure 1.1. Sterile saline has been introduced into the endometrial cavity. This acts to distend the cavity and as a negative contrast agent. Several endometrial polyps can now be identified.

When the scan is complete, the catheter is removed, and the patient advised to remain supine for 5 minutes to reduce the chance of a vagal reaction after the procedure.

1.3.1.1 Indications for HS

The indications for HS are:

- thickened endometrium;
- poor views of the endometrium, due to axial position of uterus, large myomas distorting the cavity;
- preoperative localisation, size and relation to cavity of submucous fibroids/endometrial polyps to plan hysteroscopic surgery.

1.3.1.2 Complications of the Procedure

Failure of the procedure usually occurs as a result of cervical stenosis, or in the presence of multiple large fibroids. The problems encountered with a patulous cervix may be overcome by using either a balloon catheter or infusing the saline solution faster. Overall failure rates ranging from 1.8[10] to 4.6%[11] are quoted.

There is no evidence to support the theoretical concern that instillation of fluid into the uterine cavity, either at hysteroscopy or HS, may promote dissemination of endometrial carcinoma.[12]

1.3.2 Endometrial Assessment

Transvaginal ultrasonography is a highly sensitive method for detecting endometrial abnormalities.[3,13,14]

In the assessment of postmenopausal bleeding, the finding of a regular endometrial echo with a thickness of less than 5 mm has been shown to have a high negative predictive value for the presence of pathology.[15] However, the premenopausal endometrium is a dynamic structure, and wide variations in the endometrial thickness have been associated with pathology.[16] The most consistent measurements are taken in the early proliferative phase when the endometrium is at its thinnest and most echolucent. With all measurements of the endometrial echo, it is important to visualise it as a three-dimensional structure, so as to avoid missing focal irregularities. Three-dimensional ultrasound has been shown to have a role in the assessment of congenital uterine abnormalities,[17] and it may be that it can also improve the visualisation of acquired conditions of the uterine cavity.

The endometrial outline should be regular and uninterrupted, whatever the thickness. A thick, secretory endometrium on unenhanced TVS will often disguise endometrial pathology. In contrast, a periovulatory "triple line" endometrium will offer the best unenhanced views of the uterine cavity. Transvaginal ultrasonography affords good myometrial/endometrial interface definition. This is important in the assessment of suspected endometrial carcinoma.

1.3.2.1 Endometrial Polyps

These tend to be hyperechoic or cystic structures distorting the endometrial echo. Colour Doppler may demonstrate a single feeding blood vessel to the structure.

1.3.2.2 Uterine Leiomyomas

The ultrasound appearances of leiomyomas are varied. Before the menopause they tend to be a well-defined heterogeneous or hypoechoic structure. Transvaginal ultrasonography is used in conjunction with abdominal scanning to ensure pedunculated subserosal fibroids are not missed. Submucosal fibroids project into the uterine cavity and distort the endometrium. Their accurate classification allows selection for transcervical resection in appropriate cases. Fedele et al[3] demonstrated the sensitivity of TVS for the diagnosis of submucosal fibroids to be 100%, with a sensitivity of 94%. Hysteroscopy (outpatient) performed on the same population had a sensitivity and specificity of 100% and 96% respectively in their diagnosis. The only criticism of TVS in this study was its apparent inability to differentiate endometrial polyps from submucosal fibroids. All the scans were performed in the secretory phase of the cycle. Endometrial polyps tend to be hyperechoic structures, easily masked by a thick secretory endometrium. By performing the scans during the proliferative phase, the distinction between intracavity fibroids and polyps is easier to make (Figure 1.3). The positive predictive value was as high as 92%.[1]

1.3.2.3 Adenomyosis

The presence of diffuse or focal endometrial tissue within the myometrium can result in abnormal vaginal bleeding. Classically its diagnosis has been established only after histological assessment at hysterectomy. Transvaginal ultrasound has a variable diagnostic rate. Fedele et al[18] reported a sensitivity and specificity of 80% and 74% respec-

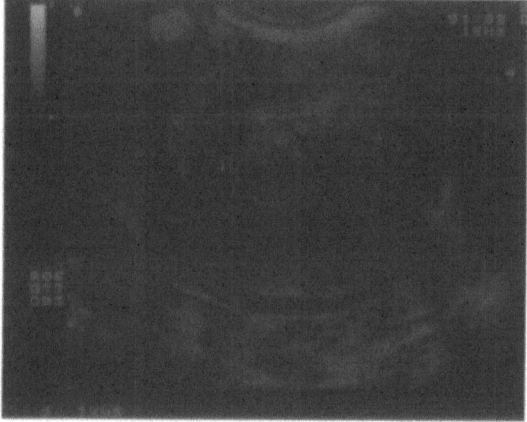

Figure 1.3 Sagittal view of the uterus, demonstrating a large, intracavity fibroid. This has been delineated further with saline hydrosonography.

tively for the detection of diffuse adenomyosis, and 87% and 98% for focal lesions.

1.3.2.4 Coexistent Pathology

Transvaginal ultrasonography allows an assessment to be made not only of the endometrium, but also of the myometrium and adnexae. One study has shown that of 93 patients attending a clinic, complaining of abnormal uterine bleeding, 14% had adnexal pathology.[19]

1.4 Conclusions

An accurate assessment of abnormal uterine bleeding is essential, not only for the exclusion of malignancy, but also for the accurate preoperative assessment of intracavity pathology. Transvaginal ultrasound is highly predictive in the diagnosis of the normal endometrium, and as up to 60% of women complaining of abnormal vaginal bleeding will have no underlying cause, more invasive diagnostic techniques can be avoided. These patients can then be reassured and offered medical or surgical therapies (Figure 1.4). Within the one-stop clinic, unenhanced pelvic ultrasound will act as a triage for further outpatient investigations – either hysteroscopy or HS, along with endometrial biopsy to allow for accurate preoperative diagnosis. The combination of these techniques has allowed the management of women with menstrual disorders to be optimised.

References

1. Schwarzler P, Concin H, Bosch H et al (1998) An evaluation of sonohysterography and diagnostic hysteroscopy for the assessment of intrauterine pathology. Ultrasound Obstet Gynecol 11:337–342
2. Indman PD (1995) Abnormal uterine bleeding. Accuracy of vaginal probe ultrasound in predicting abnormal hysteroscopic findings. J Reprod Med 40:545–548
3. Fedele L, Bianchi S, Dorta M et al (1991) Transvaginal ultrasonography versus hysteroscopy in the diagnosis of uterine submucosal myomas. Obstet Gynecol 77:745–748
4. Kadir RA, Economides DL, Sabin CA et al (1998) Frequency of inherited bleeding disorders in women with menorrhagia. Lancet 14(351):485–489
5. Holst J, Koskela O, Von Schoultz B (1983) Endometrial findings following curettage in 2018 women according to age and indications. Ann Chir Gynaecol 72:274–277
6. Stock R, Kanbour A (1975) Prehysterectomy curettage. Obstet Gynecol 45:537–541
7. Granberg S, Wikland M, Karlsson B et al (1991) Endometrial thickness as measured by endovaginal ultrasonography for identifying endometrial abnormality. Am J Obstet Gynecol 164:47–52
8. Dijkhuizen F, Brolmann H, Potters A et al (1996) The accuracy of transvaginal ultrasonography in the diagnosis of endometrial abnormalities. Obstet Gynecol 87:345–349

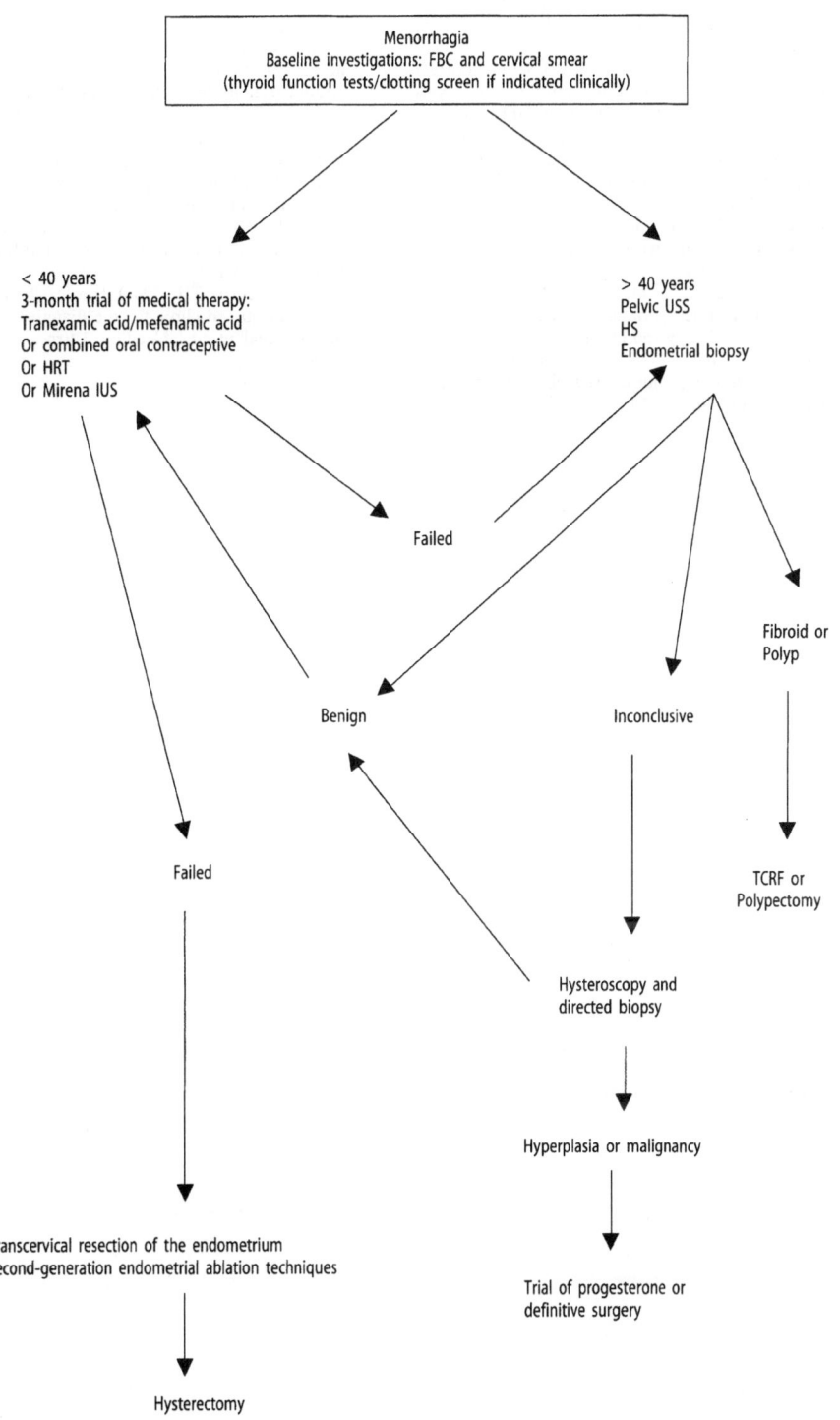

Figure 1.4 Ultrasound-based management of women with menorrhagia. FBC, Full blood count; HRT, hormone replacement therapy; IUS, intrauterine system; USS, ultrasound Scan; HS, hydrosonography; TCRF, transcervical resection of fibroids

9. Timmerman D, Deprest J, Bourne T et al (1998) A randomized trial on the use of ultrasound or office hysteroscopy for endometrial assessment in postmenopausal patients with breast cancer who were treated with tamoxifen. Am J Ob Gyn 1:62–70

10. Bernard JP, Lecuru F, Darles C et al (1997) Saline contrast sonohysterography as first-line investigation for women with uterine bleeding. Ultrasound Obstet Gynecol 10:121–125

11. Widrich T, Bradley LD, Mitchinson AR et al (1996) Comparison of saline infusion sonography with office hysteroscopy for the evaluation of the endometrium. Am J Obstet Gynecol 174:1327–1334

12. De Vore G, Schwartz P, Morris J (1982) Hysterography: a five year follow-up in patients with endometrial carcinoma. Obstet Gynecol 60:369–372

13. Mendelson EB, Bohm-Velez M, Joseph N et al (1988) Endometrial abnormalities: evaluation with transvaginal sonography. Am J Radiology 150:139–142

14. Smith P, Bakos O, Heimer G et al (1991) Transvaginal ultrasound for identifying endometrial abnormality. Acta Obstet Gynecol Scand 70:591–594

15. Granberg S, Wikland M, Karlsson B et al (1991) Endometrial thickness as measured by endovaginal ultrasonography for identifying endometrial abnormality. Am J Obstet Gynecol 164:47–52

16. Dijkhuizen F, Brolmann H, Potters A et al (1996) The accuracy of transvaginal ultrasonography in the diagnosis of endometrial abnormalities. Obstet Gynecol 87:345–349

17. Jurkovic D, Geipel A, Gruboeck K et al (1995) Three dimensional ultrasound for the assessment of uterine anatomy and detection of congenital anomalies: a comparison with hydrosonography and two-dimensional sonography. Ultrasound Obstet Gynecol 5:233–237

18. Fedele L, Bianchi S, Dorta M et al (1992) Transvaginal ultrasonography in the diagnosis of diffuse adenomyosis. Fert Steril 58:94–97

19. Jones K, Bourne TH (2001) The feasibility of a 'one stop' ultrasound-based clinic for the diagnosis and management of abnormal uterine bleeding. Ultrasound Obstet Gynecol 17:517–21

Chapter 2

Role of Hysteroscopy

Rudi Campo and Yves Van Belle

2.1 Introduction

Abnormal uterine bleeding in general, and menorrhagia in particular, is one of the most frequent reasons for patients to consult their gynaecologist.[1] The knowledge that the objective measurement of menstrual bleeding will be less than 80 ml per period (the definition of menorrhagia) in more than half of cases does not release the gynaecologist from a standardised diagnostic management.[2] This is important to avoid undertreatment, such as reassurance without correct diagnosis, as well as overtreatment, which would be a hysterectomy in the absence of organic uterine pathology. Important features deciding on the clinical value of a diagnostic procedure are simplicity, safety, patient compliance, cost–benefit relationship and accuracy.

Endoscopic techniques for diagnosis and treatment of various pathologies have gained importance in medicine, especially over the last years. The major advantage lies in the direct optical visualisation of body cavities, combined with the possibility of surgical treatment during the same procedure.

Although hysteroscopy has always been recognised as the gold standard for the diagnosis of intrauterine pathology, the conventional technique using a 5 mm single-flow hysteroscope and CO_2 gas as distension medium frequently resulted in patient intolerance and insufficient visualisation.[3,4] Thus, conventional hysteroscopy has not been generally accepted as an ambulatory, well-tolerated office procedure.

If office diagnostic hysteroscopy could be performed as easily as a vaginal ultrasound, it would play a key role in the diagnosis of abnormal uterine bleeding and would be a primary investigation tool for the infertile woman, as well as the ideal screening method for endometrial changes in patients taking hormone replacement therapy or anti-oestrogens as adjuvant treatment.[5,6] Furthermore, it would be helpful in the interpretation of uncertain findings in other indirect diagnostic techniques such as ultrasound, magnetic resonance imaging, blind biopsy or hystero-salpingography.

Hysteroscopy allows us to make a correct and complete diagnosis before entering the operation room and will avoid unnecessary surgery, such as dilatation and curettage (D&C), for a significant number of patients.

We believe that, with the development of a new generation of mini-hysteroscopes, the requirements for the above hypothesis are practically fulfilled. Hysteroscopy can now be performed in daily practice without any form of anaesthesia and with excellent patient compliance. With the use of video equipment, every finding can be documented and archived in an appropriate way (video documentation, videoprint or direct archiving of images in the computer).

The perfect imaging of the mini-hysteroscopes, the possibility of documentation and high patient compliance should guarantee the wide application of diagnostic hysteroscopy in an office environment, although the technique requires training and is characterised by a slow learning curve.

2.2 Hysteroscopy: Instrumentation and Technique

2.2.1 Instrumentation

2.2.1.1 Mini-hysteroscopic Optical System

The Circon ACMI mini-hysteroscopic system (Figure 2.1) is a combination of a 30° rigid, 3.5 mm

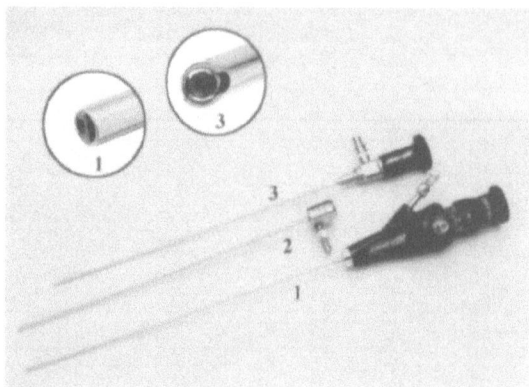

Figure 2.1 Instrumentation: fibre–optic, 2.4 mm single–flow semi–rigid 12° hysteroscope (*1*); outer sheath, 3.5 mm for single–flow use with rigid optic and continuous flow with fibre–optic (*2*); rigid optic, 2.7 mm 30° mini-hysteroscope (*3*).

total diameter, single-flow hysteroscope and a 12° semi-rigid, 2.4 mm, single-flow fibrescope. For continuous-flow purposes, the telescopes are interchangeable and the 2.4 mm semi-rigid fibrescope can be inserted in the 3.5 mm outer sheath. The gynaecologist can choose the instrument configuration that he or she finds most suitable for the situation. The advantages of the semi-rigid fibrescopes are the smaller total diameter, the superior brightness and the instrument lifetime. The advantages of the rigid optical system are the larger field and angle of view and the superior resolution.

2.2.1.2 Distension Medium

For outpatient diagnostic hysteroscopy, we use solutions such as Ringer's lactate, saline or Hartman's solution. A pressure cuff installed between 80 and 150 mm mercury delivers the necessary pressure for distension of the cavity. Physiological solutions have the advantage of being less irritating and painful than CO_2 gas.[7] In contrast to CO_2 gas, delicate structures will not collapse in a fluid distension medium, resulting in a more accurate diagnosis of subtle lesions.

2.2.1.3 Hardware: Video Camera, Printer, Xenon Light Source

With the use of video equipment, all the findings can be documented and archived in an appropriate way (video documentation, videoprint or direct archiving of images in the computer). For optimal visualisation and image quality, a high-performance light source is mandatory.

2.2.1.4 Documentation

The findings are documented with four images on a videoprint and on a pre-designed registration form, on which the physician collects details of clinical findings, patient compliance and possible complications.

2.2.1.5 Items not Necessary for Diagnostic Hysteroscopy

If the patient is not anaesthetised, a tenaculum is unnecessary, as the cervix has to be grasped only in rare cases. Grasping of the cervix is always necessary when a diagnostic hysteroscopy is conducted under general or regional anaesthesia, because of the relaxation of the pelvic floor.

In cases of cervical stenosis, we would recommend the use of an instrument with a small diameter, rather than the Hegar dilator – for instance the 2.4 mm semi-rigid hysteroscope.

There is no evidence that local anaesthesia improves patient satisfaction and compliance during the procedure. On the contrary, the application of local anaesthesia increases the operating time and the risks associated with the procedure.[8,9]

2.2.2 Procedure

A routine vaginal examination and a vaginal ultrasonography are performed to assess the size and position of the uterus and to exclude major uterine and adnexal pathology. The examination is scheduled in an office environment, preferably during the follicular phase of the cycle. The aim is to differentiate normal from abnormal cervical and/or intrauterine findings.

The patient lies in a gynaecological position, with her partner at her side if possible (Figure 2.2). The gynaecologist uses sterile gloves and, after having assembled the instruments, checks the flow and pressure of the distension medium and the presence of air bubbles in the tubing system. After disinfection of the vagina with an aqueous solution and inserting a speculum, the hysteroscope is introduced in the external cervical ostium. The speculum is removed and, after opening the inflow, the path of the cervical channel becomes visible. Slowly and under direct vision, the instrument is moved forwards. The passage through the cervical channel is generally the most difficult part of the examination. When passing through the internal cervical ostium, resistance often has to be overcome before the uterine cavity is reached. By slowly turning the instrument along its axis, the tubal ostia are clearly

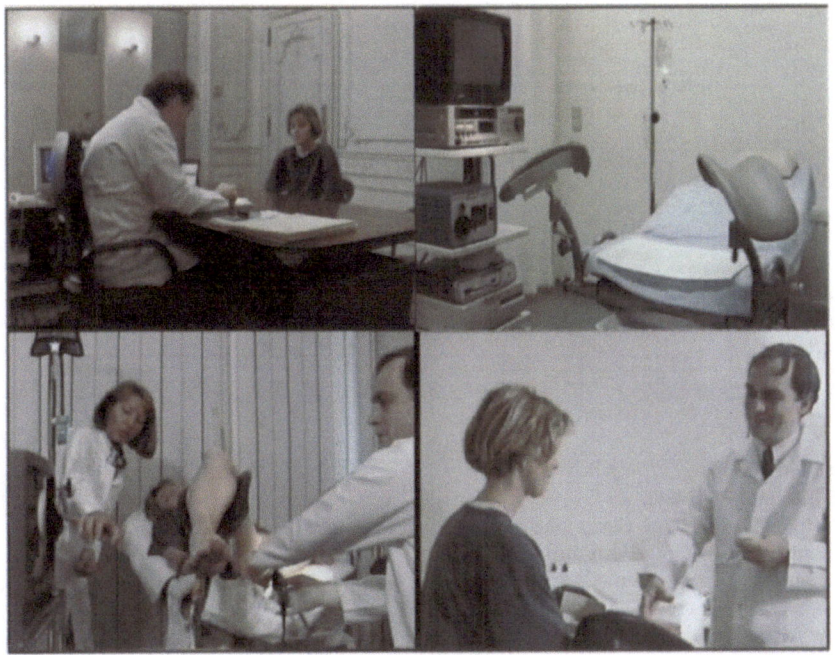

Figure 2.2 Mini–hysteroscopy is an office procedure.

visible with the 12° or 30° optic. Documentation of the form of the cavity and the aspect of the endometrium is necessary. The cervical channel is mainly inspected while slowly moving the instrument back. In cases of traumatic instrument handling, vision will be disturbed immediately by bleeding, resulting in the so-called Japanese flag image (Figure 2.3). The entire examination does not usually last longer than a few minutes and can be conducted in an outpatient setting without any form of anaesthesia.

Antibiotics are given only to patients with endometrial changes, such as hypervascularisation or a strawberry-like pattern.

Contraindications to perform an office mini-hysteroscopy are symptomatic vaginal, uterine or

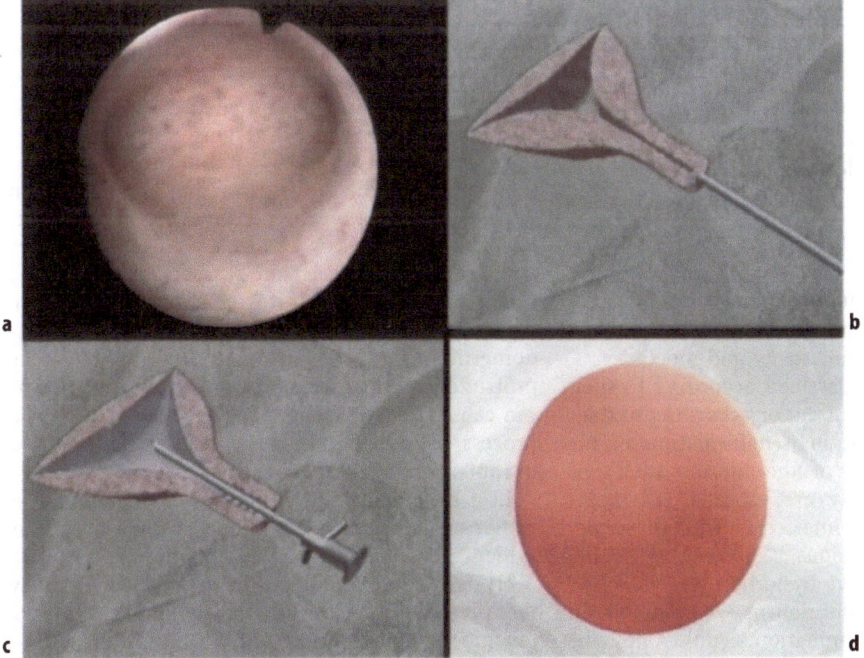

Figure 2.3 Procedure. **a** Normal uterine cavity. **b, c** Atraumatic insertion. **d** Bleeding resulting in the Japanese flag image.

Table 2.1. Indications for office hysteroscopy in normal gynaecological population between 1982 and 1989 (maximum two indications per patient possible)

Indications	No.	%
Abnormal uterine bleeding	2969	67.9
Pre-perimenopausal	2506	57.4
Postmenopausal	463	10.6
Oligo-amenorrhoea	136	3.1
Dysmenorrhoea	36	0.8
Infertility	254	5.8
Suspicion of pathology	976	22.4
Clinical examination	384	8.8
Hysterosalpingography	79	1.8
Ultrasound	200	4.6
Blind biopsy	313	7.2
Total	4371	100

Table 2.2. Hysteroscopic findings in a normal gynaecological population (1982–1989) (conventional instrumentation)

Hysteroscopic findings	No.	%
Total	4204	100
Normal	2492	59.3
No diagnosis	101	2.4
Abnormal	1611	38.3
A. Cervix	422	10
B. Cavum		
1. Congenital disorders	70	1.7
2. Acquired disorders	1119	26.6
2.1 Major lesions	455	10.8
Polyp/myoma	446	98
Partial or total cavity occlusion	9	2
2.2 Subtle lesions	664	15.8
Mucosal elevation	441	67
Endometrial synechia	70	10
Diffuse polyposis	60	9
Hypervascularisation	52	8
Necrotic	28	4
Exophytic	13	2

adnexal infections, menstrual bleeding, an evolutive pregnancy or severe uterine haemorrhage.

The atraumatic insertion technique can easily be performed in virgins without placing a speculum and without rupture of the hymen. The distension medium is warmed to 37°C and the vagina, cervix, cervical channel and uterine cavity are explored progressively.

2.3 Hysteroscopy in Patients with Abnormal Uterine Bleeding

2.3.1 Incidence

Uterine bleeding disorders are the most frequent indication for diagnostic hysteroscopy in a standard gynaecological population. Between 1982 and 1989 we documented consecutively every office hysteroscopy performed in our institution on a pre-designed registration form. In total, 4371 indications from 4204 office hysteroscopies were registered during that period and in 67.9% (2969) one of the two possible indications to perform the procedure was abnormal uterine bleeding (Table 2.1).

2.3.2 Findings

The direct visualisation of the endometrium offers far more possibilities than blind techniques or indirect interpretation of the uterine cavity and mucosa.

The findings can be classified according to their origin, congenital or acquired, or according to their size. Lesions that result in a deformation of the normal pear-like shape of the uterine cavity or totally fill up this cavity are classified as major pathology. Changes not interfering with the cavity form are called subtle lesions.

In our 4204 consecutive hysteroscopies we could establish sufficient visualisation in 3743 patients. In 101 patients the examination could not be

performed due to major discomfort or visualisation problems. In 360 cases a cervical stenosis did not permit an examination. The incidence of the different findings is shown in Table 2.2.

2.3.2.1 Major Lesions

Major lesions that cause menorrhagia are intracavity myomas and large polyps. In the case of a deformation of the cavity, the tubal ostia will serve as landmarks for correct orientation of the pathology.

A polyp is usually described as a pear-like tumour, projecting from the surrounding tissue and covered by normal-looking mucosa. It is soft tissue and has a similar colour to the endometrium. A senile polyp often contains cystic structures covered by a thin mucosa (Figure 2.4b).

Submucous myomas have a firm consistency, and their angle with the surrounding endometrium varies, depending on the percentage of its intramural part. They are covered by a thin mucosal layer and prominent vessels can be seen on the surface (Figure 2.4a). According to their size and location, myomas influence the vascularisation of the endometrium and the myometrium.[10] When they protrude into the uterine cavity, myomas or polyps can cause reactive changes in the endometrium by a process of local irritation, resulting in a so-called intrauterine device effect (Figure 2.4c).

In a histological study, Bolck demonstrated that in 88% of patients with uterine fibroids there was evidence of a pathological endometrium.[11]

Hysteroscopic examination can identify exactly the presence and intrauterine proportion of the myoma. In combination with an ultrasound exam-

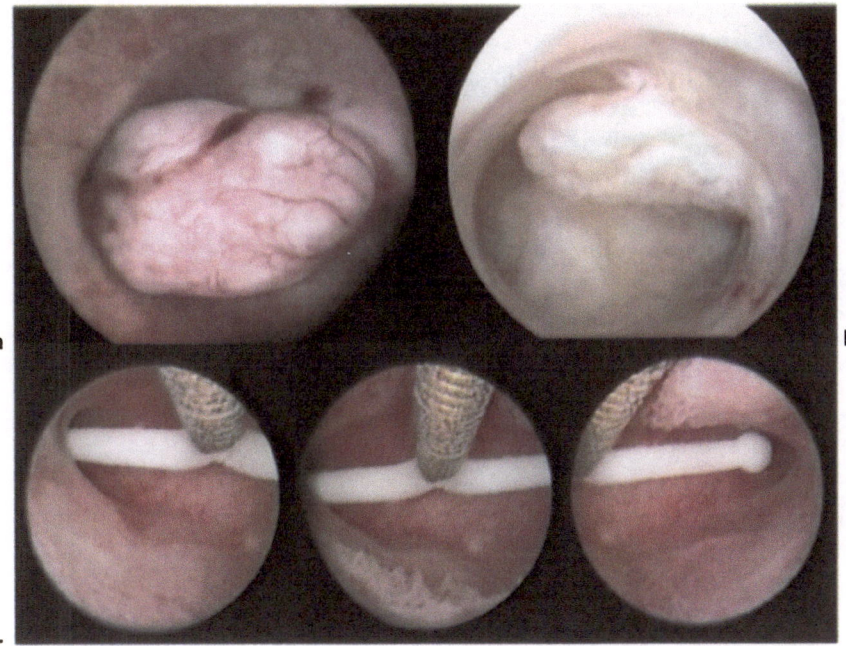

a   b   c

Figure 2.4 Myomas and polyps. **a** Pedunculated myoma with reddish surrounding endometrium. **b** Senile polyp with normal surrounding endometrium. **c** Intrauterine device with reddish endometrium similar to that in **a**.

ination, the myomatous changes in the myometrium can be documented.

For the treatment of intrauterine polyps and myomas, it is now generally accepted that the transcervical hysteroscopic approach is the standard. As reported by Hucke et al, women with an intrauterine myoma and suffering from objective menorrhagia are cured after total removal of the myoma.[12]

2.3.2.2 Subtle Lesions

Close inspection of the endometrium, with specific attention to the vascular pattern, is necessary to distinguish normal (functional or atrophic) mucosa from abnormal mucosal changes.

Atrophic mucosa appears pale, is usually 1 mm thick and, as it is very fragile, distension usually causes the formation of petechiae.

Very little is known about the hysteroscopically detectable subtle endometrial changes such as small polyps, marked and moderate mucosal elevations, endometrial hypervascularisation and diffuse polyposis (Figure 2.5b).

Localised aberration of the vascular architecture of the endometrium could be an important lesion, and its visualisation is only possible by hysteroscopy.

Generalised hypervascularisation of the endometrium is often seen in the presence of a large intrauterine or intramural myoma, but can also been seen as a solitary finding (Figure 2.5d). It is our experience that endometrial hypervascularisation,

defined as a significantly increased amount of vessels in the proliferative phase or a reddish endometrium in which the white openings of the glands produce the typical strawberry-like pattern (Figure 2.5c), can be diagnosed only by hysteroscopic visualisation. Neither cervical microbiology nor histology seems to have any diagnostic value in those cases.

The discovery of necrotic tissue can indicate blood clots, fibrin deposits or decidual casts. Exophytic lesions usually indicate a carcinoma.

2.3.2.3 Correlation with Histology?

In our view direct visualisation of the endometrium is far superior to blind or indirect interpretation of the uterine mucosa. Using fractionated curettage, which is still often conducted as a sole measure, intrauterine polyps, myomas or early stages of endometrial carcinomas might escape diagnosis.[13,14] In cases of endometrial carcinoma, a preoperative staging via hysteroscopy is possible with great accuracy.[15,16] However, this does not mean that hysteroscopy equals histology.

An atrophic, pale endometrium with small petechiae (due to the distension of the cavity) will indeed be recognised easily, even by the inexperienced hysteroscopist. The correct diagnosis of a functional endometrium can easily be made just by looking at the vascular pattern and the glandular openings.

Abnormal mucosal changes such as hypervascularisation, moderate or marked elevations, diffuse

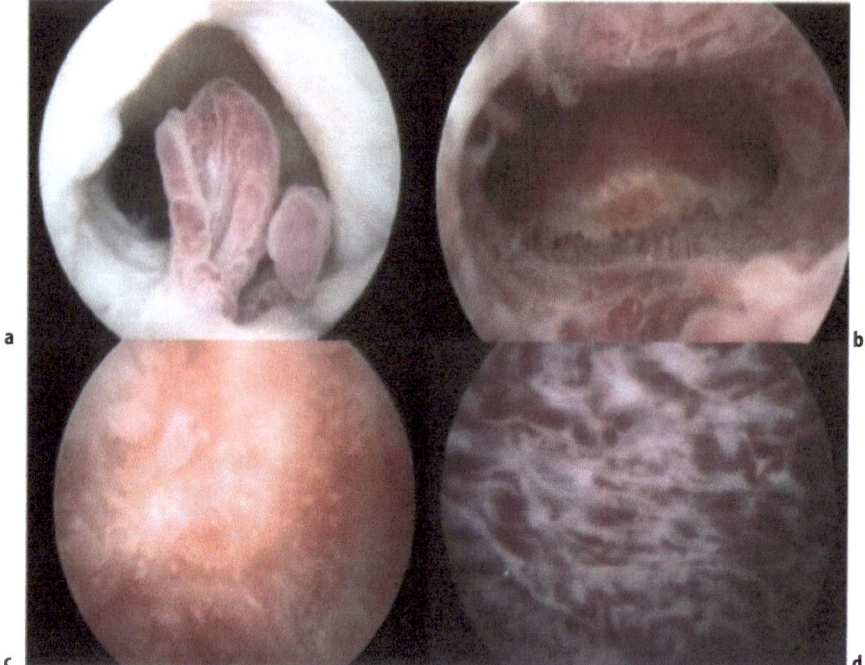

Figure 2.5 Subtle lesions.
a Cervical polyp.
b Diffuse polyposis. **c** Hypervascularisation, strawberry-like pattern. **d** Hypervascularisation, significantly increased amount of vessels.

polyposis or exophytic-necrotic lesions should always be the subject of histological examination.

Irregular, exophytic lesions featuring anarchic vascularisation will mostly be confirmed as being carcinomatous.

More difficult to interpret are the moderate or marked mucosal elevations. They correlate with a large variety of histological diagnoses. In those cases it has been proven that the eye-directed biopsy for histological examination is absolutely necessary to establish a correct diagnosis.

2.3.2.4 Technique of Tissue Biopsy for Histological Examination

The aim of office hysteroscopy is to differentiate normal from abnormal findings. In cases of uncertainty or evident pathology, the hysteroscopic procedure should always be accompanied by tissue sampling for histological analysis.

The sampling may be performed in one of three ways, depending on the hysteroscopic findings (generalised lesion, localised lesion or major pathology).

In the case of a generalised lesion, a representative sample of the endometrium is taken with a 3 mm diameter hand-suction curette (pipelle de Cornier). This procedure can easily be done at the same time as the diagnostic hysteroscopy.

In the case of marked or moderate mucosal elevation, localised abnormal vascular patterns, or in the presence of a small polyp, biopsy under direct vision or resection of the polyp should be performed.

The new mini-hysteroscopic instrumentation already offers rigid optical systems with double-flow sheath and a maximal total diameter of 5.5 mm, accessible for 15 French instrumentation. The fibre-optics offer the same possibilities with an instrument of total diameter less than 4 mm. With this instrumentation set-up, the procedure can be performed in an office environment without major patient discomfort.

For major pathology such as large polyps, myomas and complicated or combined pathology, where continuous flow and possibly diathermy are required, we prefer hospitalisation with the availability of loco-regional or general anaesthesia to establish a diagnosis and perform the treatment in the same procedure.

2.4 Feasibility of Office Hysteroscopy

Office hysteroscopy is only slowly gaining acceptance. The reason appears to be the false perception of low patient tolerance. Recently, new mini-hysteroscopic instruments have been developed that allow a virtually pain-free examination with more than adequate visual information about the uterine cavity.

In order to score objectively the pain associated with office hysteroscopy and to analyse the variables influencing it, a multicentre randomised controlled

Table 2.3. Office hysteroscopy: pain score and failure rate in a multicentre randomised trial

Pain score	≥ One vaginal delivery	No vaginal delivery
3.5 mm	1.2 (n = 65)	1.7 (n = 46)
5.0 mm	2.8 (n = 63)	3.3 (n = 48)
$p < 0.000001$		

Failures	≥ One vaginal delivery	No vaginal delivery
3.5 mm	0 (0%)	5 (5%)
5.0 mm	25 (40%)	19 (40%)
chi^2 $p < 0.05$		

study aims to enrol 600 patients. The study is stratified for instrumentation (3.5 mm versus 5.0 mm), previous experience of the surgeon (trainee versus experience of more than 1000 office procedures) and previous vaginal delivery (one or more versus no vaginal delivery). Patients who have had cervical surgery are not included in the study. Every examination is documented on a pre-designed form and on a videoprint in a standardised way. Immediately after the procedure the patients are asked to score the pain from 0 to 10 on a visual analogue scale.

The procedure is classified as a failure when the patient does not tolerate the pain or when the surgeon cannot visualise the uterine cavity sufficiently for appropriate diagnosis. Sufficient visualisation is agreed only if a third party can confirm the diagnosis on the videoprint documentation.

So far, 222 patients have been included in the study. The pain score was significantly lower in the 3.5 mm hysteroscopic system group (Table 2.3). There were relatively more procedural failures in the 5.0 mm group (Table 2.3). There was a tendency for the pain score to be lower in patients who had delivered vaginally at least once, but this effect did not reach significance.

2.5 Risks of Office Hysteroscopy

Analysis of the first 4204 outpatient hysteroscopies performed with a standard 5 mm hysteroscope and CO_2 gas as distension medium shows that seven complications were recorded, none of which required hospitalisation (Table 2.4).

Although CO_2 gas has been generally used as a distension medium, reports on embolism can seldom be found in the literature.[17] Experience, combined with reduction of the instrument diameter and a change of distension medium to the non-irritating saline solution, probably explain why no further complications have been recorded during office hysteroscopy since 1989.

2.6 Conclusions

The results of the interim analysis on the feasibility of hysteroscopy in an office environment show that the vast majority of patients tolerate office hysteroscopy without analgesia very well. Depending on the obstetric history, the average pain score for the 3.5 mm hysteroscope ranged from 1.2 to 1.7 on a scale of 10.

A prospective, randomised, blinded study was conducted by Tur Kaspa et al[18] to compare the use of a balloon catheter for performing hysterosalpingography with the use of a traditional metal cannula. Their findings show that both the balloon catheter and the traditional metal cannula provoke significantly more pain (3.8 ± 2.0 and 5.6 ± 2; on a scale of 1–10) than an office hysteroscopy using the 3.5 mm hysteroscope. Those findings would suggest that hysteroscopy is a less invasive examination than hysterosalpingography or contrast sonography, which uses a similar balloon catheter.

In addition, the low failure rates, even in patients with primary infertility and postmenopausal status, suggest that mini-hysteroscopic instruments are the instruments of choice. Even without assistance, the procedure usually takes no longer than 5 minutes.

The high patient compliance, the low failure rate and low complication rate observed during mini-hysteroscopy enable us to integrate hysteroscopy as a first-line diagnostic procedure in daily gynaecological practice. With the mini-hysteroscopic system it is easier to insert the scope in an atraumatic way, thus preventing artefacts and iatrogenic pathology. Furthermore, this equipment offers a continuous flow system in cases of uterine bleeding, without enlarging the total instrument diameter.

The use of saline as a distension medium improves the diagnostic capacity for subtle endometrial lesions and reduces pain and irritation. In a prospective study, Nagele et al demonstrated that the use of CO_2 during office hysteroscopy increased patient discomfort during the examination compared with the use of saline distension medium.[7]

The technique is certainly not more difficult than a contrast sonography and the information gathered by direct visualisation remains the gold standard.

The diagnostic work-up in abnormal uterine bleeding is standardised by a thorough anamnesis, clinical examination, vaginal sonography and blood sampling for evaluation of haematology, endocrinology and coagulation parameters. Frequently a decision about treatment, expectant management or more invasive procedures such as D&C is taken at this phase.

Introducing the ambulatory mini-hysteroscopy with or without direct tissue biopsy in a first-line diagnostic model provides both gynaecologist and patient with appropriate and valuable information

Table 2.4. Complications in 4204 conventional office hysteroscopies (1982–1989)

Complications	No.	%
Fundal perforation	2	
Prolonged vagal reaction	4	
Epileptic insult	1	
Infections	0	
Total	7	0.16

regarding the possible intrauterine causes of abnormal uterine bleeding.

An explanation of the diagnostic findings to the patient and her partner before surgery or medical treatment has the benefit of obtaining fully informed consent. In addition, if the findings are of doubtful clinical significance, the evolution can be evaluated by a repeat procedure and the effect of surgery or drug treatment on the evolution of the disease can be more readily controlled by a second-look procedure.

Based on data in the current literature and on our own experience, hospital admissions for D&C can be avoided in more than 50% of women who undergo (mini)-hysteroscopy for abnormal uterine bleeding. The office setting provides not only a major cost saving, but also a less alienating environment for the patient. The resulting increase in effectiveness and cost-benefit along with decreased patient morbidity could be very significant.

With the use of video equipment, all the findings can be documented and archived in an appropriate way (video documentation, videoprint or direct archiving of images in the computer). In addition, patient compliance is greatly increased by instant video-feedback.

The perfect imaging of the mini-hysteroscopes, the possibility of documentation and the high patient compliance should guarantee the wide application of diagnostic hysteroscopy in an office environment, although the technique requires training, is characterised by a slow learning curve and in most countries lacks adequate reimbursement as an office procedure.

Mini-hysteroscopy plays a key role in the diagnosis of abnormal uterine bleeding; it is a primary investigation tool in infertility work-up; it is the ideal screening method for endometrial changes in patients taking hormone replacement therapy or anti-oestrogen adjuvant treatment;[5,6] and it is helpful in the interpretation of uncertain findings in other diagnostic techniques such as ultrasound, magnetic resonance imaging, blind biopsy or hysterosalpingography.

In the diagnosis of pathology such as myomas, polyps, synechiae or subtle endometrial lesions, mini-hysteroscopy remains an extremely valuable tool to help interpret the sonographic findings or to identify the problem in the case of negative sonography. Both transvaginal sonography and mini-hysteroscopy have their place in first-line office diagnostic procedures.

References

1. Hallberg L, Högdall AM, Nilsson L et al (1966) Menstrual blood loss: a population study. Acta Obstet Gynecol Scand 45:320–351
2. Bayer SR, De Cherney AH (1993) Clinical manifestations and treatment of dysfunctional uterine bleeding. Am Med Assoc 269:1823–1828
3. Campo RL, Schlösser HW (1998) Uteriner Faktor der weiblichen Sterilität/Infertilität. In: Diedrich K (ed) Endokrinologie und Reproduktionsmedizin III, ch 8: Urban & Schwarzenberg, München-Wien-Baltimore, pp 138–158
4. Valle RF (1981) Hysteroscopic evaluation of patients with abnormal uterine bleeding. Surg Gynecol Obstet 153:521–526
5. Neven P, De Muylder X, Van Belle Y et al (1994) Tamoxifen and the uterus: women given this drug need careful assessment. Br Med J 309:1313–1314
6. Neven P, De Muylder X, Van Belle Y et al (1997) Longitudinal hysteroscopic follow-up during tamoxifen treatment (letter). Lancet 351(9095):36
7. Nagele F, Bournas N, O'Connor H et al (1996) Comparison of carbon dioxide and normal saline for uterine distension in outpatient hysteroscopy. Fertil Steril 65(2):305–309
8. Clark S, Vonau B, Macdonald R (1996) Topical anaesthesia in outpatient hysteroscopy. Gynaecol Endosc 5:141–144
9. Ezeh UO, Vercellini P (1995) Outpatient hysteroscopy – paracervical block. Fertil Steril 64:221–222
10. Deligdisch L (1970) Endometrial changes associated with myomata uterus. J Clin Pathol 23:676
11. Bolck F (1961) Die Pathologie der Uterusmyome. Arch Gynecol 195:166
12. Hucke J, Campo R, Debruyne P et al (1992) Die hysteroskopische Resektion submuköser Myome. Geburtsh u Frauenheilk 52:214–218
13. Brooks PG, Serden SP (1988) Hysteroscopic findings after unsuccessful dilatation and curettage for abnormal uterine bleeding. Am J Obstet Gynecol 158:1354–1357
14. Word B, Gravlee LC, Widemann GL (1958) The fallacy of simple uterine curettage. Obstet Gynecol 12:642–649
15. Cronje HS, Deale CJC (1988) Staging of endometrial cancer by hysteroscopy. S Afr Med J 73:716–717
16. Joelsson I, Levine RU, Moberger G (1971) Hysteroscopy as an adjunct in determining the extent of carcinoma of the endometrium. Am J Obstet Gynecol 111(5):696–702
17. Ghimouz A, Loisel B, Kheyar M et al (1996) Carbon dioxide embolism with transient blindness associated with hysteroscopy. Ann Fr Anesth Reanim 15:192–195
18. Tur Kaspa I, Seidman DS, Soriano D et al (1998) Hysterosalpingography with a balloon catheter versus a metal cannula: a prospective, randomized, blinded comparative study. Hum Reprod 13(1):75–7

Chapter 3

Hysteroscopic Fibroid Resection

Sjoerd de Blok

3.1 Introduction

Myomas are the most common benign neoplasms of the uterine wall. It is estimated that fibroids can be found in about 25% of women over 35 years, although exact figures are unknown. The growth of fibroids depends on hormonal stimulation, so they are seldom found before puberty or after the menopause. In daily clinical practice, fibroids are a disease of the fourth and fifth decades.

Fibroids are composed of smooth muscle cells and connective tissue; they are usually more or less round in shape and embedded in a pseudocapsula, making hysteroscopic and laparoscopic peeling possible. Fibroids may be left untreated if they do not cause symptoms. Depending on the size and the vascular supply, fibroids can degenerate, become calcified or become infarcted with central haemorrhage. In classical gynaecology, fibroids may be subdivided according to their location in the uterine wall: subserous, intramural or submucous. With the introduction of diagnostic hysteroscopy, it is now possible to visualise intracavity (submucous) fibroids.

Menstrual disorders can first be controlled with the use of drugs that regulate the ovarian–uterine axis. The only drugs that have more or less specific actions on fibroids are gonadotrophin-releasing hormone (GnRH) analogues. However, these have several side-effects, including rapid regrowth of fibroids after therapy is stopped. Gonadotrophin-releasing hormone analogues are used to reduce the size and vascular architecture of the fibroids prior to surgical treatment. Antagonists have an important role, resulting in a 35% reduction of volume within 3 weeks of treatment.

Hysteroscopy has been developed as a superior technique for the diagnosis and treatment of intracavity pathology with the introduction of new generations of instruments.[1,2]

In 1978, Neuwirth first described the possibility of hysteroscopic resection of fibroids using a urological resectoscope and 32% dextran 70 as distension medium.[3] Hallez et al introduced the use of continuous-flow hysteroresectoscopy with low-viscosity fluid distension in 1987.[4] These studies clearly demonstrated use of the hysteroresectoscope as an alternative to hysterectomy for the control of menorrhagia.

Long-term follow-up studies showing success rates of 91–96% with no need for further medical intervention for menstrual disorders have established hysteroscopic resection as an indispensable and effective tool for the treatment of intrauterine fibroids.[5-7]

In this chapter, clinical guidelines will be described for the use of hysteroscopic resection of intrauterine fibroids in daily gynaecological practice.

3.2 Symptomatology, Diagnosis and Imaging

Fibroids can be asymptomatic and detected by routine gynaecological examination or ultrasonography. In 20–50% of affected women, fibroids cause symptoms of menstrual disorder, pain and mechanical effects on other organs adjacent to the uterus, depending on the size, number and location.

Between 5 and 10% of patients with fibroids have a submucous localisation. In general, submucous fibroids are considered to be responsible for menstrual disorders and reproduction failure, although there are no evidence-based data in the literature for the latter.

Menstrual disorders are associated with submucous localisation of fibroids causing direct mechanical lesions to the endometrium opposite the submucous fibroid or as a result of interaction with the vascular architecture of the endo- and myometrium. Submucous fibroids are found significantly more often in patients with menorrhagia in combination with dysmenorrhoea, compared with patients with menorrhagia or metrorrhagia alone.[7]

Hysteroscopy has developed into an indispensable tool for the diagnosis of intrauterine pathology in the past decade. In the clinical work-up of patients with suspected intrauterine pathology, the first step will be a transvaginal ultrasound scan to find pathology of the uterine wall or the uterine cavity. Dilatation and curettage is considered obsolete for the diagnosis of intrauterine disorders in patients with persistent abnormal uterine bleeding.[8–12]

In two-thirds of patients with abnormal uterine bleeding, no anomalies are found with hysteroscopy. These patients are classified as suffering from dysfunctional uterine bleeding, which needs hormonal therapy or endometrial ablation. With the introduction of transvaginal ultrasonography for the depiction of abnormal endometrium and intracavity pathology, patients who will benefit from hysteroscopy can be selected in the office, followed by an office hysteroscopy. The sensitivity of transvaginal sonography for intrauterine pathology is greater than 95% and the specificity for the distinction of polyps and fibroids is greater than 85% (Figure 3.1).[13,14] The interpretation of the intramural extension of a submucous fibroid with transvaginal ultrasonography remains difficult. Due to the artefact of distension of the uterine cavity during hysteroscopy, the impression with transvaginal ultrasonography on the depth of intramural extension cannot be confirmed in most cases. The possibility of hysteroscopic resection can be judged only during diagnostic hysteroscopy.

With hysterosalpingography (HSG), fibroids can be visualised in the uterine cavity as a filling defect, but there are few data concerning HSG investigation in patients with abnormal uterine bleeding. Even in cases with known intrauterine fibroids, HSG

provides poor intracavity visualisation and reasonable visualisation of the lining of the cavity and the degree of distortion, which can also be caused by intramural fibroids.

The definitive diagnosis of submucous fibroids is made with diagnostic hysteroscopy, preferably performed in an ambulant office setting with continuous-flow hysteroscopy, preventing poor visibility in patients suffering from abnormal uterine bleeding. During diagnostic hysteroscopy, submucous fibroids can be mapped and classified.

The European Society for Hysteroscopy has adapted a hysteroscopic classification, which takes into account the intramural extension and enables a prognosis on the resection of submucous fibroids to be made (Table 3.1, Figures 3.2 and 3.3).

Occasionally, intramural extension is hard to predict with hysteroscopy; in these cases magnetic resonance imaging is superior to transvaginal sonography in distinguishing transmural fibroids and submucous fibroids, showing a sharp demarcation between normal myometrium and the fibroid pseudocapsula in T2-weighted sections.

Transmural fibroids cannot be resected with the hysteroscope because of the high chance of perforation of the uterine wall. Type II fibroids can be

Table 3.1. European Society for Hysteroscopy classification of submucous fibroids according to intramural extension[2]

Type 0	Pedunculated, no intramural extension
Type I	> 50% Intracavitary, < 50% intramural extension
Type II	< 50% Intracavitary, > 50% intramural extension

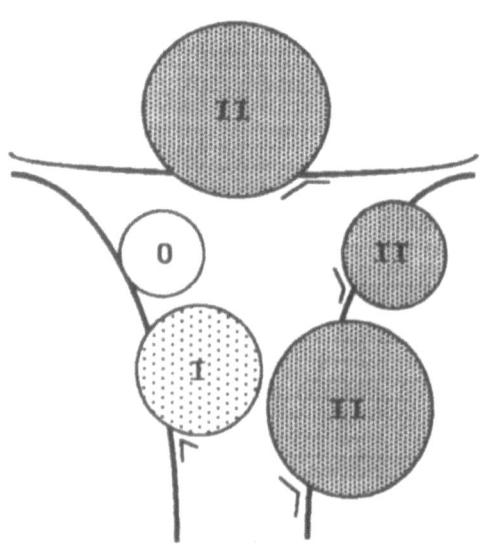

Figure 3.2 Schematic classification of submucous fibroids. Type 0, pedunculated; type I, > 50% intracavitary; type II, < 50% intracavitary.

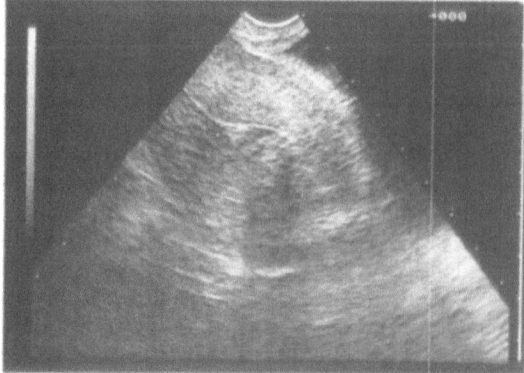

Figure 3.1 Transvaginal ultrasound scan, showing a submucous fibroid.

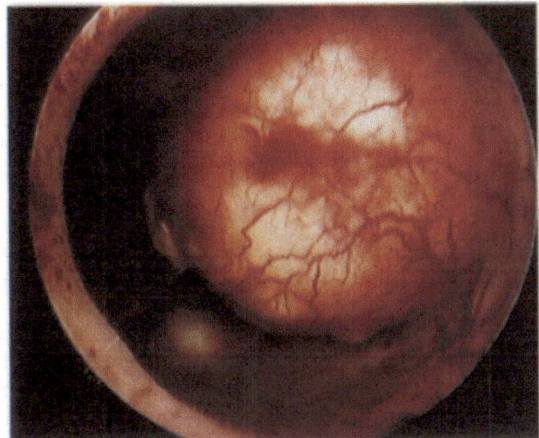

Figure 3.3 Hysteroscopic image, showing an example of a type 0 fibroid.

resected only if an adequate amount of normal myometrium is located behind the submucous fibroid (Figure 3.4).

3.3 Hysteroscopic Resection

3.3.1 Technique

The optimal technique for the treatment of submucous fibroids is with the use of a specially designed hysteroresectoscope for high-frequency electroendosurgery.

A standard hysteroresectoscope has a spring-loaded passive working element mounted with a 90° loop-wire electrode in a continuous-flow sheath system with a 12° wide-angle telescope. For fluid distension, low-viscosity fluids are recommended, such as sorbitol 4 or 5%, glycine, purisole or glucose 5%. These low-viscosity fluids are electrolyte-free for the use of monopolar electrodes and are isotonic to enhance safety if resorption occurs.

Distension during hysteroresection is preferably performed with specially designed hysteropump systems, which keep a preselected intrauterine pressure below 150 mmHg and adaptation of flow maximised at 450 ml per minute. These systems provide optimal visualisation during resection.[2]

The vascular architecture of the myometrium shows an increase of diameter of vessels from the basal lamina of the endometrium to the subserous areas. This anatomical architecture explains why resorption becomes significant when entering the myometrium with the resectoscope. During resection of fibroids with intramural extension, this fact is responsible for resorption and fluid overload.

The technique of fibroid resection consists of placing the cutting loop wire behind the fibroid and cutting under permanent visual control to prevent accidental perforation. Cutting is performed with pure cutting current or monitored automatically by the HF unit, depending on which brand is used. The pseudocapsula of the fibroid can be recognised as

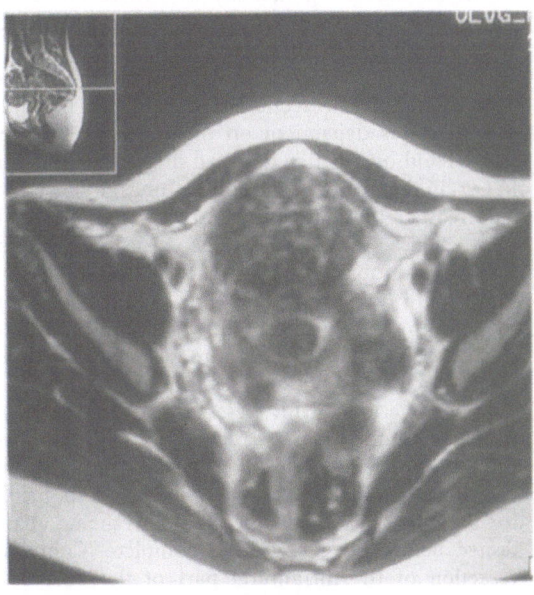

a

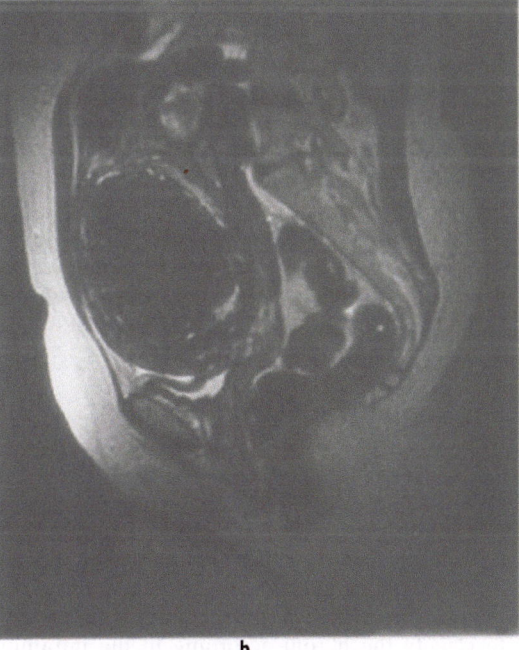

b

Figure 3.4 a Transverse section with magnetic resonance imaging, showing a type I fibroid; hysteroresection is possible. **b** Midsagittal section with magnetic resonance imaging, showing a transverse submucous fibroid on the anterior uterine wall; hysteroresection is impossible.

pink healthy myometrium so that a complete resection can be achieved.

To reduce operation time, preparation of fibroids with a GnRH analogue for 2 or 3 months is recommended. Fibroids and submucous fibroids will shrink up to 30% in diameter on ultrasound with this preparation.[15] It is not known whether use of GnRH analogues significantly influences operation time, fluid overload or efficacy of the procedure. As a result of fluid overload, a second or even sometimes a third procedure may be needed to achieve complete resection. The need for multiple procedures is dependent on the intramural extension.[6] Fluid overload is detected first by a reduction in CO_2 in the expired air from the lungs, followed by a decrease of blood pressure and oxygenation. When these signs are detected, the anaesthetist must respond appropriately. Constant electronic measuring of fluid loss is essential, and should appear on the monitor. Another technique is to add alcohol to the distension fluid and measure the expired volume of alcohol as a function of resorption.

Fluid overload with resection of submucous fibroids is more closely related to the depth of intramural extension of the fibroids than to the operation time.[16] Fluid overload may be responsible for the hysteroresectoscopic procedure being abandoned before the resection is complete. Complete resection of the intramural part of the fibroid is essential to prevent recurrence of abnormal uterine bleeding within half a year.[7]

3.3.2 Results

Long-term follow-up data on hysteroscopic resection of fibroids for the treatment of submucous fibroids show excellent results of 90–95% success for the restoration of normal menstrual bleeding at 5–9 years. These studies only described the resection of fibroids as a single procedure, without concomitant endometrial resection.

3.4 Conclusions

Submucous fibroids cause menorrhagia rather than metrorrhagia. Suspected submucous fibroids are best investigated using transvaginal ultrasonography. If confirmed with this procedure, the final diagnosis is made with an outpatient diagnostic hysteroscopy by an endoscopist who is fully trained to classify the fibroid according to the intramural extension. Dilatation and curettage is considered obsolete for the removal or diagnosis of submucous fibroids. If no certain prediction can be made with diagnostic hysteroscopy and ultrasonography about

the intramural extension or the presence of a transmural fibroid, a magnetic resonance scan is indispensable before safe resection can be offered to the patient. Preparation of the fibroids with GnRH analogues to facilitate endoresection is advised, but the benefits of this treatment have not been proven scientifically.

Specialised instruments designed for hysteroscopic resection should be used. Special attention must be given to the fluid overload, which is related to the depth of intramural extension of the submucous fibroids, rather than to operating time. Constant monitoring of fluid balance is mandatory for safe surgery. The fluid balance must be indicated on the monitor. The operating room staff must be trained in signs of fluid overload and adequate management.

Long-term follow-up results show that hysteroscopic endoresection is a superior technique for the treatment of menorrhagia caused by submucous fibroids. The role of fibroid resection in infertility is anecdotal and lacks evidence-based data.

References

1. Wamsteker K, de Blok S (1998) Diagnostic hysteroscopy: technique and documentation. In: Sutton C, Diamond MP (eds) Endoscopic surgery for gynaecologists 2nd edn. WB Saunders, London, pp 511–524
2. Wamsteker K, Blok S de, Emanuel MH (1992) Instrumentation for transcervical hysteroscopic endosurgery. Gynaecol Endosc 1:59–67
3. Neuwirth RS (1978) A new technique for and additional experience with hysteroscopic resection of submucous fibroids. Am J Obstet Gynecol 131:91–94
4. Hallez JP, Netter A, Cartier R (1987) Methodical intrauterine resection. Am J Obstet Gynecol 156:1080–1084
5. Derman SG, Rehnstrom J, Neuwirth RS (1991) The long term effectiveness of hysteroscopic treatment of menorrhagia and leiomyomas. Obstet Gynecol 63:703–708
6. Blok S de, Dijkman AB, Hemrika DJ (1995) Transcervical resection of fibroids (TCRM): results related to hysteroscopic classification. Gynaecol Endosc 4:243–246
7. Emanuel MH, Wamsteker K, de Kruiff J (1993) Transcervical hysteroscopic resection of submucous fibroids for abnormal uterine bleeding: results regarding the degree of intramural extension. Obstet Gynecol 82:736–740
8. Emanuel MH, Verdel MJC, Stas H et al (1995) An audit of true prevalence of intrauterine pathology; the hysteroscopical findings controlled for patient-selection in 1202 patients with abnormal uterine bleeding. Gynaecol Endosc 4:237–241
9. Gimpelson RJ, Pappold HO (1988) A comparative study between panoramic hysteroscopy with directed biopsies and dilatation and curettage. A review of 276 cases. Am J Obstet Gynecol 158:489–492
10. Brooks PG, Serden SP (1988) Hysteroscopic findings after unsuccessful dilatation and curettage for abnormal uterine bleeding. Am J Obstet Gynecol 158:1354–1357
11. Stock RJ, Kanbour A (1975) Prehysterectomy curettage. Obstet Gynecol 45:537–541
12. Grimes DA (1982) Dilatation and curettage: a reappraisal. Am J Obstet Gynecol 142:1–6
13. Fedele L, Bianchi S, Dorta M et al (1991) Transvaginal ultrasonography versus hysteroscopy in the diagnosis of uterine submucous myomas. Obstet Gynecol 77:745–748.

14. Emanuel MH, Verdel MJC, Wamsteker K et al (1995) A prospective comparison of transvaginal ultrasonography and diagnostic hysteroscopy in the evaluation of patients with abnormal uterine bleeding: clinical implications. Am J Obstet Gynecol 172:547–552

15. Donnez J, Nisolle M, Grandjean P et al (1993) The place of GnRH agonists in the treatment of endometriosis and fibroids by advanced endoscopic techniques. Br J Obstet Gynaecol 13:69–71

16. Emanuel MH, Wamsteker K (1997) An analysis of fluid-loss during transcervical resection of submucous myomas. Fertil Steril 68:881–886

Chapter 4

Transcervical Resection of the Endometrium: Results and Complications

Olav Istre

4.1 Introduction

Transcervical resection of the endometrium (TCRE) and of fibroids (TCRF) are alternatives to hysterectomy in the treatment of dysfunctional bleeding. The operation is more likely to be successful if patients are carefully selected. Patients who consider TCRE must be aware that further childbearing cannot be considered.[1]

The indications for TCRE are gradually evolving. In 1987, the indications were described by DeCherney: contraindication for general anaesthesia, refusal to undergo a hysterectomy and haemorrhagic dis-orders.[2] In 1991, it was agreed that TCRE was indicated for abnormal menstrual bleeding justifying a hysterectomy, which usually meant that conservative therapy had been unsuccessful or had failed.[1,3-5] The uterus had to be smaller than 12 weeks of amenorrhoea, fibroids had to be submucous and smaller than 5cm in diameter on ultrasound scan or hysteroscopy. Women with other gynaecological diseases such as endometriosis or uterine prolapse were advised against TCRE, because of the likelihood of further surgery.[4]

Today, more women are aware of the new possibilities and the absolute prerequisite of severe symptoms justifying hysterectomy is no longer valid. Furthermore, many women suffering from anaemia and menorrhagia can avoid long-term oral drug treatment, which is often associated with adverse effects and poor patient compliance.

4.2 Histology

Any malignancy must be ruled out. A preoperative cervical smear and histological samples from the uterine cavity using either the Pipelle or Vabra

method are mandatory.[6] These sampling techniques provide an adequate specimen for histological analysis and a correct diagnosis.[7,8]

Removal of the endometrium has gained popularity in Europe because it allows double-checking of the endometrial histology. Malignancies of the endometrium have been detected in specimens obtained from the resection. In studies on women with irregular and postmenopausal bleeding who had been investigated preoperatively, four patients were found to have a carcinoma of the endometrium after TCRE.[9,10] Most endometrial cancers are diagnosed in postmenopausal women and the incidence reaches a peak in women aged between 65 and 74 years of age. Ninety-five per cent of all new endometrial cancers detected are found in women aged more than 50 years (Norwegian Cancer Registry, 1987).

Women with atypical or adenomatous hyperplasia should not undergo a TCRE because of the risk of later malignancy. The preinvasive nature of atypical endometrial hyperplasia is well established, with a risk for malignant transformation of 23% over 11 years.[11] However, cystic glandular hyperplasia without atypia is not a contraindication for operation. Women with cervical dysplasia should be treated in the usual way and this is not a contraindication to TCRE.

4.3 Fibroids

Submucous fibroids are the most frequent cause of menorrhagia. Their incidence in menorrhagia is estimated to be around 20% when diagnosed by bimanual palpation.[12] Transvaginal ultrasonography (TVS) is a more accurate diagnostic method.[13] The use of fluid instillation enhances the specificity for and the mapping of fibroids.[14] Hysteroscopy can be used to detect uterine fibroids in a substantial number of patients with menorrhagia.[15,16]

In our series of 360 patients, all referred by general practitioners for abnormal bleeding and undergoing TCRE, fibroids were detected in 120 (33%). It is generally agreed that the uterus should be smaller than 12 weeks amenorrhoea, the hysterometry should be less than 12 cm and the maximum size of intracavity fibroids should not exceed 5 cm for TCRF.[4] These limitations are imposed by the equipment; both the resectoscope and the electrical sling would be too small for handling larger uteri or fibroids. However, in most cases, larger uteri or larger or multiple fibroids would create additional symptomatology in these patients, which would justify another surgical approach, including hysterectomy.[17] The location of the fibroid is another important aspect because complete resection improves long-term outcome after TCRE and TCRF as a treatment for uterine bleeding.[18] In cases of marked intramural extension, different techniques such as abdominal myomectomy could be applied. Therefore, it is essential to have accurate knowledge about the size, number and localisation of fibroids preoperatively.

4.4 Ultrasound

Transvaginal ultrasonography is a non-invasive, accurate and cost-effective procedure, which has become an important investigation in modern gynaecological practice.[19] Preoperative selection of suitable cases with TVS may improve the success rate after TCRF even further, thereby avoiding additional surgery. A preoperative ultrasound scan was performed in our patients and three parameters were assessed.

The anterior/posterior (AP) diameter of the uterus was measured, giving an accurate indication of its size. Smaller transverse and AP diameters of the uterus appear to predict a more successful outcome. Significant reductions in the AP diameter were measured in the successful group when assessed 3 months postoperatively.[19] Peroperative problems with irrigation solution were more pronounced in patients with AP diameter > 55 mm (hysterosalpingography).

The maximum thickness of the endometrium (double layer) was measured on a midline sagittal uterine section at the level of maximum AP dimension of the uterus. A double layer < 8.29 mm was more likely to lead to amenorrhoea 1 year after TCRE (hysterosalpingography).

A classification system has been developed for submucous fibroids on TVS. Pedunculated submucous fibroids without intramural extension are classified as type 0 fibroids. Type I is when the submucous fibroid is sessile and the intramural part is less than 50%. With an intramural extension of 50% or more, the fibroid is classified as type II (Figure 4.1). The degree of intramural extension can be assessed by observing the angle of the fibroid with the endometrium at the attachment to the

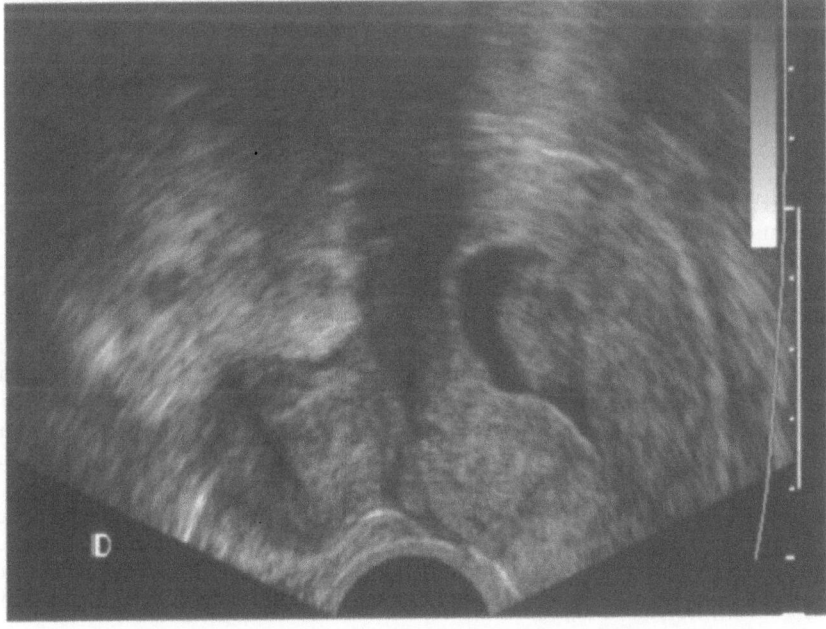

Figure 4.1 Transvaginal ultrasound scan showing subserous, intramural (type II) and submucous (type I) fibroids.

uterine wall.[18] Types II and I require a different technique, which often needs to be repeated. Knowledge of the type of fibroid is essential preoperatively, so that the operator is aware of what kind of problems to expect.

4.5 Pelvic Pain

A large indistinct group of patients suffer from pelvic pain. Three indications account for over half of the hysterectomies performed in the USA: leiomyomas, dysfunctional uterine bleeding and pelvic relaxation. A variable degree of pain was an additional indication for these hysterectomies.[20] Pelvic pain originating outside the uterus, from endometriosis or adhesions, for example, requires another approach to both diagnosis and treatment. Both diagnosis and differentiation of the reasons behind the pain may be difficult; however, TCRE or TCRF is beneficial, whether or not menorrhagia is accompanied by dysmenorrhoea.[4] Our own results indicate the same tendency: menstrual pain is reduced after TCRE. However, pain that is not accompanied by dysmenorrhoea should be treated in the usual manner.

4.6 Age

Transcervical resection of the endometrium is an irreversible treatment and should be offered only to patients who have finished childbearing. This usually means that only patients older than 25 years should be offered TCRE or TCRF: 25 years is the age for legal sterilisation in Scandinavian countries. The prevalence of menorrhagia is lowest in young women and highest in women in their 50s; parity is also a factor that may increase the tendency of bleeding disorders.[21]

In our study of 350 patients undergoing TCRE, the mean age was 44.3 (6.78), range 27–85 years (O. Istre, thesis ISBN 1996, 82-91675-05-81). Thirteen of these patients were more than 55 years of age; the histological results were six with hyperplasia, four with polyps, one secretory, one proliferative and one atrophic. These findings are in accordance with those of Brooks et al, who performed TCRE in 26 patients aged 50 years and older.[22] Thirteen of the patients were on hormone replacement therapy and suffered from metrorrhagia; 23 of the 26 patients became amenorrhoeic.[22] In my opinion, therefore, there should be no older age limit for the performance of TCRE.

4.7 Operative Complications

4.7.1 Perforation

The most dangerous complication during hysteroscopic surgery is perforation, as adjacent organs may be damaged. In larger series of TCRE, the incidence of perforation is limited. Magos reported four perforations in 250 patients and Rankin reported two perforations in 400 patients.[4,10] In our series of 375 patients, there were nine perforations, significantly more occurring during the first 50 consecutive operations.[3]

In cases of perforation during hysteroscopy, laparotomy seems to be unnecessary; when our patients were observed in the ward, no complications apart from the perforation were observed. Bowel injury is the most serious complication after TCRE. It is believed to be a result of direct damage with the resectoscope on the bowel surface,[23,24] although most reports of bowel injury result from ablation techniques such as rollerball and Nd:YAG lasers.[25,26] During ablation techniques there is immediate visible thermal injury of at least 5 mm depth, which is increased when the energy source is maintained at the same spot for long periods.[27-29]

During hysteroscopic surgery in our patients, an intrauterine pressure of about 100 mmHg is used to achieve sufficient distension of the cavity, and the intestines are probably flushed away in cases of perforation, with immediate cooling of the resection sling.[3] Finishing the operation after a perforation can be difficult, but in the absence of major intra-abdominal trauma, the perforation can be sutured by laparoscopy and the resection continued.[30]

4.7.2 Absorption of Irrigation Media

Another complication of TCRE is the transurethral resection of the prostate (TURP) syndrome, which is a clinical entity related to massive absorption of the irrigating solution.[31,32] Although toxic effects of glycine and its metabolites may contribute to the syndrome, absorption of water with dilutional hyponatraemia, water intoxication, cerebral oedema and cardiac overload are considered the main characteristics.[33-36] Absorption of the irrigating medium is presumably related to the intrauterine pressure applied during the procedure.

In our patients, a maximum pressure of about 100 mmHg was applied to the infusion system, but it is difficult to assess the intrauterine pressure because of a decrease in pressure along the infusion line and the application of suction to the effluent. Although the actual pressure probably exceeded the low levels recommended during resection of the prostate,[32] the venous systems of the prostate and the myometrium are not comparable. The results of our study suggest that, with adequate peroperative control, pressures up to 100 mmHg can be applied within the uterine cavity without occurrence of marked TURP syndrome-like complications, as shown by serum sodium levels immediately after TCRE (Figure 4.2).

In our studies, we have demonstrated minor changes in the coagulation parameters, with more marked changes after absorption of significant amounts of the glycine solution. While the observed decrease in the levels of thrombocytes, haptoglobin and fibrinogen may be explained in part by simple dilution, absorption of the hypo-osmotic glycine solution (about 200 mOsmol/l) may have caused some degree of haemolysis as well. Moreover, the increased levels of D-dimers probably reflect activated coagulation states associated with continuous and latent formation of thrombin and the onset of reactive fibrinolysis. Such changes are common after major operative procedures and seem to occur after TCRE as well. However, these changes appear to have limited clinical implications. Other papers have demonstrated positive fibrinogen split product in cases of glycine absorption and recommend limiting the input pressure.[37]

During TCRE using 1.5% glycine as irrigation solution, about one in three patients experiences post-surgical nausea.[38] These patients had all absorbed significant amounts of glycine together with the water solvent, leading to high plasma levels of glycine, ranging from 5000 to 18 000 micromoles per litre (normal plasma levels of glycine 110–330 micromoles per litre). Glycine is the simplest amino acid and undergoes a variety of metabolic reactions, largely of synthetic nature. Conversion to serine is one of the dominating pathways when there is

excess glycine available.[39] Thus, the finding that the plasma serine level of the patients with nausea is high several hours after surgery is most likely explained by conversion of glycine to serine. The secondary excess of serine may interact with cystathionine, leading to increased cysteine. Increased serum levels of nine amino acids, including glycine, are found after TCRE (Table 4.1). The high plasma levels of glycine and its secondary products may be responsible for some of the toxic symptoms observed after absorption of the irrigating glycine solution during TCRE. This absorption probably occurs mainly into vessels opened during the procedure, as no significant correlation between the peroperative glycine deficit and the operation time or the total amount of glycine used could be demonstrated in our study, in line with previous findings from our group.[40]

Patients with a glycine deficit of 1000 ml or more, or a decrease in serum sodium levels of 10 mmol/l or more, all experienced nausea and had a diagnosis of cerebral oedema on computed tomography scan (Figure 4.3). The results suggest that discrete cerebral oedema may contribute to the development of postoperative nausea in patients undergoing transcervical surgery with significant absorption of the glycine irrigating solution.

Table 4.1. Changes in plasma levels of amino acids after transcervical resection of the endometrium

Increasing	Decreasing	No change
Alanine	Proline	Histidine
Aminobutyrate	Methionine	Lysine
Asparagine	Isoleucine	Phenylalanine
Cysteine	Leucine	Tryptophan
Glutamine	Tyrosine	Valine
Glutamate	Ornithine	1-Methylhistidine
Glycine	3-Methylhistidine	Hydroxyproline
Serine	Arginine	Homocysteine
Taurine	Threonine	Phosphoetanolamine
		Citrulline

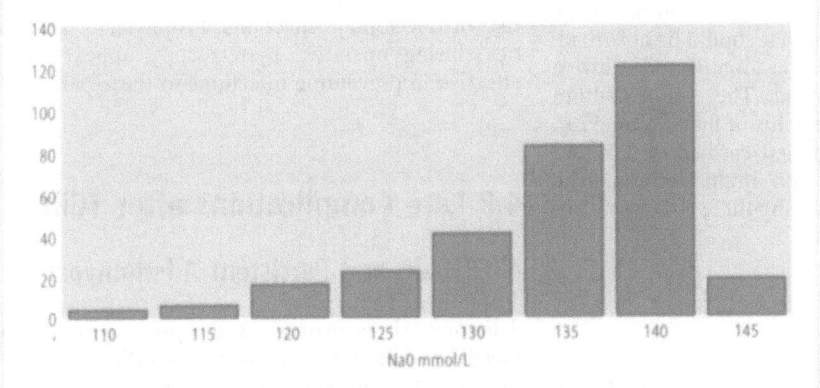

Figure 4.2 Serum sodium levels immediately after transcervical resection of the endometrium in 302 patients.

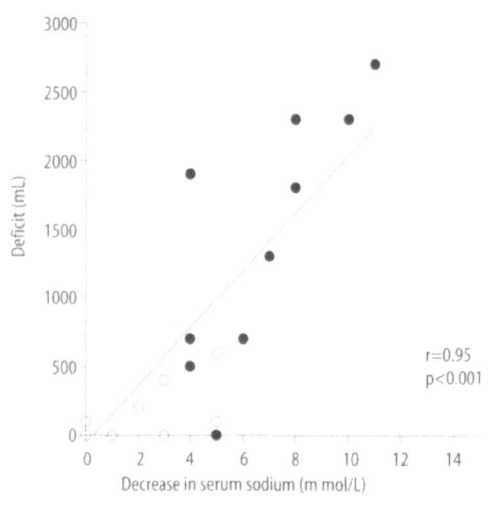

r=0.95
p<0.001

Decrease in serum sodium (m mol/L)

Figure 4.3 Decrease in serum sodium levels and glycine deficit after transcervical resection of the endometrium. The black circles represent patients with oedema.

4.7.3 Irrigation Solutions: The Future

Although glycine 1.5% has traditionally been used for resectoscopic procedures, alternative irrigating solutions should now be actively sought. Moreover, the data available demonstrate that careful monitoring of the inflow pressure and the fluid absorption during hysteroscopic surgery is mandatory.

New hysteroscopes and resectoscopes with continuous-flow designs have greatly facilitated diagnostic and therapeutic hysteroscopy. Saline is the ideal distending medium for hysteroscopic procedures in which mechanical or bipolar instruments are used; 5% mannitol may be the safest medium for traditional resectoscopic surgery. Regardless of the medium chosen, careful fluid monitoring is essential.[41]

Bipolar equipment for hysteroscopic surgery is being developed as a second-generation tool in the treatment of fibroids, polyps and menorrhagia. Insufficient data exist to be able to recommend the maximum quantity of fluid that should be absorbed. However, theoretical consideration would allow a higher deficit to be accepted. The serum sodium level will be stable, but the bolus of fluid volume can create high pressure to the left cardiac system and subsequently pulmonary and brain oedema. The volume of saline allowed during these circumstances remains to be determined.[42]

4.7.4 Haemorrhage

Peroperative heavy bleeding is uncommon during TCRE. Of 250 patients, Magos reported only one who required uterine tamponade.[4] In Rankin's series of 400 consecutive patients, four had excessive bleeding necessitating uterine tamponade.[10] In a survey of the British Society for Gynaecological Endoscopy, heavy bleeding was encountered per- or postoperatively in eight of 4038 patients.[43]

In our study, peroperative heavy bleeding was encountered in 19 patients, necessitating tamponade using a Foley catheter chariere 24 filled with 30 ml saline. The high number of tamponades compared with other publications[4,10] may be because of cautious handling by the operator. On the other hand, tamponade will certainly result in a better postoperative haemoglobin concentration. The preoperative haemoglobin level in our study was 12.5 mmol/l, decreasing to 10.4 mmol/l in the 19 patients treated with tamponade, compared with 12.5 decreasing to 11.6 in patients not treated with tamponade.

4.7.5 Infections

Postoperative infection was defined as pain, odour, fever > 38°C and increase in laboratory infection parameters. Infection was encountered in 18 (4.8%) of 370 patients in our series. Five of these patients were readmitted to hospital and treated with antibiotics, and the other 13 were treated on an outpatient basis. Peroperative antibiotic prophylaxis was not given.

In the British Society for Gynaecological Endoscopy survey, only 39 (1%) patients had postoperative infections; antibiotic prophylaxis was not mentioned in the survey.[43] As the questionnaire was only sent to the surgeons, the number of infections may have been underestimated. Some of the minor infections may have been treated by the local GP without the gynaecologist's knowledge. Although the incidence of postoperative infection is modest, in my opinion it would not justify peroperative antibiotic prophylaxis. However, patients who have a history of pelvic inflammatory disease may be at risk of developing infections. Prophylactic antibiotics during operative hysteroscopy appear to be effective in preventing infections in these patients.[44]

4.8 Late Complications after TCRE

4.8.1 Pain and Persistent Adenomyosis

Adenomyosis is defined as the presence of endometrial glands in the myometrium with no connection to the endometrial mucosa. In our study, adenomyosis was found in the resected uterus in 94

(35.3%) of 271 patients not exposed to hysterectomy or repeated resection. In the hysterectomy (n = 21) and repeated resection (n = 31) groups, adenomyosis was found in 46%, and intolerable pain was the main indication for hysterectomy or repeated resection when TCRE had failed.

There were no differences in the bleeding pattern between the groups with or without adenomyosis before and after the operation. By contrast, there were significant differences in the degree of preoperative pain in these groups. In patients with adenomyosis, 77% complained of dysmenorrhoea preoperatively. In the group without primary adenomyosis, 44% complained of dysmenorrhoea prior to the operation. Pain 1 year after TCRE was reduced to 11% and 13% respectively in these groups. It is difficult to understand why pain improves after TCRE, but reductions in bleeding intensity and pain often go together.

Of 164 patients operated on 24–60 months previously who received a questionnaire about satisfaction with the result of the operation, only five (3%) reported de novo pain or pain that was worse than before the operation.

It is possible that only minimal adenomyosis (adenomyosis subbasalis grade I), within one low-power field from the basalis, is treated by TCRE.[45] The resectoscope removes 4 mm of the endometrium and myometrium, thus removing all grade I adenomyosis. Our data are in agreement with those of other authors, that adenomyosis is not associated with adverse effects after TCRE.[1] By contrast, many cases of treatment failures, repeated resection or subsequent hysterectomy showed evidence of more extensive invasion (grade II and III adenomyosis).

The incidence of adenomyosis after hysterectomy has been reported to range from 20 to 60%, as pathologists have different interpretations of adenomyosis. Some authors have found that 40% of women undergoing TCRE have superficial adenomyosis.[46] More than 60% of patients with detectable adenomyosis suffer from meno/metrorrhagia and 30% complain of severe dysmenorrhoea – the classical symptom complex.[47] These observations agree with our observations, combinations of pain and bleeding problems being the main symptoms in patients with adenomyosis.

Adenomyosis has been described as being diagnostically elusive because of the difficulty in clinical identification and the unknown aetiology. Hysterectomy still remains the mainstay of diagnosis and treatment. Resectoscopic treatment has been proposed in some mild forms of adenomyosis to avoid hysterectomy. It is important to adopt standard histological criteria for adenomyosis.[44,48,49] The chips removed with the resectoscope provide excellent specimens for histological examination. Thus, resection may offer an opportunity to make a

reliable diagnosis of adenomyosis.[48] For this purpose, however, the resected specimens should be sliced perpendicular to the mucosal surface after fixation, preferentially in transverse sections, and oriented when embedded in paraffin. If treated in this way, the carefully resected specimens will almost always constitute a useful tissue preparation for diagnostic purposes, obviously superior to the tissue fragments normally obtained by conventional curettage.[49]

4.8.2 Tubal Patency and Pregnancy after TCRE

Hysteroscopic sterilisation using electrocoagulation would be appropriate during TCRE. Previous investigation showed an overall bilateral tubal occlusion rate of 80%, confirmed by hysterosalpingography (Figure 4.4).[45] In the 1970s there was great interest in methods to occlude the fallopian tubes at their uterotubal ostia. The potential advantages of a transcervical operation are elimination of an abdominal incision and possible adhesions. Electrocoagulation of the uterotubal ostia fell into disfavour because of failure to occlude the ostia, arising from difficulties in locating the ostia, and problems with irrigation medium, current and equipment; this operation is best performed postmenstrually.[50]

We investigated tubal patency after TCRE by means of hysterosalpingography and found open tubes in six patients (> 10%).[51] In a case report of a pregnancy after TCRE, the patient remained amenorrhoeic for 18 months postoperatively until an unexpected pregnancy occurred. Information about tubal coagulation with the rollerball ablation technique is lacking.[46] The risk of pregnancy after TCRE appears to be minimal, although patients cannot be assured that this is a sterilisation procedure.

Reduced endometrium, fibrosis and granulomatous inflammation are additional factors leading to a decreased possibility for implantation. However, the potential for an unpredictable outcome in a subsequent pregnancy is prominent,[47,52] therefore many authors recommend a sterilisation procedure to be performed during the initial operation.[1,53]

4.8.3 Haematometra and Pain after TCRE

Obstruction of the lower parts of the uterine cavity would lead to pain and haematometra if hormonally active endometrium were present.[54] The value of TVS in diagnosing the cause of postoperative pain caused by haematometra is obvious.[19] Appropriate treatment would be dilatation of the cervix or second-look resection with removal of residual endometrium. Fluid in the cavity without pain was

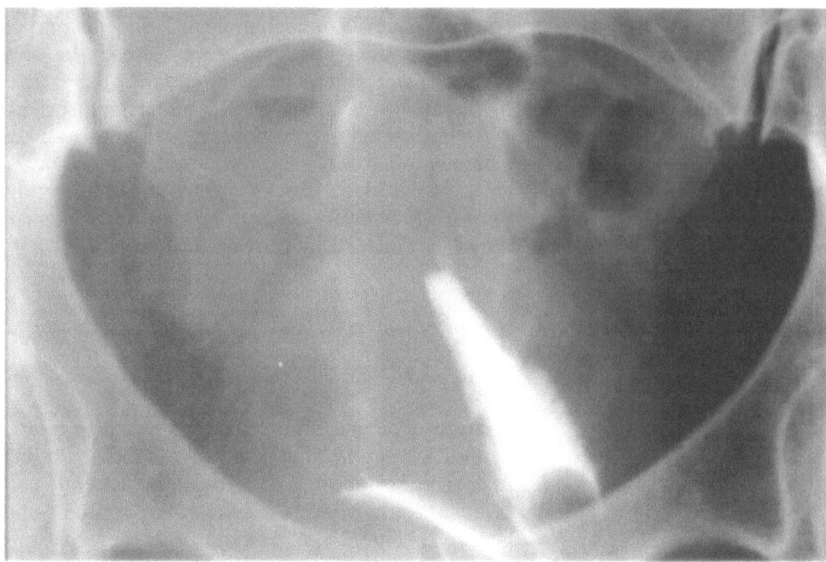

Figure 4.4 Hysterosalpingography examination of a uterine cavity with tubal occlusion 6 months after transcervical resection of the endometrium.

confirmed in ten of our patients postoperatively. In another five patients the fluid in the uterus was accompanied by pain. It is difficult to decide by ultrasound whether or not the fluid is haematometra coming from active endometrial tissue, but it is more likely that patients with pain have small active endometrial glands. Moreover, TVS is useful in assessing cyclical postoperative pain and helping to differentiate between haematometra and adenomyosis, thus selecting further surgery. Haematometra will probably benefit from dilatation and hysterectomy is the treatment of choice in cases of adenomyosis.[19] Follow-up after endometrial resection revealed a subgroup of women who developed late onset of pain with or without bleeding. Medroxyprogesterone acetate given at the time of surgery offers an advantage in terms of patient satisfaction.[55]

before presenting at admission with moderate bleeding of 3 weeks' duration.[56] Vaginal ultrasound examination may be of diagnostic value in such cases. A positive relationship between endometrial thickness and endometrial cancer has been established; no endometrial abnormalities have been found when the endometrium is less than 5 mm.[57] However, the case reported above was a patient with a high risk for developing endometrial cancer and the procedure was a rollerball ablation. Until now no cases of malignancies of the endometrium have been reported in patients who have undergone TCRE. However, bleeding after TCRE should not be assumed to be a result of treatment failure: endometrial carcinoma must be included in the differential diagnosis. In addition, a progestogen should be added to a regimen of oestrogen replacement.

4.8.4 Endometrial Cancer after TCRE

Occlusion of the lower part of the cavity and cervical canal may result in haematometra and pain, and subsequently delay the diagnosis of endometrial cancer. Cervical stenosis, fibrotic changes or synaechiae may obstruct the access to the cavity in some patients, and may cause delay of the normal symptoms when malignancy of the possible remnants of the endometrium takes place. A major concern voiced by critics of TCRE is the possibility that cryptic endometrial adenocarcinoma may develop after ablation.

One case of endometrial cancer following coagulation with the rollerball has been reported. The patient remained amenorrhoeic for 5 years

4.9 Long-term Follow-up

4.9.1 Repeated Resection

In our series, 693 patients had operations for menstrual bleeding disorders. During the 11-year follow-up period, 118 of these underwent repeat resection and 85 had a hysterectomy, either because of a failure of the repeated procedure or for other reasons.

The patient survey included a letter to 583 patients. Patients not receiving a letter were: 15 who were missing from the national registry; ten who had died during the follow-up period; 85 who had undergone a hysterectomy (the reasons were analysed but they did not receive a letter). The first letter achieved a response rate of 87%. A second letter sent to the 73 patients who did not answer the first letter resulted in a total response from 555 (95%) of the 583 patients.

During the study period, 188 patients underwent a combined fibroid and endometrial resection and 480 patients had endometrial resection in a normal uterus. There were differences between these patients with respect to age, dysmenorrhoea and previous sterilisation. In addition, adenomyosis was found in the histology specimen of some patients at the primary operation.

Of the repeated resections, 33 (17.5%) took place in the 188 combined fibroid and endometrial resection group. Repeated resection was necessary in 86 (17.9%) of the 480 patients with no fibroids. However, pain was the major indication for repeat resection in both groups (33.3% and 47.7% respectively).

In the fibroid group, 68% of the patients suffered from preoperative dysmenorrhoea, compared with 46% in the non-fibroid group (p = 0.048) who underwent a repeat operation. However, perioperative findings of adenomyosis did not indicate a significantly higher incidence of repeat operation, nor did previous laparoscopic sterilisation (33% in the fibroid group and 48% in the non-fibroid group).

Of the 33 patients in the fibroid group (n = 188) who had repeat treatment, 12 (36%) ended up with a hysterectomy. In the non-fibroid group (n = 480), 86 patients had a repeat operation; of these, 21 (24%) eventually needed a hysterectomy. In most cases we found signs of cornual haematometra on TVS. Three patients had hysterectomy for reasons unrelated to the endometrial ablation procedure (two ovarian cysts and one ovarian cancer). The difference in rates of hysterectomy after repeat operation between the fibroid and the non-fibroid group is not significant with these small numbers.

4.9.2 Discussion

Pelvic pain and dysmenorrhoea are common symptoms in patients who are diagnosed as having uterine fibroids.[58] In our study, 65% of patients complained of menstrual pain.

The strategy of performing combined myoma resection with endometrial ablation in women with symptomatic fibroids and bleeding is to reduce all subsequent surgery rates compared with endometrial ablation alone.[59] In the fibroid group, 33 (17%) of 188 patients underwent repeated resection and the major indication was pain/bleeding (19 patients). It was possible to treat 12 of these with a repeat operation. In the majority of patients an intracavity fibroid had undergone incomplete resection at the first attempt as a result of surgical difficulties. There were other cases of undetected fibroids found on vaginal ultrasound. It is important to carry out a detailed preoperative evaluation in these cases. Persistence of symptoms such as bleeding and pain might be caused by other fibroids. The mechanism of their effect on menstrual blood loss is poorly understood, but may involve abnormalities of local venous drainage,[60] as well as local changes in blood supply and the coagulation/fibrinolysis system.[61,62] However, removal of submucous fibroids results in normalisation of the bleeding pattern in the majority of patients.[63]

In our study, adenomyosis was found in 26% of patients in the fibroid group and 30.6% in the non-fibroid group. Adenomyosis was diagnosed when endometrial tissue was detected more than 3 mm below the endomyometrial interface in sections cut perpendicular to the long axis of the resected tissue strips, thus avoiding artefacts secondary to oblique sections. The finding of adenomyosis in the primary specimens did not significantly affect the incidence of later repeat resection or failure after the second resection. However, with long-term follow-up, a significant failure rate became evident, requiring a repeat hysteroscopic procedure or a hysterectomy. Deep adenomyosis is a major cause of these failures.[64]

Our diagnosis of adenomyosis did not provide any information regarding deep adenomyosis; only the 3–4 mm of the myometrial/endometrial lining was investigated. It is likely that deep adenomyosis is the aetiological factor, as adenomyosis was present in 60% of hysterectomy specimens after failed treatment. Some authors have claimed that endometrial resection might induce adenomyosis.[65] However, remnants of endometrium not removed in the primary operation, which become occluded by the scarred uterus, might be the explanation for haematometra embedded in the myometrium.[51]

Sterilisation was a predictor of pain after TCRE. Of the 118 patients who had repeated TCRE operations, 45% had been sterilised, compared with a lower incidence in the primary operations. It is possible that some of these patients experienced the postablation tubal sterilisation syndrome, caused by medial tubal accumulation of blood originating from residual cornual endometrium, as described after rollerball coagulation.[66]

After repeated endometrial resection, hysterectomy was necessary in 12 (36%) of 33 patients in the fibroid group and in 21 (24.4%) of 86 patients in the non-fibroid group. The repeated operation was therefore a wasted operation in more than one-fifth of these patients. How could we avoid these unnecessary operations? Correct selection of patients is mandatory, using all available preoperative investigative modalities, including TVS, hysteroscopy and magnetic resonance imaging to obtain a clear picture of the uterus. One surgical technique is to ensure removal of the endometrium in the cornual area to avoid relapses due to painful haematometra. Another technique is partial ablation, defined as ablation of only the anterior or posterior endometrial wall and avoidance of the cornual areas. This avoids formation of intrauterine adhesions that may lead to haematometra.[67]

Adjuvant treatment with the levonorgestrel intrauterine system may inhibit growth of the remnant of endometrium left behind after endometrial resection; however, this needs to be proven in clinical practice.

4.10 Conclusions

Surgical training is important when TCRE is performed. A significant number of operative complications can be anticipated in the first 20 procedures, and those performing TCRE for the first time would be wise to seek supervision. The learning curve seems to flatten out, with little improvement in patient outcome when 100 procedures have been completed.

Transvaginal ultrasound helps to identify uterine pathology and prognostic factors. Submucous fibroids make no difference to the clinical outcome of TCRE, while the preoperative endometrial thickness does have a significant impact on the likelihood of achieving amenorrhoea after 1 year. The data suggest that there may be a useful role for agents that produce endometrial atrophy preoperatively, or that TCRE should be performed in the immediate postmenstrual phase of the cycle (5–10 days).

Postoperative hyponatraemia and nausea after TCRE are correlated with the deficit of the irrigant fluid, but not with the operation time or the total amount of irrigant fluid used. We recommend that serum sodium should be measured during the postoperative period in patients with nausea and vomiting.

Glycine, nine other amino acids and ammonia showed increased postoperative plasma levels, which were correlated with the absorption of the amount of irrigating glycine solution and the development of hyponatraemia. Minor activation of fibrinolysis and haemolysis were also seen.

Nausea after TCRE with glycine 1.5% for irrigation may be partly explained by direct toxic effects of glycine and its secondary metabolites, in addition to the effects of water intoxication and hyponatraemia. Alternatives to glycine for creation of near-isotonic irrigating solutions are indicated.

Patients with a glycine deficit of 1000 ml or more, or a decrease of serum sodium of 10 mmol/l or more, all experienced nausea and cerebral oedema on computed tomography scan. The results suggest that discrete cerebral oedema may contribute to the development of postoperative nausea in patients undergoing transcervical surgery with significant absorption of the glycine irrigating solution.

Indomethacin administered at induction of anaesthesia reduces the number of patients in need of opiate analgesia after TCRE, while the need for treatment of nausea remains unaffected. Indomethacin does not seem to interfere with the spontaneous normalisation of hyponatraemia secondary to absorption of the irrigating solution.

Tissue destruction and increase in uterine surface temperature are minimal during TCRE, and the procedure provides excellent histological material. Careful coagulation/resection in the cornual and isthmic regions is recommended.

The uterine cavity is narrow and fibrotic after TCRE, but still accessible for diagnostic procedures such as hysteroscopy. In the majority of patients, variable amounts of endometrium were found at second-look hysteroscopy and histological examination of biopsies.

Our data support the view that tubal sterilisation and TCRE should be performed simultaneously. An alternative would be to advise women to continue their normal contraceptive practice.

Repeated endometrial resection is possible in selected cases with pain and haematometra. Repeat resection is difficult and subsequent hysterectomy will occur in more than one-quarter of the patients. In other words, three-quarters of patients will avoid a hysterectomy.

References

1. Ke RW, Taylor PJ (1991) Endometrial ablation to control excessive uterine bleeding. Hum Reprod 6:574–580
2. DeCherney AH, Diamond MP, Lavy G et al (1987) Endometrial ablation for intractable uterine bleeding: hysteroscopic resection. Obstet Gynecol 70:668–670
3. Istre O, Schiotz H, Sadik L et al (1991) Transcervical resection of endometrium and fibroids. Initial complications. Acta Obstet Gynecol Scand 70:363–366
4. Magos AL, Baumann R, Lockwood GM et al (1991) Experience with the first 250 endometrial resections for menorrhagia [published erratum appears in Lancet 1991 Jan 1; 337(8753):1362] [see comments]. Lancet 337:1074–1078
5. McLucas B (1991) Intrauterine applications of the resectoscope. Surg Gynecol Obstet 172:425–431
6. Chambers JT, Chambers SK (1992) Endometrial sampling: When? Where? Why? With what? Clin Obstet Gynecol 35:28–39
7. Stovall TG, Ling FW, Morgan PL (1991) A prospective, randomized comparison of the Pipelle endometrial sampling device with the Novak curette. Am J Obstet Gynecol 165:1287–1290
8. Stovall TG, Solomon SK, Ling FW (1989) Endometrial sampling prior to hysterectomy [published erratum appears in Obstet Gynecol Jul;74(1):105]. Obstet Gynecol 73:405–409
9. Hallez JP, Perino A (1988) Endoscopic intrauterine resection: principles and technique. Acta Eur Fertil 19:17–21.
10. Rankin L, Steinberg LH (1992) Transcervical resection of the endometrium: a review of 400 consecutive patients. Br J Obstet Gynaecol 99:911–914

11. Norris H, Connor M, Kurrmann R (1986) Preinvasive lesions of the endometrium. Clin Obstet Gynecol 13(4):725–728

12. Rybo G (1986) Variation in menstrual blood loss. Research and Clinical Forums 4:357–374

13. Fedele L, Bianchi S, Dorta M et al (1991) Transvaginal ultrasonography versus hysteroscopy in the diagnosis of uterine submucous myomas. Obstet Gynecol 77:745–748

14. Goldstein SR (1994) Use of ultrasonohysterography for triage of perimenopausal patients with unexplained uterine bleeding. Am J Obstet Gynecol 170:565–570

15. Fraser IS (1990) Hysteroscopy and laparoscopy in women with menorrhagia. Am J Obstet Gynecol 162:1264–1269

16. Valle RF (1991) Hysteroscopy. Curr Opin Obstet Gynecol 3:422–426

17. Altchek A (1992) Management of fibroids. Curr Opin Obstet Gynecol 4:463–471

18. Wamsteker K, Emanuel MH, de Kruif JH (1993) Transcervical hysteroscopic resection of submucous fibroids for abnormal uterine bleeding: results regarding the degree of intramural extension. Obstet Gynecol 82:736–740

19. Khastgir G, Mascarenhas LJ, Shaxted EJ (1993) The role of transvaginal ultrasonography in pre-operative case selection and post-operative follow up of endometrial resection. Br J Radiol 66:600–604

20. Easterday C, Grimes D, Riggs J (1983) Hysterectomy in the United States. Obstet Gynecol 62:203–212

21. Rybo G (1966) Menstrual blood loss in relation to parity and menstrual pattern. Acta Obstet Gynecol Scand Suppl 45:7

22. Brooks PG, Serden SP (1992) Endometrial ablation in women with abnormal uterine bleeding aged fifty and over. J Reprod Med 37:682–684

23. Sullivan B, Kenney P, Seibel M (1992) Hysteroscopic resection of fibroid with thermal injury to sigmoid. Obstet Gynecol 80:546–547

24. Pittrof R (1991) Near fatal uterine perforation during TCRE. Lancet 338:197–198

25. Kivnick S, Kanter MH (1992) Bowel injury from rollerball ablation of the endometrium [see comments]. Obstet Gynecol 79:833–835

26. Perry C, Daniell JF, Gimpelson RJ (1990) Bowel injury from the Nd:Yag endometrial ablation. J Gynecol Surg 6:199–203

27. Indman PD, Brown WW (1992) Uterine surface temperature changes caused by electrosurgical endometrial coagulation. J Reprod Med 37:667–670

28. Indman PD, Soderstrom RM (1990) Depth of endometrial coagulation with the urologic resectoscope. J Reprod Med 35:633–635

29. Indman PD (1991) High-power Nd:YAG laser ablation of the endometrium. J Reprod Med 36:501–504

30. Broadbent JA, Molnar BG, Cooper MJ et al (1992) Endoscopic management of uterine perforation occurring during endometrial resection. Br J Obstet Gynaecol 99:1018

31. Harrison R, Boren J, Robison H (1956) Dilutional hyonatremia shock: another concept of the transurethral prostatic resection reaction. J Urol 75:95–110.

32. Madsen P, Madsen R (1965) Clinical and experimental evaluation of different irrigation fluids for transurethral surgery. J Invest Urol 3:122–129

33. Hoyt H, Goebel J, Shoenbrod J (1958) Types of shock-like reaction during transurethral resection and relation to acute renal failure. J Urol 79:500–505

34. Henderson D, Middelton R (1980) Coma from hyponatraemia following transurethral resection of the prostate. Urology 15:267–271

35. Shepard RL, Kraus SE, Babayan RK et al (1987) The role of ammonia toxicity in the post transurethral prostatectomy syndrome. Br J Urol 60:349–351

36. Perier C, Frey J, Auboyer C et al (1988) Accumulation of glycolic acid and glyoxylic acid in serum in cases of transient hyperglycinemia after transurethral surgery. Clin Chem 34:1471–1473

37. Goldenberg M, Zolti M, Seidman DS et al (1994) Transient blood oxygen desaturation, hypercapnia, and coagulopathy after operative hysteroscopy with glycine used as the distending medium. Am J Obstet Gynecol 170:25–29

38. Istre O, Skajaa K, Schjoensby AP et al (1992) Changes in serum electrolytes after transcervical resection of endometrium and submucous fibroids with use of glycine 1.5% for uterine irrigation. Obstet Gynecol 80:218–222

39. Huxtable RJ (1989) Taurine and the oxidative metabolism of cystine: biochemistry of sulfur. Plenum Press, New York, pp 693–734

40. Istre O, Jelium E, Skajaa K et al (1995) Changes in amino acids, ammonium, and coagulation factors after transcervical resection of the endometrium with a glycine solution used for uterine irrigation. Am J Obstet Gynecol 172:939–945

41. Indman PD (2000) Instrumentation and distension media for the hysteroscopic treatment of abnormal uterine bleeding. Obstet Gynecol Clin North Am 27(2):305–15

42. Vilos GA (1999) Intrauterine surgery using a new coaxial bipolar electrode in normal saline solution (Versapoint): a pilot study. Fertil Steril 72:740–743

43. MacDonald R, Phipps JH, Singer A (1992) Endometrial ablation: a safe procedure. Gynaecological Endoscopy 1:7–9

44. McCausland VM, Fields GA, McCausland AM et al (1993) Tuboovarian abscesses after operative hysteroscopy. J Reprod Med 38:198–200

45. Cooper JM (1992) Hysteroscopic sterilization. Clin Obstet Gynecol 35:282–298

46. Mongelli JM, Evans AJ (1991) Pregnancy after transcervical endometrial resection [letter]. Lancet 338:578–579

47. Wood C, Rogers P (1993) A pregnancy after planned partial endometrial resection. Aust NZ J Obstet Gynaecol 33:316–318

48. Granberg S, Wikland M (1991) Ultrasound in the diagnosis and treatment of ovarian cystic tumours. Hum Reprod 6:177–185

49. Noren H, Granberg S, Friberg LG (1991) Endometrial cancer stage II: 190 cases with different preoperative irradiation. Gynecol Oncol 41:17–21

50. Darabi KF, Roy K, Richart RM (1978) Collaborative study on hysteroscopic sterilization procedures: final report. In: Sciarra JJ, Zatuchni GI, Spiedel JJ (eds) Risks, benefits and controversies in fertility control. Harper Row, Hagerstown, MD, p 181

51. Istre O, Skajaa K, Holm Nielsen P et al (1993) The second-look appearance of the uterine cavity after resection of the endometrium. Gynaecological Endoscopy 2:189–191

52. Friedman A, DeFazio J, DeCherney A (1986) Severe obstetric complications after aggressive treatment of Asherman syndrome. Obstet Gynecol 67:864–867

53. Hill DJ, Maher PJ (1992) Pregnancy following endometrial ablation. Gynaecological Endoscopy 1:47–49

54. Hill DJ, Maher PJ, Davison GB et al (1992) Haematometra – a complication of endometrial ablation. Aust NZ J Obstet Gynaecol 32:285–286

55. Jacobs S, Blumenthal N (1994) Endometrial resection follow up: late onset of pain and the effect of depot medroxyprogesterone acetate. Br J Obstet Gynaecol 101:605–609

56. Copperman AB, DeCherney AH, Olive DL (1993) A case of endometrial cancer following endometrial ablation for dysfunctional uterine bleeding. Obstet Gynecol 82:640–642

57. Granberg S, Wikland M, Karlsson B et al (1991) Endometrial thickness as measured by endovaginal ultrasonography for identifying endometrial abnormality. Am J Obstet Gynecol 164:47–52

58. Shaw RW (1998) Gonadotrophin hormone-releasing hormone analogue treatment of fibroids. Baillieres Clin Obstet Gynaecol 12:245–268

59. Goldfarb HA (1999) Combining myoma coagulation with endometrial ablation/resection reduces subsequent surgery rates. JSLS 3:253-260

60. Farrer-Brown G, Beilby JOW, Tarbit MH (1971) Venous changes in the endometrium of myomatous uteri. Obstet Gynecol 38:743-751

61. West CP, Lumsden MA (1989) Fibroids and menorrhagia. Baillieres Clin Obstet Gynaecol 3:357-374

62. Christiansen JK (1993) The facts about fibroids. Presentation and latest management options. Postgrad Med 94:129-134, 137

63. Broadbent JA, Magos AL (1995) Menstrual blood loss after hysteroscopic myomectomy. Gynaecological Endoscopy 4:41-44

64. McCausland V, McCausland A (1998) The response of adenomyosis to endometrial ablation/resection. Hum Reprod Update 4:350-359

65. Yuen PM (1995) Adenomyosis following endometrial rollerball ablation. Aust NZ J Obstet Gynaecol 35:335-336

66. Townsend DE, McCausland V, McCausland A et al (1993) Post-ablation-tubal sterilization syndrome. Obstet Gynecol 82:422-424

67. McCausland AM, McCausland VM (1999) Partial rollerball endometrial ablation: a modification of total ablation to treat menorrhagia without causing complications from intrauterine adhesions. Am J Obstet Gynecol 180:1512-1521

Chapter 5

Laparoscopic Subtotal Hysterectomy

Marie Ellström

5.1. Introduction

The role of laparoscopic surgery is to be a substitute for abdominal surgery without creating new indications when using this new technique. It is therefore not possible to discuss laparoscopic subtotal hysterectomy (LSH) without commenting on the ongoing discussion about benefits and hazards of preserving the cervix.

Historically, subtotal abdominal hysterectomy (SAH) was the preferred method for hysterectomy, due to less operative morbidity. After the introduction of modern anaesthetic principles and antibiotics in the mid-1940s, total abdominal hysterectomy (TAH) was recommended, mainly to eradicate the risk of cervical stump cancer. Today, the frequency of subtotal hysterectomy in the western world varies. In the Nordic countries, subtotal hysterectomy accounts for 20–27% of all hysterectomies performed for benign disorders.[1,2] In other countries, such as the UK and the USA, the figure is less than 1%.[3,4] The current interest in a more conservative approach to hysterectomy could possibly be due to the introduction of the laparoscopic technique. Subtotal hysterectomy seems to be easier to perform using the laparoscopic rather than the vaginal approach. This is in contrast to the previous discussion where total laparoscopic hysterectomy (TLH) has been questioned by advocates of vaginal hysterectomy (VH). Unfortunately, there is little evidence that can be used when comparing subtotal with total hysterectomy. The only thing that can be agreed upon (without randomised controlled trials) is the case for SAH in emergency situations, when surgical dissection is difficult and the anatomy is gravely distorted.

When looking for an answer to the question of which method to recommend, subtotal or total hysterectomy, it is important to focus on the long-term outcomes and on the impact on quality of life. If no differences are found between the two surgical procedures in a long-term perspective, the short-term clinical effects should be considered.

5.2 Subtotal Hysterectomy Compared to Total Hysterectomy

5.2.1 Sexuality

Discussion has focused on the existence of an internal orgasm and the role of the cervix in this event.[5] Some authors have claimed that a large segment of the pelvic plexus of parasympathetic and sympathetic nerves may be at risk when removing the cervix, leading to a reduction in sexual satisfaction.[6] Most advocates of subtotal hysterectomy refer to the studies by Kilkku and co-workers, in which patients undergoing total and subtotal abdominal hysterectomies were compared in this respect. One of the studies showed that the frequency of orgasms was less impaired in patients undergoing SAH compared to TAH. The study was not randomised, however, which makes it open to bias.[7] In contrast, 30% of the patients undergoing a Wertheim–Meigs radical operation, where the autonomic nerves in the pelvic plexus are extensively compromised, were still able to experience regular orgasms.[8]

Randomised studies comparing sexuality after endometrial ablation and TAH or VH have not revealed any difference in several parameters measuring sexuality.[9,10] A non-randomised study investigating outcomes of sexuality comparing LSH, TAH and VH did not show any differences in outcome.[11] Most data tend to suggest that the surgical approach is of no importance for the woman's postoperative sexuality when undergoing hysterectomy. These results support the suggestion that orgasm is a central experience, in which extragenital and psychological factors play the most important part.[8] We have to remember, however, that our instruments for measuring this complex outcome are blunt and we may not be able to monitor accurately the concept of sexuality. When asked open questions about the meaning of sexuality, the majority of women defined this as expressions of a partner relationship, sometimes contradicting the answers to questionnaires concerning frequency of desire.[12]

5.2.2 Bladder and Bowel Dysfunction

Another claimed advantage of performing subtotal hysterectomy is less disturbance of bladder and bowel function. Some studies show a negative impact on bladder function after TAH,[13] whereas other studies show a lesser degree of bladder disturbance after TAH compared with before surgery.[14] Prospective non-randomised studies have shown a greater reduction of symptoms such as incontinence and sensation of residual urine after SAH compared with TAH.[15] These findings have not been supported by the few randomised studies published, in which no differences have been found comparing SAH with TAH or endometrial ablation in these respects.[16,17] Concerning the impact on bowel function, to our knowledge there are no studies comparing subtotal and total hysterectomy. In fact, there is no consensus as to what extent TAH has a negative impact on bowel function.[3]

5.2.3 Prevention of Prolapse

Several advocates of subtotal hysterectomy claim that the cervix plays a role as the anchor of the pelvic floor, thus making it important for prevention of prolapse.[6] One of the few studies performed monitoring this aspect, however, indicates the opposite, with an increased risk of vault prolapse after SAH.[18]

5.2.4 Risk of Stump Cancer

The reappraisal of subtotal hysterectomy is mainly the result of the cervical screening programme, which has lowered the incidence of stump cancer to 0.1–0.3% of women with the cervix left in place.[19,20] The low frequency of cervical cancer in well-screened populations in most developed countries enables us to discuss aspects of quality of life when comparing subtotal and total hysterectomy.

5.2.5 Other Long-term Effects

Persistent bleeding occurs in about 10% of women after LSH.[21] A well-informed patient will not regard this as a complication. This will, however, necessitate adding gestagens if the patient needs hormone replacement therapy.

Persistent postoperative dyspareunia and abdominal pain have been emphasised as complications when patients with known or unknown endometriosis/adenomyosis have undergone LSH.[22] This finding has led some authors to regard endometriosis/adenomyosis as a relative contraindication to subtotal hysterectomy. The same problem has been noted in patients with endometriosis/adenomyosis after endometrial ablation.[23]

5.2.6 Short-term Results

Subtotal abdominal hysterectomy is perceived as a technically easier procedure with a reduced risk of bleeding, infection and damage to the ureter and bladder compared with TAH. Conformational data supporting this statement are lacking, however. There are few non-randomised data suggesting a lower risk of infection and postoperative haematoma after SAH compared with TAH.[24]

5.3 Laparoscopic Subtotal Hysterectomy

5.3.1 Definitions and Terminology

To be able to compare different surgical approaches, Munroe and Parker have suggested a classification system for subtotal hysterectomy (Table 5.1).[25] The established term for a subtotal hysterectomy performed with the laparoscopic technique is laparoscopic subtotal hysterectomy. Several variants of LSH have also been described in the literature. For the sake of convenience, the term LSH is used in this chapter to describe all laparoscopic operations conserving the cervix, including classical intrafascial supracervical hysterectomy. For the same reasons, the term total laparoscopic hysterectomy, which is normally used to describe a total hysterectomy that is performed exclusively by the laparoscopic route, will be used in this chapter to describe all operations that combine laparoscopic and vaginal surgery (including laparoscopic-assisted vaginal hysterectomy) when a total hysterectomy is performed.

5.3.2 Surgical Technique

Semm was the first person to describe the technique of subtotal hysterectomy performed by laparoscopy; he named it classical intrafascial supracervical

Table 5.1. Classification system for subtotal hysterectomy as suggested by Munro and Parker[25]

Type ST I	Uterine arteries are not specifically dissected or occluded
Type ST II	Uterine arteries are occluded but not divided
Type ST III	One or both uterine arteries are occluded and divided
Subtype A	Cervical canal is left intact
Subtype B	Cervical canal is electrodesiccated
Subtype C	Cervical canal is partly or totally excised

hysterectomy.[26] The technique includes both a laparoscopic and a vaginal approach. The first laparoscopic step includes the dissection of the uterus from the pelvic wall down to the isthmus, initially leaving the uterine arteries intact. Thereafter, coring of the cervix is performed from the vaginal approach, to ablate the transformational zone, using a special coring device. The operation is completed laparoscopically when amputating the corpus uteri and securing the cervical stump with pre-made ligatures. The amputate is then morcellated and extracted.

A purely laparoscopic technique for subtotal hysterectomy was described shortly after Semm's report.[27] This technique includes dissection down to the level of the uterine arteries using bipolar diathermy or staples, after which the uterus is amputated and the cervical canal desiccated.

The most time-consuming part of performing an LSH is the removal of the uterus from the abdominal cavity. Different devices with electromechanical morcellators of varying diameters have been constructed. The harmonic scalpel has also been used to transsect the uterine muscles, as have different electrosurgical instruments (scissors, spoons). The uterus is removed from the abdominal cavity through the persisting cannulas or by extension of the abdominal incisions. Sometimes culdotomy is done, extracting a preferably small uterus intact by the vaginal approach.

5.3.3 Short-term Results

There are limited published data regarding short-term results after LSH. The cases are few and they are presented as descriptive or observational data. In the observational studies, LSH is often compared retrospectively with previously reported TLHs or with consecutively treated cases at the same unit (Table 5.2).[28-34] The data are not always analysed statistically and are influenced by the general problems for studies comparing surgical methods, i.e. lack of definitions of when an operation starts and ends, no attempt to blind the patients or investigators, and the obvious risk of bias as a result of patients' and doctors' expectations.

The operating time reported for LSH in observational studies varies from 106 to 229 minutes and the differences in operating time may reflect variations in surgical training and experience, or different definitions of operative time. Only some of the studies have indicated that LSH is less time-consuming than TLH. The fact that the removal of the uterine body from the abdominal cavity when performing an LSH is time-consuming may explain the apparent lack of difference in operative time.

Hospital stay is reported to be 4–34 hours and convalescence 7–22 days after LSH. Traditions and different economic incitement for the patients to leave hospital and go back to work often influence outcome measures such as hospital stay and convalescence. All comparative studies show a shorter hospital stay in the LSH group, although a statistically significant difference was noted in only two of them.[28, 34]

Table 5.2. Short-term clinical results. Cases published in observational studies. LSH, Laparoscopic subtotal hysterectomy; TLH, total laparoscopic hysterectomy.

Author	Operation	Number of patients	Operation (min)	Hospital stay (hours)	Convalescence (days)
Lyons[28]	LSH	50	118	18	7
	TLH	50	145	37	22
Schwartz[29]	LSH	20	229	14	6
	TLH[a]	232	185	60	18
Richards[30]	LSH	20	127	34	
	TLH	21	117	46	
Lalonde[31]	LSH	20	106	26	22
	TLH	20	124	41	24
Mettler[32b]	LSH	113	118	412	
	TLH	22	200	515	
Dong[33]	LSH	102	176		
	TLH	419	160		
Milad[34]	LSH	27	181	24	
	TLH	105	220	48	

[a] Average results obtained from 12 previously published studies.
[b] The numbers are approximated from figures in the article.

The most important short-term outcome when comparing surgical techniques is the complication rate. It is also one of the most difficult aspects to monitor. The first problem is the lack of consensus on how to define complications and therefore the huge difficulties in comparing materials. The second problem is that of study groups that are too small. This is one of the most frequently discussed problems in the surgical science literature. Economic and practical considerations still make us publish studies that lack the statistical power to show differences in this important respect. Only two observational studies comparing LSH and TLH[32] has enough patients to perform comparisons of complication rates. These studies reported a higher rate of complications associated with TLH.

5.3.4 The Gold Standard

If there is an indication for subtotal hysterectomy, the laparoscopic approach seems to be a feasible alternative to abdominal surgery, although subtotal hysterectomy by the transvaginal route has been described.[35] To support this statement, LSH has to be compared with the conventional surgical technique, i.e. the gold standard, SAH.

Parallel to performing randomised trials comparing total laparoscopic and abdominal hysterectomy,[36-39] our group in Gothenburg has performed a study comparing short-term clinical results after LSH and SAH. Women scheduled for abdominal hysterectomy due to benign disorders with a maximum width of the uterus < 11 cm, as measured by transvaginal ultrasound, and wishing to have a subtotal hysterectomy, were randomised to undergo either LSH or SAH. Seventy patients were randomised. Three patients withdrew as they changed their minds about having surgery. One patient wanted to have an SAH instead of the procedure she was assigned to. These patients were excluded. Two patients in the SAH group were converted to TAH due to technical difficulties. Four patients in the LSH group were converted to SAH due to anaesthesiological (n = 2) and surgical difficulties (n = 2). The converted patients all remained in their randomised groups.

Patient characteristics were the same in both groups, with the exception of the width of the uterus, which was smaller in the LSH group. The weight of the uterus was the same in both groups (Table 5.3). Short-term clinical results showed longer operating time, shorter hospital stay and shorter convalescence in the laparoscopic group. These findings are in line with our earlier study comparing TAH and TLH (Table 5.4).[36] Quality-of-

Table 5.3. Patient characteristics. Values are median (range). LSH, Laparoscopic subtotal hysterectomy; SAH, subtotal abdominal hysterectomy; BMI, body mass index; NPL, number of prior laparotomies.

	LSH (n = 33)	SAH (n = 33)
Age	48 (37–58)	47 (41–56)
BMI	24.0 (19.0–33.5)	24.5 (19.0–38.1)
Parity	2 (0–5)	2 (0–4)
NPL	0 (0–2)	0 (0–3)
Uterus width (cm)	6.8 (3.3–11.0)	8.0 (4.0–13.0)*
Uterus length (cm)	6.9 (4.0–11.5)	8.0 (5.0–16.0)
Uterus weight (g)	163 (74–468)	181 (40–803)

* $p < 0.05$.

life measurements with the Medical Outcome Trust 36-Item Short-Form Health Survey questionnaire (SF-36) showed a faster return to normal life in the LSH group compared with the SAH group (Figure 5.1). This is in line with the results obtained when comparing TLH and TAH.[39] The total complication rate is shown in Table 5.5. No difference in bleeding, estimated by the change in the erythrocyte volume fraction 2 days after surgery, was noted. One patient in each group received blood transfusion. No major complications occurred. The limited patient material makes it impossible to draw any conclusions about the differences in the complication rate between the two operative techniques.

Table 5.4. Time in the operating theatre, length of hospital stay and convalescence. Values are median (range). LSH, Laparoscopic subtotal hysterectomy; SAH, subtotal abdominal hysterectomy. *p < 0.001

	LSH (n = 33)	SAH* (n = 33)
Anaesthesia (min)	170 (102–225)	120 (65–273)
Surgery (min)	130 (79–175)	80 (44–222)
Hospital stay (days)ᵃ	2.0 (1–5)	3.0 (2–6)
Convalescence (days)	11.0 (0–28)	35.0 (24–55)

ᵃ Number of postoperative days.

Table 5.5. Complications. LSH, Laparoscopic subtotal hysterectomy; SAH, subtotal abdominal hysterectomy.

	LSH (n=33)	SAH (n=33)
Haematoma		
Vaginal cuff	0	2
Abdominal wall	1	1
Infections		
Pyrexia	1	0
Wound infection	0	1
Pyelonephritis	0	1
Cystitis	0	1

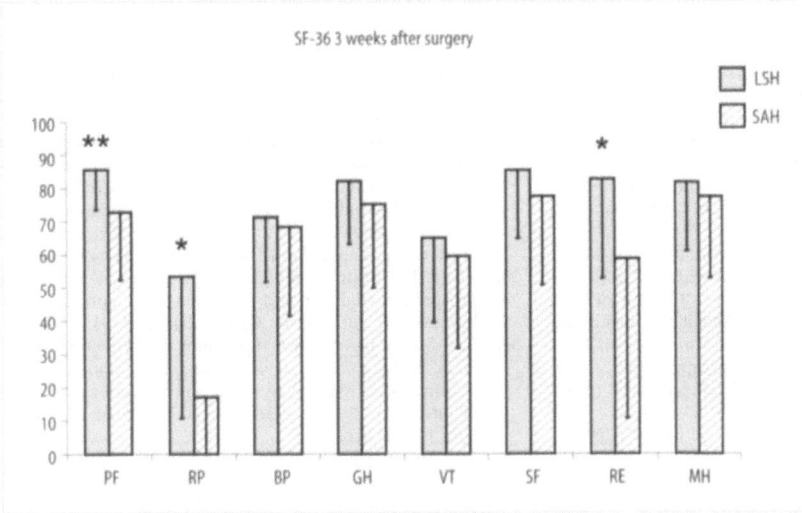

Figure 5.1 Postoperative health status and quality of life assessed 3 weeks after surgery using the Medical Outcome Trust 36–Item Short–Form Health Survey questionnaire (SF–36). LSH, Laparoscopic subtotal hysterectomy (n = 23); SAH, subtotal abdominal hysterectomy (n = 20); PF, physical functioning; RP, role limitation as a result of physical problems; BP, bodily pain; GH, general mental health; VT, vitality; SF, social functioning; RE, role limitation as a result of emotional problems; MH, mental health. The scoring algorithm produces a scale from 0 (poor health) to 100 (good health). Mean and one–tailed standard deviation are shown. *$p < 0.05$, **$p < 0.01$.

5.4 Conclusions

The need to perform as little surgery as possible and not to remove healthy organs when not indicated seems to be the strongest argument for leaving the cervix in place. Other possible advantages or disadvantages have yet to be proved when comparing subtotal hysterectomy with total hysterectomy.

When the decision is made to perform a subtotal hysterectomy, LSH should be considered. Our randomised study indicates the same short-term advantages with the laparoscopic technique as do randomised studies comparing TLH and TAH. Register studies have indicated that major complications, such as damage to the urinary tract, may be more frequently associated with TLH compared with TAH.[40] Whether this increased risk of complications also applies when performing LSH, or if it can be avoided due to the comparatively larger distance to adjacent organs, remains to be shown.

References

1. Virtanen H (1994) Sequelae of operations related to uterine removal. Thesis, Turku University, Turku
2. The hospital discharge registry (1996) Centre for Epidemiology, Swedish Medical Board, Stockholm
3. Wessey M, Villard-Mackintosh L, McPherson K et al (1992) The epidemiology of hysterectomy: findings in a large cohort study. Br J Obstet Gynecol 99: 402–407
4. Sills E, Saini J, Applegate M et al (1998) Supracervical and total abdominal hysterectomy trends in New York State: 1990–1996. J Urban Health 75:903–910
5. Masters W, Johnson V (1966) Human sexual response. Little, Brown and Co, Boston
6. Hasson H (1993) Cervical removal at hysterectomy for benign disease. Risks and benefits. J Reprod Med 38:781–789
7. Kilkku P (1983) Supravaginal uterine amputation vs hysterectomy. Effects on libido and orgasm. Acta Obstet Gynecol Scand 62:147–152
8. Eicher W (1994) Totale und subtotale Hysterektomie. Arch Gynecol Obstet 255:S359–S366
9. Alexander A, Naji A, Pinion S et al (1996) Randomised trial comparing hysterectomy with endometrial ablation for dysfunctional uterine bleeding: psychiatric and psychosocial aspects. BMJ 312:280–284
10. Crosignani P, Vercellini P, Apolone G et al (1997) Endometrial resection versus vaginal hysterectomy for menorrhagia: long-term clinical and quality of life outcomes. Am J Obstet Gynecol 177:95–101
11. Strauss B, Jakel I, Koch-Dorfler M et al (1996) Psychiatric and sexual sequelae of hysterectomy – a comparison of different surgical methods. Geburtshilfe Frauenheilkd 56:473–481
12. Helström L, Sörbom D, Bäckström T (1995) Influence of partner relationship on sexuality after subtotal hysterectomy. Acta Scand Obstet Gynecol 74:142–146
13. Parys B, Haylen B, Hutton J et al (1989) The effect of simple hysterectomy on vesicourethral function. Br J Urol 64:594–599
14. Virtanen H, Makinen J, Tenho T et al (1993) Effects of abdominal hysterectomy on urinary and sexual symptoms. Br J Urol 72:868–872
15. Kilkku P (1985) Supravaginal uterine amputation versus hysterectomy with reference to subjective bladder symptoms and incontinence. Acta Obstet Gynecol Scand 64:375–379
16. Lalos O, Bjerle P (1985) Early and late effects of subtotal and total hysterectomy on bladder function. Arch Gynecol 237:140–144
17. Bhattacharya S, Mollison J, Pinion S et al (1996) A comparison of bladder and ovarian function two years following hysterectomy or endometrial ablation. Br J Obstet Gynaecol 103:898–903
18. Virtanen H, Mäkinen J (1993) Retrospective analysis of 711 patients operated on for pelvic relaxation in 1983–1989. Int J Gynecol Obstet 42:109–115
19. Kilkku P, Gronroos M (1982) Preoperative electrocoagulation of the endocervical mucosa and later carcinoma of the cervical stump. Acta Obstet Gynecol Scand 62:265–267
20. Storm H, Clemmensen I, Manders T et al (1992) Supravaginal uterine amputation in Denmark 1978–1988 and risk of cancer. Gynecol Oncol 45:198–201

21. van der Stege J, van Beek J (1999) Problems related to the cervical stump at follow-up in laparoscopic supracervical hysterectomy. JSLS 3:335–336

22. Ewen S, Sutton C (1995) Advantages of laparoscopic supracervical hysterectomy. Bailliere's Clin Obstet Gynaecol 4:707–714

23. Garry R, Shelley-Jones D, Mooney P et al (1995) Six hundred endometrial laser ablations. Obstet Gynecol 85:24–29

24. Nathorst Böös J, Fuchs T, von Schoultz B (1992) Consumer's attitude to hysterectomy. The experience of 678 women. Acta Gynecol Scand 71:230–234

25. Munro M, Parker W (1993) A classification system for laparoscopic hysterectomy. Obstet Gynecol 82:624–629

26. Semm K (1991) Hysterektomie per laparotomiam der per pelviskopiam ohne Kolpotomy. Geburtshilfe Frauenheilkd 51:996–1003

27. Pelosi M, Pelosi M 3d (1992) Laparoscopic supracervical hysterectomy using a single umbilical puncture (minilaparoscopy). J Reprod Med 37:777–784

28. Lyons T (1993) Laparoscopic supracervical hysterectomy. A comparison of morbidity and mortality results with laparoscopically assisted vaginal hysterectomy. J Reprod Med 38:763–767

29. Schwartz R (1994) Laparoscopic hysterectomy. Supracervical vs assisted vaginal. J Reprod Med 39:625–630.

30. Richards S, Simpkins S (1995) Laparoscopic supracervical hysterectomy versus laparoscopic-assisted vaginal hysterectomy. J Am Ass Gynecol Laparosc 2:431–435

31. Lalonde C, Daniell J (1995) Early outcomes of laparoscopic-assisted vaginal hysterectomy versus laparoscopic supracervical hysterectomy. J Am Gynecol Laparosc 2:S24–S28

32. Mettler L, Semm K (1997) Subtotal versus total laparoscopic hysterectomy. Acta Obstet Gynecol Scand 76:88–93.

33. Dong HK, Do H, Min H et al (1998) Comparison of classic intrafascial supracervical hysterectomy with total laparoscopic and laparoscopic-assisted vaginal hysterectomy. J Am Gynecol Laparosc 5:253–259

34. Milad M, Morrison K, Sokol A et al (2001) A comparison of laparoscopic supracervical hysterectomy vs laparoscopically assisted vaginal hysterectomy. Surg Endosc 15:286–288

35. Hefni M, El-Toukhy T (2000) Vaginal subtotal hysterectomy and sacrospinous colpopexy: an option in the management of uterine prolapse. Am J Obstet Gynecol 183:494–495

36. Olsson JH, Ellström M, Hahlin M (1996) A randomised prospective trial comparing laparoscopic and abdominal hysterectomy. Br J Obstet Gynaecol 103:345–350

37. Ellström M, Bengtsson A, Tylman M et al (1996) Evaluation of tissue trauma after laparoscopic and abdominal hysterectomy: measurements of neutrophil activation and release of interleukin-6 cortisol and C-reactive protein. J Am Coll Surg 182:423–430

38. Ellström M, Fagevik Olsén M, Olsson JH et al (1998) Pain and pulmonary function following laparoscopic and abdominal hysterectomy: a randomized study. Acta Obstet Gynecol 77:923–928

39. Ellström M, Ferraz-Nunez J, Olsson JH et al (1998) A randomized trial with a cost-consequence analysis after laparoscopic and abdominal hysterectomy. Obstet Gynecol 91:30–35

40. Härkki Siren P, Sjöberg J, Tiitinen A (1998) Urinary tract injuries after hysterectomy. Obstet Gynecol 92:113–118

Chapter 6

Vaginal Hysterectomy

Michel R. Cosson, Rechad Rajabally, Denis Querleu and Gilles Crépin

6.1 Introduction

Hysterectomy remains the most frequent surgical intervention carried out on women. Initially, the operation was performed for critical, life-threatening conditions. The increase in the number of indications has been paralleled by a spectacular decline in mortality and complication rates. The choice of hysterectomy as a therapeutic procedure will depend on the patient's age, her wishes for pregnancy and desire to preserve her uterus. Conservative surgical treatment is possible in almost all cases. For most patients, removal of the uterus is more likely to be accepted if it is unavoidable or necessary because of failure of conservative forms of treatment.

The widening spectrum of indications has led to interventions being performed to improve patients' "comfort" and quality of life, such as for menorrhagia. Nevertheless, arguments persist as to the best way to reach this goal. Surgeons often differ in their preferred route for hysterectomy: some favour the vaginal route, while others prefer the classic laparotomy or, more recently, laparoscopic approach. Vaginal hysterectomy is associated with fewer complications and shorter hospitalisation and recovery periods than the abdominal approach. However, abdominal hysterectomy is more commonly performed than vaginal hysterectomy.[1] It is therefore necessary to assess the various complications related to vaginal access compared with the laparoscopic and abdominal routes before evaluating the extent to which the vaginal route should be performed. Finally, we will discuss some technical aspects of surgery that should be considered to reach this goal.

6.2 Costs and Complications of Vaginal Hysterectomy

6.2.1 Mortality and Operative Complication Rates

Wingo published the most important recent study on the subject in 1985, in which he analysed figures released by the Commission on Professional and Hospital Activity from 1979 to 1980.[1] After exclusion of hysterectomies carried out during pregnancy or for malignant conditions, the mortality rate was 2.7/10 000 after vaginal hysterectomy (n = 177 684) compared with 8.6/10 000 after abdominal hysterectomy (n = 286 163).

Vaginal hysterectomy has a lower mortality rate than abdominal hysterectomy because the former is associated with fewer thromboembolic complications. There are no large-scale figures available concerning laparoscopic hysterectomy but the morbidity, operative and postoperative complication rates are close to those for vaginal hysterectomy.

These studies[2-4] show that, on the whole, there is less operative bleeding during vaginal hysterectomy. Bladder injury appears to be more frequent, but the frequency of bowel injury is approximately the same in both routes and injury to the ureter is more frequent during abdominal or laparoscopic hysterectomy.

Postoperative bleeding rates vary considerably from one surgical team to another, but seem to be higher after vaginal hysterectomy.[5,6] Our own results do not confirm this finding. Postoperative ileus, bowel obstruction and thromboembolic complications are more frequent after abdominal hysterectomy.

Complications related to laparoscopic hysterectomy are difficult to evaluate because studies published so far have included only a limited number of cases and several different operative techniques have been used. Laparoscopic-assisted hysterectomy gives rise to only a few complications, but studies using laparoscopic hysterectomy reveal a high rate of operative complications.[7-9] In his series in 1992, Liu noted 1.8% of cases had bladder injuries, 0.8% had bowel injuries and 2% of the procedures failed.[7] Professor Bruhat's team from Clermond-Ferrand have published their 4 years of experience from 1990 to 1993.[10] Of 691 procedures, 2.5% of the indications were for endometrial carcinoma and 0.9% for prolapse; 46.1% of the hysterectomies were performed laparoscopically. Bladder (1.6%) and ureteral (0.6%) injury rates were higher than those found in the literature for both abdominal and vaginal hysterectomies, even though no bowel injuries were noted.[8,11,12] These results are confirmed by Chapron.[13] In 4.4% of cases, failure of laparoscopic hysterectomy resulted in a vaginal approach and in 6.9% of cases, conversion to laparotomy was necessary. In a recent review of the literature, Munro noted an even higher rate of major complications, with an average of 3.2% (146/4502).[8] The average laparotomy rate was 2.5%. Nevertheless, complication rates with this technique are rapidly declining for experienced operators. Referring to his series of 222 laparoscopic hysterectomies, Chapron reported only around 1% of bladder injuries and no lesions affecting the ureters or intestinal tract.[13] This figure therefore seems close to the results obtained with the other surgical routes.[8,11,12]

6.2.2 Costs and Morbidity Related to Vaginal Hysterectomy

The results of the randomised studies published so far allow comparison, for similar indications, of the various advantages and disadvantages of the different routes. They also allow the choice of the best possible route for the easier indications in patients with no associated pathology and small uterine volume.

Given the limited number of cases in these studies, the only comparable end-points are the respective lengths of the procedure, hospitalisation and the recovery period, the amount of peroperative bleeding and postoperative infectious complications. These results cannot be used to compare events such as serious per- and postoperative complications. To our knowledge, no study has established reliable figures concerning the costs of these complications. Short of a nationwide inquiry, evaluation of indirect

costs will prove to be extremely difficult. An estimate of both direct and indirect costs, which differ considerably from one social security system to another, has never been established satisfactorily on a large enough sample of patients.

In an attempt to compare the different techniques used for hysterectomy, we will use the respective lengths of operation and of hospitalisation, both of which are directly related to the hospital costs.

All the studies to date show longer operative times for laparoscopic-assisted hysterectomy or if the intervention is performed entirely by laparoscopy. Our own experience confirms this finding: performing a simple vaginal hysterectomy is faster than doing an abdominal hysterectomy when both options are possible (Table 6.1). All the studies confirm that hospitalisation is longer after abdominal hysterectomy (Table 6.2).

Several others report shorter hospitalisation periods after laparoscopic hysterectomy compared with simple vaginal hysterectomy. However, it is worth noting that all the studies involved were carried out on a retrospective basis. Laparoscopic hysterectomies performed on a single-day hospitalisation, outpatient basis were compared with vaginal hysterectomies, for which this scheme had not been proposed to the patients concerned. Several authors have recently suggested performing vaginal hysterectomies as outpatient procedures in selected cases.[5,14]

Summit performed 27 vaginal hysterectomies and 26 laparoscopic hysterectomies as outpatient procedures.[14] Only two patients who required conversion to laparotomy were hospitalised for more than 12 hours. In accordance with our results, it therefore seems reasonable to consider that these two techniques have similar lengths of hospitalisation.[5] To our knowledge, the costs related to the length of the recovery period after hysterectomy have never been evaluated, so we have taken these into account in our assessment of the different routes.

The average convalescence period after vaginal or laparoscopic hysterectomy is around 3 weeks, compared with 6 weeks after an abdominal hysterectomy (Table 6.3).[5,12,15,16] The only prospective study on this topic revealed comparable convalescence times after laparoscopic and vaginal hysterectomies.[16]

Table 6.1. Length of operative time. LAVH, Laparoscopic-assisted vaginal hysterectomy; VH, vaginal hysterectomy; AH, abdominal hysterectomy

	LAVH	VH	AH
Nezhat[12]	131 min	99 min + prolapse	66 min
Casey[23]	112 min	90 min	115 min
Cosson[6]	123 min	66 min	76 min
Johns[24]	102 min	63 min	82 min
Richardson[16]	134 min	81 min	
Summit[14]	120 min	64 min	

Table 6.2. Length of hospital stay. LAVH, Laparoscopic-assisted vaginal hysterectomy; VH, vaginal hysterectomy; AH, abdominal hysterectomy

	LAVH	VH	AH
Cosson[6]	4.2 days	4.1 days	6.6 days
Nezhat[12]	2.3 days	3 days	3.3 days
Casey[23]	2.5 days	3.3 days	4.3 days
Johns[24]	1.8 days	1.7 days	2.8 days
Summit[14]	HV + LA 53 / 55 = 12 H		

Table 6.4. Global hospital costs ($) related to hysterectomies. LAVH, Laparoscopic-assisted vaginal hysterectomy; VH, vaginal hysterectomy; AH, abdominal hysterectomy

	LAVH	VH	AH
Summit[14]	7905	4891	
Nezhat[12]	7161	4868	4926
Without cure of prolapse		4868	
Reusable bipolar trocars	4669		
Johns[24]	6431	5879	6552
Boike[17]	12469	7881	10626

Several authors have compared hospital costs according to surgical route employed (Table 6.4). In a randomised study carried out in 1992, Summit compared vaginal and laparoscopic-assisted vaginal hysterectomies and calculated an average cost of $4891 for a vaginal hysterectomy compared with $7905 for a laparoscopic-assisted procedure.[14] Use of an automatic endoGIA stapler during laparoscopy resulted in an extra $400 in costs.

The type of equipment used has a major influence on the costs of hysterectomy: In France, laparoscopic hysterectomy performed without the use of automatic staplers, laser or single trocars and that does not take into account the expense generated by the use of sterilising equipment, costs €103, compared with €62 for the abdominal procedure.[5] Use of disposable trocars increases the costs of laparoscopic hysterectomy by €548. The use of prosthetic devices such as endoclips, endoGIA staplers and FLC 60 with cartridges, while improving the safety and speed of the procedure, also adds another €1124 to the expenses. The use of laser increases the cost by the same amount.

Summit[14] and Boike[17] reported a 40–50% increase in costs when performing laparoscopic hysterectomy. Nezhat[12] noted hospital costs of $7161 for a laparoscopic-assisted vaginal hysterectomy, which could be reduced to $4669 with the use of bipolar coagulation and reusable trocars. This figure is then close to the estimated expenses for the abdominal and vaginal routes.

A more precise estimate requires re-evaluation of these figures, taking into account costs related to the recovery period. As we have seen above, the time needed for convalescence is reduced by half after a vaginal or laparoscopic procedure when compared with the abdominal route.

Table 6.3. Length of convalescence. LAVH, Laparoscopic-assisted vaginal hysterectomy; VH, vaginal hysterectomy; AH, abdominal hysterectomy

	LAVH	VH	AH
Nezhat[12]	3 weeks		6 weeks
Phipps[15]	2 weeks		6 weeks
Richardson[16]	No difference between LAVH and VH		

Automatic equipment is particularly costly, especially if laser and disposable trocars are used at the same time. Their use undoubtedly speeds up the procedure and can reduce blood loss, but a 12 mm trocar is necessary and this is associated with a higher incidence of urinary tract injuries involving the bladder and ureters.

6.2.3 Conclusion: Priority should be for Vaginal Route Whenever Possible

Combining shorter hospitalisation, convalescence and operative times, vaginal hysterectomy is undoubtedly the least costly intervention. It should therefore be recommended to trainee surgeons as the standard procedure, whenever possible.

Laparoscopic assistance is useful as it will allow hysterectomy to be performed vaginally in patients with adnexal pathology or pelvic adhesions resulting from infections, surgical interventions or endometriosis.[5] This procedure is longer and more costly and should be indicated only if it can help to avoid a laparotomy. Non-disposable equipment should be used whenever possible and bipolar coagulation is preferable to automatic staplers in order to reduce costs. In these cases, laparoscopic-assisted hysterectomy will cost 20% more than vaginal hysterectomy. Hospital expenses for abdominal hysterectomy are similar to those for the laparoscopic and vaginal routes, but the longer hospitalisation and convalescence periods result in a considerable increase in costs.

6.3 Indications for the Various Surgical Routes

6.3.1 Review of the Literature

Although the indications in some cases cannot be contested, the extent to which each route should be used has not yet been determined. The vaginal approach is advocated in 20–90% of cases, according to different authors.

Comparison between the percentages of abdominal, vaginal and laparoscopic hysterectomies noted in the literature is difficult, as most of these series include interventions performed for cases of cancer or prolapse. In these series, the percentage of vaginal hysterectomies often reflects the rate of indications for prolapse. Experienced vaginal surgeons perform 60–80% of hysterectomies vaginally, including cases of prolapse.[5]

6.3.1.1 Large Uterine Volume

While evaluating the influence of uterine volume on complications during vaginal hysterectomy, Gitsch noted a higher incidence of peroperative bleeding when morcellation was needed.[18] Draca[19] and Kovac[4] noted no increase in morbidity after vaginal hysterectomy requiring reduction of uterine volume.

6.3.1.2 History of Previous Surgical Interventions

According to Tyrone, morbidity rates are not increased after vaginal hysterectomy in patients who have previously undergone pelvic surgery.[20] Previous conisation does not generate more complications during vaginal hysterectomy.[18]

6.3.1.3 Adnexectomy during Vaginal Hysterectomy

Gitsch reported no increase in the rate of complications if adnexectomy was performed during vaginal hysterectomy[18] but he gave no indication as to the number of cases in which adnexectomy was effected. In a series of 138 vaginal hysterectomies, Ballard noted that adnexectomy was possible by the same route in about two-thirds of cases (90 patients) without a rise in the level of morbidity or of peroperative complications.[21] Analysing the results after 740 vaginal hysterectomies, Sheth noted that adnexectomy was feasible in 94% of cases without risk of excessive blood loss or ureteral injuries.[22] Failure to remove the adnexa occurs more frequently in patients who are obese or nulliparous, who have a large uterine volume or reduced uterine mobility, or if there is a pathological process affecting the tubes and the ovaries.

If removing the adnexa proves to be difficult or impossible during vaginal hysterectomy (two cases in our experience), the procedure can always be completed subsequently by laparoscopy. We believe that the decision to remove the adnexa during vaginal hysterectomy should not lead to the systematic performance of a laparoscopic hysterectomy beforehand.[5]

Likewise, uterine volume alone should not be regarded as an obstacle to the performance of a vaginal procedure. Previous pelvic surgery should lead to an anticipated, systematic laparoscopy only if a major or complicated procedure was performed.

6.3.2 Our Experience

A prospective study was conducted at the Clinique Universitaire de Gynécologie – Obstétrique et Pathologie de la Reproduction, Pavillon Paul Gellé of Roubaix from 31 March 1991 to 31 March 1996. During this 5-year period, choice of the surgical route was determined as follows:

- priority was given to simple vaginal hysterectomy in all cases where the procedure seemed possible;
- laparoscopic assistance in cases of associated adnexal pathology or if pelvic adhesions were thought to be present;
- hysterectomy completed entirely by laparoscopy was reserved for patients with a moderately enlarged uterus and poor vaginal access;
- abdominal hysterectomy for all other cases.

Hysterectomies were performed on 1151 women for benign pathology with no associated prolapse. Nine hundred and eighteen interventions (79.8% of the cases) were effected vaginally and 119 (10.3% of the cases) required laparoscopic assistance. Abdominal hysterectomies were performed on 114 patients (9.9%) (Table 6.5). Operators frequently resorted to the use of techniques for reducing the uterine volume during vaginal hysterectomy (49% of the 918 cases). The indications for laparoscopic-assisted vaginal hysterectomies and abdominal hysterectomies are noted in Table 6.5. Mean uterine weight was 800 g for the abdominal route, 240 g for the vaginal route and 170 g for the laparoscopic-assisted procedure.

Table 6.5. Indications for laparoscopic and abdominal hysterectomies. AH, Abdominal hysterectomy; LAVH, laparoscopic-assisted vaginal hysterectomy

	AH (n = 114)	LAVH (n = 119)
Adhesions	2	73
Adhesions and volume	62	
Adnexal pathology	6	37
High uterine volume and limited vaginal access	32	6
Failure of vaginal hysterectomy	12	3

Postoperative complications required repeat interventions in six cases:

- acute bowel obstruction after abdominal hysterectomy because of undiagnosed perforation during intervention; the injured segment of the intestine was resected;
- wound infection after abdominal hysterectomy;
- four cases of postoperative haemorrhage after vaginal hysterectomy; reintervention was by laparoscopy in three cases and the vaginal route in the fourth.

No deaths were reported in our series. Use of the laparoscopic or abdominal routes is significantly higher in nulliparous or primigravid women and for those with endometriosis, previous pelvic surgery or caesarean section, or with uterine weights more than 600 g. Mastering the vaginal hysterectomy procedure and in particular the techniques of morcellation or volume reduction allows for conversion from an abdominal to a vaginal approach in certain cases. Several publications in the literature show similar results. High percentages of vaginal hysterectomies are always associated with correspondingly high percentages of volume reduction procedures.[2,4,5]

Failure to complete the procedure vaginally, leading to conversion to the abdominal route, occurred in 12 cases. This figure of 1.3% is comparable to results found in the literature. Four patients (0.4%) had postoperative haemorrhage after vaginal hysterectomy and subsequent reintervention. This complication rate is lower than that of Dargent, who reported a 4.3% reintervention rate for postoperative bleeding after vaginal hysterectomy.[2] His indications, however, also included cases of prolapse. In spite of our favoured use of the vaginal route, our per- and postoperative complication rates were not much higher than those found in other publications (Table 6.6), where laparotomy rates were higher.

6.3.3 Discussion

Taken on an individual basis, an enlarged uterus, previous pelvic surgery or caesarean section,

endometriosis or nulliparity do not constitute contraindications to the vaginal route.

We can therefore reasonably consider that hysterectomy can be performed vaginally in eight patients out of ten. In "borderline" cases combining moderate enlargement of the uterus, suspected pelvic adhesions and average vaginal access, clinical examination will appreciate the degree of uterine mobility or "relaxation". The extent of descent of the uterus is also assessed by traction on the cervix. Uterine volume should be compared with vaginal access if the uterus displays no mobility or downward displacement by traction on the cervix. Prior to a decision, an ultimate examination can be carried out after induction of anaesthesia just before the start of the operation. Full explanations should always have been given to the patient and she should be informed of a possible change in the surgical route during the procedure.

Some authors have suggested more widespread use of both laparoscopic-assisted and total laparoscopic hysterectomy when faced with a "difficult" vaginal approach. Our results show that surgeons who are familiar with the vaginal route can continue without these procedures and in cases where they do resort to laparoscopy, this can help to avoid a laparotomy.

If the guidelines given above are followed, the indications for abdominal hysterectomy will be restricted to cases of failure in completion of a vaginal approach, patients with very large uteri or those who have both an enlarged uterus and a history of major pelvic surgery.

6.4 Technique for Standard Vaginal Hysterectomy

6.4.1 Simple Vaginal Hysterectomy

There are four steps involved in performing a vaginal hysterectomy: (1) dissection of the anterior cul-de-sac and entrance in the pouch of Douglas to expose the broad ligament; (2) progressive clamping of the uterosacral and cardinal ligament to allow

Table 6.6. Peroperative complications for all surgical routes combined

	Bladder injuries	Bowel injuries	Total peroperative complications	Total no. of reinterventions	Mortality
Dargent[2]	18	3	21	36	3
(n = 894)	2%	0.33%	2.33%	4%	0.33%
Dicker[3]	12	6	18	20	2
(n = 1851)	0.65%	0.32%	0.97%	1.08%	0.10%
Kovac[4]	12	0	12	3	1
(n = 902)	1.20%		1.20%	0.33%	0.11%
Cosson[6]	9	7	16	6	0
(n = 1151)	0.78%	0.60%	1.3%	0.50%	

exposure of the uterine pedicle and selective suturing; (3) posterior delivery of the uterus after reduction of volume if necessary with morcellation techniques – clamping and suture ligation of the tubo-ovarian and round ligament are then possible; (4) closure of the vaginal cuff and suspension by suturing it to the uterosacral ligament.

A Museux tentaculum is used to grasp the cervix and allow traction on the cervix. When there are no contraindications, we inject 100 ml of serum beneath the vaginal mucosa around the cervix to facilitate dissection and reduce blood loss. The serum is composed of half sterile saline solution and adrenaline. The bladder is dissected from the cervix and the lower anterior uterine segment. Peritoneal incision is extended laterally to the uterosacral ligaments.

The operation proceeds by successively clamping, cutting and ligating the cardinal and uterosacral ligaments. The uterine pedicles are then identified and selectively secured. The anterior cul-de-sac should be opened before clamping the uterine pedicles. If the vesicovaginal peritoneal reflection is not easily identified, it may be preferable to delay entry. Identification and incision of the anterior cul-de-sac may be easier when exposed by the finger in the posterior cul-de-sac.

After removal of the uterus, the remaining portion of the upper part of the broad ligament is clamped, cut and double ligated. If removal of the uterus is not possible at this time, reduction of uterine volume should be performed, as described in the next section.

Peritoneal closure is not necessary. In some cases a continuous absorbable suture allows all the pedicles to be covered with peritoneum.

The vaginal vault is suspended by suturing the uterosacral and ovarian ligaments. The suture is first placed through the vagina and tied. A running suture unites the vaginal vault and the two ligaments. The suture runs to the opposite side, taking the vagina, and the same procedure is performed on the other ligaments and vaginal angle.

The bladder is drained at the end of the procedure. After simple hysterectomy, a bladder catheter or vaginal packing is not necessary.

6.4.2 Reduction of Uterine Volume

Many procedures have been described to allow reduction of uterine volume. They are all contra-indicated if uterine malignancy is suspected.

The procedures involve ligation of both uterine arteries and entering of the peritoneal cul-de-sac. After ligation of the uterine vessels, bleeding is reduced to the blood supply through the ovarian arteries. All the procedures have to be performed under direct vision to avoid accidental injury to a loop of intestine or the bladder. They are time consuming but allow safe removal of the uterus in most cases.

The methods described include hemisection, amputation of the cervix, myomectomy, morcellation of the uterus fundus or of a large fibroid, and myometrial coring. We never use amputation of the cervix as it does not help to reduce the volume of the uterus fundus. When there are suspected adhesions of the uterus fundus, we prefer to perform an intramyometrial coring. In all other cases, the procedure begins with hemisection of the cervix and progressive bisection of the corpus. Cervical tenaculum on the cervix are used for traction, while the uterine corpus is reduced by myomectomy or morcellation of the myomas. Traction allows a progressive exposition of the uterine corpus and further bisection on the midline. Even a very large uterus can be removed safely with these procedures. However, success depends on the volume of the uterus, the vaginal access and the experience of the operator.

We performed a retrospective study comparing abdominal and vaginal hysterectomies for patients with very large uteri weighing over 500 g. The patients were comparable except for their parity. Peroperative blood loss and mean operative duration were comparable for the two routes. Length of stay in hospital and postoperative pain were significantly less after the vaginal route. These results suggest that, even for very large uteri, the vaginal route is preferable to the abdominal route, when possible.

In our experience, surgical procedures for reduction of uterine volume are always necessary for uteri weighing over 300 g. These procedures are necessary for the vaginal surgeon who wants to reduce his laparotomy rate for hysterectomies.

6.5 Conclusions

Mastering the vaginal approach will enable a hysterectomy to be performed by this route in about 80% cases, requiring a procedure for reduction in uterine volume such as morcellation in around 50% of patients. In experienced hands, previous pelvic surgery or caesarean sections do not contraindicate the use of the vaginal route. Laparoscopic assistance is useful in 10% of cases, allowing the operation to be performed vaginally instead of having to resort to laparotomy. This is particularly useful in cases of associated adnexal pathology or suspected pelvic adhesions. The abdominal approach is restricted to large uteri in which the fundus is above the umbilicus and which may be associated with pelvic adhesions.

Reduction of postoperative thromboembolic complications and shortened hospital stays are among the expected benefits of the vaginal approach. Minimal postoperative discomfort and rapid recovery will result in a faster return to work, thereby decreasing costs for the social welfare system. The patient will appreciate having no surgical scar for both aesthetic and functional reasons, especially if simple vaginal hysterectomy is performed. Reduced mortality and morbidity rates are directly related to a limitation, within reasonable limits, of the abdominal approach. Laparoscopic assistance and volume reduction procedures can be helpful in reaching this goal. Insufficient use of the vaginal route inevitably leads to additional laparoscopic procedures and higher costs, with no obvious benefits for the patient.

From our point of view, the vaginal route should be considered as the standard procedure and presented as such to gynaecological surgeons during their training in university teaching hospitals. The abdominal approach should nevertheless not be disregarded as it can still prove to be useful in difficult situations.

References

1. Wingo PA, Huezo CM, Rubin GL et al (1985) The mortality risk associated with hysterectomy. Am J Obstet Gynecol 152:803-808
2. Dargent D, Rudigoz RD (1980) L'hysterectomie vaginale: notre experience des années 1970 à 1979 (556 opérations). J Gyn Obstet Biol Reprod 2:895-908
3. Dicker RC, Greespan JR, Strauss LT et al (1982) Complications of abdominal and vaginal hysterectomy among women of reproductive age in the United States. Am J Obstet Gynecol 144:841-848
4. Kovac RS (1986) Intramyometrial coring as an adjunct to vaginal hysterectomy. Obstet Gynecol 67:131-136
5. Coppenhaver EH (1962) An analysis of indications and complications among 1000 operations. Am J Obstet Gynecol 84:123-128
6. Cosson M, Querleu D, Subtil D et al (1996) The feasibility of vaginal hysterectomy. Eur J Obstet Gynecol 64:95-99
7. Liu CY (1992) Laparoscopic hysterectomy: report of 215 cases. Gyn Endosc 1:73-77
8. Munro MG, Deprest J (1995) Laparoscopic hysterectomy: does it work? A bicontinental review of the literature and clinical commentary. Clin Obstet Gynecol 38(2):401-425
9. Reich H, De Caprio JR, McGlynn F (1989) Laparoscopic hysterectomy. J Gynecol Surg 5:213-215
10. Mage G, Masson FN, Canis M et al (1995) Laparoscopic hysterectomy. Curr Opin Obstet Gynecol 7:283-289
11. Nezhat F, Nezhat C, Gorbon S et al (1992) Laparoscopic versus abdominal hysterectomy. J Reprod Med 3:247-250
12. Nezhat C, Bess O, Admon D et al (1994) Hospital cost comparison between abdominal, vaginal and laparoscopic assisted vaginal hysterectomies. Obstet Gynecol 83:713-716
13. Chapron C, Dubuisson JB, Ansquer Y (1996) Is total laparoscopic hysterectomy a safe surgical procedure? Hum Reprod 11(11):2422-2424
14. Summit RL Jr, Stovall TG, Lipscomb GH et al (1993) Randomised comparison of laparoscopy-assisted vaginal hysterectomy with standard vaginal hysterectomy in outpatient setting. Obstet Gynecol 80(6):895-901
15. Phipps JH, John M, Nayak S (1993) Comparison of laparoscopically assisted vaginal hysterectomy and bilateral salpingo-oophorectomy with conventional abdominal hysterectomy and bilateral salpingo-oophorectomy. Br J Obstet Gynaecol 100:698-700
16. Richardson RE, Bournas N, Magos AL (1995) Is laparoscopic hysterectomy a waste of time? Lancet 345:36-41
17. Boike GM, Elfstrand E, Delpriore G et al (1993) Laparoscopically assisted vaginal hysterectomy in a university hospital: report of 82 cases and comparison with abdominal and vaginal hysterectomy. Am J Obstet Gynecol 168:1690-1697
18. Gitsch G, Berger E, Tatra G (1991) Complications of vaginal hysterectomy under "difficult" circumstances. Arch Gynecol Obstet 249:209-212
19. Draca D (1986) Vaginal hysterectomy by means of morcellation. Eur J Obs Gyn Reprod Biol 22:237
20. Wilcox LS, Coonin LM, Strauss LT et al (1994) Hysterectomy in the United States, 1988-1990. Obstet Gynecol 83:849-855
21. Ballard LA, Walters MD (1996) Transvaginal mobilization and removal of ovaries and fallopian tubes after vaginal hysterectomy. Obstet Gynecol 87:35-39
22. Sheth SS (1991) The place of oophorectomy at vaginal hysterectomy. Br J Obstet Gynaecol 98:662-666
23. Casey MJ, Garcia-Padial J, Johnson C et al (1994) A critical analysis of laparoscopic assisted vaginal hysterectomies compared with vaginal hysterectomies unassisted by laparoscopy and transabdominal hysterectomies. J Gynecol Surg 10:7-14
24. Johns DA, Carrera B, Jones J et al (1995) The medical and economic impact of laparoscopically assisted vaginal hysterectomy in a large, metropolitan, not-for-profit hospital. Am J Obstet Gynecol 172:1709-1715

Chapter 7

Laparoscopic Myomectomy

Jean-Bernard Dubuisson, Arnaud Fauconnier and Charles Chapron

7.1 Introduction

The technique of laparoscopic myomectomy (LM) only appeared recently, with the first cases being described for subserous fibroids in the 1980s.[1,2] Since the beginning of the 1990s, several teams in Europe and the USA have reported their experience with LM for interstitial fibroids.[3–6] Although there is still some hesitation, use of LM is becoming more widespread and the large number of studies addressing the subject show that the technique has reached maturity.[3,5–27] It has been the subject of several prospective randomised studies,[16,28,29] one of which compared the LM technique with laparotomy.

Our own team has considerable experience in the use of LM: between March 1989 and July 1998 we carried out 373 procedures. The purpose of this chapter is to focus on the operative technique and to describe the advantages, limitations and risks involved.

7.2 Procedures for Myomectomy using Laparoscopy

Four different myomectomy procedures using laparoscopy can be described: intraperitoneal myomectomy; myomectomy assisted by laparoscopy (LAM); laparoconversion; and diagnostic laparoscopy.

7.2.1 Intraperitoneal Myomectomy

This is complete myomectomy with all the phases being carried out by laparoscopy (hysterotomy, enucleation and suture of the hysterotomy).

7.2.2 Myomectomy Assisted by Laparoscopy

In 1994 Nezhat defined a myomectomy procedure that is midway between laparotomy and laparoscopy: LAM.[30] In the initial description by this author, laparoscopy was used solely to treat any associated lesions (adhesions) and to help expose the myoma(s); enucleation, extraction and suture of the hysterotomy were carried out by mini-laparotomy. Our method of LAM is a little different, consisting of carrying out only the hysterotomy suture and extraction of the fibroid by mini-laparotomy; with enucleation of all the fibroids achieved totally by laparoscopy.

7.2.3 Conversion to Laparotomy

In this category we include all operations where recourse to laparotomy is required, when the initial phase of myomectomy had been started by laparoscopy. Conversion may be needed due to technical difficulties (cleavage of the fibroid cannot be achieved, difficulties with achieving haemostasis), or for complications connected with the myomectomy (haemorrhage) or not (anaesthesia complication, for example).

7.2.4 Diagnostic Laparoscopy

The term diagnostic laparoscopy includes all myomectomies that use laparoscopy to assess the characteristics of the fibroids and decide whether laparoscopic myomectomy is feasible or not, but for which none of the operative steps for the actual myomectomy is carried out by laparoscopy. It also includes all procedures carried out by laparoscopy and aimed at allowing satisfactory exploration of the pelvis and fibroids (adhesiolysis).

By LM, we mean all myomectomy procedures for which at least the first step for myomectomy was started by laparoscopy. The term thus covers all laparoconversions, intraperitoneal myomectomies and LAM. In our work almost all LM are in fact intraperitoneal myomectomies.

Alternatives have been proposed for LM, such as use of pneumosuspension[31] and myolysis techniques.[32–34]

7.3 Operative Technique

7.3.1 Principles

The LM technique we use in our institution comprises four main phases: hysterotomy and revelation of the fibroid; enucleation; suture of the myomectomy site; and extraction of the fibroid.[35]

The main difficulties with the operation, as with myomectomy by laparotomy, are the risk of peroperative haemorrhage and the prevention of postoperative adhesions. Use of the laparoscopic route for the myomectomy also raises certain problems connected with this approach: the fibroids are more difficult to access than with laparotomy; enucleation of the fibroids must be as bloodless as possible; and one of the crucial points is the method for obtaining a good quality scar.

Use of the LM technique is therefore based on several basic principles. The principles of microsurgery must be applied to the technique: avoidance of intraperitoneal contamination; use of fine and atraumatic instruments; avoidance of tissue dessiccation; gentle and atraumatic manipulation and grasping of the pelvic organs. These precautions make it possible to minimise postoperative adhesions.

With LM, each fibroid must be excised via its own hysterotomy; it is not possible to apply the same technique as with myomectomy by laparotomy,[36,37] that is, removing all the myomas present on the uterus via the same hysterotomy.

A distinct cleavage plane separates the fibroid from the adjacent myometrium. This cleavage plane is bound by a pseudocapsule made up of compressed muscular fibres and diverted uterine vessels.[38] Vascularisation of the fibroid is plurifocal through the cleavage plane by means of a multitude of small nourishing vessels and there is no true vascular pedicle.[39] Dissection must always take place

along this cleavage plane for two reasons: preservation of healthy adjacent myometrium is one of the conditions for obtaining a good-quality uterine scar, and to help avoid damaging the perimyomatous vessels, which are often the subject of dilatation due to compression by the fibroid,[40] but may be the origin of considerable haemorrhage. Another advantage with the laparoscopic approach is that the small nourishing vessels can be viewed clearly, thus permitting elective coagulation.

Electrocautery must be used as sparingly as possible to achieve haemostasis of the edges and seat of the myomectomy. Certain cases of uterine rupture after LM[6,41,42] suggest that the use of electrocautery may induce necrosis of the myometrium, resulting in a secondary fistula. Furthermore, electrocautery is responsible for delayed healing,[43] which could also adversely affect the solidity of the myomectomy scar.

Suture of the hysterotomy must always respect a certain number of principles; indeed, any technical deficiency when carrying it out may result in uterine rupture during a subsequent pregnancy.[41] Apart from pedunculated fibroids or certain sessile subserous fibroids with a narrow implantation base, the myomectomy sites must always be sutured. In the experience of certain teams at the beginning, when no suture was carried out, the resulting scars were fine or dehiscent.[44,45] The suture must always take up the full depth of the edges of the hysterotomy and result in total contact over the whole of the myomectomy site in order to avoid secondary constitution of a haematoma deep inside the myometrium. This kind of haematoma can cause weakness in the scar tissues and the constitution of a secondary fistula.[20,36,44]

The uterine suture does not necessarily have to use several planes, despite the recommendation of certain authors.[46,47] Suture of the uterine serosa is unnecessary and could increase the risk of postoperative adhesions.[43,48–50] Sometimes it is necessary to make a suture in two or three planes if the uterine cavity has been broached or if the myomectomy site is very deep. It is possible to make this type of suture in several planes by laparoscopy;[20,22,51] however, if this proves difficult, there should be no hesitation in using a mini-laparotomy to complete it successfully.

7.3.2 Instrumentation

In addition to the standard instrumentation for any operative laparoscopy, certain specific instruments are useful when carrying out LM. Short curved monopolar scissors enable incision of the myometrium and section of the tracti between the fibroid and myometrium. Other instruments are useful when making the intra- or extracorporeal sutures: needle holders, atraumatic forceps with no slot or claws, suture pusher. A strong grasping forceps specifically for fibroids (Museux forceps type) means that efficient traction can be exerted on the myoma.

Ideally an electric morcellation device such as the Steiner morcellator[52] allows fibroids over 4 cm to be extracted by the suprapubic port: in our experience this device proved easy to use after a learning phase, and has enabled us to reduce considerably the duration of our operations. The relatively high cost of this device is compensated for by a quick amortisation as a result of the shorter operation times.[53]

7.3.3 Installation

The patient lies in the following position: thighs spread with abduction providing access to the vagina; buttocks protruding generously over the edge of the table to allow manipulation of the uterus with an intrauterine cannula. The main surgeon stands to the patient's left, with the first assistant opposite and the second assistant between the patient's legs.

Injection of undiluted methylene blue into the uterine cavity at the beginning of the operation makes it possible to see when dissection of intramural fibroids is coming close to the endo-metrium and to know when the uterine cavity is broached peroperatively. The uterus is then cannulated, enabling it to be manipulated during the operation.

Two 5 mm lateral trocars and one 12 mm midline trocar are inserted in the suprapubic position. The position of the trocars should be adapted whenever possible to the size and location of the fibroids. Generally speaking, the two lateral trocars should be placed relatively high and outside the epigastric vessels so that good accessibility is provided for myomas in various locations and to ensure that the surgeon has sufficient scope for movement when carrying out the sutures.

7.3.4 Incision of the Myometrium and Exposure of the Fibroid

The hysterotomy is direct, lined up with the fibroid. The direction may be either sagittal or transverse. We tend to use sagittal hysterotomies because they are easier to suture. The myometrium is incised using low-voltage monopolar current in section mode in order to safeguard the myometrium as far as possible. Haemostasis of the intramyometrial vessels is carried out progressively (and preventively, if possible) using mono- or bipolar current. Identification of the avascular plane surrounding the fibroid is helped by the magnifying effect of the laparoscopic images. The fibroid is easy to recognise by its smooth appearance and pearly white colour, which contrasts with the adjacent myometrium. In addition, the fibroid is firm to the touch, different from the myometrium, and this can be felt via the laparoscopic instruments.

7.3.5 Enucleation

Dissection of the fibroid should run inside the avascular plane, leaving the pseudocapsule around the outside and the uterine vessels pushed back. Dissection is easier if the following manoeuvre is used: the myoma is grasped with a strong grasping forceps and pulled hard towards the anterior abdominal wall or upwards; at the same time the surgeon or his assistant exerts traction in the opposite direction using the endouterine cannula or by pushing on the edges of the hysterotomy with an instrument. This dissection proceeds from the superficial areas inwards, and always under visual control in order to identify the fine tracti adhering to the fibroid. The tip of a blunt instrument is used (curved scissors or bipolar forceps) to press against the fibroid. The tracti adhering to the fibroid are coagulated (as close as possible to the fibroid), then sectioned.

Some authors recommend the use of "atraumatic" dissection instruments (harmonic scalpel, ultrasonically activated laparosonic coagulating shears, aquadissector, laser).[17,24,54,55] The use of such instruments is supposed to improve preservation of the adjacent myometrium. The ultrasonically activated laparosonic coagulating shears are reputed to make dissection of the fibroid easier than with standard instruments.[20] We have no experience of this instrument in our institution.

The bed of the myomectomy is usually free from haemorrhage at the end of dissection if care has been taken to follow the avascular cleavage plane; there is no need to take further steps for haemostasis.

7.3.6 Hysterotomy Suture

We use fine resorbable suture, diameter 00 gauge, mounted on a curved needle with atraumatic tip. The suture is usually carried out in a single plane. We use single, separate knots, tied in or outside the body. These stitches go through the whole thickness of the edges of the hysterotomy, and through the uterine serosa. They are placed sufficiently close for the edges to be approximated completely, yet far enough apart to avoid making the myometrium too fragile.

When the myomectomy is located deeply, or the uterine cavity has been opened, we suture along a deep plane with a few single stitches deep in the myometrium, and along a superficial plane, taking in the serosa and the superficial part of the myometrium. The superficial plane can be dealt with using a running suture or with individual stitches. When suturing the deep plane, it can sometimes be difficult to take the needle through the thickness of the defect. In this case it can be an advantage to use a U-shaped transfixing stitch, the "belt stitch",[44] running through the uterine serosa and taking in the whole thickness of the edges of the myomectomy. One or two of these stitches are sufficient to ensure that all the deep part of the hysterotomy is brought into contact. When the uterine suture proves difficult to carry out, it is essential to know when to stop and use a mini-laparotomy for the suture.

7.3.7 Extraction of the Fibroid

Various methods are possible for extraction: direct extraction; standard intra-abdominal morcellation; electric morcellation; extraction via posterior colpotomy; extraction via mini-laparotomy. Direct suprapubic extraction is appropriate only for fibroids measuring less than 3 cm. Extraction takes place through the midline suprapubic incision, which may be enlarged if needed. For ports larger than 10 mm, it is important to close the abdominal wall correctly in order to avoid incisional hernias.[56–58] Standard morcellation is carried out either with the scissors or with the monopolar electrode, and is appropriate for small fibroids (less than 4 or 5 mm diameter). Electric morcellation uses the Steiner morcellator.[52] This device has proved easy to use and without danger, but the position of the blade in the device must be under perfect control at all times to avoid any risk of damaging any neighbouring organs. Posterior colpotomy also allows large fibroids to be extracted.[17] Some authors have suggested that postoperative adhesions involving the colpotomy scar are possible,[5,20] but we have not found any increase in this risk in our study on adhesions after LM.[49] Since the advent of the electric morcellator, we hardly ever use a posterior colpotomy to extract fibroids.

7.4 Results of Laparoscopic Myomectomy

7.4.1 Advantages of Laparoscopic Myomectomy

It is now accepted that the technique is both feasible and reproducible, as can be seen from the large numbers of teams who now use LM and have reported their experience.[3,5–27] Analysis of these series of LM, together with the experience gained in our own institution,[59] enable us to state that this technique does not involve a higher risk of peroperative or immediate postoperative complications as compared with myomectomy via laparotomy. Furthermore, two controlled studies suggest that the risk of peroperative haemorrhage and the risk of postoperative complications are reduced.[10,60]

From the cosmetic point of view, the absence of a scar is very much appreciated by our patients. As for function, the fact that the patients are more comfortable has been proved by a clinical trial: there is less postoperative pain after LM and the hospital stay is shorter.[16]

Laparoscopic myomectomy could reduce the risk of adhesions after myomectomy. In our study on second-look after LM, we observed that there was a 36% rate of adhesions in the 45 patients who underwent the check; if only adhesions involving the adnexa were taken into account, the rate was 24%.[49] These rates are low in comparison with those observed at second-look after myomectomy via laparotomy, which reach nearly 90%, with nearly two-thirds of the cases showing involvement of the adnexa.[61–64] Two controlled studies also suggest a lower risk of adhesions after LM.[9,60] This reduction in postoperative adhesions presents a particular advantage when the myomectomy is carried out in a context of infertility because it could help to improve the fertility of the patients.

The results of LM relative to fertility have been assessed.[65] In our series of 91 infertile patients, we observed a cumulative conception rate of 44% at 2 years. This rate was 70% when no other factor was found for infertility other than the fibroid. These results are comparable to those of the series of myomectomy via laparotomy, which in our opinion justifies preferential use of the laparoscopic approach whenever the fibroids are medium-sized and few in number. However, there has been no randomised clinical trial to validate this proposal.

7.4.2 Limits and Risks of LM

Laparoscopic myomectomy, particularly in the case of interstitial fibroids, is nevertheless a difficult technique, which requires surgeons who are highly experienced in laparoscopic surgery.[35,59] Moreover, it takes time and the operations do seem to last longer than with laparotomy.[60]

We consider that the maximum size of fibroids operated by LM should not exceed 8 cm and that no more than three fibroids should be removed in total.[66] In practice, we do sometimes go beyond these limits and some teams have also reported carrying out LM for far larger fibroids, up to 16 cm.[7,26] However, using LM for large fibroids can lead to difficulties in obtaining cleavage of the fibroids for several reasons: the growth of certain fibroids results in reorganization of the myomatous tissues and neighbouring myometrium, making the attachments of the fibroids more dense and difficult to cleave; the depth of the site of the fibroid hampers access for the instruments and visibility of the tissues to be dissected; the larger fibroids have a more highly developed vascularisation, which results in an increased risk of peroperative haemorrhage; and finally, the time required for electric morcellation increases considerably with the size of the fibroid. When we first started using the technique, we planned to use luteinising hormone-releasing hormone analogues preoperatively to reduce the size of the fibroids. This proved to be inefficient because the tissue reorganisation induced by the analogues resulted in the cleavage plane around the fibroid becoming less distinct.

To date, five cases of uterine rupture during pregnancy have been reported after LM, in particular one in our institution.[18,41,42,67,68] These accidents raise the question of the quality of the scars after LM and some authors[30,69] consider that the laparoscopic route is not satisfactory to make solid sutures of the myometrium if there is a deep defect.

We have several arguments to counter these criticisms. Although experience with pregnancies after myomectomy via laparotomy shows that uterine rupture is rare (no case in the largest series published),[70-72] observations of uterine rupture after laparotomy are nevertheless reported regularly in the literature.[45,73-76] Cases of rupture have also been reported after hysteroscopy.[77]

At present there is no knowledge concerning the real incidence of rupture after LM, because only the cases themselves are reported. The incidence is probably low, because in our population, for example, we observed a single case of rupture for 92 pregnancies after LM (unpublished data).

There is probably a publication bias connected with the newness of the technique for LM. This kind of bias could explain the number of cases reported in the literature over a short period. With myomectomy via laparotomy, observations of uterine rupture are reported only when the particular circumstances under which they occur make them interesting enough to publish.

It took a long time to arrive at a good suture technique by laparoscopy. In the beginning, some teams (including ours) did not immediately apply certain principles for making the uterine sutures, which have since become clear. Some authors did not systematically suture the myomectomy sites[6] at the beginning of their experience. In addition, our observation[41] suggests that electrocautery plays a part in the secondary development of parietal necrosis resulting in a fistula.

At the present time, although suturing by the intraperitoneal route remains a technically difficult technique requiring surgeons skilled in laparoscopic surgery, we agree with other teams[20,22,44] in considering that provided the technique is meticulous, the uterine suture can be carried out satisfactorily by the purely laparoscopic route. Nevertheless we remain vigilant and this is one of the reasons why, when there is a desire for pregnancy, we propose systematically to take a second look by laparoscopy, which enables the appearance of the uterine scars after LM to be assessed.

7.5 Conclusions

Laparoscopic myomectomy enables subserous and interstitial fibroids to be treated surgically using minimally invasive techniques. Analysis of the advantage/risk ratio for this operation as compared with the use of laparotomy for myomectomy supports its use for medium-sized fibroids ($<$ 8 cm) when few in number. Laparoscopic myomectomy appears to present particular advantages when operating in a context of infertility, because it may reduce the risk of postoperative adhesions.

For good-quality healing to be obtained, the surgeons need to be experienced in laparoscopic surgery techniques and the principles for making uterine sutures defined for myomectomy via laparotomy must be applied.

References

1. Kolmorgen K (1989) [Ovariectomy by laparoscopy]. Zentralbl Gynakol 111(9):613–617
2. Semm K, Mettler L (1980) Technical progress in pelvic surgery via operative laparoscopy. Am J Obstet Gynecol 138 (2):121–127

3. Daniell JF, Gurley LD (1991) Laparoscopic treatment of clinically significant symptomatic uterine fibroids. J Gynecol Surg 7:37–40

4. Dubuisson JB, Lecuru F, Foulot H et al (1991) Myomectomy by laparoscopy: a preliminary report of 43 cases. Fertil Steril 56(5):827–830

5. Hasson HM, Rotman C, Rana N et al (1992) Laparoscopic myomectomy. Obstet Gynecol 80(5):884–888

6. Nezhat C, Nezhat F, Silfen SL et al (1991) Laparoscopic myomectomy. Int J Fertil 36(5):275–280

7. Adamian LV, Kulakov VI, Kiselev SI et al (1996) Laparoscopic myomectomy in treatment of large myomas. J Am Assoc Gynecol Laparosc 3(4)(Suppl):S1

8. Andrei B (1996) Myomectomy by pelvicoscopy. Int Surg 81 (3):271–275

9. Bulletti C, Polli V, Negrini V et al (1996) Adhesion formation after laparoscopic myomectomy. J Am Assoc Gynecol Laparosc 3(4):533–536

10. Carter JE, McCarus S, Baginiski L et al (1996) Laparoscopic outpatient treatment of large myomas. J Am Assoc Gynecol Laparosc 3(4)(Suppl):S6

11. Cittadini E (1998) Laparoscopic myomectomy: the Italian experience. J Am Assoc Gynecol Laparosc 5(1):7–9

12. Daraï E, Deval B, Darles C et al (1996) Myomectomie: coelioscopie ou laparotomie. Contracep Fertil Sex 24 (10):751–756

13. Dubuisson JB, Chapron C (1994) Laparoscopic myomectomy. Operative procedure and results. Ann NY Acad Sci 734:450–454

14. Keckstein J, Karageorgieva E, Darwish A et al (1994) Laparoscopic myomectomy: sonographic follow-up and second-look laparoscopy for the evaluation of a new technique. J Am Assoc Gynecol Laparosc 1(4)(Pt 2):S16

15. Kolmorgen K (1995) [Laparoscopic myomectomy]. Zentralbl Gynakol 117(12):659–662

16. Mais V, Ajossa S, Guerriero S et al (1996) Laparoscopic versus abdominal myomectomy: a prospective, randomized trial to evaluate benefits in early outcome. Am J Obstet Gynecol 174(2):654–658

17. Mangeshikar PR (1995) New instrumentation and technique for laparoscopic myomectomy. J Am Assoc Gynecol Laparosc 2(4)(Suppl):S29

18. Mecke H, Wallas F, Brocker A et al (1995) [Pelviscopic myoma enucleation: technique, limits, complications]. Geburtshilfe Frauenheilkd 55(7):374–379

19. Mettler L, Alvarez-Rodaz E, Semm K (1995) Myomectomy by laparoscopy: a report of 482 cases. Gynaecol Endosc 4:259–264

20. Miller CE, Johnston M, Rundell M (1996) Laparoscopic myomectomy in the infertile woman. J Am Assoc Gynecol Laparosc 3(4):525–532

21. Montevecchi L, Bagnini C, Campo S et al (1995) Laparoscopic myomectomy. J Am Assoc Gynecol Laparosc 2(4) (Suppl):S34

22. Ostrzenski A (1997) A new laparoscopic myomectomy technique for intramural fibroids penetrating the uterine cavity. Eur J Obstet Gynecol Reprod Biol 74(2):189–193

23. Parker WH, Rodi IA (1994) Patient selection for laparoscopic myomectomy. J Am Assoc Gynecol Laparosc 2(1):23–26

24. Reich H (1995) Laparoscopic myomectomy. Obstet Gynecol Clin North Am 22(4):757–780

25. Seinera P, Arisio R, Decko A et al (1997) Laparoscopic myomectomy: indications, surgical technique and complications. Hum Reprod 12(9):1927–1930

26. Stringer NH (1996) Laparoscopic myomectomy in African-American women. J Am Assoc Gynecol Laparosc 3(3):375–381

27. Wood EC, Maher P (1995) New strategies for endoscopic myomectomy. J Am Assoc Gynecol Laparosc 2(4)(Suppl):S60–61

28. Mais V, Ajossa S, Piras B et al (1995) Prevention of de-novo adhesion formation after laparoscopic myomectomy: a randomized trial to evaluate the effectiveness of an oxidized regenerated cellulose absorbable barrier. Hum Reprod 10 (12):3133–3135

29. Zullo F, Pellicano M, De Stefano R et al (1998) A prospective randomized study to evaluate leuprolide acetate treatment before laparoscopic myomectomy: efficacy and ultrasonographic predictors. Am J Obstet Gynecol 178(1)(Pt 1):108–112

30. Nezhat C, Nezhat F, Bess O et al (1994) Laparoscopically assisted myomectomy: a report of a new technique in 57 cases. Int J Fertil Menopausal Stud 39(1):39–44

31. Chang FH, Soon YK, Lee CL et al (1996) Laparoscopic removal of a large leiomyoma using airlift gasless laparoscopy. J Am Assoc Gynecol Laparosc 3(4)(Suppl):S7

32. Goldfarb H (1995) Laparoscopic coagulation of myomas (myolysis). Obstet Gynecol Clin N Am 22:807–819

33. Nisolle M, Smets M, Malvaux V et al (1993) Laparoscopic myolysis with the Nd Yag laser. J Gynecol Surg 9:95–98

34. Olive DL, Rutherford T, Zreik T et al (1996) Cryomyolysis in the conservative treatment of uterine fibroids. J Am Assoc Gynecol Laparosc 3(4)(Suppl):S36

35. Dubuisson JB, Chapron C, Fauconnier A et al (1997) Laparoscopic myomectomy and myolysis. Curr Opin Obstet Gynecol 9(4):233–238

36. Bonney V (1931) The technique and results of myomectomy. Lancet 220:171–173

37. Buttram VC, Reiter R (1981) Uterine leiomyomata: etiology, symptomatology and management. Fertil Steril 36:433–445

38. Vollenhoven BJ, Lawrence AS, Hely DL (1990) Uterine fibroids: a clinical review. Br J Obstet Gynaecol 97:285–298

39. Acien P, Quereda F (1996) Abdominal myomectomy: results of a simple operative technique. Fertil Steril 65(1):41–51

40. Farrer-Brown G, Beilby J, Tarbit MH (1971) Venous changes in the endometrium of myomatous uteri. Obstet Gynecol 38:743

41. Dubuisson JB, Chavet X, Chapron C et al (1995) Uterine rupture during pregnancy after laparoscopic myomectomy. Hum Reprod 10(6):1475–1477

42. Harris WJ (1992) Uterine dehiscence following laparoscopic myomectomy. Obstet Gynecol 80(3):545–546

43. Elkins TE, Stoval TG, Warren J et al (1987) A histologic evaluation of peritoneal injury and repair. Obstet Gynecol 70:225–228

44. Hasson H (1996) Laparoscopic myomectomy. Infertil Reprod Med Clin N Am 7(1):143–159

45. Palerme G, Friedman E (1966) Rupture of the gravid uterus in the third trimester. Am J Obstet Gynecol 94(4):571–576

46. Davids AM (1957) Myomectomy in the relief of infertility and sterility and in pregnancy. Surg Clin North Am 37:563

47. Verkauf BS (1992) Myomectomy for fertility enhancement and preservation. Fertil Steril 58(1):1–15

48. Buckman R, Buckman P, Hufnagel H et al (1976) A physiologic basis for the adhesion free healing of deperitonealized surfaces. J Surg Res 21:67–76

49. Dubuisson JB, Fauconnier A, Chapron C et al (1998) Second-look after laparoscopic myomectomy. Hum Reprod 13 (8):2102–2106

50. MacDonald M, Elkins TE, Wortham GF et al (1988) Adhesion formation and prevention after peritoneal injury and repair in the rabbit. J Reprod Med 33:436–439

51. Dubuisson JB, Chapron C, Chavet X et al (1995) Traitement coeliochirurgical des volumineux fibromes utérins. Technique opératoire et résultats. J Gynecol Obstet Biol Reprod 24 (7):705–710

52. Steiner R, Wight E, Tadir Y et al (1993) Electrical device for removal of tissue from the abdominal cavity. Obstet Gynecol 81:471–474

53. Carter JE, McCarus SD (1997) Laparoscopic myomectomy. Time and cost analysis of power vs manual morcellation. J Reprod Med 42(7):383–388

54. Starks GC (1988) CO2 laser myomectomy in an infertile population. J Reprod Med 33(2):184–186

55. Stringer NH, Strassner HT (1996) Pregnancy in five patients after laparoscopic myomectomy with the harmonic scalpel. J Gynecol Surg 12:129–133

56. Boike GM, Miller CE, Spirtos NM et al (1995) Incisional bowel herniations after operative laparoscopy: a series of nineteen cases and review of the literature. Am J Obstet Gynecol 172(6):1726–1733

57. Chang FH, Soong YK, Cheng PJ et al (1995) Laparoscopic repair of bowel herniation through previous cannula insertion sites. J Am Assoc Gynecol Laparosc 2(4):489–492

58. Kurtz BR, Daniell JF, Spaw AT (1993) Incarcerated incisional hernia after laparoscopy. A case report. J Reprod Med 38 (8):643–644

59. Dubuisson JB, Chapron C, Lévy L (1996) Difficulties and complications of laparoscopic myomectomy. J Gynecol Surg 12:159–165

60. Stringer NH, Walker JC, Meyer PM (1997) Comparison of 49 laparoscopic myomectomies with 49 open myomectomies. J Am Assoc Gynecol Laparosc 4(4):457–464

61. Diamond MP (1996) Reduction of adhesions after uterine myomectomy by Seprafilm membrane (HAL-F): a blinded, prospective, randomized, multicenter clinical study. Seprafilm Adhesion Study Group. Fertil Steril 66(6):904–910

62. Myomectomy Adhesion Multicenter Study Group (1995) An expanded polytetrafluoroethylene barrier (Gore-Tex surgical membrane) reduces post-myomectomy adhesion formation. Fertil Steril 63(3):491–493

63. Tulandi T, Murray C, Guralnick M (1993) Adhesion formation and reproductive outcome after myomectomy and second-look laparoscopy. Obstet Gynecol 82:213–215

64. Ugur M, Turan C, Mungan T et al (1996) Laparoscopy for adhesion prevention following myomectomy. Int J Gynaecol Obstet 53(2):145–149

65. Dubuisson J, Fauconnier A, Chapron C et al (2000) Reproductive outcome after laparoscopic myomectomy in infertile women. J Reprod Med 45:23–30.

66. Dubuisson JB, Chapron C (1996) Laparoscopic myomectomy today. A good technique when correctly indicated. Hum Reprod 11(5):934–935

67. Friedmann W, Maier RF, Luttkus A et al (1996) Uterine rupture after laparoscopic myomectomy. Acta Obstet Gynecol Scand 75(7):683–684

68. Pelosi M, Pelosi MA (1997) Spontaneous uterine rupture at thirty-three weeks subsequent to previous superficial laparoscopic myomectomy. Am J Obstet Gynecol 177(6):1547–1549

69. Tulandi T, Youssef H (1997) Laparoscopy assisted myomectomy of large uterine myomas. Gynaecol Endosc 6:105–108

70. Brown AB, Chamberlain R, Te Linde RW (1956) Myomectomy. Am J Obstet Gynecol 71:759–763

71. Davids A (1952) Myomectomy: surgical technique and results in series of 1150 cases. Am J Obstet Gynecol 63:592–604

72. Finn WF, Muller PF (1950) Abdominal myomectomy: special reference to subsequent pregnancy and to the reappearance of fibromyomas of the uterus. Am J Obstet Gynecol 60:109

73. Garnet J (1964) Uterine rupture during pregnancy. Obstet Gynecol 23:898

74. Georgakopoulos P, Bersis G (1981) Sigmoido-uterine rupture in pregnancy after multiple myomectomy. Int Surg 66:367–368

75. Golan D, Aharoni A, Gonon R et al (1990) Early spontaneous rupture of the post myomectomy gravid uterus. Int J Gynaecol Obstet 31:167–170

76. Quakernack K, Bordt J, Nienhaus H (1980) [Placenta percreta and rupture of the uterus]. Geburtshilfe und Frauenheilkunde 40(6):520–523

77. Yaron Y, Shenhav M, Jaffa A et al (1994) Uterine rupture at 33 week's gestation subsequent to hysteroscopic perforation. Am J Obstet Gynecol 170:786–787

Part II

The Postmenopausal Endometrium

Contents

Summary

Only a small proportion of women with postmenopausal bleeding have significant endometrial pathology. The role of ultrasonography in these patients is its high negative predictive value for the absence of pathology. If the endometrial thickness is less than 5 mm, the risk of endometrial cancer is minimal (approximately 1.4%). An increased endometrial thickness in these patients is a relatively non-specific finding and demands further investigation. Hysteroscopy is indicated in these patients when the ultrasound scan is inconclusive or when there is persistent bleeding irrespective of the ultrasound findings. Outpatient biopsy techniques compare favourably with dilatation and curettage for the detection of endometrial pathology, but share the same risks as any blind procedure. The use of outpatient biopsies should be linked to the use of ultrasound both for patient selection and quality control. If there is doubt about the diagnosis, hysteroscopy is warranted.

Ultrasound can be used to assess the endometrium of women taking hormone replacement therapy (HRT); however, the examination should be performed in the immediate postmenstrual phase. The endometrial thickness in women taking continuous combined and sequential therapy should be similar, and an endometrial thickness of more than 5 mm considered abnormal irrespective of the bleeding pattern. The assessment of the endometrium of women taking tamoxifen therapy poses particular diagnostic problems. The relative merits of ultrasonography, hydrosonography and hysteroscopy are discussed. While ultrasound may play a role in the assessment of such women, hysteroscopically directed biopsies are needed to exclude pathology in women with abnormal bleeding.

Key Points

- Transvaginal ultrasonography has a high negative predictive value for the presence of endometrial pathology. A cut-off value for endometrial thickness of < 5.0 mm can be used to define normality
- An increased endometrial thickness is a non-specific finding and warrants further investigation in symptomatic women
- Hydrosonography and colour Doppler can decrease the number of false-positive test results from ultrasound
- Outpatient biopsy techniques compare well with dilatation and curettage for the detection of endometrial pathology
- For women taking sequential HRT, an ultrasound scan should be performed on day 5–10 of the cycle
- The endometrial thickness during the immediate postmenstrual phase of sequential therapy should be < 5.0 mm and the same as the endometrium of women taking continuous combined HRT
- The use of hydrosonography or hysteroscopy is needed in women taking tamoxifen therapy to discriminate between the common finding of glandulocystic endometrium and glandulocystic polyps
- The endometrial thickness of women taking tamoxifen therapy is often increased. A cut-off value of < 8.0 mm seems reasonable given current information
- Hysteroscopically directed biopsies are needed for women who present with abnormal bleeding while taking tamoxifen

Chapter 8

Postmenopausal Bleeding: Ultrasound and Hydrosonography versus Hysteroscopy

Dirk Timmerman

8.1 Introduction

Postmenopausal bleeding is a common complaint of women referred to a gynaecologist. It is usually defined as uterine bleeding in postmenopausal women not taking exogenous hormonal treatment or bleeding at an unexpected time during cycle replacement therapy. The first aim of the management of these patients is to exclude the presence of endometrial cancer. In many western countries, endometrial cancer is the most common gynaecological malignancy. Survival is generally good, as most cases present at an early stage with abnormal vaginal bleeding. Ninety per cent of patients with endometrial cancer are postmenopausal. Endometrial cancer is found in 10–15% of women with postmenopausal bleeding. Other causes of postmenopausal bleeding include exogenous oestrogens (30%), atrophic endometritis or vaginitis (30%), endometrial or cervical polyps (10%), endometrial hyperplasia (5%) and other diseases such as uterine sarcoma, trauma and cervical cancer (10%).[1] Around 5% of endometrial cancers are found in patients without any vaginal bleeding. Occasionally, a pyometrium or endometrial cells on a Papanicolaou smear in asymptomatic postmenopausal women are the first signs of endometrial cancer. The risk of endometrial cancer is strongly related to exposure to unopposed oestrogens. Oestrogen replacement therapy, obesity and oestrogen-secreting tumours are considered as risk factors, whereas oral contraceptives, progesterone therapy and early menopause reduce the risk.

A special group of patients at risk consists of postmenopausal breast cancer patients treated with tamoxifen. Tamoxifen has been shown to reduce mortality in breast cancer patients and it is currently the hormonal treatment of choice. It has been estimated that nearly one million women are on tamoxifen treatment in the USA and this number is likely to increase. Furthermore, tamoxifen was approved by the Food and Drug Administration in 1998 as a prophylactic agent against breast cancer. This has led to an increased interest in the potential side-effects of this drug. It is well established that tamoxifen can induce endometrial hyperplasia and polyps. These endometrial polyps can display a wide range of appearances.[2] The possible association between tamoxifen and the occurrence of endometrial cancer (two- to threefold risk) has been reviewed previously.[3]

Despite a false-negative rate of 2–6%,[4] the histopathological diagnosis obtained at dilatation and curettage (D&C) was long considered to be the "gold standard" for distinguishing between benign and malignant endometrium. It is now usually done in conjunction with hysteroscopy to eliminate the "blind nature" of the procedure. Several methods have been developed to reduce the need for D&C under general anaesthesia in order to reduce associated cost and morbidity. Three types of specialised investigation are commonly used in patients presenting with postmenopausal bleeding: outpatient endometrial biopsy, ultrasound and hysteroscopy. Each method of assessment has advantages and disadvantages, and the choice of method should be made accordingly.

The use of outpatient endometrial biopsy (e.g. with a Pipelle device) or aspiration methods (e.g. Vabra suction) is convenient. No special expertise or equipment is needed, and the procedure can be performed quickly. The presence of endometrial cancer can be demonstrated in 88–97% of cases. However, the introduction of endometrial biopsy methods has never led to a significant decrease of the number of D&C procedures performed, because most clinicians judge them to be insufficiently reliable to exclude the presence of endometrial cancer in patients with postmenopausal bleeding. These "blind" procedures cannot sample all of the endometrium, and endometrial polyps may be missed. In a study on 433 perimenopausal patients with abnormal uterine bleeding, non-directed office biopsy alone would have potentially missed the diagnosis of focal lesions such as polyps, submucous myomas and focal endometrial hyperplasia in up to 80 patients (18%).[5] In this study, Goldstein and colleagues proposed a clinical algorithm based on unenhanced transvaginal sonography followed by saline infusion (hydrosonography) for selected patients. Their approach consisted of either no endometrial sampling, non-directed sampling or directed sampling, depending on whether the ultrasound-based triage revealed no anatomical abnormalities, globally thickened endometrial tissue or focal abnormalities, respectively.

8.2 Ultrasound

8.2.1 Endometrial Thickness and Doppler

Transvaginal sonography is used to assess endometrial thickness, endometrial and myometrial homogeneity or heterogeneity, and abnormalities of endometrial morphology. When using ultrasound, a thin hyperreflective endometrial line can be seen in most postmenopausal women. This atrophic endometrium is characterised by a maximal total (double layer) endometrial thickness of less than 5 mm.[6] The mean endometrial thickness is higher (between 4 and 8 mm) in women on hormone replacement therapy compared with postmenopausal women not taking exogenous hormones (between 1 and 3 mm). In patients with postmenopausal bleeding, (1) an endometrial line that cannot be clearly visualised, (2) a measurement greater than 5 mm or (3) high echogenicity or irregularities in endometrial morphology, whereby one area is thicker than another, indicate the need for further investigation. The false-negative rate of transvaginal sonography for the detection of pathology is comparable with other existing techniques, such as D&C,[7] and in experienced hands transvaginal sonography is a very reliable tool to exclude endometrial cancer.[4,8] If only patients with postmenopausal bleeding and an endometrial thickness of more than 4 mm were to be referred for hysteroscopy and/or D&C, it may be possible to reduce the number of operative procedures by about 50%. However, a surprisingly high rate of endometrial cancer has been reported in some studies among patients with postmenopausal bleeding associated with an endometrial thickness of less than 5 mm (15/212) (9–11). Although many recent papers (Table 8.1) advise limitation of D&C to patients with postmenopausal bleeding associated with an endometrial thickness 5 mm at ultrasonography, we continue to recommend that office

Table 8.1. Prevalence of endometrial cancer in patients with postmenopausal bleeding in relation to (double layer) endometrial thickness (ET) at transvaginal sonography (from Timmerman and Vergote,[7] with permission). NR, Not recorded

	ET < 5 mm	ET ≥ 5 mm	Mean ET (mm) in endometrial cancer
Nasri and Coast 1989	0/37	7/63	24.4 (11.5–38)
Osmers et al 1990	0/46	13/57	NR
Goldstein et al 1990	0/11	1/19	NR
Nasri et al 1991	0/51	6/42	22.2 (83–8)
Granberg et al 1991b	0/150	18/55	18.2 (9–35)
Smith et al 1991	0/22	4/23	18.2 (14–22)
Ghirardini et al 1991	0/30	5/8	NR
Bourne et al 1991a[a]	0/NR	17/NR	20 (6–41)
Dørum et al 1993	3/54	12/45	20 (2–30)
Kurjak et al 1993a[a]	0/NR	35/NR	NR
Karlsson et al 1993[a]	0/ ≤ 57	15/ ≥ 48	NR (5–NR)
Sladkevicius et al 1994[a]	0/NR	23/NR	24 (7–56)
Dhont and Beghin 1994	0/34	12/48	NR
Emanuel et al 1995[a]	0/NR	7/NR	14.3 (9–20)
Karlsson et al 1995	0/518	114/620	21.2 (5–68)
Van den Bosch et al 1995[a]	0/NR	6/NR	22.5 (13–35)
Malinova and Pehlivanov 1995[a]	0/ ≤ 35	57/ ≥ 83	18.4 (7–40)
Schramm et al 1995	10/74	19/121	11 (0–20)
Seelbach-Göbel et al 1995	2/86	37/146	23.6 (NR)
All	15/1113	248/1247	

[a] Not included for statistical analysis (insufficient data).
Overall prevalence of endometrial carcinoma: 11.1%.
Transvaginal sonography (5 mm cut-off): sensitivity 94.3%; specificity 52.4%; positive predictive value 19.9%; negative predictive value 98.6%; accuracy 57.0%.

endometrial sampling be performed in patients presenting with postmenopausal bleeding and with an endometrial thickness of less than 5 mm (Figure 8.1). From the review of reported studies (Table 8.1), it may be concluded that in patients presenting with postmenopausal bleeding, endometrial cancer will be found in 11%. If the subsequent transvaginal sonography reveals an endometrial thickness of 5 mm or more, this figure rises to 20%. With an endometrial thickness of less than 5 mm, the risk for endometrial cancer in patients with postmenopausal bleeding is only 1.4%. If one is prepared to take this small risk of missing endometrial cancer in patients presenting with postmenopausal bleeding, the initial step of taking an office endometrial biopsy in all patients could be omitted, as proposed by many authors. Such a policy would certainly reduce the cost of the investigation. However, cost savings may differ considerably among countries.

The problems affecting the accuracy of transvaginal sonography include polypoid growths of endometrial cancer and the presence of adenomyosis and myomas deforming the uterine anatomy and volume. The latter pathological conditions can increase the false-positive results of the technique. On the other hand, further investigation is indicated if it is not possible to measure the endometrial thickness with transvaginal sonography in symptomatic women. Otherwise, cases of endometrial cancer will be missed and this in turn will result in a fall of the sensitivity of ultrasound.

The initial reports on the use of spectral analysis of colour Doppler signals from the uterine artery were promising, but more recent reports suggest that the contribution of a Doppler examination to the differential diagnosis in women with postmenopausal bleeding is very limited.[12] On the other hand, colour Doppler imaging can be very useful to evaluate endometrial pathology (Timmerman et al., unpublished data). Endometrial polyps often have a clearly visible vascular pedicle (Figure 8.2), while submucous myomas are characterised by a circular blood flow (Figure 8.3), and endometrial cancer commonly has irregular feeding neovascularisation in the subendometrial myometrium (Figure 8.4).

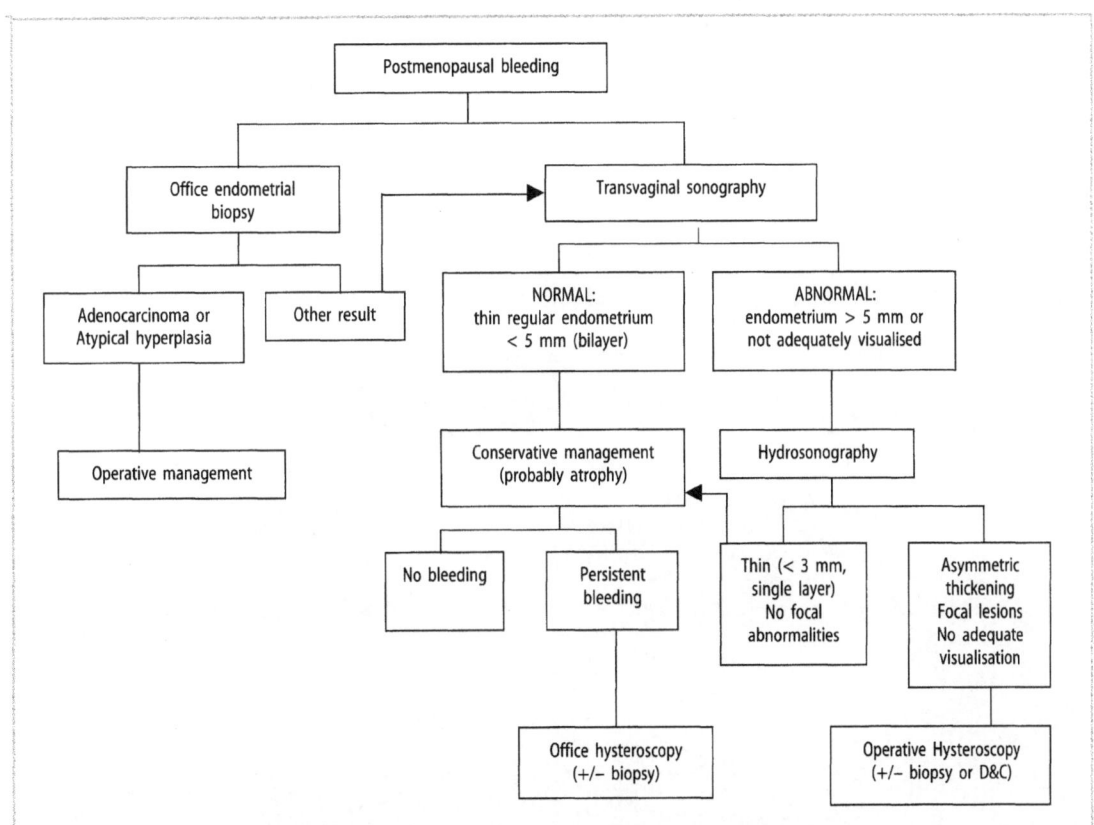

Figure 8.1 Algorithm for triage of women with postmenopausal bleeding

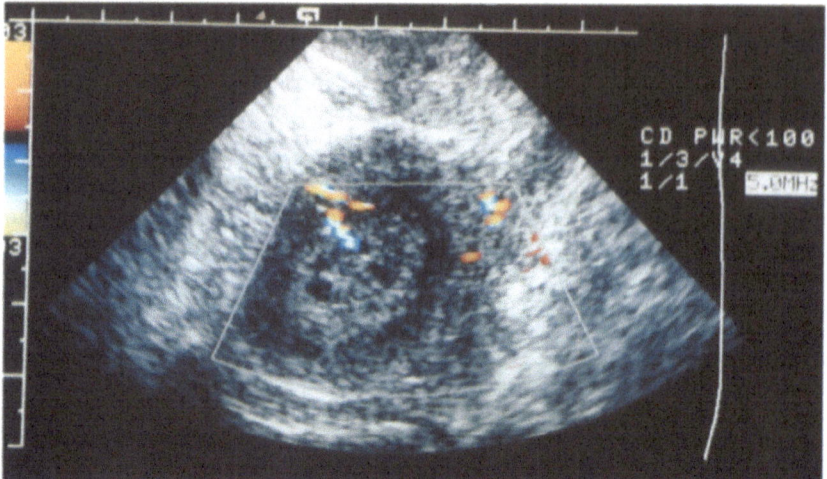

a

Figure 8.2a Clearly visible vascular pedicle in an endometrial polyp.

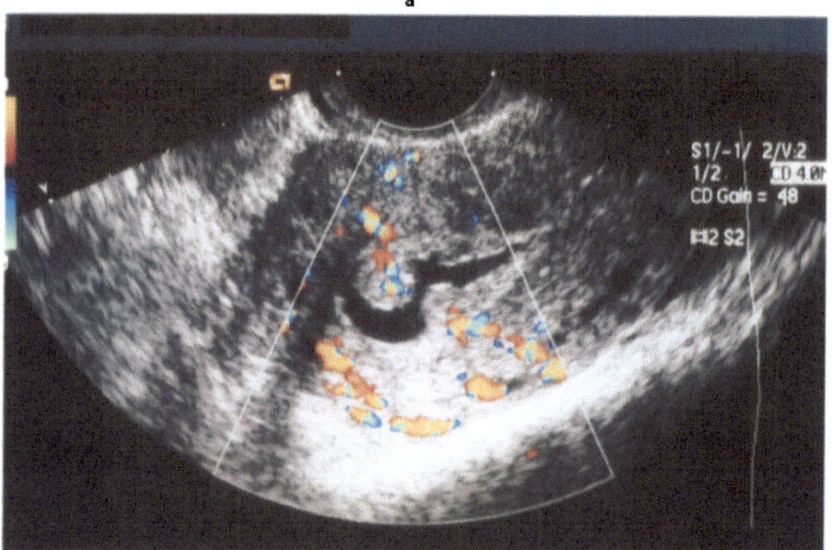

b

Figure 8.2b Two polyps with vascular pedicles visualised with hydrosonography.

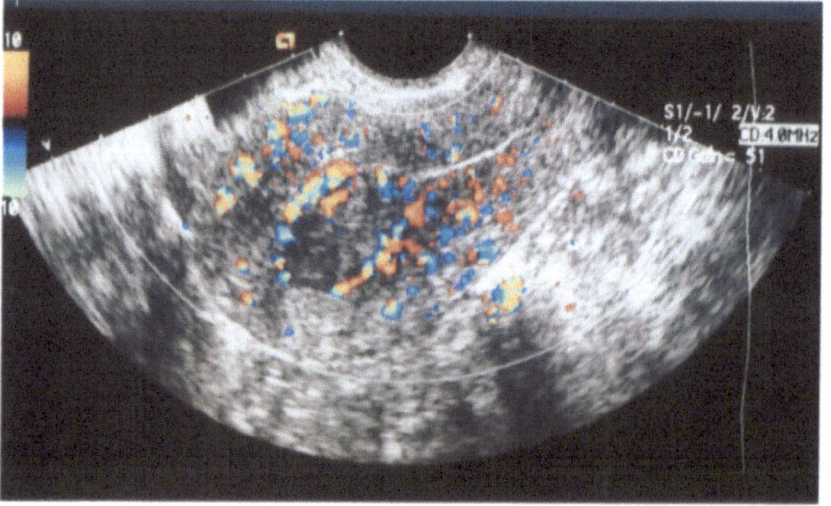

Figure 8.3 Submucous myoma characterised by a circular blood flow.

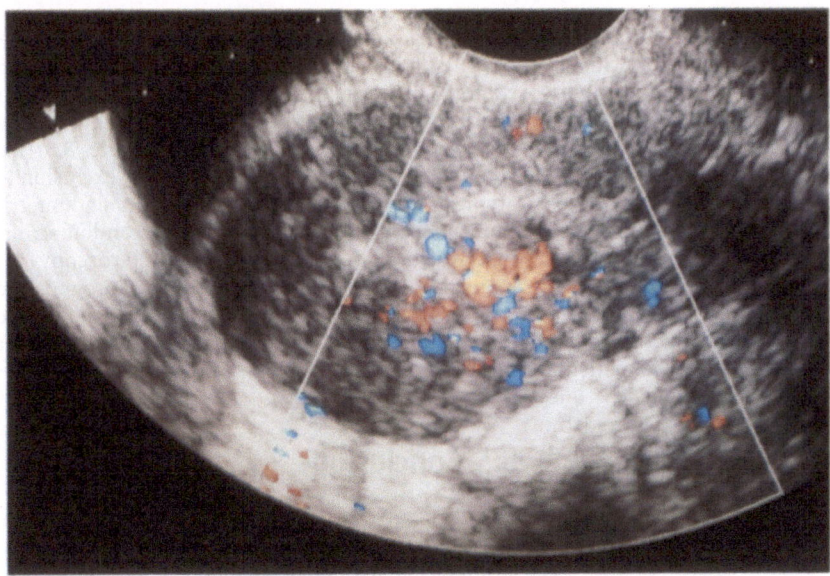

Figure 8.4 Stage I endometrial cancer with irregular feeding neovascularisation in the subendometrial myometrium of the posterior uterine wall.

8.2.2 Differential Diagnosis

It should be noted that abnormal ultrasonographic findings always warrant further investigation leading to histopathological diagnosis.

Endometrial hyperplasia is characterised by a highly reflective, thick endometrium, which is often homogeneous, but sometimes cystic with echo-free areas. There is an intact halo surrounding the endometrium. An ultrasound based differentiation of different forms of hyperplasia or endometrial cancer is not possible.

Treatment with tamoxifen or hormone replacement therapy will often lead to a very thick endometrium with or without the presence of cysts. If polyps are suspected, hydrosonography can be used.

Endometrial polyps are suspected if there is distortion of the midline of the endometrium. They are easily visualised with sonohysterography.

In patients presenting with endometritis, the presence of intrauterine free fluid is common, but the clinical presentation will nearly always lead to a correct diagnosis.

Uterine sarcoma (mixed Müllerian tumour or endometrial stromal sarcoma) can result in a thickened hyperechoic endometrium, an enlarged uterus without an intact halo surrounding the endometrium, and the presence of a polypoid endometrial tumour.

In cases of adenomyosis, an asymmetrical uterine enlargement, a distorted endometrial and myometrial echo texture, and occasionally small cystic areas have been described. In contrast with fibroids there are no circular feeding arteries around the adenomyomatous lesion which has no distinct contour.

8.3 Hydrosonography

Using a negative-contrast agent (e.g. normal saline solution), hydrosonography can improve the diagnostic performance of transvaginal sonography.[13,14] In this technique, sterile saline (3–20 ml) is injected into the uterine cavity under ultrasound control using a balloon catheter or an intrauterine insemination catheter. It can be used as a secondary test in patients with a thickened endometrial line at transvaginal sonography, to distinguish between intracavity polyps or fibroids and endometrial thickening (hyperplasia or carcinoma).[15-17] This may allow appropriate preoperative triage for operative hysteroscopy. If the endometrium is thin at hydrosonography and if no focal abnormalities are visualised, conservative management is appropriate in patients with postmenopausal bleeding. Hydrosonography is easy to learn, and is well tolerated by patients. In a prospective controlled study on 100 postmenopausal patients with abnormal uterine bleeding, the combination of endometrial biopsy and transvaginal sonography with hydrosonography was positively correlated with surgical findings in > 95% of the patients.[18] No patients with endometrial hyperplasia or cancer were misdiagnosed.

After treatment with tamoxifen, the endometrial appearance at transvaginal sonography typically changes from a postmenopausal atrophic (1–3 mm) endometrium into a characteristic endometrial pattern: it thickens and becomes hyperechogenic, with or without the presence of cysts. The junctional area is irregular and not clearly defined. In most of these cases, hysteroscopy shows only an apparent atrophic endometrium with many cysts. The histological findings are most often consistent with an atrophic endometrium. Hydrosonography is very useful to discriminate between globally thickened endometrium and polyps or other endometrial irregularities.

In a randomised, cross-over study in asymptomatic postmenopausal breast cancer patients, who had taken tamoxifen (20 or 40 mg/day) for at least 6 months, we compared the screening effectiveness and acceptability of transvaginal sonography (with hydrosonography if the endometrial thickness was > 4 mm) with office hysteroscopy.[19] Two patients had endometrial cancer (one primary, one secondary to breast cancer: both only detected by transvaginal sonography). Twenty-six patients had at least one polyp. The sensitivity for polyps and the specificity of transvaginal sonography were 85 and 100%, respectively. The corresponding values for office hysteroscopy were 77 and 92%. Significantly more patients preferred ultrasound to hysteroscopy (p < 0.001). We therefore conclude that transvaginal sonography (plus hydrosonography) is more effective and acceptable than office hysteroscopy for detecting endometrial abnormalities in women taking tamoxifen.

8.4 Hysteroscopy

The main advantages of hysteroscopy are direct visualisation of the endometrial cavity and the possibility of obtaining directed biopsies. Diagnostic hysteroscopy was found to be superior to D&C in 276 patients with abnormal bleeding in making an accurate diagnosis of pathological conditions in the uterine cavity.[20] In 45 women with postmenopausal bleeding, hysteroscopy had higher specificity but lower sensitivity for the detection of endometrial pathology compared with transvaginal sonography.[21] In this study, hysteroscopy failed to detect two out of four endometrial cancers. In a report comparing hydrosonography and office hysteroscopy in patients presenting with abnormal uterine bleeding, significantly more patients preferred transvaginal sonography to office hysteroscopy.[22] Hysteroscopy cannot be used to screen for extra-uterine pathology and sometimes fails to detect endometrial polyps[13] and cancers.[23,24] Furthermore, the procedure requires specialised equipment and is operator dependent. It cannot be used in patients with cervical stenosis, and is difficult in patients with active bleeding. It is difficult to find studies comparing state-of-the-art hysteroscopy with state-of-the-art transvaginal sonography. Office hysteroscopy is certainly useful when transvaginal sonography is not informative, when it reveals

asymmetric endometrial abnormalities, or when patients with a normal transvaginal sonography exhibit persistent postmenopausal bleeding. Operative hysteroscopy enables a minimally invasive resection of endometrial polyps (Figure 8.5) and submucous myomas, and a reliable exclusion of atypical endometrial hyperplasia or endometrial cancer in patients with an irregular endometrium. Finally, the debate whether hysteroscopy (or hydrosonography) could worsen the prognosis of endometrial cancer by retrograde seeding of malignant cells has not ended yet, but several publications are reassuring in this regard.

8.5 Conclusions

Transvaginal sonography is a reliable technique to exclude the presence of endometrial cancer or other endometrial pathology in patients presenting with postmenopausal bleeding. It is inexpensive and well tolerated by the patients. Hydrosonography and colour Doppler imaging can decrease the number of false-positive results. When transvaginal sonography is not informative, when it reveals asymmetric endometrial abnormalities, or when patients with a normal transvaginal sonography exhibit persistent postmenopausal bleeding, office hysteroscopy or other investigations are indicated. Because both transvaginal sonography and office hysteroscopy have limitations, any abnormal sonographic or hysteroscopic finding warrants further investigation (e.g. operative hysteroscopy) in order to reach the correct histopathological diagnosis.

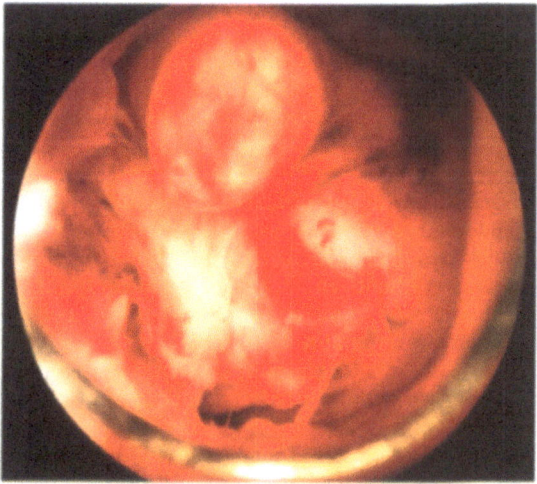

Figure 8.5 Operative hysteroscopy enables the resection of benign endometrial polyps.

References

1. Hacker NF (1994) Uterine cancer. In: Berek JS, Hacker NF (eds) Practical gynecologic oncology, 2nd edn. Williams and Wilkins, Baltimore, pp 285–326
2. Timmerman D, Deprest J, Vergote I (1997) Tamoxifen-induced endometrial polyp [reply]. N Engl J Med 336:1389–1390
3. Assikis VJ, Neven P, Jordan VC et al (1996) A realistic clinical perspective of tamoxifen and endometrial carcinogenesis. Eur J Cancer 32A:1464–1476
4. Granberg S, Wikland M, Karlsson B et al (1991) Endometrial thickness as measured by endovaginal ultrasonography for identifying endometrial abnormality. Am J Obstet Gynecol 164:47–52
5. Goldstein SR, Zeltser I, Horan CK et al (1997) Ultrasonography-based triage for perimenopausal patients with abnormal uterine bleeding. Am J Obstet Gynecol 177:102–108
6. Nasri MN, Shepherd JH, Setchell ME et al (1991) The role of vaginal scan in measurement of endometrial thickness in postmenopausal women. Br J Obstet Gynaecol 98:470–475
7. Timmerman D, Vergote I (1997) Endometrial cancer and uterine sarcoma. In: Brosens I, Wamsteker K (eds) Diagnostic imaging and endoscopy in gynecology: a practical guide. WB Saunders, London, pp 199–212
8. Karlsson B, Granberg S, Wikland M et al (1995) Transvaginal sonography of the endometrium in postmenopausal women to identify endometrial abnormality – a Nordic multi-center study. Am J Obstet Gynecol 172:1488–1494
9. Dørum A, Kristensen GB, Langebrekke A (1993) Evaluation of endometrial thickness measured by endovaginal ultrasound in women with postmenopausal bleeding. Acta Obstet Gynecol Scand 72:116–119
10. Schramm Th, Kürzl R, Schweighart C et al (1995) Endometriumkarzinom und Vaginalsonographie: Untersuchungen zur diagnostischen Validität. Geburtsh Frauenheilk 55:65–72
11. Seelbach-Göbel B, Rempen A, Kristen P (1995) Transvaginaler Ultraschall am Endometrium in der Postmenopause. Geburtsh Frauenheilk 55:59–64
12. Sladkevicius P, Valentin L, Marsál K (1994) Endometrial thickness and Doppler velocimetry of the uterine arteries as discriminators of endometrial status in women with postmenopausal bleeding: a comparative study. Am J Obstet Gynecol 171:722–728
13. Bourne TH, Lawton F, Leather A et al (1994) Use of intracavity saline instillation and transvaginal ultrasonography to detect tamoxifen-associated endometrial polyps. Ultrasound Obstet Gynecol 4:73–75
14. Gaucherand P, Piacenza JM, Salle B et al (1995). Sonohysterography of the uterine cavity: preliminary investigations. J Clin Ultrasound 23:339–348
15. Parsons A, Lense JJ (1993) Sonohysterography for endometrial abnormalities: preliminary results. J Clin Ultrasound 21:87–95
16. Goldstein SR (1994) Use of ultrasonohysterography for triage of perimenopausal patients with unexplained uterine bleeding. Am J Obstet Gynecol 170:565–570
17. Cohen JR, Luxman D, Sagi J et al (1994) Sonohysterography for distinguishing endometrial thickening from endometrial polyps in postmenopausal bleeding. Ultrasound Obstet Gynecol 4:227–230
18. O'Connell LP, Fries MH, Zeringue E et al (1998) Triage of abnormal postmenopausal bleeding: a comparison of endometrial biopsy and transvaginal sonohysterography versus fractional curettage with hysteroscopy. Am J Obstet Gynecol 178:956–961
19. Timmerman D, Deprest J, Bourne TH et al (1998) A randomized trial on the use of ultrasonography and office hysteroscopy for endometrial assessment in postmenopausal patients with breast cancer who were treated with tamoxifen. Am J Obstet Gynecol 179:62–70
20. Gimpelson RJ, Rappold HO (1988) A comparative study between hysteroscopy with directed biopsies and dilatation and curettage. A review of 276 cases. Am J Obstet Gynecol 158:489–492
21. Cacciatore B, Ramsay T, Lehtovirta P et al (1994) Transvaginal sonography and hysteroscopy in postmenopausal bleeding. Acta Obstet Gynecol Scand 73:413–416
22. Widrich T, Bradley LD, Mitchinson AR et al (1996) Comparison of saline infusion sonography with office hysteroscopy for the evaluation of the endometrium. Am J Obstet Gynecol 174:1327–1334
23. Townsend DE, Fields G, McCausland A et al (1993) Diagnostic and operative hysteroscopy in the management of persistent postmenopausal bleeding. Obstet Gynecol 82:419–421
24. Colafranceschi M, Bettocchi S, Mencaglia L et al (1996) Missed hysteroscopic detection of uterine carcinoma before endometrial resection: report of three cases. Gynecol Oncol 62:298–300

Chapter 9

Endometrial Sampling Techniques

Thierry Van den Bosch and Axel Vandendael

9.1 Introduction

Since its introduction by Récamier in 1843 till the early 1990s, dilatation and curettage (D&C) has been the standard diagnostic approach for the detection of endometrial disease. In 1935, Novak developed the first outpatient sampling curette, obviating the need for general anaesthesia. In the following decades, other outpatient endometrial sampling devices became available. More recently, hysteroscopy and vaginal ultrasonography have completed the diagnostic arsenal for the detection of endometrial disease.

The first section of this chapter compares different endometrial sampling methods. The second section discusses the indications for endometrial assessment.

9.2 Methods of Endometrial Sampling

Different sampling methods to evaluate the endometrial lining are used: extrauterine sampling for cytological examination and intrauterine sampling for cytological and/or histological evaluation.

9.2.1 Extrauterine Sampling

The cytologist reports the presence or absence of exfoliated endometrial cells on cervical or cervicovaginal smear. Endometrial cells should be absent in the second half of the menstrual cycle and after the menopause. If endometrial cells are present, they are evaluated with special attention to cellular atypia. Overall, a low diagnostic accuracy for endometrial disease of about 50% (range 18–66%) is found.[1] Sampling the vaginal pool, the ectocervical area or the endocervical canal have a similar diagnostic accuracy.[2] If normal endometrial cells are seen on screening, endometrial carcinoma is found in 5.7–11.2%.[3,4] If atypical or malignant endometrial cells are reported, malignancy is present in 64–100%.[5,6] Larson[7] evaluated cervical cytology in 164 women with endometrial cancer: 12.8% showed atypical endometrial cells and 23.9% malignant cells (giving a sensitivity of 42.7% and 29.9% respectively). Extrauterine sampling is of limited value as a screening method for endometrial pathology, although a cervical smear may alert the clinician to possible endometrial disease.

9.2.2 Intrauterine Sampling

9.2.2.1 Intrauterine Cytology

Intrauterine cytology sampling can be obtained by "flushing" the uterine cavity (e.g. with a Gravlee jet washer or Isaacs cell sampler) or by "scraping" the endometrial wall using a small device (e.g. Endopap, Endocyte). The processing is similar to that of cervical cytology and thus relatively inexpensive. The thicker devices like the Gravlee jet washer may necessitate cervical dilatation and have been replaced by thinner disposable samplers (e.g. Endopap). Failure to introduce the Endopap because of cervical stenosis has been reported in up to 10% of cases. The diagnostic accuracy for malignant endometrial lesions ranges from 66 to 97%.[1] The sensitivity for endometrial carcinoma ranges from 58 to 94%.[8,9] The positive predictive value for endometrial disease ranges from 43.6 to 66.7%, and from 93.7 to 96.4% for malignant lesions. The frequent occurrence of false positives indicates that the clinician should not rely on endometrial cytology, but must await histology before proceeding with hysterectomy for alleged endometrial malignancy.[10]

9.2.2.2 Intrauterine Histology

Intrauterine sampling methods for histological examination can be divided into three groups: (1) D&C, (2) office sampling and (3) selective endometrial biopsy under hysteroscopic guidance.

9.2.2.2.1 Dilatation and Curettage. This was the most common elective operation in the UK in 1989. The aim of D&C is to obtain sufficient endometrial tissue by scraping the uterine cavity with a curette to exclude organ pathology. Although a transient reduction of menstrual blood loss has been observed in the first postoperative cycle in women with menorrhagia, D&C has only incidental therapeutic properties. Disadvantages of the procedure include the fact that it is performed blind. Stock[11] found that in 60% of cases, less than half the endometrial surface was sampled during the procedure. Focal intrauterine lesions may thus be missed.[11–14] Another disadvantage is that it is an invasive procedure, performed under general anaesthesia. Grimes[15] reported a 1.7% complication rate, mainly uterine perforation (0.9%), infection (0.4%) and haemorrhage (0.4%).

9.2.2.2.2 Office Sampling. In office sampling, endometrial tissue is yielded by negative pressure (aspiration; e.g. Vabra aspirator, Pipelle de Cornier, Z-sampler) and/or scraping (e.g. Sharman and Kevorkian curette) through a specially designed device introduced through the cervical canal into the uterine cavity. The most commonly used devices are the Novak curette, the Vabra aspirator, and more recently the Pipelle de Cornier and the Z-sampler. The Pipelle de Cornier and the Z-sampler are easy to use, relatively inexpensive, and cause less patient discomfort than Vabra or Novak sampling.[16,17] In up to 10% of cases, the procedure may not be feasible due to cervical stenosis. As for D&C, office sampling methods are blind procedures. Vabra, Novak and Pipelle share a similar accuracy in the detection of endometrial disease, and compare well with D&C.[15] Although the endocavity surface is always incompletely sampled, most office biopsies give sufficient information for proper evaluation of the endometrial status. Malignant and hyperplastic endometrial tissue is probably more friable and thus more prone to be aspirated during sampling; endometrial polyps, however, are generally missed.[18,19] The results of office sampling are more reliable if matched with ultrasound findings of the endometrial lining performed before sampling: if a thickened endometrial lining is visualised on ultrasound, and the sampling yielded only atrophic tissue, a lesion most likely has been missed.

9.2.2.2.3 Hysteroscopy. Hysteroscopy with selective endometrial sampling has become the procedure of choice in evaluating intrauterine pathological conditions. Gimpelson[20] demonstrated its superiority to D&C. Diagnostic hysteroscopy can usually be performed without anaesthesia, or after local infiltration of the cervix. Although some authors[21,22] state that if hysteroscopy reveals an atrophic endometrium, endometrial biopsy is not needed, others[23] report a limited concordance between the hysteroscopy and histology, emphasising the importance of endometrial sampling after hysteroscopic evaluation. The biopsies taken with forceps used in office hysteroscopy are relatively small, and may be insufficient for proper histological evaluation in up to 20%.[24] An office sampler or a formal curettage (in case of general anaesthesia) may be indicated to obtain sufficient tissue.

Seeding of malignant cells into the abdominal cavity after hysteroscopy has been observed in women with endometrial carcinoma.[25] There is no evidence so far that prognosis is worsened by hysteroscopy.[26]

9.3 Indications for Endometrial Assessment

9.3.1 Asymptomatic Population

Screening for endometrial malignancy (in analogy with cervical cancer screening) in an asymptomatic population has not been proven useful so far. The opportunity for screening depends on the following conditions: (1) the incidence of the disease screened for, (2) the prognosis of the disease, (3) the curability of the disease in its early or pre-cancerous stage, and (4) the availability of an easy, cheap and painless screening method. Endometrial malignancy is the most common gynaecological cancer in the USA, with an incidence of 1.7 per 1000. The incidence of endometrial cancer is extremely low in young women (1 : 100 000 in women younger than 36 years). Screening in young women is therefore not defensible. Endometrial cancer is more likely in older women (relative risk, RR = 3), in the obese (RR = 10–23), and in women on unopposed oestrogen therapy (RR = 4–30). The 5-year survival of patients with early endometrial cancer is excellent, but shows a steep decline in more advanced stages. Atypical endometrial hyperplasia may be considered a pre-cancerous disease and can be cured medically in some cases, and surgically in all cases. The following screening methods may be considered: endometrial sampling, progesterone challenge test, vaginal ultrasound. Endometrial sampling is an easy, relatively cheap diagnostic tool, but remains an invasive procedure. Its use is warranted only in women at high risk for endometrial disease. A progesterone challenge test as screening in apparently normal menopausal women has been advocated:[27] if the patient had uterine bleeding, endometrial pathology was demonstrated in 22–100% of cases. Ultrasound may be better suited as a screening method in selecting "high-risk" women.[28,29] Endometrial sampling could be performed as a second step in cases of abnormal ultrasound findings.

9.3.2 Symptomatic Population

9.3.2.1 Postmenopausal Bleeding

Endometrial sampling is mostly performed in women presenting with abnormal uterine bleeding. Postmenopausal uterine bleeding in women without hormone replacement therapy (HRT) has long been considered an absolute indication for biopsy. Feldman,[30] using a statistical model with different risk factors, demonstrated that office endometrial sampling was the most cost-effective initial evaluation for postmenopausal bleeding. Feldman, however, did not include ultrasound in her model.

In half the menopausal women presenting with uterine bleeding, no intrauterine lesion is present. There is clearly a need for a better selection of patients at risk for endometrial pathology to lower the need for endometrial sampling. By using vaginal ultrasound to evaluate and measure the endometrial lining, it has been demonstrated that the need for endometrial sampling may be reduced by 50%: if the endometrial lining is thin and regular, the risk for benign or malignant endometrial disease is extremely low.

9.3.2.2 Hormone Replacement Therapy

The diagnosis of endometrial disease in women on HRT is less clearly established. Padwick[31] reported that in cases of regular bleeding induced on or after day 11 of progestogen, endometrial disease was unlikely. A change in menstrual pattern may be an indication for endometrial investigation. Sturdee[32] could not confirm any correlation between bleeding pattern and occurrence of endometrial pathology.

The question is whether endometrial sampling is warranted before the start of HRT. Because the risk for carcinoma is about 0.1%, most authors do not recommend endometrial biopsy in women without abnormal bleeding.

Vaginal ultrasound may be of benefit before the initiation of HRT to make sure that the endometrial

lining is thin and regular. During HRT, the timing of the ultrasound examination is important if a sequential HRT scheme is used: during the oestrogen-only phase of the cycle, a "follicular" three-layer pattern is mostly observed, making the diagnosis of focal lesions easier. Since focal lesions are common, Nagele[33] recommends hysteroscopy in women with abnormal bleeding on HRT.

9.3.2.3 Tamoxifen

Women on tamoxifen therapy have an increased risk for endometrial disease (RR = 2.3–6.4).[34,35] Some authors have suggested periodic endometrial sampling. As most tamoxifen-induced endometrial pathologies are focal lesions, blind sampling may prove less appropriate. The use of hysteroscopy with selective biopsy has been advocated. It is unclear if all women taking tamoxifen should undergo hysteroscopy on a regular basis. The use of vaginal ultrasound is limited by the frequent occurrence of pseudohyperplasia (false impression of thickened endometrial lining). Hydrosonography may be a better screening method to identify those patients at risk for endometrial pathology.[36,37]

9.3.2.4 Women in Reproductive Years

In younger women, life-threatening endometrial pathology is unusual.[38] In women aged 35 or less presenting with abnormal uterine bleeding, the aetiology is most likely dysfunctional. Medical treatment and clinical follow-up without histological diagnosis is justifiable. In case of failure of medical therapy, further investigation is warranted. Ash[38] reported that if the dysfunctional uterine bleeding shows a regular pattern, the risk for organic lesion is less than 1%, and endometrial biopsy is not warranted; if the menstrual pattern is irregular, lesions are more likely (14%), indicating further endometrial investigation. An ultrasound examination to detect myomas or polyps may be the most appropriate next diagnostic step. Office endometrial sampling is useful in the diagnosis of maturation defects, endometritis, hyperplasia or malignancy.

In women over age 35, endometrial disease becomes more prevalent, and the clinician must have a higher level of suspicion in the diagnostic approach.

9.3.2.5 Subfertility Investigation

Endometrial sampling is also used in subfertility investigation, mostly for "dating" the endometrium to exclude luteal insufficiency. The endometrium serves as a bioassay to evaluate ovarian function. In case of insufficient progesterone production, the maturation of the endometrium will be hampered. However, endometrial sampling poorly predicts pregnancy outcome. Some authors suggest the superiority of serial measurement of progesterone in the second phase of the cycle.[39]

Kaminski[40] reported a 0.6% risk of sampling the implantation site at endometrial sampling in the luteal phase. Although none of the three reported cases had an evolutive gestation, the authors conclude on the relative safety of the procedure in subfertility investigation.

9.4 Conclusions

In the last decade, there has been a significant evolution in the diagnostic approach of endometrial disease from D&C under general anaesthesia towards office procedures: office endometrial sampling, office hysteroscopy and vaginal ultrasonography. Today there remains no place for the classical D&C without hysteroscopy.

Before proceeding with office sampling, ultrasound evaluation should be considered an essential step in endometrial investigation: first, to select the patient at risk of endometrial disease in whom endometrial sampling is warranted; secondly, as "quality control" of the endometrial sampling. If insufficient tissue has been sampled in a woman with a thickened endometrial lining, a lesion most probably has been missed, and further investigation is indicated.

If there is still doubt about the diagnosis after initial investigation, hysteroscopy with selective endometrial sampling is the investigation of choice.

In a setting with no ultrasound or hysteroscopy facilities, there is still a place for blind office sampling in the diagnostic work-up. The clinician must be aware of its limitation, and rely on a rigorous clinical follow-up in case of initial negative findings.

References

1. Kawada CY, An-Foraker SH (1979) Screening for endometrial carcinoma. Clin Obstet Gynecol 22:713–728
2. Van den Bosch T, Vandendael A, Wranz PA et al (1998) Cervical cytology in menopausal women at high risk for endometrial disease. Eur J Cancer Prevention 7:149–152
3. Ng ABP, Reagan JW, Hawliczek S et al (1974) Significance of endometrial cells in the detection of endometrial carcinoma and its precursors. Acta Cytol 18:356–361
4. Cherkis RC, Patten SF, Andrews TJ et al (1988) Significance of normal endometrial cells detected by cervical cytology. Obstet Gynecol 71:242–244
5. Mitchell H, Giles G, Medley G (1993) Accuracy and survival benefit of cytological prediction of endometrial carcinoma on routine cervical smears. Int J Gynecol Pathol 12:34–40
6. Zucker PK, Kasdon EJ, Feldstein ML (1985) The validity of Pap smear parameters as predictors of endometrial pathology in menopausal women. Cancer 56:2256–2263
7. Larson DM, Johnson KK, Reyes CN et al (1994) Prognostic significance of malignant cervical cytology in patients with endometrial cancer. Obstet Gynecol 84:399–403
8. Karlsson B, Granberg S, Wikland M et al (1993) Endovaginal scanning of the endometrium compared to cytology and histology in women with postmenopausal bleeding. Gynecol Oncol 50:173–178
9. Palermo VG, Blythe JG, Kaufman RH (1985) Cytologic diagnosis of endometrial adenocarcinoma using the Endo-Pap sampler. Obstet Gynecol 65:271–275
10. Van den Bosch T, Vandendael A, Wranz PAB (1996). Endopap^R versus Pipelle^R sampling in the diagnosis of postmenopausal endometrial disease. Eur J Obstet Gynecol 64:91–94
11. Stock RJ, Kanbour A (1975) Prehysterectomy curettage. Obstet Gynecol 45:537–541
12. Word B, Gravlee LC, Wideman GL (1958) The fallacy of simple curettage. Obstet Gynecol 12:642–648
13. Stovall TG, Solomon SK, Ling FW (1989) Endometrial sampling prior to hysterectomy. Obstet Gynecol 73:405–409.
14. Van den Bosch T, Cornelis A (1998) Endometrial malignancy missed by office sampling. Aust NZ J Obstet Gynaecol 38:1–2
15. Grimes DA (1982) Diagnostic dilatation and curettage: a reappraisal. Am J Obstet Gynecol 142:1–6
16. Eddowes HA, Codling BW (1990) Pipelle: a more acceptable technique for outpatient endometrial biopsy. Br J Obstet Gynaecol 97:961–962
17. Silver MM, Miles P, Rosa C (1991) Comparison of Novak and Pipelle endometrial biopsy instruments. Obstet Gynecol 78:828–830
18. Townsend DE, Fields G, McCausland A et al (1993) Diagnostic and operative hysteroscopy in the management of persistent postmenopausal bleeding. Obstet Gynecol 82:419–421
19. Van den Bosch T, Vandendael A, Van Schoubroeck D et al (1995) Combining vaginal ultrasonography and office endometrial sampling in the diagnosis of endometrial disease in postmenopausal women. Obstet Gynecol 85:349–352
20. Gimpelson RJ, Rappold HO (1988) A comparative study between panoramic hysteroscopy with directed biopsies and dilatation and curettage. Am J Obstet Gynecol 158:489–492
21. Loffer FD (1989) Hysteroscopy with selective endometrial sampling compared with D&C for abnormal uterine bleeding: the value of a negative hysteroscopic view. Obstet Gynecol 73:16–20
22. Downes E, Al-Azzawi F (1993) The predictive value of outpatient hysteroscopy in a menopause clinic. Br J Obstet Gynaecol 100:1148–1149
23. Pungetti D, Dimicco R, Mattucci M et al (1990) A comparative study between panoramic hysteroscopy and endometrial biopsy. Analysis of 150 cases. Acta Eur Fertil 21:201–203
24. Marty R, Amouroux J, Haouet S et al (1990) The reliability of endometrial biopsy performed during hysteroscopy. Int J Gynecol Obstet 34:151–155
25. Romano S, Shimoni Y, Muralee D et al (1992) Retrograde seeding of endometrial carcinoma during hysteroscopy. Case report. Gynecol Oncol 44:116–118
26. Mencaglia L (1995) Hysteroscopy and adenocarcinoma. Obstet Gynecol Clin N Am 22:573–579
27. Macia M, Novo A, Ces J et al (1993) Progesterone challenge test for the assessment of endometrial pathology in asymptomatic menopausal women. Int J Gynecol Obstet 40:145–149
28. Osmers RGW, Kuhn W (1994) Endometrial cancer screening. Curr Opin Obstet Gynecol 6:75–79

29. Goldstein SR (1996) The routine use of ultrasound in the gynecological visit. Ultrasound Obstet Gynecol 8:369–370

30. Feldman S, Berkowitz RS, Tosteson ANA (1993) Cost-effectiveness of strategies to evaluate postmenopausal bleeding. Obstet Gynecol 81:968–975

31. Padwick ML, Pryse-Davies J, Whitehead MI (1986) A simple method for determining the optimal dosage of progestin in postmenopausal women receiving estrogens. N Eng J Med 315:930–934

32. Sturdee DW, Barlow DH, Ulrich LG et al (1994) Is the timing of withdrawal bleeding a guide to endometrial safety during sequential oestrogen-progestagen replacement therapy? Lancet 344:979–982

33. Nagele F, O'Connor H, Baskett TF et al (1996) Hysteroscopy in women with abnormal uterine bleeding on hormone replacement therapy: a comparison with postmenopausal bleeding. Fertil Steril 65:1145–1150

34. van Leeuwen FE, Benraadt J, Coebergh JWW et al (1994) Risk of endometrial cancer after tamoxifen treatment of breast cancer. Lancet 343:448–452

35. Fornander T, Cerdermark B, Mattsson A et al (1989) Adjuvant tamoxifen in early breast cancer: occurrence of new primary cancers. Lancet i:117–119

36. Tepper R, Beyth Y, Altaras MM et al (1997) Value of sonohysterography in asymptomatic postmenopausal tamoxifen-treated patients. Gynecol Oncol 64:386–391

37. Timmerman D (1997) Ultrasonography in the assessment of ovarian and tamoxifen-associated endometrial pathology. Acta Biomedica Lovaniensia 163, Leuven University Press

38. Ash SJ, Farrell SA, Flowerdew G (1996) Endometrial biopsy in DUB. J Reprod Med 41:892–896

39. Jordan J, Craig K, Clifton DK et al (1994) Luteal phase defect: the sensitivity and specificity of diagnostic methods in common clinical use. Fertil Steril 62:54–62

40. Kaminski PF, Lyon DS (1990) Implications of sampling the implantation site in the endometrial biopsy for infertility. J Reprod Med 35:208–210

Chapter 10

Monitoring Hormone Replacement Therapy

Enrico Ferrazzi, Umberto Omodei, Cristina Ruggeri and Giuseppe Perugino

10.1 Introduction

Transvaginal ultrasonography (TVS) provides a valuable tool for the diagnosis of a wide range of gynaecological disorders, including those of the endometrium and the myometrium.[1] The ability of TVS to show changes of endometrial thickness in abnormal endometrium has been well established. The Nordic trial[2] and the Italian multicentre trial[3] provided independent evidence that in patients with postmenopausal bleeding without hormone replacement therapy (HRT) – 787 and 930 patients, respectively – an endometrial thickness $\leq$ 4 mm safely excludes endometrial cancer as a possible cause of bleeding and accurately predicts atrophy in more than 80% of cases. According to Osmers,[4] endometrial lesions and thickenings that turned out to be asymptomatic cancers were of a lower stage than cancers diagnosed in symptomatic postmenopausal women. The effects of drugs known to cause proliferative changes of the endometrium, such as tamoxifen, can be monitored by TVS.[5] The use of intracavity instillation of saline allows accurate diagnosis of polyps already suspected by simple transvaginal scanning.[6] There is therefore considerable potential for the use of TVS examination of the endometrium in patients taking HRT.

Clinical practice is far from taking advantage of this diagnostic tool. For many years, HRT monitoring has been influenced by the study of Padwick et al,[7] which speculated that bleeding on or after day 11 of prostestogen administration could be taken as reassurance of effective endometrial protection. However, Padwick's study recruited only a small number of women, among whom no cases of endometrial cancer were observed. This "rule of thumb" method has been scientifically questioned since the early 1980s.[8] Recently, however, a large multicentre study carried out by the United Kingdom

Collaborative Group[9] provided unquestionable evidence that there is no correlation between postmenopausal bleeding and endometrial lesions. In fact, this study showed that 37 out of 65 cases of complex hyperplasia and four out of eight cases of atypia occurred in women who had regular bleeding after 11 days of progesterone administration. Because the bleeding pattern can no longer be considered a predictor of abnormal histology in postmenopausal women on HRT, there is a need to develop clear guidelines based on objective criteria to manage these women clinically. Moreover, although there is a lower risk of endometrial cancer associated with the use of a combined oestrogen-prostestogen regimen than with unopposed oestrogens, results from Beresford et al[10] do not support the optimistic view of an overall lower risk of endometrial cancer being associated with combined therapy compared with no therapy. The overall relative risk, estimated on the basis of a meta-analysis of patients on oestrogen plus progesterone for at least 10 days, was 0.8 (95% confidence interval 0.6–1.2).[11] Beresford's data hold that this relative risk can increase up to 1.9.

10.2 Challenging the Endometrial Changes of HRT with TVS

This research and clinical background, added to the increasing number of women on HRT in western countries, has led to many research and clinical protocols to evaluate the possible role of TVS in monitoring the possible unwanted effects of this preventive therapy. Until recently, however, only a few studies had been published addressing the issue of ultrasonographic evaluation of the endometrium in women receiving HRT.[12–17]

Changes in the thickness and echogenicity of the endometrium in postmenopausal women on HRT

67

have been reported consistently. Lin and colleagues[12] observed that continuous combined oestrogen and progestogen was associated with endometria less than 8 mm in 85% of cases, whereas half of those on unopposed oestrogens showed endometria thicker than 8 mm. Cyclic progestogens and oestrogens produce an endometrium of varying thickness, which increases to 8 mm, mimicking the natural cyclic variation. The authors tentatively concluded that postmenopausal women receiving HRT who are found to have an endometrium ≥ 8 mm should undergo further investigation in the form of endometrial biopsy. Similar changes were observed by Bonilla-Musoles.[15] These studies observed that sequential combined therapy is associated with a thicker endometrium, and that unopposed oestrogen therapy is more likely to cause a thicker endometrium, hiding hyperplastic changes. In these studies, no attention was paid to the phase of the cycle in which sonography should be used to monitor hormonally induced endometrial changes.

This biological bias was addressed by Deborah Levine in 1995. Women on sequential therapy, examined at random during the cycle, showed the largest variation of endometrial thickness. The greatest mean thickness in this group of 40 women was 8.3 ± 3.9 mm and the mean change during the cycle was 4 mm, ranging from 0 to 13 mm. The expected effect of progestogen was measured by ultrasound imaging of the endometrium. In 33 women on continuous combined hormonal replacement, Dören[14] found that the endometrial thickness was 2.8 ± 1.8 mm, compared with 4.2 ± 5.6 in 22 control women who received no hormones.

The action of progestogen is both physical – shedding of endometrial tissue as a consequence of withdrawal – and metabolic. Progesterone is responsible for a reduction in DNA synthesis, nuclear oestrogen receptor content, and changes in intracellular protein production. The duration of progestogen action is critical and 10 days are necessary, although the first two effects described are achieved from the sixth day. We believe that results of studies using all possible HRT treatments and different timings of sonographic scanning add to the confusion in a field in which TVS is regarded suspiciously. Under these "random" conditions, as reported by Holbert,[18] the endometrial thickness ranges from 1 to 14 mm in patients with combined HRT and from 1 to 15 mm in patients with sequential HRT.

The role of oestrogen and progestogen and the timing of the sonographic examination were eventually addressed by Ylöstalo et al,[17] who followed 54 postmenopausal women for 1 year from the start of HRT. An endometrial sample was taken prior to starting therapy and again 1 year later. All women received a cyclical progestogen (10 mg daily) for 12 days during each calendar month. The mean

endometrial thickness prior to starting HRT was 2.8 ± 1.1 mm; 1 year later, during the progestogen phase of the cycle, it was 4.2 ± 1.7 mm; and 2–4 days after the start of withdrawal bleeding it was 3.1 ± 1.5 mm. Transvaginal sonography accurately identifies the overall trophic effect of HRT on the endometrium and the role of progestogen.

10.3 Possible Protocol for HRT Monitoring: Multicentre Study

The primary aim of the study designed in our centres was to define a range of endometrial thickness in both symptomatic and asymptomatic women on HRT at increased risk for endometrial abnormalities. Postmenopausal patients were recruited from outpatient menopause clinics, the only selection criteria being the duration of postmenopausal amenorrhoea (> 9 months) and the duration of HRT (> 6 months). Women were excluded if they had had an endometrial biopsy within 8 weeks or were bleeding at the time of examination. In women on sequential oestrogen plus progestogen therapy, great attention was paid to the timing of TVS examination, which was always performed immediately after the withdrawal bleeding between the fifth and tenth day from the last progestogen tablet. This schedule allowed us to measure the endometrium when, under normal conditions, it is supposed to be at its minimal thickness. The maximum endometrial thickness was measured in a longitudinal plane, from one endometrial–myometrial interface to another. This TVS measurement excludes intracavity fluid, but includes any other tissue. A hysteroscopy with endometrial biopsy was performed when the endometrial thickness was > 4 mm, always within 5 days from TVS examination. Because of the hormonal-induced "physiological" endometrial thickening, this 4 mm threshold was even more important for postmenopausal women receiving hormonal supplementation. The choice of hysteroscopy as the "gold standard" for assessment of endometrial pathology was suggested by several studies investigating the specificity and sensitivity of hysteroscopy in comparison with other techniques.[19] For many years, the most widely used technique for obtaining endometrial samples was dilatation and curettage. However, this procedure proved to have a false-negative rate between 2 and 6% for diagnosing endometrial cancer and hyperplasia.[20–24]

One hundred and ninety women gave their informed consent to enter the study. Table 10.1 summarises the ages of the women at the time of study and at the start of the menopause. Ultrasonographic uterine mean longitudinal diameter ($\pm$ SD)

Table 10.1. Age at study and age at menopause (n = 190)

	Age (years)	Age at menopause (years)
Mode	56	50
25	53	47
75	59	52

Table 10.2. Distribution of patients according to HRT regimen

HRT regimen	No. of patients	%
Group 1 (sequential HRT)	138	72.5
1a Cyclic sequential (oral)	17	8.9
1a Cyclic sequential (transdermal)	57	30.0
1b Continuous sequential (oral)	32	16.8
1b Continuous sequential (transdermal)	32	16.8
Group 2 (combined HRT)	52	27.5
2a Continuous combined (oral)	31	16.3
2a Continuous combined (transdermal)	11	5.8
2b Cyclic combined (oral)	10	5.2
Total	190	100

was 70 ± 14 mm. Ninety-seven fibroids (41%) were observed in this series.

Women were enrolled in one of two groups according to the HRT regimen they were following: women in group 1a received either 0.625 mg conjugated oestrogens for 21/25 days and 5/10 mg medroxyprogestogen acetate (MPA) for 12 days, or transdermal 17β-oestradiol patches (0.05 mg/day for 21 days/cycle) and 10 mg MPA for 12 days/cycle. Women in group 1b received continuously either oral oestrogens (0.625 mg conjugated oestrogens daily) or transdermal oestrogens (0.05 mg/day), plus 5/10 mg MPA for 12 days/cycle.

Group 2a included patients on a continuous combined regimen, either oral (0.625 mg conjugated oestrogens daily) or transdermal (0.05 mg daily) oestrogens. All were receiving 2.5–5 mg MPA daily. Group 2b included women following a cyclic combined regimen with 0.625 mg conjugated oestrogens and 5 mg MPA administered daily.

One hundred and thirty-eight women were receiving oestrogen plus progestogen in a sequential combined regimen and 52 women were receiving the two drugs in a continuous combined regimen (Table 10.2).

The mean endometrial thickness in the whole series was 3.4 mm (range: 0.7–9.2 mm). Table 10.3 shows the results of the ultrasonographic measurements in the two groups. In women on a sequential combined regimen (group 1) the mean endometrial thickness was calculated from measurements obtained between the fifth and tenth days after the progestogen phase. The difference in endometrial growth between the groups was not significant and no differences were observed according to the method of oestrogen administration. Endometrial thickness did not increase with the duration of use of HRT.

Twenty-eight patients (9.6%) had an endometrial thickness > 4 mm; all underwent hysteroscopy with endometrial biopsy. Histological examination revealed endometrial atrophy in 39%, endometrial polyps in 25%, simple hyperplasia in 11% and proliferative/secretive endometrium in 25%. When we compared the histological results with the clinical data of these patients, we found that the incidence of endometrial abnormalities was 22% among women with unscheduled bleeding and 42% in asymptomatic women. If we had taken the bleeding pattern as a guide for selection of patients requiring endometrial sampling, we would have missed 80% of all endometrial pathologies. Moreover, all the cases of endometrial hyperplasia were observed in asymptomatic patients. The regular or irregular bleeding in patients on sequential HRT in this series was not correlated with the histology of the endometrium, as expected from the larger meta-analysis by Grady.[11]

10.4 Conclusions

The findings of this series support the clinical feasibility of our monitoring protocol: patients taking sequential combined HRT should be examined from the fifth to the tenth day after the progestogen phase. Consideration of patients with an endometrium ≥ 5 mm for an invasive diagnostic procedure should be independent of their bleeding pattern. This simple protocol can be used when the timing of an ultrasound scan is carefully chosen. Random office examinations are a predictable waste of time and money, and invasive procedures or time-consuming counselling and re-scanning can be avoided. This safe cut-off can be adopted in the evaluation of the endometrium without significantly increasing the number of invasive procedures.

The invasive diagnostic procedures deserve further discussion. Hysteroscopy is the gold standard for any

Table 10.3. Endometrial thickness according to HRT regimen (sequential combined versus continuous combined)

	No. of cases	Endometrial thickness (mm, mean)	Standard deviation	Range	p <
Sequential combined	138	3.6	1.5	0.7–9.2	n.s.
Continuous combined	52	3.0	1.8	0.7–6.0	n.s.

scientific study on monitoring HRT. However, we believe that the results achievable by hydrosonography suggest that this minimally minor invasive office procedure could be undertaken in women in whom the endometrium is thicker than 5 mm. In cases in which the increased thickness is caused by homogeneous thickening, a simple cytological examination can be performed; in cases in which the lesion is focal or intracavitary, a diagnostic or operative hysteroscopy should be performed.

The time interval between the beginning of HRT and sonographic scanning is still under investigation. In our study, TVS was performed after at least 6 months of HRT. According to our experience, patients could be screened ultrasonographically 1 year before they start taking HRT. If we speculate further, we could assume that progestogen-induced endometrial bleed or endometrial biopsy in high risk cases would allow us to use HRT more safely. Transvaginal ultrasonography can be used to detect irregular or thickened endometria; medical or minimally invasive surgical therapy could remove focal areas of abnormally stimulated endometrium in the last years before menopause. In our view a history of regular or irregular bleeding and bimanual pelvic examination are of little value in the management of patients taking HRT.

References

1. Bourne T (1995) Evaluating the endometrium of postmenopausal women with transvaginal sonography. Ultrasound Obstet Gynecol 6:75–80
2. Karlsson B, Granberg S, Wickland M et al (1995) Transvaginal ultrasonography of the endometrium in women with postmenopausal bleeding – a Nordic trial. Am J Obstet Gynecol 172:1488–1494
3. Ferrazzi E, Torri V, Trio D et al (1996) Sonographic endometrial thickness: a useful test to predict atrophy in patients with postmenopausal bleeding: an Italian multicenter study. Ultrasound Obstet Gynecol 7:315–321
4. Osmers RGW, Osmers M, Khun W (1995) Prognostic value of transvaginal sonography in asymptomatic endometrial cancers. Ultrasound Obstet Gynecol 6:103–107
5. Achiron R, Lipitz S, Silvan E et al (1995) Changes mimicking endometrial neoplasia in postmenopausal tamoxifen treated women with breast cancer: a transvaginal Doppler study. Ultrasound Obstet Gynecol 6:116–120
6. Bourne TH, Lawton F, Leather A et al (1994) Use of intracavitary saline instillation and transvaginal ultrsonography to detect tamoxifen-associated polyps. Utrasound Obstet Gynecol 4:73–75
7. Padwick ML, Pryse-Davies J, Whitehead MI (1986) A simple method for determining the optimal dosage of progestin in postmenopausal women receiving estrogens. N Engl J Med 315:930–934
8. Paterson MEL, Wade EL, Sturdee DW et al (1980) Endometrial disease after treatment with estrogens and progestogens in the climacteric. Br Med J 1:822–829
9. Sturdee DW, Barlow DH, Ulrich LG et al (1994) Is the timing of withdrawal bleeding a guide to endometrial safety during sequential oestrogen-prostestogen replacement therapy? Lancet 343:979–982
10. Beresford SAA, Weiss NS, Voigt LF et al (1997) Risk of endometrial cancer in relation to use of oestrogen combined with cyclic progestagen in postmenopausal women. Lancet 349: 458–462
11. Grady D, Gebretsadik T, Ernster V et al (1995) Hormone replacement therapy and endometrial cancer risk: a metaanalysis. Obstet Gynecol 85:304–313
12. Lin MC, Gosink BB, Wolf SI et al (1991) Endometrial thickness after menopause: effect of hormone replacement. Radiology 180:427–432
13. Levine D, Gosink BB, Johnson LA (1995) Change in endometrial thickness in postmenopausal women undergoing hormonal replacement therapy. Radiology 197:603–608
14. Dören M, Süselbeck B, Schneider HPG et al (1997) Uterine perfusion and endometrial thickness in postmenopausal women on long-term continuous combined estrogen and progestogen replacement. Ultrasound Obstet Gynecol 9:113–119
15. Bonilla-Musoles F, Ballester MJ, Martì MC et al (1995) Transvaginal color Doppler assessment of endometrial status in normal postmenopausal women: the effect of hormone replacement therapy. J Ultrasound Med 14:503–507
16. Varner RE, Sparks JM, Cameron CD et al (1991) Transvaginal sonography of the endometrium in postmenopausal women. Obstet Gynecol 78:195
17. Ylöstalo P, Granberg S, Bäckström AC et al (1996) Uterine findings by transvaginal sonography during percutaneous estrogen treatment in postmenopausal women. Maturitas 23:313–317
18. Holbert TR (1997) Transvaginal ultrasonographic measurement of endometrial thickness in postmenopausal women receiving estrogen replacement therapy. Am J Obstet Gynecol 176:1334–1339
19. Gimpelson RJ, Rappold HO (1988) A comparative study between panoramic hysteroscopy with directed biopsies and dilatation and curettage. Am J Obstet Gynecol 158:489–492
20. Stock R, Kanbour A (1975) Prehysterectomy curettage. Obstet Gynecol 45:537–541
21. Stoval T, Solomon S, Ling F (1989) Endometrial sampling prior to hysterectomy. Obstet Gynecol 73:405–409
22. Mencaglia L, Valle RF, Perino A et al (1990) Endometrial cancer and its precursors: early detection and treatment. Int J Gynecol Obstet 31:107–116
23. Holst J, Koskela O, von Schoultz B (1983) Endometrial findings following curettage in 2018 women according to age and indications. Ann Chir Gynaecol 72:274–277
24. Lidor A, Ismajovich B, Confino E et al (1986) Histopathological findings in 226 women with postmenopausal bleeding. Acta Obstet Gynecol Scand 65:41–42

Chapter 11

Endometrial Surveillance of Tamoxifen Patients

Patrick Neven

11.1 Introduction

Tamoxifen is the most important anti-breast cancer drug in clinical use and has the potential to be used as a chemopreventive breast cancer agent. Although many women retain an atrophic endometrial layer, tamoxifen intake can lead to extensive benign cystic atrophia of the human endometrium, to endometrial hyperplasia and endometrial polyp formation. Based on a critical review of the literature, it is now clear that tamoxifen increases the risk of endometrial cancer in postmenopausal women.

Screening breast cancer patients on tamoxifen for endometrial abnormalities is feasible and uterine morbidity related to tamoxifen intake is preventable. Although screening may increase drug compliance, it may not be cost-beneficial. Uterine safety, however, becomes important when only a small benefit of the treatment is to be expected, as in healthy women using tamoxifen for breast cancer prevention – an indication recently approved by the Food and Drug Administration (FDA).

The aim of this chapter is to discuss methods and guidelines for detecting endometrial side-effects of tamoxifen and to provide the clinician with a current opinion on timing and frequency of screening patients taking tamoxifen for the development of endometrial cancer.

Those who advocate screening should start with pretreatment uterine assessment using transvaginal ultrasonography (TVS) or outpatient hysteroscopy. Symptom-free women with a normal pretreatment uterine cavity can be screened annually with TVS 2–3 years after the start of tamoxifen. Hysteroscopy or hydrosonography will be required if there is endometrial thickening; in contrast a thin regular endometrium as measured by TVS has a high negative predictive value and is reassuring.

Newer compounds, such as raloxifene, have a similar selective oestrogen receptor modulator (SERM) profile to tamoxifen, but have a neutral effect on the uterus. This has recently been proven by 5 years of endometrial follow-up data, and longer endometrial safety data will hopefully confirm these early findings. Potential benefits of the newer SERMs are being investigated in ongoing studies.

11.2 The Clinical Importance of Tamoxifen

Breast cancer is the leading cause of cancer deaths among women. It is clear that most breast cancers depend on oestrogens for growth and progression. Results from epidemiological studies have clearly indicated that female hormones are associated with breast cancer.

Consequently, therapies designed to reduce serum oestrogen levels or to block the effects of oestrogens on cancer cells are used to improve disease-free survival of breast cancer patients. Beatson in 1896 observed that bilateral oophorectomy could cause regression of advanced breast cancer in premenopausal women.[1] Nowadays, endocrine therapies are the major treatment modality for the management of breast cancer. The first non-steroidal oestrogen, stilboestrol, was developed in 1938; at high doses, it inhibited breast tumour growth. Successive chemical modifications of the weakly oestrogenic stilbene nucleus led to the development of a class of less toxic molecules with anti-oestrogenic anti-breast cancer properties, called the triphenylethylenes.[2] One of these, tamoxifen, was synthesised in 1966,[3] at about the same time as Toft and Gorski[4] discovered the oestrogen receptor, a possible biochemical marker for the hormone-dependency of breast tumours.

Tamoxifen inhibits oestrogen-induced cell growth predominantly by competitive blockade of the oestrogen receptor. In 1986, tamoxifen was approved for adjuvant treatment in early-stage disease because of its efficacy in preventing the

71

progression of metastatic disease from advanced breast cancer and its general lack of toxicity. It also prevents occult metastatic disease from early breast cancer and is now established as the front-line endocrine treatment for breast cancer in more than 110 countries; there are more than 10 million women-years of experience. The worldwide overview on tamoxifen as an adjuvant for breast cancer therapy from the Early Breast Cancer Trialists' Collaborative Group, published in 1998[5] and updated in September 2000, showed that tamoxifen treatment in postmenopausal women reduced mortality by almost 25% and recurrence of breast cancer by 50%. Because of its very low toxicity, the general recommendation is to prescribe 20 mg daily for 5 years. Whether longer would be better is the subject of ongoing trials such as the ATLAS and aTTom studies.

Tamoxifen has tissue-specific oestrogenic or anti-oestrogenic properties. Whereas the molecule is an anti-oestrogen in the breast, it mainly behaves as an oestrogen in other tissues. One hypothesis suggests that tamoxifen may have stronger oestrogen agonist properties in the liver, uterus and bone because these tissues have proteins that augment transcription via a binding region on the oestrogen receptor. This capability of tamoxifen to maintain bone mineral density in postmenopausal women[6] and to reduce serum cholesterol levels and in particular low-density lipoproteins, with a decreased incidence of myocardial infarction,[7] has stimulated current trials exploring the use of tamoxifen as a prophylactic agent in healthy women at high risk of developing breast cancer. Thousands of women in the USA, Europe and Australia are participating in such trials. In a placebo-controlled trial from the USA (National Surgical Adjuvant Breast and Bowel Project-P1, NSABP-P1), with an average follow-up of 3.6 years, tamoxifen reduced oestrogen receptor-positive breast cancer risk in all age groups by 45%; this effect was increased with age (35% < 49 years versus 53% > 60 years) and with a longer duration of tamoxifen treatment.[8] Recently, the FDA approved tamoxifen for breast cancer prevention for those at risk.

In Europe, this is not yet the case because interim results from Italian and British chemoprevention trials showed no evidence of a beneficial effect. There are several possible explanations for this. The NSABP-P1 trial was conducted on 13 388 women, whereas both the British (2471) and Italian (5408) studies were smaller.[9,10] The degree of risk and age were different in all these studies. In the American trial, the placebo group had an average annual incidence of 6.7/1000, whereas this was only 2.5/1000 in the Italian group. Results from the International Breast Cancer Intervention Study, currently in the process of data managing, will soon provide additional evidence concerning the value of tamoxifen as a breast cancer chemopreventive agent.

In the future, millions of women, even those with a low probability of breast cancer, may be taking tamoxifen for an indefinite period.

11.3 Tamoxifen-induced Endometrial Changes

Up to 30% of women taking tamoxifen have some degree of gynaecological symptoms: vaginal dryness and discharge are most often quoted. Increasing attention has been paid to the relationship between tamoxifen and endometrial changes.

Asymptomatic postmenopausal breast cancer patients and those who have vaginal bleeding on tamoxifen 20 mg daily are more likely to have benign endometrial and endocervical polyps and a hyperplastic endometrial layer than a matched control group with postmenopausal vaginal bleeding but no breast cancer, not taking tamoxifen.[11] Case reports of endometrial cancer with tamoxifen treatment are similar. Although there is evidence that some endometrial cancers reported in patients on tamoxifen had been present before the women started taking the drug, or were related to other risk factors, such as obesity and past oestrogen replacement therapy,[12,13] the few well-designed studies adequately controlling for background risks clearly show a carcinogenic effect of tamoxifen on the human endometrium. Three randomised clinical trials indicated that women treated with tamoxifen for breast cancer are at increased risk for developing endometrial cancer.[14-16] These three trials were large studies in which the subjects were restricted to postmenopausal women with follow-up times of at least 4.5 years. In our literature review, using all reported endometrial cancers from placebo-controlled trials with tamoxifen, we found a twofold increase in the incidence rate of endometrial carcinoma risk in tamoxifen-treated patients (0.79% versus 0.37%).[17] Therefore, tamoxifen was classified by the International Agency for Research on Cancer as a human endometrial carcinogen.[18] Although most clinicians agree that long-term tamoxifen users have an increased risk of endometrial cancer, this risk should not be overestimated and does not alter the risk-benefit ratio for breast cancer patients on tamoxifen.

The endometrial effect of tamoxifen does not seem to differ in healthy postmenopausal women. Healthy postmenopausal women assigned to receive either tamoxifen or placebo, with a mean follow-up time of 22 months, had histological evidence of abnormal endometrium (39% in the tamoxifen group versus 10% in the control group), although all changes were benign.[19] In a close to normal postmenopausal population participating in a placebo-controlled breast cancer chemoprevention trial with tamoxifen (the NSABP-P1 study), tamoxifen intake led to a 2.5-fold excess risk of endometrial carcinoma.[8] Other studies have recently highlighted the endometrial effect of tamoxifen, even for high-grade and aggressive endometrial cancers.[20-25] The increased risk of endometrial cancer in this group of women on tamoxifen has caused concern over the safety of long-term tamoxifen treatment. This potential side-effect is particularly important if large groups of healthy women are exposed to anti-oestrogens for the prevention of breast cancer and protection against osteoporosis and cardiovascular disease.

11.4 Ultrasonographic and Hysteroscopic Images

The best way to evaluate the effect of tamoxifen on the endometrium is to evaluate the uterine cavity prior to tamoxifen intake and at regular intervals thereafter. This method also allows exclusion of pretreatment endometrial abnormalities. In a prospective hysteroscopic follow-up study, we found that nine out of 16 breast cancer patients on tamoxifen underwent some endometrial changes.[26] Most were benign changes such as pseudo- and real polyps and endometrial hyperplasia. There was one case of a newly developed endometrial cancer. Other ultrasonographic follow-up studies have reported an irregularly thickened endometrium with a typical Gruyère cheese appearance in up to 75% of tamoxifen users (Figure 11.1).

Some sonographic and hysteroscopic images are pathognomonic for tamoxifen-induced endometrial lesions such as polyps. In cases with a thickened endometrium on TVS, only hysteroscopy and hydrosonography are able to differentiate between two of the typical endometrial effects of tamoxifen, namely pseudopolypoid glandulocystic endometrium (Figure 11.2) and glandulocystic polyps (Figure 11.3).

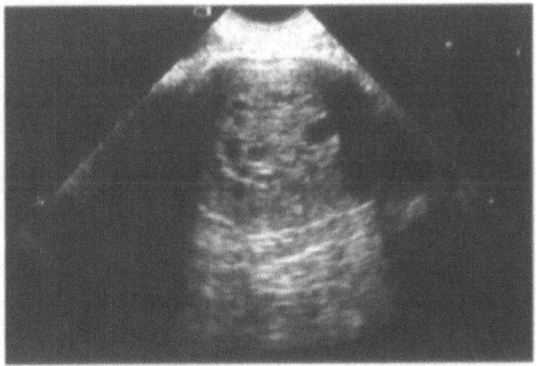

Figure 11.1 An irregularly thickened endometrium with a typical Gruyère cheese appearance.

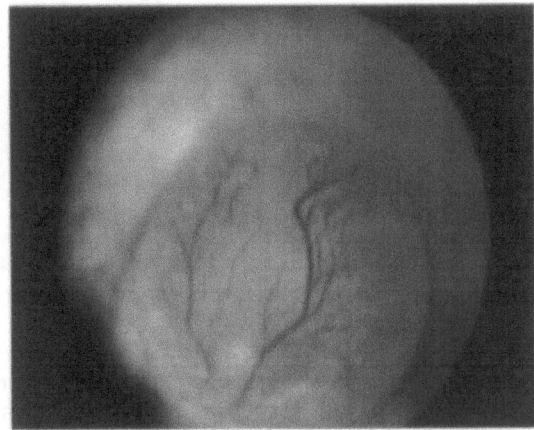

Figure 11.2 Hysteroscopic image of pseudopolypoid glandulocystic endometrium.

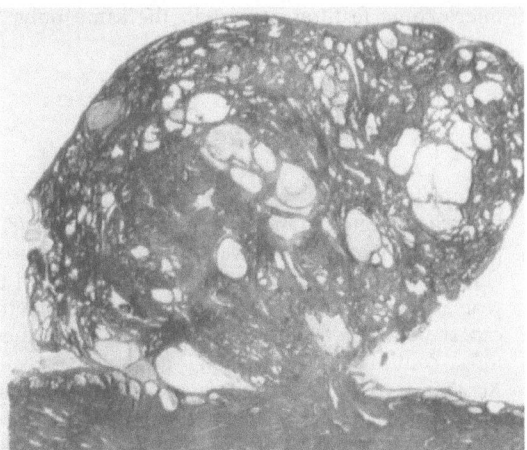

Figure 11.3 Histopathological image of a glandulocystic polyp.

In pseudopolypoid glandulocystic endometrium, hysteroscopy shows a smooth white but hypervascularised endometrial layer with many scattered protuberances. When such a protuberance is opened, there is a thin atrophic endometrium overlying a cystic dilated gland, which is an oedematous stroma. On hydrosonography (Figure 11.4), there is an empty cavity, with the Gruyère cheese appearance in the subepithelial layer of the endometrium. Histologically, this endometrium typically shows periglandular stromal condensation, epithelial metaplasias and proliferative activity, sometimes with varying degrees of cytological atypia.

On hydrosonography, the glandulocystic structure of polyps is free floating and surrounded with saline (Figure 11.5); on hysteroscopy, the endometrium surrounding the polyp is mostly not thin and regular. The majority of endometrial polyps occur on a background of simple endometrial hyperplasia; however, the neighbouring endometrium may be atrophic. Microscopically, the polyps are charac-

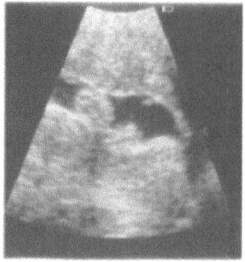 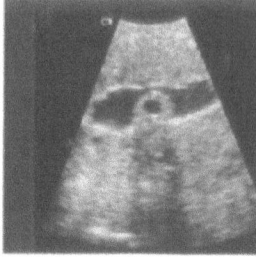

Figure 11.4 Hydrosonographic of pseudopolypoid glandulocystic endometrium.

terised by patchy periglandular condensation of stroma, proliferative activity in epithelial and stromal cells and an admixture of epithelial metaplasias, including squamoid and mucinous metaplasias. It is highly unlikely that these three microscopic features coexist in the same polyp in women not using tamoxifen.

11.5 Is screening worthwhile?

Endometrial polyps and "hyperplastic" lesions in tamoxifen-treated women, traditionally thought to be premalignant, rarely evolve into invasive cancers. Only an extra two to three asymptomatic women per year and per 1000 women will develop endometrial cancer because of tamoxifen. Many clinicians therefore continue to question general screening. According to some, screening may do more harm than good in terms of unnecessary interventions, subsequent complications, increased cost and no advantage to the patient. This notion is supported by: (1) the huge discrepancy between the high rates of asymptomatic endometrial lesions and the fairly low frequency of symptomatic endometrial cancers; and (2) the fact that although aggressive screening would most probably lead to early diagnosis, there is, to date, no evidence that this would confer a survival advantage. Endometrial cancer is a slowly progressing

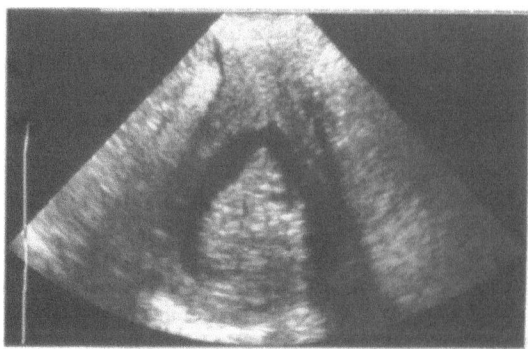

Figure 11.5 Hydrosonographic image of a glandulocystic polyp.

malignancy with high 5-year survival rates, in contrast to breast cancer relapse, which results in a significant increase in morbidity and death. Others believe that the value of routine screening should be determined by prospective studies.

From a histopathological and biological behaviour point of view, endometrial cancers in tamoxifen users do not appear to be different from those developing in women not using tamoxifen,[16] but not all agree on this.[23-25] There is, however, enough evidence that the main purpose of a screening programme for endometrial cancer in tamoxifen users – lowering mortality related to endometrial cancer – is unlikely to be fulfilled.[27]

In some cases, however, there is a need to consider prevention rather than cure. Those using tamoxifen as a chemopreventive drug will request it because the potential endometrial cancer risk with long-term use is very low. Offering endometrial surveillance in this group will improve compliance and is the only way forward. The new generation of anti-oestrogens, the SERMs, have less proliferative or have anti-oestrogenic effects on the human endometrium. Their protective effect against myocardial infarction, bone fractures and breast cancer is still under investigation, but preliminary results are as promising as those for tamoxifen. In a recently presented placebo-controlled trial, involving healthy postmenopausal women (mean age 66.5 years) at increased risk for osteoporosis (Multiple Outcomes of Raloxifene Evaluation trial), raloxifene markedly reduced bone fracture risk and the risk of newly diagnosed mainly oestrogen-receptor-positive breast cancer; 74% of the women were followed-up for an average of 33 months. Raloxifene decreased the incidence of endometrial cancer by more than half (relative risk, $RR = 0.38$).[28]

11.6 Monitoring Techniques

Transvaginal ultrasonography and hysteroscopy have been advocated as the most applicable techniques to screen asymptomatic women on tamoxifen. We notify the patient and her general practitioner about the "polypogenic" effect of tamoxifen on the endometrium, which in some cases may lead to abnormal vaginal bleeding. In experienced hands, hydrosonography is equally valuable, with a similar detection rate for intrauterine lesions.[29]

In asymptomatic women, a "wait and see" policy is an option, but a diagnosis is required in cases of abnormal vaginal bleeding. Direct visualisation of the uterine cavity using a hysteroscope with guided endometrial biopsies is the only method to obtain such a diagnosis. Polyps and localised endometrial changes are easily missed with blind intrauterine procedures. Small patches of atypical hyperplasia within the polyp and polyp-cancers can be diagnosed only once the polyp has been removed and examined histologically.

In asymptomatic women on tamoxifen, TVS is of limited value as a tool for endometrial assessment and can be misleading. However, it is a valuable method for the visualisation of all uterine layers (e.g. fibroids) and the ovaries; ovarian pathology is not uncommon in breast cancer patients, and tamoxifen-induced ovarian cysts have been reported. In tamoxifen users, as in those using hormone replacement therapy,[30] TVS has an excellent negative predictive value. Pathology is unlikely if there is a very thin (< 5 mm) endometrial line in an asymptomatic postmenopausal women. Small, probably clinically irrelevant pathology will be missed, but overall, ultrasound is a sensitive test. Unfortunately, tamoxifen thickens the endometrium abnormally in up to 75% of asymptomatic women without any pathological significance.[31] Tamoxifen-induced endometrial changes result in a ultrasonographically unique picture of an irregularly echogenic endometrium that is attributed to cystic glandular dilatation, stromal oedema and oedema and hyperplasia of the adjacent myometrium.[32] Therefore, the positive predictive value of TVS is low. In these cases, the only way to obtain a correct diagnosis is to do additional tests, such as hydrosonography, endometrial blood flow studies and hysteroscopy.

Hydrosonography was first described by Randolph et al in 1986, when they injected saline into the uterine cavity through a thin flexible cervical catheter and observed the intrauterine contours using an abdominal ultrasound probe.[33] Using a transvaginal probe, this technique accurately delineates the uterine cavity, providing a contrast medium as well as a distending agent, and facilitating a more precise measurement of endometrial thickness. This technique will easily detect free-floating polyps and localised endometrial thickening,[34] but in comparison with hysteroscopy, the interpretation of a shadow remains less accurate, in which case a guided biopsy may be necessary. However, it has been proven that, in experienced hands, hydrosonography and outpatient hysteroscopy are equally effective.[29]

Doppler flow studies have been investigated as an endometrial surveillance test in women on tamoxifen therapy, but changes are not specific enough to detect endometrial pathology.[35] Tamoxifen induces significant reductions of the impedance to blood flow in the endometrial and subendometrial vasculature, regardless of the presence or absence of endometrial pathology. This is probably due to dilatation of the existing vascular bed.

11.7 Screening Guidelines

11.7.1 Consensus Meeting Guidelines

In an earlier study, we found a close relationship between the total (cumulative) dose of tamoxifen and the appearance of benign endometrial lesions;[36] this relationship was later confirmed for endometrial cancers.[13] To evaluate the numbers of years the uterine cavity can be left without screening, we performed another longitudinal hysteroscopic follow-up study. We further evaluated the effect of duration of tamoxifen intake and the appearance of endometrial lesions in 57 postmenopausal women on tamoxifen.[37] All had an atrophic endometrium and an empty uterine cavity and were evaluated regularly by means of outpatient panoramic hysteroscopy using CO_2 as distension medium. Although there was no comparative cohort of non-tamoxifen-exposed breast cancer patients to differentiate background events that may be unrelated to tamoxifen, we found that during the 3 years following the finding of a normal baseline endometrium, postmenopausal women on tamoxifen 20 mg daily did not develop endometrial hyperplasia or endometrial cancer. However, benign endometrial polyps and glandulocystic endometria did appear during this period. Although more women participating in such a longitudinal endometrial follow-up are needed to confirm our findings, on the basis of this study we concluded that, with a hysteroscopically normal uterus at the start of therapy (i.e., an empty uterus with an atrophic endometrium), atypical endometrial hyperplasia or cancer is unlikely to be found in the first 2–3 years. Therefore, women who are concerned about potential uterine side-effects should, ideally, be screened prior to tamoxifen use.

At a recent international meeting in Brussels, organised by the Flemish Gynaecological Oncology Group, it was agreed that one should start with pretreatment uterine assessment using TVS or outpatient hysteroscopy.[38,39] In the absence of pretreatment endometrial pathology, asymptomatic long-term tamoxifen users are followed up on a yearly basis, starting after 2–3 years of treatment because of the effect of cumulative doses. Hysteroscopy or hydrosonography will be required if there is endometrial thickening because the only value of TVS is in detecting a normal finding (Table 11.1). The participants agreed that screening breast cancer patients on tamoxifen for endometrial cancer is unlikely to be cost-beneficial and that women without breast cancer who are being treated with tamoxifen within a chemopreventive trial should be monitored closely for the development of endometrial hyperplasia or cancer.

Table 11.1. Endometrial surveillance of patients taking tamoxifen. TVS, transvaginal ultrasonography; HS, hydrosonography; ET, endometrial thickness

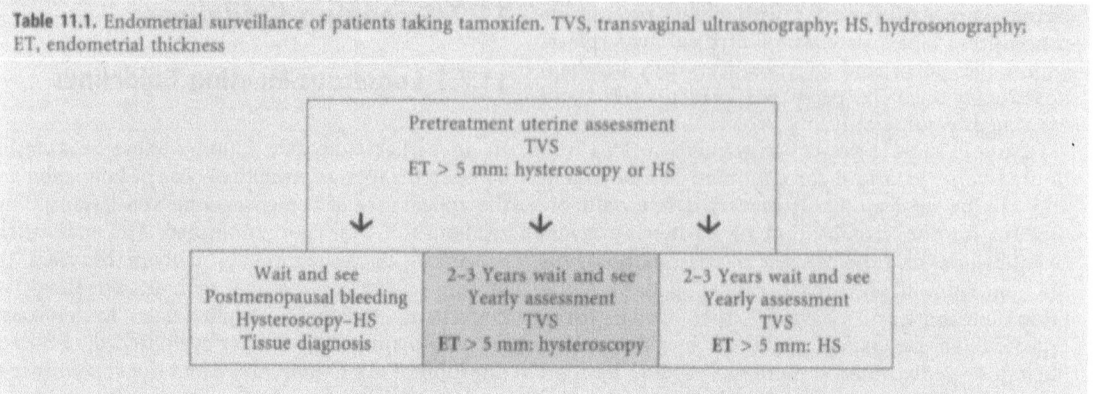

11.7.2 American College of Obstetricians and Gynecologists' Guidelines

These recommendations (published in 1996 and updated in 2000)[40] for women taking tamoxifen are as follows:

(1) Women with breast cancer should have annual gynaecological examinations, including PAP tests and bimanual and rectovaginal examinations.
(2) Any abnormal bleeding, including bloody discharge, spotting, or any other gynaecological symptoms, should be evaluated thoroughly. Any bleeding or spotting should be investigated by biopsy.
(3) Practitioners should be alerted to the increased incidence of endometrial malignancy. Screening procedures or diagnostic tests should be performed at the discretion of the individual gynaecologist.
(4) Women without breast cancer who are being treated with tamoxifen within a chemopreventive trial should be monitored closely for the development of endometrial hyperplasia or cancer.
(5) If atypical hyperplasia develops, use of tamoxifen should be discontinued, and dilatation and curettage or other appropriate gynaecological management should be instituted within an appropriate interval.
(6) If tamoxifen therapy must be continued, hysterectomy should be considered in women with atypical endometrial hyperplasia.
(7) Tamoxifen use may be reinstituted following hysterectomy for endometrial carcinoma in consultation with the physician responsible for the woman's breast care.

11.8 Conclusions

The association between long-term tamoxifen use and endometrial pathology, including endometrial cancer, is a real one. This adverse reaction is acceptable in the context of the expected benefits of tamoxifen for breast cancer; screening for endometrial abnormalities is unlikely to be cost-beneficial. However, screening becomes an important issue because of the troublesome endometrial effect of tamoxifen in healthy women considering this treatment for postmenopausal health, to obtain protection against breast cancer, osteoporosis and myocardial infarction.

Several methods for detecting gynaecological side-effects on tamoxifen have been discussed. Simple TVS may be sensitive, but should be considered a nonspecific procedure. Hysteroscopy and hydrosonography in cases of endometrial thickening are more specific but consequently, treatment of all visible lesions will undoubtedly lead to a high ratio of benign/malignant lesions.

References

1. Beatson GT (1896) On the treatment of inoperable cases of carcinoma of the mamma: suggestions for a new method of treatment, with illustrative cases. Lancet ii:104–107, 162–165
2. Walpole AL, Patterson E (1949) Synthetic oestrogens in mammary cancer. Lancet ii:783–786
3. Harper MJK, Walpole AL (1966) Contrasting endocrine activities of cis and trans isomers in a series of substituted triphenylethylenes. Nature 212:87
4. Toft D, Gorski J (1966) A receptor molecule for estrogens: isolation from the rat uterus and preliminary characterisation. Proc Natl Acad Sci USA 55:1574–1581
5. Early Breast Cancer Trialists' Collaborative Group (1998) Tamoxifen for early breast cancer: an overview of the randomized trials. Lancet 351:1451–1467
6. Love RR, Mazess RB, Barden HS et al (1992) Effects of tamoxifen on bone mineral density in postmenopausal women with breast cancer. N Eng J Med 326:852–856
7. Love RR, Wiebe DA, Newcomb PA et al (1994) Effects of tamoxifen on cardiovascular risk factors in postmenopausal women after 5 years of treatment. J Natl Cancer Inst 86:1534–1539
8. Fisher B, Constantino JP, Wickerham DL et al (1998) Tamoxifen for prevention of breast cancer: report of the National Surgical Adjuvant Breast and Bowel Project-P1 study. J Natl Cancer Inst 90:1371–1388
9. Veronesi U, Maisonneuve P, Costa A (1998) Prevention of breast cancer with tamoxifen: preliminary findings from the Italian randomised trial among hysterectomised women. Italian Tamoxifen Prevention Study. Lancet 352:93–97
10. Powles T, Eeles R, Ashley S (1998) Interim analysis of the incidence of breast cancer in the Royal Marsden Hospital tamoxifen randomised chemoprevention trial. Lancet 352:98–101

11. Neven P, De Muylder X, Van Belle Y et al (1989) Tamoxifen and the uterus and endometrium. Lancet i:375–376
12. Berlière M, Charles A, Galant C (1998) Uterine side effects of tamoxifen: a need for systematic pretreatment screening. Obstet Gynecol 91:40–44
13. Jackson TL, Duffy SRG (2000) On behalf of the ATAC Trialists Group. Baseline endometrial sub-protocol data. Eur J Cancer 3655:S69
14. Fornander T, Cedermark B, Mattsson A et al. (1989) Adjuvant tamoxifen in early breast cancer: occurrence of new primary cancers. Lancet ii:117–120
15. Andersson M, Storm HH, Mouridsen HT (1991) Incidence of new primary cancers after adjuvant tamoxifen therapy and radiotherapy for early breast cancer. J Natl Cancer Inst 83:1013–1017
16. Fisher B, Constantino JP, Redmond CK et al (1994) Endometrial cancer in tamoxifen-treated breast cancer patients: findings from the National Surgical Adjuvant Breast and Bowel Project B-14. J Natl Cancer Inst 86:527–537
17. Assikis VJ, Neven P, Jordan VC et al (1996) A realistic clinical perspective of tamoxifen and endometrial carcinogenesis. Eur J Cancer 32A:1464–1476
18. International Agency for Research on Cancer (1996) Some pharmaceutical drugs. IARC monographs on the evaluation of carcinogenic risks to humans, vol 66. IARC, Lyon
19. Kedar RP, Bourne TH, Powles TJ et al (1994) Effects of tamoxifen on uterus and ovaries of postmenopausal women in a randomized breast cancer prevention trial. Lancet 343:1318–1321
20. Ismail SM (1999) Gynaecological effects of tamoxifen. J Clin Pathol 52:83–88
21. Bernstein L, Deapen D, Cerhan JR (1999) Tamoxifen therapy for breast cancer and endometrial cancer risk. J Natl Cancer Inst 91:1654–1662
22. Cohen I, Bernheim J, Azaria R (1999) Malignant endometrial polyps in postmenopausal breast cancer tamoxifen-treated patients. Gyn Oncol 75:136–141
23. Bergman L, Beelen MLR, Gallee MPW (2000) Risk and prognosis of endometrial cancer after tamoxifen for breast cancer. Lancet 356:881–887
24. McCluggage WG, Abdulkader M, Price JH (2000) Uterine carcinosarcoma in patients receiving tamoxifen. A report of 19 cases. Int J Gyn Cancer 10:280–284
25. Deligdisch L, Kalir T, Cohen CJ (2000) Endometrial histopathology in 700 patients treated with tamoxifen for breast cancer. Gyn Oncol 78:181–186
26. Neven P, De Muylder X, Van Belle Y et al (1990) Hysteroscopic follow-up during tamoxifen treatment. Eur J Obstet Gynaecol Rep Biol 35:235–238
27. Barakat RR (1999) Screening for endometrial cancer in patients receiving tamoxifen for breast cancer. J Clin Oncol 17:1967–1968
28. Cummings SR, Norton L, Eckert S (1998) Raloxifene reduces the risk of breast cancer and may decrease the risk of endometrial cancer in postmenopausal women. Two-year findings from the Multiple Outcomes of Raloxifene Evaluation (MORE) trial. Proc ASCO 17:3
29. Timmerman D, Deprest J, Bourne TH et al (1998) A randomized trial on the use of ultrasonography or office hysteroscopy for endometrial assessment in postmenopausal patients with breast cancer who were treated with tamoxifen. Am J Obstet Gynecol 179:62–70
30. Langer RD, Pierce JJ, O'Hanlan KA et al (1997) Transvaginal ultrasonography compared with endometrial biopsy for the detection of endometrial disease. N Engl J Med 337:1792–1798
31. Perrot N, Guyot B, Antoine M et al (1994) The effects of tamoxifen on the endometrium. Ultrasound Obstet Gynecol 4:83–84
32. Goldstein SR (1994) Unusual ultrasonographic appearance of the uterus in patients receiving tamoxifen. Am J Obstet Gynecol 170:447–451
33. Randolph J, Ying Y, Maier D (1986) Comparison of real time ultrasonography, hysterosalpingography and laparoscopy/hysteroscopy in the evaluation of uterine abnormalities and tubal patency. Fertil Steril 46:828–832
34. Parsons A, Lense J (1993) Sonohysterography for endometrial abnormalities: preliminary results. J Clin Ultrasound 21:87–95
35. Achiron R, Lipitz S, Sivan E (1995) Changes mimicking endometrial neoplasia in postmenopausal, tamoxifen-treated women with breast cancer. A transvaginal Doppler study. Ultrasound Obstet Gynecol 6:116–120
36. De Muylder X, Neven P, De Somer M et al (1991) Endometrial lesions in patients undergoing tamoxifen therapy. Int J Gynecol Obstet 36:127–130
37. Neven P, De Muylder X, Van Belle Y et al (1998) Longitudinal hysteroscopic follow-up during tamoxifen treatment. Lancet 351:36
38. Neven P, Vergote I (1998) Should tamoxifen users be screened for endometrial lesions? Lancet 351:155–157
39. Vergote I, Neven P (1998) Tamoxifen and the uterus: potential uterine risks of anti-oestrogens. Eur J Cancer 34:S4
40. American College of Obstetricians and Gynecologists Committee Opinion no 232 (2000) Tamoxifen and endometrial cancer. ACOG, Washington DC

Part III

Endometrial Malignancy

Contents

Summary

The potential role of ultrasonography once a diagnosis of endometrial cancer has been made is for preoperative staging of the disease. The difficulties associated with this are discussed. There are few good data relating to the ability of ultrasound to assess myometrial invasion and very little regarding prediction of cervical involvement. The relative merits of magnetic resonance imaging (MRI) and computed tomography (CT) scanning are described; however, no one technique offers a significant diagnostic advantage. The use of contrast agents may significantly improve the performance of MRI in this context. The aim of all these approaches is to predict the likelihood of lymph node involvement; however, the therapeutic advantage of lymphadenectomy in these patients is uncertain. This section outlines these controversies.

The role of laparoscopy in the management of endometrial cancer is largely confined to assisting surgical staging of the disease. The same number of lymph nodes can be removed laparoscopically as at laparotomy. The introduction of laparoscopic lymphadenectomy has made vaginal hysterectomy an attractive option for women with early-stage endometrial cancer.

Key Points

- Ultrasonography, MRI and CT scanning offer similar diagnostic performance for the prediction of the depth of myometrial invasion
- The presence of fibroids makes an assessment of tumour invasion difficult
- Ultrasonography may have a role in predicting minimal or no myometrial invasion
- There are insufficient data to suggest that ultrasound can predict cervical involvement
- The yield of lymph nodes obtained by a laparoscopic approach compares favourably with laparotomy
- Laparoscopy can be used for lymphadenectomy and permits a shift away from laparotomy to vaginal hysterectomy for women with stage one endometrial cancer

Chapter 12

Ultrasound Staging of Endometrial Cancer

Gerardo Zanetta

12.1 Introduction

According to the guidelines of the International Federation of Obstetrics and Gynaecology and TNM, the staging of endometrial cancer relies on clinical examination, curettage or hysteroscopy, cystoscopy, proctoscopy, pyelogram and imaging of the lungs and skeleton.[1] Diagnostic imaging of the uterus is not yet considered the basis for changing the clinical stage.

Based on this definition, the role of ultrasound for the staging of endometrial cancer could be dismissed within a few lines. Nevertheless, the treatment of cancers of the corpus uteri is currently the subject of clinical debate.

Hysterectomy represents the cornerstone of treatment and surgical staging, but some details remain to be defined. Are different modalities relevant for the outcome of the patient (radical hysterectomy versus extrafascial hysterectomy; vaginal versus abdominal approach in selected patients)? Is there a role for neoadjuvant chemotherapy or radiation before surgery in patients with locally advanced disease? Is it possible, based on preoperative grading and tumour imaging, to tailor the operation? In this respect, diagnostic imaging, and ultrasound in particular, may offer a relevant contribution.

The main field of investigation for ultrasound in the preoperative assessment of endometrial cancer is the definition of myometrial invasion. When transvaginal ultrasound appeared in clinical practice, some pioneers described the potential of this new technique in defining the thickness of the endometrium.

In the 1980s and early 1990s, several studies demonstrated that a strong correlation existed between the thickness of the endometrium on ultrasound and the risk of endometrial abnormality, including cancer.[2,3] This observation stimulated large-scale studies on the use of vaginal ultrasound for the triage of women with postmenopausal bleeding. At about the same time, other authors observed that invasive endometrial cancer is often associated with interruption of the subendometrial halo.[4]

A second field of investigation is the potential of diagnostic imaging, such as magnetic resonance imaging (MRI), transvaginal ultrasound and intrauterine ultrasound, for the documentation of cervical infiltration.

Finally, a third field of investigation is the potential of colour Doppler ultrasound in describing blood flow characteristics associated with the infiltration and with lymph node spread of endometrial carcinoma.

12.2 Assessment of the Depth of Invasion with Ultrasound

Several studies have been conducted to assess the potential of ultrasound in defining preoperatively the degree of myometrial invasion.[5-20] Most studies use transvaginal probes; a few used intrauterine probes.

Different techniques have been proposed for assesing the depth of myometrial invasion. Some authors use a ratio: $R = DTE/IM$, where DTE represents the deepest tumour extension in the myometrium and IM represents the total width of the adjacent intact myometrium. A ratio of > 0.5 is designated as deep myometrial invasion. Others use a ratio originally proposed by Karlsson:[21] $R = H/DAP$, where H is the endometrial height and DAP is the anterior–posterior diameter. A myometrial invasion depth of greater than 50% is assumed when $R > 0.5$ (Figure 12.1). These differences in assessment represent a major confounding factor for the interpretation of results.

81

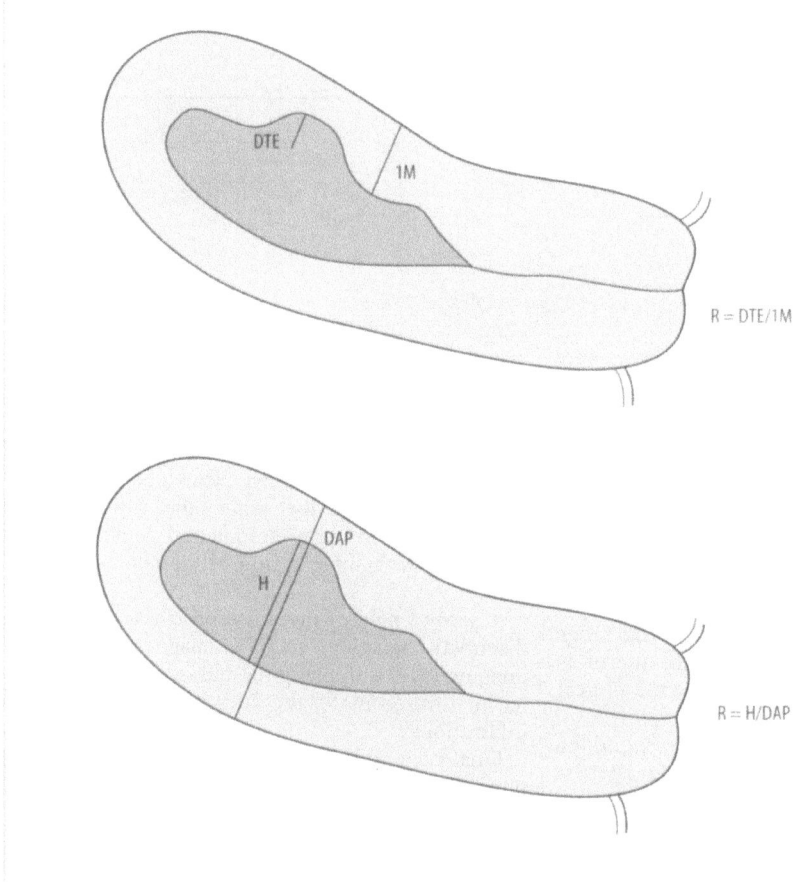

Figure 12.1 Assessment of the depth of invasion with ultrasound. R, Ratio; DTE, deepest tumour extension; IM, width of intact myometrium; H, endometrial height; DAP, anteriorposterior diameter.

Another problem in comparing such studies is the lack of homogeneity of the outcome measures. Most studies investigated the ability to predict the absence of invasion, invasion of less than 50% and invasion of more than 50% of the myometrium. Finally, a weakness of the majority of studies are the small numbers of patients involved. Furthermore, the data are often presented uncritically.

The available studies describe that transvaginal ultrasound has an accuracy of 60–100% for detecting the depth of invasion of endometrial cancer and a striking lack of homogeneity with regard to the sensitivity and specificity (Table 12.1). This probably reflects differences in equipment and study populations and, most importantly, intrinsic difficulties in the interpretation of "difficult" cases.

12.3 Assessment of the Involvement of the Cervical Canal

Only a handful of studies[5,10,12,16,22] have addressed the potential of ultrasound in predicting invasion of the cervical canal (Table 12.2). Even if sufficient patients were included in the study populations, only a few had stage II disease. Therefore, the significance of the data remains a matter of opinion. Based on the available data, an accuracy of 60–90% may be reached.

12.4 Comparison of Transvaginal Ultrasound and MRI

Some authors have compared the performance of transvaginal ultrasound and MRI in the assessment of myometrial invasion (Table 12.3). Most series are extremely small, but the majority of the studies confirm that MRI offers little advantage over transvaginal ultrasound. The results of MRI may, however, be improved significantly by the use of contrast enhancement.

A recent meta-analysis[13] compared the effectiveness of computed tomography (CT), ultrasound and MRI in staging endometrial cancer. The authors identified six studies using CT, 16 using ultrasound and 25 using MRI. According to this analysis, there

Table 12.1. Ability of transvaginal ultrasound to detect deep involvement (outer half) of the myometrium. PPV, Positive predictive value; NPV, negative predictive value

Author	No. of patients	Sensitivity (%)	Specificity (%)	PPV (%)	NPV (%)	Accuracy (%)
Cacciatore[5a]	93					92
Conte[6]	20					90
Sahakian[7]	18					100
Yamashita[8]	40	77	83			68
Del Maschio[9]	42	86	73			76
Prompeler[10]	96	93				81
Lehtovirta[11]	78	95		71	98	88
Artner[12]	69	100	100			100
Kim[13]	26	50	81			69
Weber[14]	80					85
Teefey[15]	12		1/1			
Gabrielli[16]	67	88	71	66	91	
Tsuda[17b]	20					85
Olaya[18]	50	94	84			88
Develioglu[19]	39	37	90	78	60	
Alcazar[20]	50	86	94	86	94	

[a] Transabdominal transducer; [b] intrauterine transducer.

were no significant differences in the overall performance of CT, ultrasound and MRI, but contrast-enhanced MRI performed significantly better than the other techniques in the assessment of myometrial invasion. The authors concluded that contrast-enhanced MRI offers a "one-step" examination with the highest efficacy. Nevertheless, it should be noted that MRI is more expensive, more disturbing for the patient and much less readily available in gynaecology departments than transvaginal ultrasound.

In addition, other biological characteristics of endometrial cancer should be taken into account when discussing the usefulness of diagnostic imaging. Supporters of MRI and CT scanning claim that these techniques are far superior to transvaginal ultrasound for the detection of lymph node metastases, which is reasonably true. However, a study published by Girardi et al[23] showed that only approximately 50% of metastatic nodes from endometrial cancer have a diameter greater than 10 mm and only 7% have a diameter greater than 20 mm. Lymph node metastases are found in 15–40% of endometrial cancers, depending on grade and stage. It is commonly accepted that pelvic lymph nodes should be considered suspicious at CT scan or MRI when larger than 15–20 mm. Even if a diagnostic imaging

technique has a sensitivity of 100% for enlarged nodes, CT scan and MRI may identify at most two to four enlarged nodes for every 100 patients examined.

Irrespective of the ability of diagnostic imaging to indicate the risk of lymph node metastases, several studies[24,25] have shown that macroscopic examination of the uterine specimen at surgery (in particular when combined with knowledge about the tumour grade) is a reliable and inexpensive method for evaluating the degree of invasion of endometrial cancer and allows the selection of those patients who might benefit from a lymphadenectomy. Therefore, the cost-effectiveness of any additional procedure should be considered carefully. Finally, the therapeutic role of lymphadenectomy in endometrial cancer has not been fully established.

12.5 Usefulness of Blood Flow Resistance as a Prognostic Parameter

Some authors have analysed in small populations the usefulness of blood flow characteristics in

Table 12.2. Ability of transvaginal ultrasound to predict cervical involvement. PPV, Positive predictive value; NPV, negative predictive value

Author	No. of patients	Stage II patients	Sensitivity (%)	Specificity (%)	PPV (%)	NPV (%)	Accuracy (%)
Cacciatore[5a]	93	8	75	95			93
Prompeler[10]	96	7	71				81
Artner[12]	69	9	67	100			95
Gabrielli[16]	67	11			46	91	82
Kikuchi[22b]	30	7	75	85	43	96	77
Kikuchi[22c]	30	7	75	100	100	96	87

[a] Transabdominal ultrasound; [b] intravaginal transducer; [c] intrauterine transducer.

Table 12.3. Comparison of performance between transvaginal ultrasound (TVS) and magnetic resonance imaging (MRI) in predicting deep myometrial invasion. PPV, Positive predictive value; NPV, negative predictive value

Author	No. of patients	Sensitivity TVS (%)	Specificity TVS (%)	PPV TVS (%)	NPV TVS (%)	Accuracy TVS (%)	Accuracy MRI (%)
Del Maschio[9]	42	86	73			76	83
Tsuda[17a]	20			85	85		
Yamashita[8]	40			68	68		
Kim[13]	26	50	81	69	89		

[a] Intrauterine transducer.

predicting myometrial invasion or the risk of lymph node metastases.

In 1993, Kurjak et al[4] described the usefulness of colour Doppler ultrasonography for detecting endometrial carcinoma in postmenopausal women. These authors studied 750 postmenopausal women undergoing surgery. In this group, 35 had endometrial cancer and 32 (91.4%) were detected by transvaginal colour Doppler ultrasonography. All women with blood flow detected within the endometrium and a resistance index < 0.4 had endometrial cancer, whereas no endometrial flow could be observed in 92% of hyperplastic endometria.

In 1999, Develioglu et al[19] studied 39 women with endometrial cancer and observed a strong correlation between the resistance index of the uterine artery and the risk of deep myometrial invasion. In a multiple logistic regression model, only patient age, tumour grade and resistance index of the uterine artery were independent determinants of deep myometrial invasion. These authors concluded that transvaginal ultrasound is unreliable for diagnosing the depth of myometrial invasion, but this pathological feature can be predicted with higher accuracy by combining information about age, tumour grade and uterine artery resistance index.

Other authors have studied this clinical problem from a different standpoint. Hata et al[26] found that intratumoural blood flow analysis in endometrial cancer could not provide individual tumour characteristics such as myometrial invasion, lymph node metastasis or histological subtype. However, a thicker endometrium tended to predict the presence of lymph node metastases.

12.6 Value of Preoperative Staging of Endometrial Cancer

All these studies have contributed considerably to our knowledge of endometrial cancer. But to date they have changed very little the clinical management of this disease. Hence the clinical use of preoperative ultrasound remains poorly defined. Until the roles of radical surgery and lymph node dissection are defined, preoperative staging remains of limited value, as it adds little to the clinical management of the patient.

Only approximately 15–20% of endometrial cancers are considered unsuitable for surgical resection at the time of first diagnosis; for most of these, gynaecological examination and traditional staging techniques are sufficient for the choice of therapeutic strategy.

In addition, most studies regarding preoperative staging of endometrial cancer fail to report the potential pitfall represented by the presence of uterine abnormalities concurrent with the endometrial tumour. For instance, 20–40% of women develop fibroids during their life. Some of these women will undergo surgery and will never experience endometrial cancer thereafter. However, a proportion of women with fibroids will preserve their uterus and may develop endometrial cancer. These patients will always represent a problem for the preoperative ultrasound assessment of tumour infiltration, as the results may be inaccurate and sometimes even misleading. Cacciatore et al[5] observed uterine fibroids in 28% of patients and reported that the accuracy of predicting myometrial invasion was slightly less in those women.

On the other hand, it should be emphasised that, at least in Europe, most women with endometrial cancer usually undergo endometrial sampling after an abnormal transvaginal ultrasound scan. Even those who remain sceptical about the use of preoperative diagnostic imaging for endometrial carcinoma must admit that some women are referred to the gynaecological oncologist after an ultrasound, therefore some degree of information about the presumed size of the tumour is already available, even before a formal staging has been attempted.

As for many other fields of investigation, a diagnostic tool must be of simple application in order to be useful. Regarding transvaginal ultrasonography, the available data for the staging of endometrial cancer show a lack of homogeneity of results and a disappointing variability of methods. Concerning the ability of ultrasound to detect early tumour invasion of the myometrium, it should be noted that the differential diagnosis between atypical hyperplasia and very early endometrial cancer is occasionally extremely difficult, even on direct microscopic examination. As a consequence, it seems unlikely that an indirect sign, such as interruption of the subendometrial halo, may add any information, unless in obvious cases where such information is of little clinical relevance.

Among the different prognostic factors of interest for the management of a patient with endometrial cancer, the involvement of the outer half of the myometrium is probably one of the most important, as such information may lead to differences in the radicality of surgery and may suggest the need for a lymph node dissection. The results of several studies indicate the negative predictive value of a scan suggesting only minimal or no myometrial invasion. In such cases, the information provided by endometrial sampling and transvaginal ultrasonography may be extremely useful for tailoring the surgical procedure (radical versus extrafascial; vaginal versus abdominal in severely obese women). Based on the available data, this is probably the most meaningful application of preoperative transvaginal ultrasonography today.

The use of contrast-enhanced MRI should be encouraged only in cases of poorly differentiated carcinoma, high-risk histological type, or suspicious results at transvaginal ultrasonography; this might represent a second step in preoperative staging. Such a strategy would allow an acceptable accuracy of staging with limited costs in the majority of patients and would limit the use of more expensive and troublesome techniques to a minority of selected women.

There are insufficient data to support the use of transvaginal ultrasonography to predict cervical involvement (stage II) in daily practice. The accuracy reported is in the range of 60–90%, but only a few women have been studied. As with myometrial involvement, it would be more practical to make use of the negative predictive value of this diagnostic technique, rather than speculating about subtle characteristics. Few patients with suspicious results at ultrasonography may be correctly staged by means of hysteroscopy, fractional curettage and MRI.

In the future, colour Doppler ultrasound may become an additional aid for the preoperative study of women with endometrial cancer. However, given the absence of large-scale studies in multiple institutions, this interesting technique remains a research tool.

12.7 Conclusions

Transvaginal ultrasound is a promising technique for the preoperative staging of endometrial cancer and deserves further investigation, in particular in multicentre studies. However, the lack of homogeneity of data provided by different authors and the mixture of

methods and techniques probably reflect the current absence of a consensus regarding the clinical use of the information. Each institution, based on its own philosophy of treatment, should choose its own technique (if any) and use it accordingly.

Acknowledgement

I thank my colleague Andrea Lissoni for his contribution to this chapter.

References

1. American Joint Committee on Cancer (1993) TNM Committee of the International Union Against Cancer. Handbook for staging cancer, 4th edn. JB Lippincott, Philadelphia
2. Granberg S, Wikland M, Karlsson B et al (1991) Endometrial thickness as measured by endovaginal ultrasonography for identifying endometrial abnormality. Am J Obstet Gynecol 164:47–52
3. Goldstein SR, Nachtigall M, Snyder JR et al (1990) Endometrial assessment by vaginal ultrasonography before endometrial sampling in patients with postmenopausal bleeding. Am J Obstet Gynecol 163:119–123
4. Kurjak A, Shalan H, Sosic A et al (1993) Endometrial carcinoma in postmenopausal women. Evaluation by transvaginal color Doppler ultrasonography. Am J Obstet Gynecol 169:1597–1603
5. Cacciatore B, Lehtovirta P, Wahlstrom T et al (1989) Preoperative sonographic evaluation of endometrial cancer. Am J Obstet Gynecol 160:133–137
6. Conte M, Guariglia L, Benedetti-Panici P et al (1990) Transvaginal ultrasound evaluation of myometrial invasion in endometrial carcinoma. Gynecol Obstet Invest 29:224–226
7. Sahakian V, Syrop C, Turner D (1991) Endometrial carcinoma: transvaginal ultrasonography prediction of depth of myometrial invasion. Gynecol Oncol 43:217–219
8. Yamashita Y, Mizutani H, Torashima M et al (1993) Assessment of myometrial invasion by endometrial carcinoma: transvaginal sonography vs contrast-enhanced MR imaging. AJR 161:595–599
9. Del Maschio A, Vanzulli A, Sironi S et al (1993) Estimating the depth of myometrial involvement by endometrial carcinoma: efficacy of transvaginal sonography vs MR imaging. AJR 160:533–538
10. Prompeler HJ, Madjar H, du Bois A et al (1994) Transvaginal sonography of myometrial invasion depth in endometrial cancer. Acta Obstet Gynecol 73:343–346
11. Lehtovirta P, Cacciatore B, Ylostalo P (1994) Serum CA 125 levels and sonography in the pre-operative assessment of myometrial invasion of endometrial cancer. Br J Obstet Gynaecol 101:532–535
12. Artner A, Bosze P, Gonda G (1994) The value of ultrasound in preoperative assessment of the myometrial and cervical invasion in endometrial carcinoma. Gynecol Oncol 54:147–151
13. Kim SH, Kim HD, Song YS et al (1995) Detection of deep myometrial invasion in endometrial carcinoma: comparison of transvaginal ultrasound, CT and MRI. J Comput Assist Tomogr 19:766–772
14. Weber G, Merz E, Bahlmann F et al (1995) Assessment of myometrial infiltration and preoperative staging by transvaginal ultrasound in patients with endometrial carcinoma. Ultrasound Obstet Gynecol 6:362–367
15. Teefey SA, Stahl JA, Middleton WD et al (1996) Local staging of endometrial carcinoma: comparison of transvaginal and

intraoperative sonography and gross visual inspection. AJR 166:547–552

16. Gabrielli S, Marabini A, Bevini M et al (1996) Transvaginal sonography vs hysteroscopy in the preoperative staging of endometrial carcinoma. Ultrasound Obstet Gynecol 7:443–446

17. Tsuda H, Murata K, Kawabata M et al (1997) Preoperative assessment of myometrial invasion of endometrial cancer by MR imaging and intrauterine ultrasonography with a high-frequency probe: preliminary study. J Ultrasound Med 16:545–548

18. Olaya FJ, Dualde D, Garcia E et al (1998) Transvaginal sonography in endometrial carcinoma: preoperative assessment of the depth of myometrial invasion in 50 cases. Eur J Radiol 26:274–279

19. Develioglu OH, Bilgin T, Yalcin OT et al (1999) Adjunctive use of the uterine artery resistance index in the preoperative prediction of myometrial invasion in endometrial carcinoma. Gynecol Oncol 72:26–31

20. Alcazar JL, Jurado M, Lopez-Garcia G (1999) Comparative study of transvaginal ultrasonography and CA 125 in the preoperative evaluation of myometrial invasion in endometrial carcinoma. Ultrasound Obstet Gynecol 14:210–214

21. Karlsson B, Norström A, Granberg S et al (1992) The use of endovaginal ultrasound to diagnose invasion of the endometrial carcinoma. Ultrasound Obstet Gynecol 2:35–39

22. Kikuchi A, Sultana J, Okai T et al (1997) Intrauterine sonography for preoperative assessment of cervical invasion in endometrial carcinoma. Gynecol Oncol 65:415–420

23. Girardi F, Petru E, Heyderfadai M et al (1993) Pelvic lymphadenectomy in the surgical treatment of endometrial cancer. Gynecol Oncol 49:177–180

24. Doering DL, Barnhill DR, Weiser EB et al (1989) Intraoperative evaluation of depth of myometrial invasion in stage I endometrial adenocarcinoma. Obstet Gynecol 74:930–933

25. Franchi M, Ghezzi F, Melpignano M et al (2000) Clinical value of intraoperative gross examination in endometrial cancer. Gynecol Oncol 76:357–361

26. Hata K, Hata T, Kitao M (1996) Intratumoral blood flow analysis in endometrial cancer: does it differ among individual tumor characteristics? Gynecol Oncol 61:341–344

In Memoriam to Gerardo Zanetta

In writing this memoriam we have tried to summarise the professional contribution made by a friend, a valued colleague and a thoughtful tutor. It is an almost impossible task. We have not tried to write about Gerardo as a friend or colleague – our words could not do him justice – but we wanted to document his outstanding contribution to his chosen profession.

Gerardo Zanetta was born in Monza on February 14, 1959, the youngest son of three. During time at high school he spent one year at the Maasland College, Oss (the Netherlands). This experience certainly had a lasting impression and contributed to his openness towards people and his problem-solving capacity.

He graduated cum laude in 1985 presenting his thesis, "Retroperitoneal spread of malignant tumours of the ovary at early stages", and he achieved the specialty board in Obstetrics and Gynaecology cum laude in 1989 with his second thesis that described the "Usefulness of the marker CA125 in Gynaecologic Oncology". From then onwards, Gynaecological Oncology became his mission, both clinically in caring for patients, as well as tutoring residents, and in his scientific research.

He spent two years at the Mayo Clinic (Rochester, MN) in the Departments of Gynecologic Oncology and Pathology, whilst a member of the staff at the Department of Obstetrics and Gynaecology of "San Gerardo" Hospital in Monza (1989–1997).

In 1994 he was proposed national coordinator for the project, "Use of transvaginal ultrasound and colour Doppler for non palpable adnexal masses", by the SIGO (Italian Society of Gynaecology and Obstetrics).

His clinical and scientific experience made him an international expert and an important member of international studies focusing on Gynaecologic Oncology and Ultrasound (IOTA, Action, ICON, SNAP). His papers on ovarian and cervical cancer were respected worldwide. More recently his professional life came full circle when he was appointed as chief of the Oncological Unit of the Department of Obstetrics and Gynaecology in Monza where he started his career. Gerardo prematurely left us on May 3, 2002, aged 43. We miss him greatly.

Enrico Ferrazzi, Andrea Lissoni, Dirk Timmerman

Chapter 13

Laparoscopy in Patients with Endometrial Cancer

Jan Decloedt and Ignace Vergote

13.1 Introduction

Endometrial cancer is a very common malignancy; although it is sometimes considered to be relatively benign, the commonly reported 5-year survival remains only 75%. Endometrial cancer, like pelvic carcinomas in general, metastasise to regional (pelvic) lymph nodes. The internal iliac and low para-aortic (below the level of the inferior mesenteric artery) lymph nodes are the most frequently involved regions. As current imaging modalities are suboptimal in detecting these metastases, a significant percentage of patients with clinical stage I adenocarcinoma of the endometrium will be wrongly staged.[1]

13.2 Problems with Clinical Staging

Surgical-pathological staging studies have clearly demonstrated the inaccuracy of clinical staging.[1,2] In a study by the Gynecologic Oncology Group,[1] the surgical-pathological features of 621 patients with stage I endometrial cancer were presented. All patients had a total abdominal hysterectomy, bilateral salpingo-oophorectomy, selective pelvic and para-aortic lymphadenectomy and peritoneal cytology. Seventy-four per cent of the patients had an adenocarcinoma, 25% had poorly differentiated lesions and 41% had significant myometrial invasion (middle or outer third). Five per cent of the patients had metastases to one or both ovaries and only 6% had para-aortic node metastases. Six per cent of the patients had other intraperitoneal metastases identified at the time of surgery. Tumour grade was correlated with depth of invasion and with frequency of nodal metastases. There was an excellent correlation between depth of invasion and nodal metastases. As less than 10% of the

patients with metastases to the lymph nodes had grossly enlarged nodes, the decision to perform a lymphadenectomy should not be based on intraoperative palpation of the nodal area. The study clearly confirmed that: (1) a significant number of patients with stage I disease have extrauterine disease; (2) certain patients have significant risk of lymph node metastases; and (3) histological evaluation of the regional lymph nodes is mandatory in those patients.

A more recent Gynecologic Oncology Group study[3] concentrated on the relationship between surgical-pathological risk factors and outcome in stage I and II carcinoma of the endometrium. Of the 1180 women with clinical stage I or II (occult) endometrial carcinoma, 895 with endometroid or adenosquamous carcinoma were evaluable for the study, which related surgical-pathological parameters and postoperative treatment to recurrence-free interval and recurrence site. For patients without metastasis determined by surgical-pathological staging, the greatest determinant of recurrence was grade 3 histology. Of 48 patients with histologically documented aortic node metastases, 47 had one or more of the following features: (1) grossly positive pelvic nodes, (2) grossly positive adnexal metastasis or (3) outer one-third myometrial invasion. Pelvic radiation was administered to 48% and vaginal brachytherapy alone to 10.2% of patients postoperatively; 41.8% received no adjuvant radiotherapy. None of three recurrences in the vaginal implant group were vaginal or pelvic; 7.4% of recurrences in the pelvic radiation therapy group were vaginal and 16.8% were pelvic; 18.2% of recurrences in the group with no adjuvant radiation were vaginal and 31.8% pelvic. The 5-year recurrence-free interval for patients with negative surgical-pathological risk factors (other than grade and myometrial invasion) was 92.7%; involvement of the isthmus/

cervix 69.8%; positive pelvic cytology 56%; vascular space invasion 55%; pelvic node or adnexal metastases 57.8%; and aortic node metastases or gross laparotomy findings 41.2%.

It is not clear that cervical invasion per se reduces survival, because it is more often associated with poor tumour differentiation and deep myometrial invasion. Adjuvant postoperative radiotherapy results in better local control (34.6% of vaginal/pelvic recurrences in the surgery-only group compared with 12.5% in the radiotherapy group), but the only published randomised study on the value of adjuvant postoperative radiotherapy did not show any substantial advantage in the radiotherapy arm.[4]

13.3 Vaginal Hysterectomy for Endometrial Cancer

Patients with endometrial cancer are generally managed with total abdominal hysterectomy and bilateral salpingo-oophorectomy, as it is impossible to (1) assess the peritoneal cavity, (2) perform a lymphadenectomy and (3) obtain pelvic washings using the vaginal hysterectomy technique. Vaginal hysterectomy has therefore been limited to the medically compromised patient. Bloss[5] published a series in which vaginal hysterectomy was performed on 31 patients with stage I endometrial cancer because of medical problems that placed them at high risk for morbidity and mortality from abdominal surgery. These risk factors included: (1) morbid obesity (87%), (2) hypertension (58%), (3) diabetes mellitus (35%) and (4) cardiovascular diseases (26%). It was suggested that the cure rates with vaginal and abdominal hysterectomies were comparable, while morbidity and mortality rates were significantly lower in patients undergoing vaginal hysterectomy, with a 93% 5-year survival rate. Thirty-five per cent of their patients received adjuvant radiotherapy because of deep myometrial invasion or unfavourable histology. Although Bloss et al recommended the removal of both ovaries, this procedure was performed in only 11 (35%) of their patients.

13.4 Laparoscopic Pelvic Lymphadenectomy

Laparoscopic pelvic lymphadenectomy is a new technique, first described in 1990 by Reich[6] in a patient with stage I ovarian cancer. Querleu[7] published a study of 39 patients who had the procedure for cervical cancer.

Despite the many publications on laparoscopy in patients with cervical or ovarian cancer, only a few series have been published on laparoscopy in patients with endometrial cancer.

13.4.1 Laparoscopic-Assisted Surgical Staging

The first low elective para-aortic lymphadenectomy in combination with simple vaginal hysterectomy[8] for the surgical staging and treatment of two patients with endometrial carcinomas was described by Childers and Surwit[8] in 1992. One year later, they published a first series of laparoscopic-assisted surgical staging (LASS) of endometrial cancer.[9] Fifty-nine patients with a clinical stage I adenocarcinoma of the endometrium were included. Six patients were found to have intraperitoneal disease. Of the remaining 53 patients, 29 underwent lymphadenectomy, one of whom had positive para-aortic nodes. Complications (one transected ureter during ligation of the uterine artery using the Endo-GIA and a 1.5 cm cystotomy during the laparoscopic takedown of the bladder) were related to the laparoscopic-assisted vaginal hysterectomy (LAVH) and occurred in the first quarter of their series.

The disadvantages of a single vaginal hysterectomy without LASS have been discussed previously. In his series of LASS, Childers[9] found metastatic disease in seven patients, six intraperitoneally and one retroperitoneally, which confirms the additive value of laparoscopy in patients with early-stage endometrial cancer. Two patients (6%) who should have undergone lymphadenectomy by their protocol guidelines could not have the procedure due to obesity, a well-known risk factor for endometrial cancer. Obesity is the greatest limitation to using a laparoscopic approach.[9,10]

Boitke[11] presented a retrospective non-randomised review comparing laparotomy and laparoscopy in managing stage I endometrial carcinoma. Thirty-seven patients were managed with both methods. Four procedures could not be completed laparoscopically. The same number of pelvic and para-aortic lymph nodes were removed in both groups. The median weight in the laparoscopy group was significantly less than that in the laparotomy group (63 versus 81 kg). The laparoscopy approach prolonged the procedure by 23 minutes (217 versus 194 minutes) but shortened the hospital stay by 2.6 days (2.4 versus 5 days). The association between increased weight and well-differentiated tumours was confirmed by Childers,[9] who noted an average weight of the patients who did not qualify for lymphadenectomy of 76.1 kg compared with 64.8 kg in patients who had or should have had a lymphadenectomy according to his treatment algorithm.

13.4.2 Laparoscopic-Assisted Vaginal Hysterectomy in our Series

We performed LASS and LAVH with bilateral salpingo-oophorectomy in 30 patients with clinical stage I endometrial cancer. All patients were admitted less than 24 hours before surgery. A detailed personal and family history was obtained; clinical evaluation, routine biochemistry including diabetes screening and CA 125, chest X-ray, computed tomography of the abdomen and pelvis and a transvaginal ultrasonography were performed. Mechanical bowel preparation, low molecular weight heparin and prophylactic antibiotics were administered. Written consent was obtained and patients were advised about the possible conversion to laparotomy. Surgery was performed under general anaesthesia with the patient in the dorsal lithotomy position, extending the upper legs as much as possible. The procedure we use is similar to the four-trocar technique described by Childers.[8,9] In patients at risk of complications of trocar insertion, we performed an open laparoscopy and used the 12 mm Origin balloon trocar, which has a very low complication rate in high-risk patients.[10] Secondary trocars were inserted under direct view. We routinely use a subumbilical 10 mm trocar, two lateral 10 mm trocars and a 5 mm trocar suprapubically.

The LASS procedure included a systematic and thorough inspection of the intraperitoneal cavity, pelvic washings and LAVH. The LAVH was performed with unipolar coagulation in a classical way. The uterine artery was clipped at its origin from the internal iliac artery. When indicated, the lymphadenectomy was performed after the hysterectomy. The criteria for lymphadenectomy are based on tumour grade and depth of invasion (Table 13.1). In patients with endometrial cancer stage Ia or Ib grade 1, a LAVH with peritoneal cytology was performed. A bilateral pelvic lymphadenectomy was performed in all patients with a stage Ib or Ic grade 2 endometrial cancer. The same procedure was performed in all patients with grade 3 disease, clear cell carcinoma and serous carcinoma. Only in patients with macroscopically positive lymph nodes, serosal invasion or

adnexal metastases, a para-aortic lymphadenectomy extending from below the inferior mesenteric artery was performed.

The mean age of the patients was 61 (47–76) years. Their average weight was 63 kg (44–95 kg) and average length 162 cm (151–170 cm). In three patients we converted to laparotomy. One patient with two previous caesarean sections and an anterior colporrhaphia was found to have very dense adhesions with insufficient laparoscopic visualisation. One patient developed bleeding (< 300 ml) from the external iliac vein and in one case laparotomy was performed as tumour growth through the serosa was visualised at laparoscopy. Twenty-seven patients were treated by LASS and LAVH. Eighteen of these were low-risk patients and had an inspection of the pelvic lymph nodes, peritoneal washings and LAVH and bilateral salpingo-oophorectomy. The mean operating time in this group was 175 minutes. In nine high-risk patients, a pelvic lymphadenectomy was performed. Three of these patients were found to have node metastases. The median number of nodes removed was 17 (6–31). Average operating time in the high-risk group was 225 (130–240) minutes. We had a clear learning curve (Table 13.2), with a median operating time of 200 minutes in the first 15 cases and 165 minutes in the last 15 cases.

The median decrease in haemoglobin was 1.2 g/dl (0.1–3.1), excluding two patients who received 2 units and 1 unit of packed cells intraoperatively, who had decreases in haemoglobin of 0 and 0.9 g/dl respectively. Six patients had postoperative radiotherapy. Three patients had a stage IIIc endometrial cancer (two with clear cell and/or serous tumours), two had stage IIb disease. A sixth patient had endometrial cancer stage Ic on final histology but did not have a lymphadenectomy, as the frozen section showed stage Ib. Our median follow-up is 18 (1–36) months with a 2-year disease-free survival of 95%. One patient presented with a pelvic side wall relapse 12 months after surgery. The histopathological examination at the time of primary surgery showed a serous papillary tumour with deep myometrial infiltration and positive pelvic lymph nodes. The patient received three courses of adjuvant cisplatin-doxorubicin chemotherapy and 50 Gy pelvic radiotherapy postoperatively. Two complications

Table 13.1. Leuven criteria for laparoscopic lymphadenectomy in patients with stage I endometrial cancer

Grade 3
Grade 2 with myometrial infiltration (frozen section)
Grade 1 with more than 50% myometrial infiltration
Serous or clear cell tumours

Table 13.2. Operating time (min) for the laparoscopic treatment of endometrial cancer

	Median	Range
Operating time	180	130–240
Cases 1–15	200	
Cases 15–30	165	
Low-risk group	175	
High-risk group	225	130–240

occurred in the 30 cases. One patient developed bleeding of the external iliac vein during lymphadenectomy, which was stopped after conversion to laparotomy, and one patient developed a hernia of the lateral trocar site.

No bladder or ureteral injuries occurred in our series, unlike in other series.[9,11] Before we performed laparoscopic lymphadenectomies, we trained in animal models and performed 46 procedures before switching to humans. We strongly recommend proper training and specific training in vivo in animal models before performing the procedure in patients, to avoid major complications and long operating times when starting to perform these procedures. Although the complications differ in the laparoscopic and laparotomy approaches,[11] the incidence is the same. Our median hospital stay was 4 (3–9) days, which is substantially lower than after laparotomy in Belgium (median approximately 8 days); all patients stayed 3–5 days, except one who insisted on a long hospital stay for personal reasons.

13.5 Quality of Life and Cost Considerations

Recently, Spirtos[12] published a retrospective study to determine whether the cost or quality of life associated with the surgical treatment of women with presumed early-stage endometrial cancer differed on the basis of the surgical approach chosen. He compared a group of 17 women who underwent exploratory laparotomy, total abdominal hysterectomy, bilateral salpingo-oophorectomy and pelvic and para-aortic lymphadenectomy with a group of 13 women who underwent the same surgery by laparoscopy. The patient population differed significantly with regard to weight and body mass index. The laparotomy group required significantly longer hospitalisation than the laparoscopy group (6.3 versus 2.4 days), resulting in higher overall hospital costs. Similarly, patients undergoing laparotomy took longer to return to normal activities (5.3 versus 2.4 weeks). These findings agree with the short hospital stay in the laparoscopy group in our series and in those of Boitke[11] and Childers.[9]

13.6 Conclusions

In patients with stage I endometrial carcinoma, LASS and LAVH is an attractive alternative to the traditional surgical approach, with the same surgicopathological possibilities but a significantly shorter hospital stay and postoperative recovery. Our series confirms the feasibility of the technique when performed in properly selected patients by laparoscopically trained gynaecological oncologists.

References

1. Creasman WT, Morrow CP, Bundy BN et al (1987) Surgical pathologic spread patterns of endometrial cancer: a Gynecologic Oncology Group study. Cancer 60:2035–2041
2. Shepherd JH (1989) Revised FIGO staging for gynecologic cancer. Br J Obstet Gynecol 96:889–892
3. Morrow CP, Bundy BN, Kunnan RJ et al (1991) Relationship between surgical-pathological risk factors and outcome in clinical stage I and II carcinoma of the endometrium: a Gynecologic Oncology Group study. Gynecol Oncol 40:55–65
4. Aalders J, Abeler V, Kolstad P et al (1980) Postoperative external irradiation and prognostic parameters in stage I endometrial carcinoma: clinical and histopathologic study of 540 patients. Obstet Gynaecol 56(4):419–427
5. Bloss JD, Ben-nan ML, Bloss LP et al (1991) Use of vaginal hysterectomy for the management of stage I endometrial cancer in the medically compromised patient. Gynecol Oncol 40:74–77
6. Reich H, McGlynn F, Wilie W (1990) Laparoscopic management of stage I ovarian cancer: a case report. J Reprod Med 35:601–604
7. Querleu D, LeBlanc E, Castellain B (1991) Laparoscopic pelvic lymphadenectomy in the staging of early carcinoma of the cervix. Am J Obstet Gynecol 164:579–581
8. Childers JM, Surwit EA (1992) Combined laparoscopic and vaginal surgery for the management of two cases of stage I endometrial cancer. Gynecol Oncol 45:46–51
9. Childers JM, Brzechffa PR, Hatch KD et al (1993) Laparoscopically assisted surgical staging (LASS) of endometrial cancer. Gynecol Oncol 51:33–38
10. Decloedt JF, Berteloot P, Vergote IB (1997) The feasibility of open laparoscopy in gynecologic-oncologic patients. Gynecol Oncol 66:138–140
11. Boitke GM, Lurain JR, Burke JJ (1994) A comparison of laparoscopic management of endometrial cancer with traditional. 25th Annual Meeting, Society of Gynecologic Oncologists, Orlando, Florida
12. Spirtos NM, Schlaerth JB, Gross GM et al (1996) Cost and quality-of-life analyses of surgery for early endometrial cancer: laparotomy versus laparoscopy. Am J Obstet Gynecol 174:1795–1800

Part IV

Urogynaecology

Contents

Summary

An increasing number of patients are seeking medical help for pelvic floor problems. Their problems are functional and complex, and an accurate diagnosis is essential for appropriate therapy to be implemented. Ultrasound is becoming increasingly important for the assessment of these patients. Its role in incontinence and detrusor instability is at present confined to research. In contrast, anal endosonography is a well-established method that has significantly improved our understanding of anal incontinence. Occult anal sphincter defects can be visualised by anal ultrasound and are common following vaginal delivery and particularly after instrumental procedures.

Endoscopy has for some time been used to assist needle suspensions for incontinence surgery. These operations are truly minimally invasive; different techniques have been introduced and the results that can be expected are discussed.

The Burch-type colposuspension is usually considered as the gold standard for the treatment of genuine stress incontinence and is now also performed laparoscopically. Once the learning curve has been overcome, similar cure rates can be achieved as with the open technique. Sling procedures are better in patients with sphincter deficiency, and initial experience with a laparoscopic modification of this abdominal operation is described.

Urogenital prolapse presents in a variety of ways and either the abdominal or vaginal route can be used for surgery. Laparoscopy can be used to reduce the morbidity associated with abdominal surgery, without compromising the success of the procedure. Different chapters illustrate techniques for reconstructing the middle compartment of the pelvic floor. In theory, all abdominal procedures can be mimicked by endoscopy. The best results for correction of vault prolapse are obtained by sacral colpopexy, which can now be performed by laparoscopy. In young patients, hysteropexy is preferred, conserving the uterus. An isolated enterocele repair is also possible, as visualisation of the recto-vaginal area is often better with the laparoscope than the naked eye. The technical aspects of these complex endoscopic procedures are described and outcomes discussed.

Key points

- The prevalence of anal incontinence has been reported as being 2.2% in a general population and 6.6% in the year following vaginal delivery

- 35% of primigravid and 44% of multiparous women have occult anal sphincter defects following vaginal delivery and a significant proportion develop anal incontinence

- An overlap anal sphincter repair technique produces very good results

- Needle suspensions of the bladder neck have evolved over time. They are minimally invasive and good cure rates can be achieved. They can be associated with other vaginal prolapse procedures. The number of vaginal wall sling procedures is increasing. Conceptually this fits well into the current trend in incontinence surgery to use modern approaches to revive procedures that support the mid-urethra

- Sling procedures are feasible using the endoscope, although case selection is of utmost importance

- Recent data show that colposuspension can be performed by laparoscopy, with equally good results as when the abdominal approach is used

- Enterocele repair is perfectly feasible by means of laparoscopy

- Laparoscopic sacral colpopexy mimics its abdominal counterpart, without its access-related morbidity. Endoscopic suturing skills are required. The minimal access nature of this procedure has led to a widening of its use, particularly for the older patient

- Laparoscopic hysteropexy is the method of choice for severe uterine descent, in patients where preservation of the uterus is important

Chapter 14

Anal Endosonography and Incontinence

Abdul H. Sultan

14.1 Introduction

Anal endosonography followed modification of the rectal endoprobe (B&K Medical, Gentofte, Denmark) first described in 1982 by Frentzel-Beyme[1] for imaging the prostate gland. In 1986, using the same probe, Beynon et al.[2] clarified the interpretation of endosonic appearances of normal colon and rectum. For the purposes of anal endosonography, Law and Bartram[3] modified the tip of the probe by replacing the water-filled balloon with a hard sonolucent plastic cone measuring 17 mm in diameter (Figure 14.1). The rotating endoprobe is fitted with a 7 or preferably a 10 MHz transducer (focal range 5–45 mm), which provides a 360° cross-sectional image.

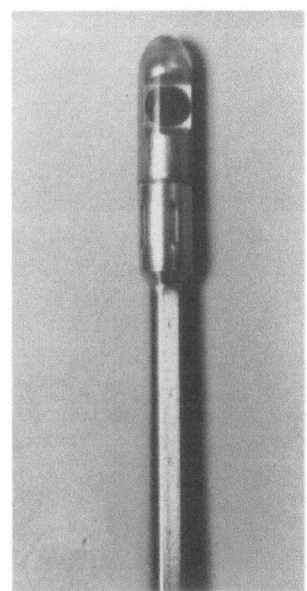

Figure 14.1 The tip of the rotating B&K Medical endoprobe covered by a hard sonolucent plastic cone.[35]

14.1.1 Technique

The subject is scanned in the left lateral position, although some prefer the prone position; no bowel preparation is necessary. The probe is covered with a condom, which has ultrasound gel applied to both surfaces. All images are orientated according to convention such that anterior lies at the top, although earlier descriptions were orientated such that anterior was to the right of the image. The probe is inserted about 6 cm into the rectum and as it is withdrawn down the anal canal, images of the puborectalis muscle, the anal mucosa and submucosa, internal anal sphincter, longitudinal muscle and external anal sphincter become visible (Figure 14.2).

14.1.2 Interpretation

The exact anatomy of the anal sphincter mechanism has remained controversial and there is still a lack of uniformity in the classification of the external anal sphincter into deep, superficial and subcutaneous components.[4,5] This inconsistency is due to the enormous anatomical variation seen not only between individuals but also between two anal canal hemispheres of the same individual.[5] Anal endosonography therefore requires in-depth knowledge of normal anatomical variants of the anal canal and a more accurate interpretation can be obtained from dynamic images. Further research has led to clarification and redefinition of previous misconceptions regarding the sonographic appearances of the various layers within the anal sphincter complex.[6] Gender differences are also important; failure to recognise that the anal sphincter is shorter anteriorly in the female has led to the erroneous diagnosis of anal sphincter defects.[4,5] The longitudinal muscle layer is not always distinguishable

93

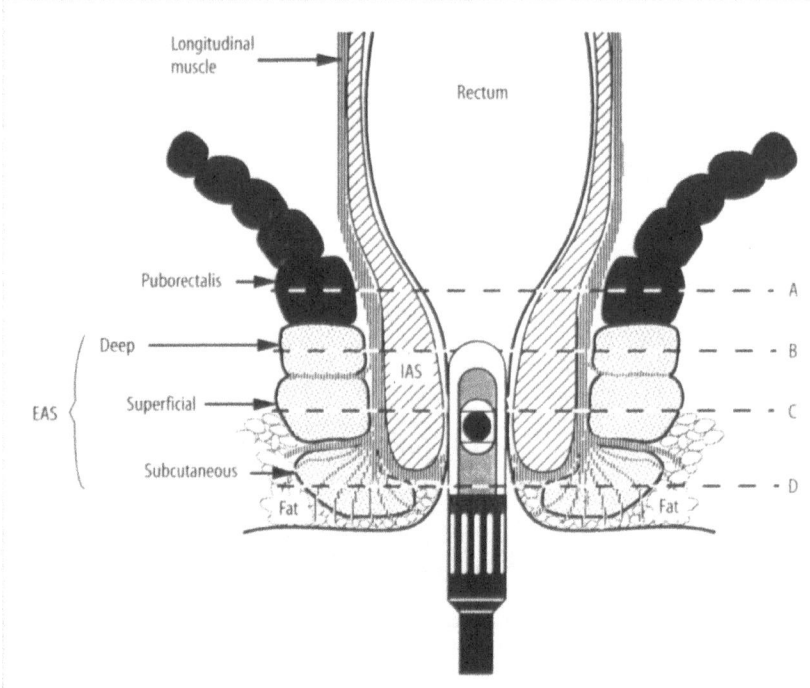

Figure 14.2 Schematic representation of a coronal section through the anorectum. As the probe is withdrawn down the anorectum, static images are taken at the four levels (A–D). IAS, Internal anal sphincter; EAS, external anal sphincter. Reprinted from: Sultan AH, Ka mm MA. Atlas of gastrointestinal motility: in health and disease. Schuster MA (ed) Williams and Wilkins, 1993.[35]

from the external sphincter and was seen in only 40% of females using the 7 MHz probe.[4,5]

Until the development of anal endosonography, defects in the striated external sphincter could only be identified by needle electromyography (EMG) "mapping" and defects in the smooth muscle of the internal anal sphincter could only be inferred by a low maximum resting anal pressure. The advent of anal endosonography, however, has enabled clear imaging of the anal sphincter muscles[3,6] (Figure 14.3). Consequently, when anal endosonography was performed in patients believed to be suffering from "neurogenic" faecal incontinence, unsuspected internal and external sphincter defects were identified. In a blinded prospective study, anal endosonography has been shown to be very accurate and superior to clinical examination, manometry or EMG mapping.[7] External sphincter defects (Figure 14.4) have been verified histologically to represent fibrosis,[7] while the appearance of internal sphincter defects (Figure 14.4) have been validated prospectively in patients undergoing lateral internal anal sphincterotomy.[8]

14.1.3 Clinical Application

Anal endosonography has now superseded needle EMG mapping and is accepted as the "gold standard" in the diagnosis of sphincter trauma[7,8]

(Figure 14.4). Vaizey et al.[9] have also used anal endosonography to diagnose primary degeneration of the anal sphincter associated with passive faecal incontinence (see below). Other uses include diagnosis of sepsis, fistulae and malignancy.

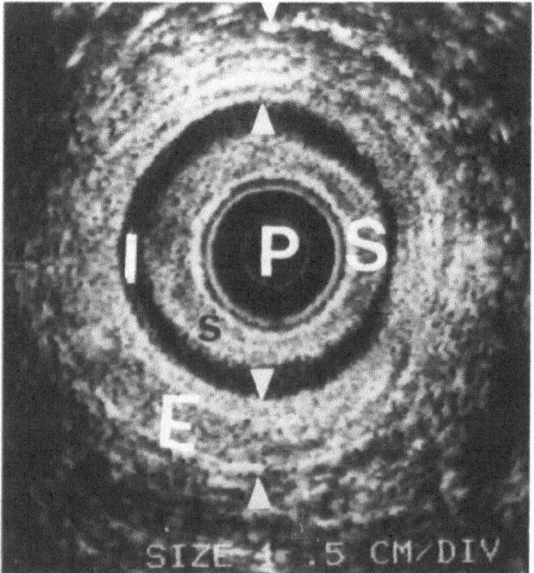

Figure 14.3 Endosonographic image of the mid-anal canal of a healthy nulliparous woman. P, Probe in anal canal; S, submucosa; I, internal sphincter; E, external sphincter within arrows.

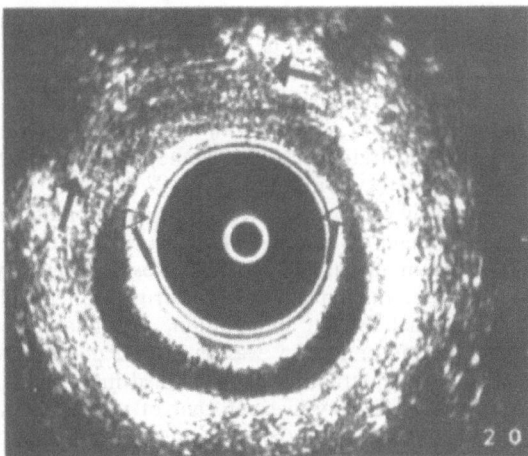

Figure 14.4 Anal endosonographic image of a 38-year-old woman who reported faecal incontinence 4 years after a traumatic forceps delivery. There is a distinct external sphincter defect (*between closed arrows*) and an internal sphincter defect (*between open arrows*).

14.1.4 Other Imaging Techniques

Vaginal endosonography using the B&K endoprobe to image the undistended anal sphincter and perianal tissues has been described previously[10] (Figure 14.5). Poen et al.[11] used vaginal endosonography in addition to anal endosonography, and reported that the diagnostic yield of faecal incontinence and perianal sepsis can be increased in 25% of patients. Other sonographic techniques include the echo gastroscope,[12] 120° sector ultrasound probe,[13] vector manometry,[13] transperineal ultrasound[14] and endoa-

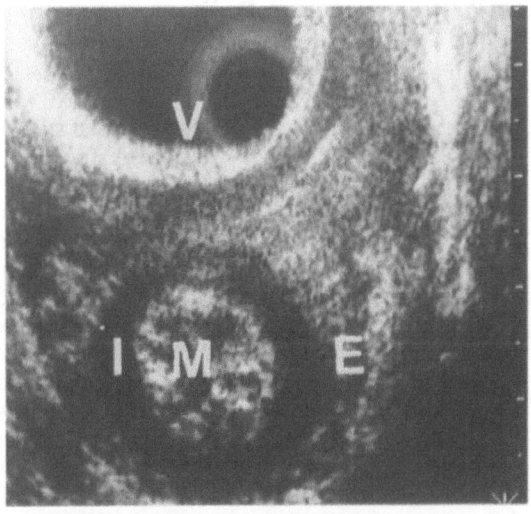

Figure 14.5 Endovaginal ultrasound[10] demonstrating the undisturbed anal sphincter in the resting state. *V*, Probe in vagina; *M*, mucosa; *I*, internal sphincter; *E*, external sphincter.

nal magnetic resonance imaging.[15] These alternative techniques do have advantages and limitations and therefore need scientific validation before acceptance into clinical practice.

14.2 Anal Incontinence

Anal incontinence is an embarrassing symptom that carries a social stigma and can have a devastating effect on a woman's quality of life. Consequently, women rarely volunteer this symptom and the true incidence is grossly underestimated. Community prevalence studies show inconsistency in definition of anal incontinence and include a heterogeneous population. One American study reported anal incontinence in 2.2% of the general population. MacArthur et al.[16] interviewed 906 women 10 months after delivery and reported a prevalence of 6.6% (including faecal urgency but excluding flatus incontinence).

Previously, the development of anal incontinence was attributed largely to pelvic nerve trauma. Prospective studies measuring EMG fibre density and pudendal nerve motor latency during pregnancy and childbirth have shown that vaginal delivery results in denervation and reinervation in up to 80% of primiparous women.[17]

Vaizey et al.[9] described primary degeneration of the internal anal sphincter smooth muscle as a discrete clinical entity causing faecal incontinence. This was identified in 45 patients (in the absence of denervation, structural damage, external sphincter weakness or sensory abnormalities) using anal endosonography to demonstrate a thin, often hyperechogenic internal sphincter with poorly defined borders (Figure 14.6). The resting anal pressure, which largely reflects internal anal sphincter (smooth muscle) function, was reduced and the median voluntary squeeze pressure, which reflects external sphincter (striated muscle) function, was within the normal range. Although no histological confirmation of the condition was provided, many of the patients were successfully treated with constipating drugs such as loperamide.

14.3 Occult Anal Sphincter Trauma

Sultan et al.[18] performed the first prospective study before and after childbirth to evaluate the prevalence of occult anal sphincter trauma and pudendal nerve damage during childbirth. Two hundred and two pregnant women were investigated with anal endosonography, manometry, perineometry and pudendal nerve terminal motor latency measure-

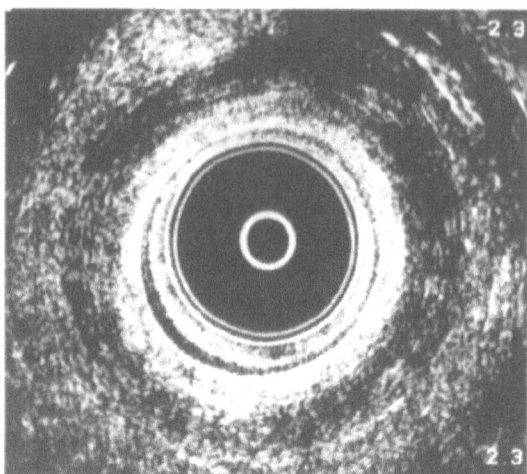

Figure 14.6 Endoanal image of a 56-year-old woman who complained of passive soiling. The internal anal sphincter is abnormally thin, measuring 0.9 mm at its maximum thickness (normal range 24 mm). The appearances are in keeping with primary degeneration of the internal sphincter.[9]

ments in the last 6 weeks of delivery and repeated 6 weeks after delivery in 150 of these women. Occult anal sphincter defects (Figure 14.4) were identified in 35% of primiparous and 44% of multiparous women following vaginal delivery. Thirteen per cent and 23% respectively developed defaecatory symptoms (faecal urgency and/or anal incontinence) after delivery. Only two of the 150 women (both primiparous) had recognised tears of the anal sphincter at the time of delivery. Internal and combined sphincter defects occurred more frequently than external sphincter defects alone. A strong association was demonstrated between the presence of any defect and the development of symptoms. As only 4% of multiparae sustained new sphincter damage following a subsequent delivery compared with 35% of primiparae, women are at greatest risk during the first vaginal delivery. Internal sphincter defects were associated with significantly lower maximum resting anal pressures and external sphincter defects with significantly lower maximum incremental squeeze pressures. These defects persisted at the 6-month follow-up examination. The single independent obstetric factor associated with anal sphincter damage was identified as forceps delivery. The 23 women delivered by caesarean section remained asymptomatic and none developed a new sphincter defect. In all but 16% of the vaginal delivery group, the abnormally prolonged pudendal nerve motor latency at 6 weeks postpartum had returned to

normal by 6 months. Furthermore, antenatally, the incidence of abnormal latencies was similar in both the nulliparous and multiparous groups. This suggests that pudendal nerve damage is largely a neuropraxia and recovers with time. No relationship was demonstrated between latency measurements and defaecatory symptoms.

Donnelly et al.[13] recruited 219 pregnant nulliparous women, of whom 184 returned for 6-week postpartum evaluation. In this prospective study, anal vector manometry was performed antenatally and postnatally but in addition, pudendal nerve terminal motor latency was measured postnatally. Anal endosonography was performed in 81 women postnatally. Twenty-five per cent of women delivered vaginally (n = 168) developed disturbance of faecal incontinence compared with none following caesarean section (n = 16). Donnelly et al. identified evidence of occult anal sphincter injury in 35% of primiparous vaginal deliveries, confirming the findings of Sultan et al. (n = 79), who reported identical findings.

Chaliha et al.[19] recruited 286 nulliparous pregnant women, of whom 161 returned for 3 months postnatal evaluation. Anal manometry and anal electrosensation were performed antenatally and postnatally but in addition, anal endosonography was performed postnatally. Twenty-four per cent of women developed defaecatory symptoms (anal incontinence or urgency) and occult anal sphincter defects were identified in 38%. Childbirth was not associated with an overall change in anal electrosensitivity.

14.4 Instrumental Delivery

Instrumental delivery is a recognised cause of perineal trauma, which in turn is associated with urinary and anal incontinence. Randomised studies have confirmed that the vacuum extractor is associated with less perineal trauma than forceps delivery.[20,21] Using anal endosonography, Sultan et al.[22] identified occult anal sphincter defects in 80% of women undergoing forceps delivery. In another small randomised study of forceps and vacuum delivery, occult anal sphincter defects were identified in 79% of forceps compared with 48% of vacuum deliveries, and anal incontinence was reported in 32% and 16% respectively.[23] Donnelly et al.[13] reported a 7.2-fold increase in incidence of disturbed anal continence associated with a change in vector symmetry index following instrumental delivery.

14.5 Recognised Anal Sphincter Disruption

The incidence of third- and fourth-degree perineal tears varies according to the technique of episiotomy practised. Recent studies suggest rates of 11% in centres where midline episiotomy is practised, compared with 0.5–2.5% in centres where mediolateral episiotomy is practised.[24] In the last decade, 11 studies[24] have evaluated outcome following anal sphincter rupture and it is evident that about one-third of women continue to suffer from anal incontinence despite primary sphincter repair. A recently published long-term study[25] has revealed that anal incontinence prevails in 40% of women 5 years after primary repair. Anal sphincter defects have been demonstrated with endosonography in about 85% following conventional end-to-end primary repair of the anal sphincter.[25,26] Persistence of defaecatory symptoms is related more to a structural sphincter defect rather than a pudendal neuropathy.[26] Colorectal surgeons prefer to perform an overlap repair of the anal sphincter when treating faecal incontinence and a successful outcome has been reported in 76–100% of patients.[27] In a prospective study, Engel et al.[28] have reported that demonstration of overlap sonographically following anterior sphincter repair is associated with a good outcome. We therefore evaluated overlap repair as a primary procedure immediately after vaginal delivery (Figure 14.7) and found that this technique was not only feasible following acute disruption, but also produced exceptionally good results.[29] A randomised study of end-to-end versus overlap repair is currently being planned.

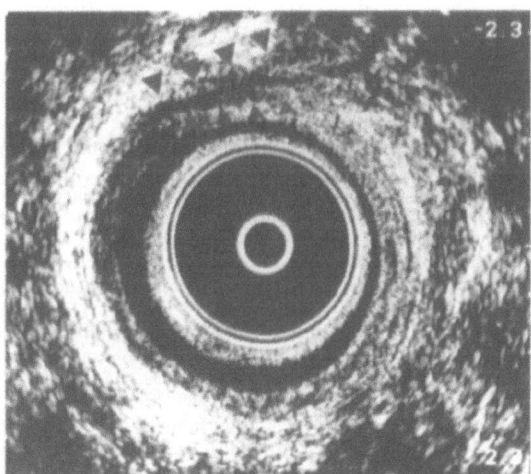

Figure 14.7 Endoanal image 3 months after a primary overlap repair of an obstetric third-degree tear. The arrows demonstrate the overlapping ends of the external anal sphincter.

14.6 Non-obstetric Trauma

Anal endosonography has also enabled a better understanding of the pathophysiology of faecal incontinence following non-obstetric injuries.

Engel et al.[30] demonstrated endosonographic evidence of internal sphincter damage in all seven subjects who experienced unwanted anal penetration, three of whom also had evidence of external sphincter dysfunction. As sexual abuse can have a devastating psychological effect, it is often undisclosed to the clinician. Therefore, unexplained internal sphincter disruption, particularly fragmented disruption, should alert the attending clinician of possible sexual abuse.

An anal stretch (Lord's) procedure has been and still is practised by some clinicians as a treatment for anal fissure and haemorrhoids. Anal incontinence has been noted in 27% of patients following this procedure and over 90% have sonographic and manometric evidence of internal anal sphincter disruption and 25% have associated external sphincter disruption.[31]

Lateral internal anal sphincterotomy, a popular surgical procedure in the treatment of anal fissure, is also associated with anal incontinence in up to 50% of patients.[32] A prospective endosonographic study has shown that, although the intention of the surgical procedure is to divide the distal one-third to one-half of the internal sphincter, in the vast majority of women the whole length of the sphincter was divided.[8]

Anal incontinence following surgical excision of haemorrhoids has been identified in 29% of patients.[33] There is now increasing evidence from anal endosonographic studies that inadvertent sphincter damage, especially of the internal sphincter, is a major contributory factor. It should be noted, however, that the sonographic appearances of haemorrhoids (Figure 14.8) can mimic an internal sphincter defect or anorectal prolapse. The true diagnosis can only be appreciated during dynamic scanning when the woman is asked to squeeze and strain.

Surgical treatment of fistula-in-ano is also associated with considerable sphincter trauma and persistent anal sphincter defects are demonstrable on anal endosonography. Up to 60% of patients can be rendered incontinent following fistula surgery.[34]

14.7 Conclusions

Anal endosonography has revolutionised our understanding and management of anal incontinence. Vaginal delivery is a major aetiological factor in the development of anal sphincter injury. The development of anal endosonography has enabled identification of occult anal sphincter trauma in

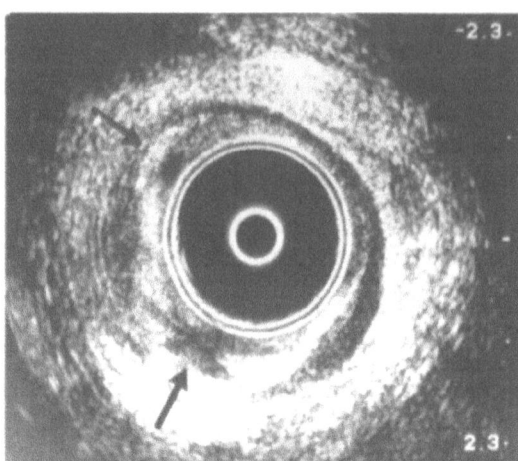

Figure 14.8 Endoanal image demonstrating haemorrhoids distorting the internal sphincter.

about of one-third of primiparous vaginal deliveries. The majority of women have persistent anal sphincter defects despite primary sphincter repair. Instrumental delivery is a major independent factor in the development of sphincter injury. However, there are many factors apart from obstetric injury that can injure the anal sphincter mechanism, such as anorectal surgery, sexual abuse, neuropathy and degeneration of the internal sphincter; these should be excluded before surgical intervention. Although anal endosonography is now regarded as the gold standard investigation, other tests such as manometry may be useful in evaluating functional compromise.

References

1. Frentzel-Beyme B (1982) Die transrektale prostatasonographie. Computertomogr Sonogr Juni 2(2):58–112
2. Beynon J, Foy DMA, Temple LN et al. (1986) The endosonic appearances of the normal colon and rectum. Dis Colon Rectum 29:810–813
3. Law PJ, Bartram CI (1989) Anal endosonography: technique and normal anatomy. Gastrointest Radiol 14:349–353
4. Sultan AH, Kamm MA, Hudson CN et al. (1994) Endosonography of the anal sphincters: normal anatomy and comparison with manometry. Clin Rad 49:368–374
5. Sultan AH (1995) The effect of childbirth on the anal sphincters as demonstrated by anal endosonography and anorectal physiology. MD Thesis, University of Natal, South Africa
6. Sultan AH, Nicholls RJ, Kamm MA et al. (1993) Anal endosonography and correlation with in vitro and in vivo anatomy. Br J Surg 80:508–511
7. Sultan AH, Kamm MA, Talbot IC et al. (1994) Anal endosonography: precision of identifying sphincter defects confirmed histologically. Br J Surg 81:466–469
8. Sultan AH, Kamm MA, Nicholls RJ et al. (1994) Internal anal sphincter division during lateral sphincterotomy. Prospective ultrasound study. Dis Colon Rectum 37:1031–1033
9. Vaizey CJ, Kamm MA, Bartram CI (1997) Primary degeneration of the internal anal sphincter as a cause of passive faecal incontinence. Lancet 349:612–615.
10. Sultan AH, Loder PB, Bartram CI et al. (1994) Vaginal endosonography: a new technique to image the undisturbed anal sphincter. Dis Colon Rectum 37:1296–1299
11. Poen AC, Felt-Bersma RJF, Cuesta MA et al. (1998) Vaginal endosonography of the anal sphincter complex is important in the assessment of faecal incontinence and perianal sepsis. Br J Surg 85:359–363
12. Meyenberger C, Bertschinger P, Zala GF et al. (1996) Anal sphincter defects in fecal incontinence: correlation between endosonography and surgery. Endoscopy 28:217–224
13. Donnelly V, Fynes M, Campbell D et al. (1998) Obstetric events leading to anal sphincter damage. Obstet Gynecol 92:955–961
14. Peschers UM, DeLancey JOL, Schaer GN et al. (1997) Exoanal ultrasound of the anal sphincter: normal anatomy and sphincter defects. Br J Obstet Gynaecol 104:999–1003
15. Stoker J, Hussain SM, Lameris JS (1996) Endoanal magnetic resonance imaging versus endosonography. La Radiologia Medica 92:738–741
16. MacArthur C, Bick DE, Keighley MRB (1997) Faecal incontinence after childbirth. Br J Obstet Gynaecol 104:46–50
17. Allen RE, Hosker GL, Smith ARB et al. (1990) Pelvic floor damage and childbirth: a neurophysiological study. Br J Obstet Gynaecol 97:770–779
18. Sultan AH, Kamm MA, Hudson CN et al. (1993) Anal sphincter disruption during vaginal delivery. N Engl J Med 329:1905–1911
19. Chaliha C, Sultan AH, Bland M (2001) Anal function: effect of pregnancy and delivery. Am J Obstet Gynecol 185:427–432
20. Johanson RB, Rice C, Doyle M et al. (1993) A randomised prospective study comparing the new vacuum extractor policy with forceps delivery. Br J Obstet Gynaecol 100:524–530
21. Bofill JA, Rust OA, Schorr SJ et al. (1996) A randomized prospective trial of the obstetric forceps versus the M-cup vacuum extractor. Am J Obstet Gynecol 175:1325–1330
22. Sultan AH, Kamm MA, Bartram CI et al. (1993) Anal sphincter trauma during instrumental delivery. A comparison between forceps and vacuum extraction. Int J Gynecol Obstet 43:263–270
23. Sultan AH, Johanson RB, Carter JE (1998) Occult anal sphincter trauma following randomized forceps and vacuum delivery. Int J Gynecol Obstet 61:113–119
24. Sultan AH (1997) Anal incontinence after childbirth. Curr Opin Obstet Gynecol 9:320–324
25. Poen AC, Felt-Bersma RJF, Strijers RLM et al. (1998) Third-degree obstetric perineal tear: long-term clinical and functional results after primary repair. Br J Surg 85:1433–1438
26. Sultan AH, Kamm MA, Hudson CN et al. (1994) Third degree obstetric anal sphincter tears: risk factors and outcome of primary repair. BMJ 308:887–891
27. Jorge JMN, Wexner SD (1993) Etiology and management of fecal incontinence. Dis Colon Rectum 36:77–97
28. Engel AF, Kamm MA, Sultan AH et al. (1994) Anterior anal sphincter repair in patients with obstetric trauma. Br J Surg 81:1231–1234
29. Sultan AH, Monga AK, Kumar D et al. (1999) Primary repair of obstetric anal sphincter rupture using the overlap technique. Br J Obstet Gynaecol 106:318–323
30. Engel AF, Kamm MA, Bartram CI (1995) Unwanted anal penetration as a physical cause of faecal incontinence. Europ J Gastroenterol Hepatol 7:65–67
31. Speakman CTM, Burnett SJD, Kamm MA et al. (1991) Sphincter injury after anal dilatation demonstrated by anal endosonography. Br J Surg 78:1429–1430
32. Khubchandani IT, Reed JF (1989) Sequelae of internal sphincterotomy for chronic fissure in ano. Br J Surg 76:431–434
33. Bennett RC, Friedman MHW, Goligher JC (1963) Late results of haemorrhoidectomy by ligature and excision. BMJ 2:216–219.
34. Kennedy HL, Zegarra JP (1990) Fistulotomy without external sphincter division for high anal fistula. Br J Surg 77:898–901
35. Sultan AH, Kamm MA (1993) Ultrasound of the anal sphincter. In: Schuster MA (ed) Atlas of gastrointestinal motility: in health and disease. Williams and Wilkins, Baltimore, pp 115–120

Chapter 15

Laparoscopic Treatment of Uterine and Vault Prolapse

Arnaud Wattiez, Reinaldo Goldchmit, Stephen Chew, Michel Canis, Gérard Mage, Jean-Luc Pouly and Maurice-Antoine Bruhat

15.1 Introduction

Urogenital prolapse is a frequent functional pathology resulting mainly from loss of tone and laxity of pelvic supports due to deliveries and ageing.[1,2] Obesity, pulmonary pathologies that increase intra-abdominal pressure and huge myomatous uteri may also be contributory.

Uterine prolapse is frequently associated with cystocele, urethrocele, rectocele and enterocele of different degrees. Urinary incontinence is also usually present.[1,2] Surgical treatment has to be durable and treat all the affected structures. Several surgical techniques exist;[3,4] the method with the least morbidity and the best long-term results should be chosen.

The technique of promontofixation was conceptualised by Freund in 1889, but it was Otto Kustner who first used this technique in 1890 to treat prolapse in menopausal women. The first operations were performed using cutaneous flaps but in 1958, Huguier and Scali first described promontofixation by laparotomy with mersylene.[5] In 1974, Scali[6] modified the technique, which consisted of two parts: an anterior component forming the subvesical support and a posterior component that assisted in promontofixation.

Both laparotomy and the vaginal approach are useful in the management of uterine prolapse. The disadvantage of open laparotomy is the difficulty in correcting a rectocele or enterocele. In the presence of the latter, the vaginal approach might offer better results but promontofixation would then be impossible. With the advent of better instrumentation and advanced endoscopic suturing techniques, investigators from our department performed our first laparoscopic promontofixation in 1991. We believe our technique offers the advantages of both open laparotomy and the vaginal approach, enabling the correction of cystoceles, stress incontinence, uterine prolapse and rectoceles. In this chapter, we will describe our technique of laparoscopic promontofixation.

15.2 Positioning of the Patient

The legs are abducted and stretched to provide easy vaginal access. The stirrups are placed relatively low in relation to the table so that the surgeon can insert the suprapubic trocars properly and manipulate the instruments freely. The buttocks are also placed at the edge of the table to allow easy manipulation of the uterus. A shoulder brace is always used with the arms fixed alongside the patient's body. Bladder drainage with a size 18 Foley's catheter is also essential.

The surgeon stands on the left, with the first assistant on the right and the second assistant between the legs to manipulate the uterus.

15.3 Placement of Trocars

As endoscopic suturing is required during the laparoscopic treatment of prolapse, correct placement of trocars to aid this suturing is essential. Four trocars are needed: one 10 mm umbilical trocar for the optics; one 10 mm trocar in the lower abdominal wall in the midline for easy introduction of needles and mesh; two 5 mm trocars in the lower abdomen, lateral to the border of the rectus abdominis muscle (approximately 3 cm medial to the anterior superior iliac spine). For the sake of ergonomics, the lower central trocar should not be lower than the horizontal line between the lateral trocars. If the distance between the lower central trocar and the umbilical trocar is less than 8 cm, the umbilical trocar is used for instumentation while another 10 mm trocar for the optics is placed above the umbilicus in the midline.

15.4 Technique

Two techniques may be used. The first involves a unilateral fixation preferably on the right side, since the rectosigmoid on the left does not allow a subperitoneal path. In the second technique, described by Scali, a bilateral fixation with two pieces of mesh is used. These two techniques have similar steps of dissection and fixation to the promontory. We prefer the second method as it offers a better support with the same operative time.

During surgery, three fundamental principles have to be observed:

- suspension of the uterus to restore its physiological position and re-creation of a solid subvesical layer;
- treatment of the urinary stress incontinence even if the patient is asymptomatic. It is an illusion to treat only the uterine prolapse, as correction of prolapse will increase the incontinence;
- posterior reconstruction of the rectovaginal support.

Treatment of uterine prolapse involves three steps:

- anterior dissection, where the mesh is placed between the bladder and vagina, passed through the broad ligament and attached to the promontory;
- posterior dissection;
- colposuspension.

15.4.1 Anterior Dissection

15.4.1.1 Preparation of Vesicouterine and Vesicovaginal Space

The uterus is first pushed up with slight retroversion by the second assistant. The first assistant provides upward traction of the prevesical peritoneum by applying a grasping forceps to the peritoneum in the midline approximately 1 cm below the uterovesical fold of peritoneum. The peritoneum is then cauterised and sectioned perpendicular to the uterus to avoid bladder damage. This combination of incision of peritoneum and the pushing up of the uterus will facilitate opening of the vesicovaginal space. The bladder is gently dissected and pushed downward. The vesicovaginal space is limited

laterally by the two vesicovaginal pillars, which tend to converge down at the level of the posterior urethra. The dissection is then carried out in the midline, as low as possible and close to the bladder neck to allow the anterior attachment of the mesh (Figure 15.1). The mesh has to be placed near the bladder neck. The pneumoperitoneum also helps this dissection, which can usually be performed without any bleeding.

15.4.1.2 Dissection of Broad Ligament

The dissection of the broad ligament occurs at the level of the isthmus but at a distance from the uterine vessels. The uterus is first slightly anteverted and displaced laterally, which aids dissection of the contralateral broad ligament. The vessels of the broad ligament are then coagulated until the posterior layer of the broad ligament is seen. A grey appearance of the posterior layer of the broad ligament indicates an absence of bowel behind it and an incision can then be made. The opening in the broad ligament is initially in the direction of the origin of the uterosacral ligaments and enlarged by divergent traction with two instruments.

The passage of the mesh through the broad ligament requires careful dissection. In the case of a unilateral attachment, the posterior layer does not have to be perforated. A tunnel within the peritoneum is made from the promontory to the right margin of isthmus, allowing an extraperitoneal pathway. Hence the mesh will remain outside the peritoneal cavity in this procedure.

In the case of bilateral mesh attachment, which we recommend, the posterior peritoneum of broad ligament must be opened.

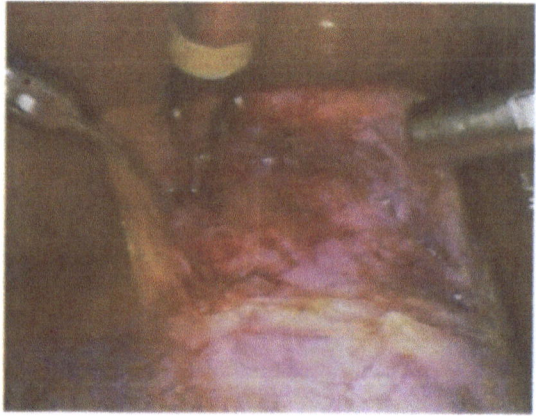

Figure 15.1 Preparation of the vesicouterine space.

15.4.1.3 Posterior Dissection

The junction of the two uterosacral ligaments is first identified and the peritoneum is cauterised and dissected 2 cm below this point. This dissection is then continued down to a point 1 cm from the fourchette. The right and left meshes are tied at the back of the uterus, with a knot.

15.4.1.4 Preparation of the Promontory

The approach to the promontory can be done only after careful identification of L5–S1, the inferior limit of the left common iliac vein and the right ureter. The patient has to be in the Trendelenburg position with the bowel pushed back. In some patients, anchoring of the bowel to the abdominal wall is necessary to afford better visualisation. To accomplish this, a needle is introduced in the left abdominal flank, passed through the mesosigmoid and brought out near the point of entry in the abdominal wall.

After identification of the right ureter and the inferior limit of the left common iliac vessels, the prevertebral parietal peritoneum is then incised vertically from the promontory and retracting the ureter laterally. The common anterior vertebral ligament is then identified and mobilised sufficiently to allow the identification of the median sacral vessels and adequate suturing. The median sacral vessels are generally not coagulated unless they interfere with suturing and cannot be displaced laterally.

The dissection is then continued vertically downwards to meet the incision on the peritoneum that opens into the rectovaginal space.

15.4.1.5 Fixation of Mesh in the Vesicovaginal Space

The mesh is introduced by the 10 mm trocar. We use mersylene mesh due to its strength and its elasticity in its longitudinal axis. It is cut in the form of a "V". The length of the mesh is estimated by pushing the uterus towards L5–S1. The mesh should not be too tight (risk of cutting through).

The larger portion of the mesh is spread out in the vesicovaginal space and the two straps of the mesh are then introduced through the window created in the broad ligament. They are tied posteriorly al the level of the isthmus of the uterus (Figure 15.2).

The mesh is then sutured to the anterior vaginal wall with mersuture 2/0 and a 23 mm needle (Ethicon, Neuilly, France) without penetrating the vagina. Extracorporeal knots are used. Six to eight sutures are usually necessary to obtain a solid

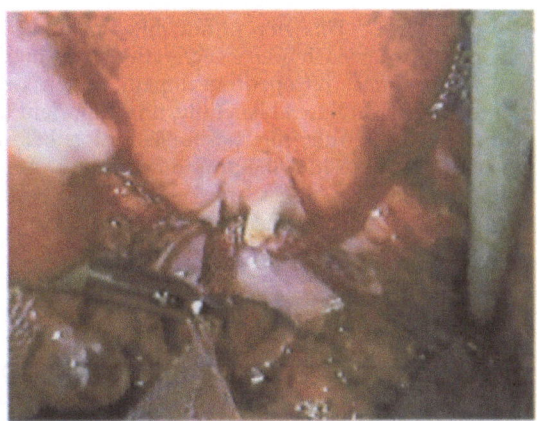

Figure 15.2 Tying of mesh over posterior aspect of uterus.

attachment (Figure 15.3). It is not necessary to obtain a perfect attachment of the mesh since infiltration by fibroblasts and fibrosis will occur.

15.4.1.6 Promontofixation

Promontofixation is accomplished by suturing the two mesh straps to the common anterior vertebral ligament at the level of the promontory with one or two sutures of ethibond 1, using a 30 mm curved needle (Ethicon). The needle should be passed carefully under direct vision to avoid any risk of spondilodiscitis and perforation of the disc (Figure 15.4). Once the two sutures are fixed, traction is applied to confirm its strength (Figure 15.5).

15.4.1.7 Peritonealisation

The peritoneum is closed from the promontory to the Pouch of Douglas using two or three separate

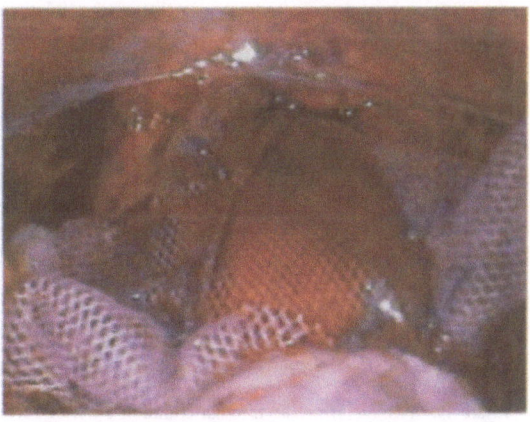

Figure 15.3 Fixation of mesh in vesicovaginal space.

Vicryl sutures.[10] This step is not difficult but it is important to avoid bowel incarceration. The mesh will have a final retroperitoneal path. When two pieces of mesh are used bilaterally, it is important to complete the retrouterine peritonealisation before fixation of the mesh to the promontory.

At the end of surgery, the uterus is correctly positioned and haemostasis secured.

15.4.2 Posterior Step

A posterior step is usually necessary. The uterus or vaginal vault is first maximally anteverted. Rectovaginal dissection is then performed, keeping in mind the need to maintain contact with the vagina. The rectum is identified with a Hegar's dilator. The dissection is continued to a point 1 cm short of the fourchette. Lateral dissection of the rectum is also necessary to identify the levator ani muscles. The mersylene mesh is then fixed to the vagina (Figure 15.6). Approximation of the levators may be accomplished with a few ethibond 1 sutures (Ethicon) (Figure 15.7). Obliteration of the Pouch of Douglas will complete the treatment of posterior prolapse.

15.4.3 Burch Colposuspension

Similar to the technique described by laparotomy, laparoscopic Burch colposuspension[7] is also performed to treat associated urinary stress incontinence or to avoid changing the vesicourethral angle due to excessive traction of the mesh towards the promontory. Asymptomatic urinary stress incontinence may become clinically evident if this step is not performed.[1,8]

We perform the laparoscopic Burch colposuspension by the transperitoneal approach. The perito-

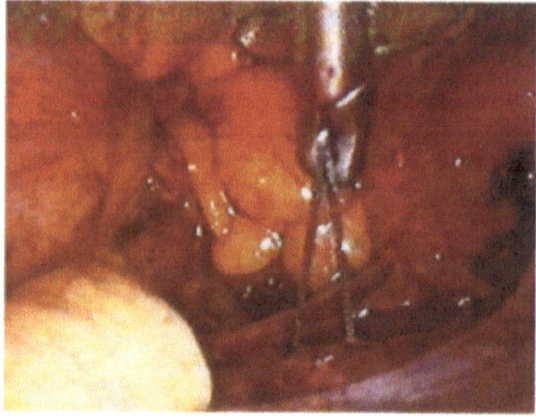

Figure 15.5 Traction of promontory suture to confirm strength.

neum is incised above the bladder dome. The assistant then applies downward traction of the peritoneum with a pair of grasping forceps. This will aid the surgeon in making a horizontal incision from one umbilical artery to the other.

The urachus is cauterised and sectioned and dissection continued vertically in the direction of the anterior abdominal wall. The umbilico-prevesical fascia is dissected and the avascular space opened up. Pneumodissection also helps this dissection to reach the cave of Retzius. Several tissue layers are successively opened while maintaining contact with the apponeuroses until adipose tissue just before the Cooper's ligament is reached. The Cooper's ligaments are then identified along with the transverse ligament of the perineum.

A finger is placed in the vagina and the portion of the lateral vaginal wall where the suture will be placed is prepared by dissecting off the superficial tissue. The combination of pushing the lateral vaginal wall with the finger while displacing the bladder medially with the bipolar forceps will bring

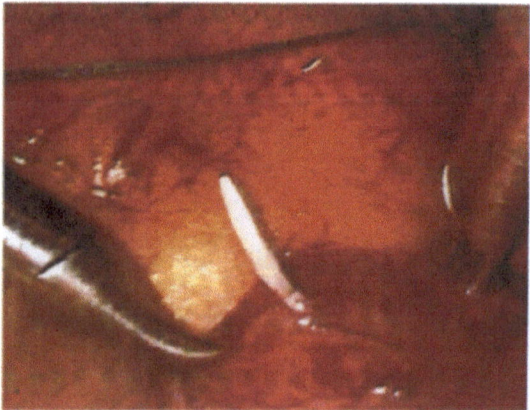

Figure 15.4 Passage of needle through common anterior vertebal ligament over promontory.

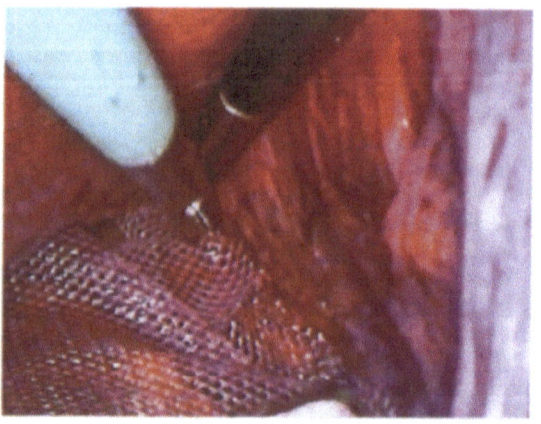

Figure 15.6 Posterior placement of mesh.

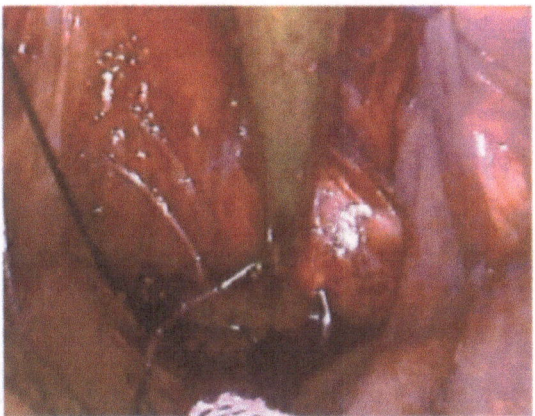

Figure 15.7 Approximation of levator ani muscles.

into view the site where the sutures will be placed. The limits of the bladder are often revealed by the presence of a vein, which must be carefully separated and coagulated if necessary.

Suturing is performed using an ethibond 0, with a 26 mm needle (Ethicon). The suture is first passed through the Cooper's ligaments from above downwards with the needle holder inserted through the left trocar. The lateral vaginal vault is then sutured with the needle passing in a medial to lateral direction. In the case of promontofixation, one suture is enough on each side and extracorporeal knotting is performed.

At the end, reperitonealisation is performed with two or three Vicryl 0 sutures to avoid bowel incarceration.

15.5 Alternative Techniques

It is also possible to treat a vault prolapse with the technique of promontofixation.[9,10] A Hegar's dilator is first placed in the vagina to help the dissection between the bladder and vagina. The rest of the operation is similar to the procedure described above, except that a linear strap of mersylene mesh (2 cm wide × 20 cm long) is used and an extra-peritoneal path of the mesh is created in this case. Two incisions are made: one on the promontory and the other at the level of the rectovaginal dissection. The mesh is then fixed anteriorly and passed to the promontory.

If a subtotal hysterectomy has to be combined with a promontofixation, the uterine cervix is preserved and used to attach the mesh. This avoids the opening of the vagina, which may theoretically diminish the risk of infection. A linear mesh is also used. For these cases we use a morcellator to remove

the uterus. Also, complete dissection of the peritoneum is not necessary. It is sufficient to just create a retroperitoneal tunnel from the promontory and leading to the cervical stump.

15.6 Complications

Several complications are associated with the laparoscopic treatment of uterine and vault prolapse.

15.6.1 Complications During Dissection

15.6.1.1 Vesicovaginal Space

The two main complications that can arise during dissection of the vesicovaginal space include bladder damage and haemorrhage. They are usually due to dissection in the wrong plane. Ureteric injury is also rare but may occur at the ureteric junction if the surgeon dissects too laterally.

15.6.1.2 Broad Ligament

Haemorrhage may occur because of adnexal or uterine vein injury. Injury to the sigmoid is rare but may occur if the sigmoid is in the Pouch of Douglas during the opening of the broad ligament. To avoid this complication, the opening of the broad ligament should be done only after excluding the presence of bowel behind it.

15.6.1.3 Rectovaginal Space

Dissection of this space is usually difficult. Haemorrhage and rectal injury may occur. To avoid these complications, principles of good traction and dissection close to the vagina should be observed.

15.6.1.4 Promontory

During dissection of the promontory, several complications are possible: bowel injury, ureteric injury (mainly the right ureter), median sacral artery or left iliac vein injury. To avoid these accidents, an accentuated Trendelenburg may be used to push back the bowel and transparietal fixation of the sigmoid may be necessary.

15.6.1.5 Posterior Peritoneum

During the dissection in the Pouch of Douglas, ureteric damage or bowel injury and haemorrhage may occur. These accidents may be avoided if the dissection is carried out from the promontory down to the rectovaginal space and paying careful attention to always keeping in contact with the peritoneum. This should minimise the chance of inadvertant injury to the surrounding structures.

15.6.1.6 Retzius Space

Dissection of the Retzius space may be complicated by bladder injury and haemorrhage. The bladder is commonly injured during the opening of the peritoneum. Haemorrhage is rarer but may occasionally occur when the urachus or the umbilical arteries are cut. Any injury to the obturator vessels or to the inferior obturator vein can result in significant bleeding. Thus, a good knowledge of the anatomy of this region is essential.

15.6.2 Complications due to Fixation

15.6.2.1 Loosely Applied Meshes and Sutures

Loose application of mesh and sutures (or staples) may occur during promontofixation. Undue laxity of the applied mesh is a common problem and may occur at the vesicovaginal attachment or at the promontory.

15.6.2.2 Infection

Although rare, infections may be severe due to the presence of the mesh (foreign body). Asepsis is essential and where possible, the needle should avoid entering the vagina during suturing. Preservation of the uterus or subtotal hysterectomy may also reduce the risk of infection since the vagina is not opened.

15.6.2.3 Urinary Complications

Urinary retention or incontinence may occur. Retention is usually due to the excessive elevation of the bladder neck. To avoid this problem, a suture should not be placed closer than 15 mm from the junction. Urodynamic studies identify patients at risk and are of great prognostic value.

Urinary incontinence may occur as the result of excessive correction of the prolapse, resulting in the opening of the urethrovesical angle.

15.7 Conclusions

A laparoscopic approach for stress incontinence and prolapse is possible.[4] Nezhat et al. demonstrated satisfactory results in a series where all the women had a vault prolapse after hysterectomy.[9]

Workers have reported that promontofixation is a sure and efficient technique for the treatment of uterine prolapse (with or without uterine preservation).[6,11] The procedure can also help reorientate the uterovaginal axis and provide the patient with satisfactory functional support. The Burch colposuspension can also effectively treat urinary incontinence while promontofixation can correct the cystocele.

Laparoscopy has the advantages of conventional treatment of prolapse and the low morbidity of the vaginal approach, i.e., less haemorrhage, less infection, less hospitalization, better postoperative recovery and more rapid return to normal activity. Based on the technique and the results obtained by laparotomy, laparoscopic promontofixation may thus represent the ideal surgery for women with complex urogenital prolapse.

References

1. DeLancey JO (1993) Anatomy and biomechanics of genital prolapse. Clin Obstet Gynecol 36:897–909
2. Norton PA (1993) Pelvic floor disorders: the role of fascia and ligaments. Clin Obstet Gynecol 36:926–938
3. Imparato E, Aspesi G, Rovetta E et al. (1992) Surgical management and prevention of vaginal vault prolapse. Surg Gynecol Obstet 175:233–237
4. Wattiez A, Boughizane S, Alexandre F et al. (1995) Laparoscopic procedures for stress incontinence and prolapse. Curr Opin Obstet Gynecol 7:317–321
5. Huguier J, Scali P (1958) La suspension posterieure de l'axe genital au disque lombo-sacre dans le traitement de certains prolapsus. Presse Med 66:781–784
6. Scali P, Blondon J, Bethoux A et al. (1974) Operations of support-suspension by upper route in the treatment of vaginal prolapse. J Gynecol Obstet Biol Reprod (Paris) 3:365–378
7. Burch JC (1961) Urethrovaginal fixation to Cooper's ligament for correction of stress incontinence, cystocele and prolapse. Am J Obstet Gynecol 81:281
8. DeLancey L (1994) Structural support of urethra as it relates to stress urinary incontinence: the hammock hypothesis. Am J Obstet Gynecol 170:1713–1720
9. Nezhat CH, Nezhat F, Nezhat C (1994) Laparoscopy sacral colpopexy for vaginal vault prolapse. Obstet Gynecol 84:885–888
10. Voltz J, Strittmatter H, Voltz E et al. (1993) Pelviscopy sacropexy in treatment of vaginal prolapse. Geburtshilfe frauenheilkd 53:705–708
11. Timmons MC, Addison WA, Addison SB et al. (1992) Abdominal sacral colpopexy in 163 women with posthysterectomy vaginal vault prolapse and enterocele. J Reprod Med 37:323–327

Chapter 16

Enterocele Repair

Jonathan-David Broome and Thierry G. Vancaillie

16.1 Introduction

An enterocele is a herniation through the vaginal support structures, of a peritoneum-lined sac containing small bowel or omentum. Most commonly, this herniation occurs posteriorly between the rectum and vagina, but theoretically, it may present anywhere along the vaginal axis. The occurrence of an enterocele in isolation is unusual, except in patients who have undergone previous hysterectomy, bladder neck surgery or pelvic floor repair. More often, it is a component of general pelvic floor relaxation with accompanying rectocele, cystocele, or uterine or vaginal vault prolapse. The diagnosis of enterocele in these circumstances can sometimes be difficult. A combined rectovaginal examination with the patient bearing down may detect a palpable loop of bowel between thumb and index finger leading to the diagnosis; however, this is not always the case and occasionally an enterocele is only discovered intraoperatively. Ultrasound assessment of the pelvic floor increases the diagnostic accuracy of prolapse, allowing proper planning of corrective surgery.

The transvaginal ultrasound diagnosis of enterocele is usually obvious due to the characteristic features of small bowel in the hernial sac. The presence of gas in the bowel lumen causes a distinctive pattern of hyper- and hypoechogenicity. Changes in the echogenicity and appearance of this pattern due to peristalsis can usually be seen. If intra- or extraluminal fluid is present, the detail of the sac contents displayed is improved substantially. The hypoechogenic wall of small bowel can be seen to surround the intraluminal fluid, low-level echoes can be seen to swirl within the fluid, and the diameter of the lumen will vary as the bowel peristalses. The small bowel peristalses frequently and contains numerous echogenic mural folds corresponding to the plicae circulares, unlike the large bowel, which can be identified by its larger luminal diameter, reduced peristalsis and less numerous haustral folds.

Transvaginal and perineal ultrasound, in experienced hands, can provide excellent views of the pelvic anatomy and the supporting structures.[1] Movement of the pelvic floor is clearly demonstrated during dynamic assessment with the patient performing Valsalva's manoeuvre. The posterior vaginal wall rotates around the anterior, inferior border of the pubic symphysis in a downward and forward direction on increasing intra-abdominal pressure. This movement occurs in all women to some degree, but is greatly exaggerated in women with prolapse. The amount of movement can be quantified as the displacement measured by ultrasound directly correlates to the degree of prolapse detected by clinical examination. The perineal probe is more suitable for dynamic assessment of prolapse compared to the transvaginal approach, as its positioning on the perineum provides an overall view of the movement of the pelvic floor without causing local distortion of the anatomy. The perineal probe is more comfortable for the patient when straining and is less likely to be displaced during raised intra-abdominal pressure.

The results of prolapse surgery are often disappointing, with many patients undergoing further surgical procedures for recurrence. Although the use of ultrasound postoperatively is mainly of academic interest, objective evaluation of surgical outcome may lead to improvements in operative techniques.

The aetiology of enterocele formation is multifactorial. Genetic predisposition is probably a major factor. Parity, obstetric and surgical damage, the loss of oestrogen at menopause and causes of a chronic increase in intra-abdominal pressure all contribute to the pathophysiological process.[2]

The symptoms associated with an enterocele are usually vague and variable. Patients often describe a feeling of pelvic heaviness or fullness and a sensation of bearing down; these are often exacerbated by standing. A mass protruding through the vulva may cause local vaginal discomfort, and in the presence of ulceration, bleeding and discharge may occur. An often overlooked symptom is the inability to have normal sexual intercourse.

Nichols[3] describes four types of enterocele (Table 16.1). The aims of surgical repair are to:

- identify the hernia sac;
- identify the defect in the support structures through which the hernia occurred;
- close the defect without tension.

The repair will result in restoration of normal vaginal depth and axis. Enterocele repair is rarely carried out in isolation; it is more commonly part of a larger intervention to correct genital prolapse.

The anatomical findings in patients presenting with an enterocele, regardless of aetiology, are thinning or rupture of the fascial structures (Denonvilliers' fascia, endopelvic fascia) and widening of the hiatus between both levator ani muscles. The difficulties encountered in achieving adequate repair of an enterocele by the vaginal approach led to the development of abdominal techniques such as the Moschcowitz, Halban and McCall procedures. Recent achievements in our understanding of the functional anatomy of the pelvic floor, combined with advances in endoscopic surgery, have led to the development of laparoscopic techniques to correct enterocele. Initial reports were related to the McCall procedure, employing excision of the hernial sac and approximation of the uterosacral ligaments.[4] Use of the carbon dioxide laser to vapourise the hernial peritoneum, causing retraction of the cul-de-sac, before approximating the uterosacral ligaments, has also been described.[5] Both these techniques employed a vaginal approach to approximate the levator muscles where necessary. More recently, laparoscopic closure of the levator hiatus has been reported.[6] In view of the anatomical defects present,

we propose that surgical correction of an enterocele consists of approximation of the levator muscles to reduce the levator hiatus, closure of fascial tears, reinforcement of the fascial tissues, where necessary using a graft, either autologous (vaginal skin) or artificial (surgical mesh), and plication of the uterosacral ligaments to close the neck of the enterocele. These procedures need not be performed exclusively by laparoscopy; indeed, the combination of defects seen in pelvic floor relaxation often requires a combined vaginal/abdominal approach.

16.2 Procedures for Enterocele Repair

16.2.1 Vaginal Approach

Repair of a defect of the posterior vaginal wall can be achieved without recourse to an abdominal approach when there is a small enterocele in the presence of a dominant rectocele, and sufficient support is identified at the level of the upper posterior vaginal wall and vaginal vault. If the defect in Denonvilliers' fascia extends from the perineal body to below the upper third of the posterior vagina, repair may be best achieved by the vaginal approach.

16.2.2 Combined Vaginal and Laparoscopic Approach

The combined approach can be employed when there is a dominant enterocele associated with a rectocele and good vaginal vault support is not available. It is used in the young patient, in whom sufficient vaginal length is desired, to correct a posterior vaginal wall defect or vaginal vault prolapse when there is an accompanying perineal defect, and also in cases where there are co-existing posterior and anterior vaginal wall defects. When maintaining vaginal length is not a priority, the laparoscopic approach can be omitted. This decision

Table 16.1. Causes of enteroceles

Cause	Location	Treatment
Congenital	Sac between posterior vaginal wall and anterior rectal wall	Excise sac, high ligation of neck, approximation of uterosacral ligaments
Pulsion	Eversion of vaginal vault	Shorten cardinal and uterosacral ligaments or culdoplasty; if ligaments poor, sacrospinous fixation or sacrocolpopexy; coincident hysterectomy often desirable
Traction	Lower eversion pulling vault into eversion	Same as above with anterior and posterior colporrhaphy
Iatrogenic	Anterior to vaginal wall or posterior, due to change in vaginal axis	Excise or obliterate sac and restore normal vaginal axis

is made intraoperatively when the surgeon estimates to have satisfactory attachment of the vagina to the vertical axis of support.

16.2.3 Laparoscopic Approach

This method of repair can be employed when there is recurrence of an enterocele or when an enterocele occurs in isolation, particularly when there is upper vaginal wall prolapse but good perineal support in patients where maintenance of vaginal length is important. Quite often these patients have previously undergone a posterior repair for rectocele. Occasionally, subclinical enterocele is identified at the time of laparoscopic bladder neck suspension, and a prophylactic laparoscopic repair can then be undertaken.

16.2.4 Use of Vaginal Skin Graft

In patients undergoing a combined vaginal and laparoscopic procedure, particularly when there is an associated rectocele and where there is sufficient vaginal mucosa, this can be harvested and used as a graft to reinforce Denonvilliers' fascia. In most cases the graft leads to inclusion cysts, which occasionally cause symptoms related to their size only. The use of vaginal skin as a graft has been promoted by Zacharin.[7]

16.2.5 Use of Vicryl Mesh Graft

In cases where support structures cannot be brought together without tension, a synthetic mesh can be used. It can also be employed for repair of recurrent enterocele and when there are combined anterior and posterior defects. Our personal preference is Vicryl mesh, which is absorbable, remaining in the body long enough to cause fibrosis, while unlikely to erode through the vaginal wall, rectum or bladder.

16.2.6 Use of Marlex or Prolene Mesh

The use of non-absorbable mesh for the repair of posterior wall defects is confined to sacrocolpopexy, where the mesh is used to connect the perineal body to the promontorium. These are cases in which the vertical axis is considered insufficient. All other defects are closed using Vicryl mesh as a tissue enhancer.

16.3 Surgical Technique

16.3.1 Combined Vaginal and Laparoscopic Approach

The procedure is started vaginally. A transverse incision is made at the posterior fourchette to isolate the perineum from the vaginal mucosa. Two parallel longitudinal incisions are made into the vaginal mucosa approximately 3 cm apart, and a strip of vaginal mucosa is separated from the underlying fascia and rectum. The dissection is continued up to the apex or posterior fornix of the vagina, where the strip of vaginal tissue is cut off and placed in saline for later use. Using sharp dissection, the lateral walls of the vagina are separated from the underlying connective tissues to expose the endopelvic fascia. The rectal pillars are invariably dissected free during this process. Dissection continues until the entire enterocele defect is exposed and the levator muscle clearly identifiable; care is taken not to open the peritoneum. Four to six sutures are used to approximate the levator muscles in front of the rectum. The sutures are loosely tied. It is not necessary to pull the muscles together, as the length of the suture line is the more important factor determining success, and any gap left will be bridged by the graft. The vaginal graft is placed mucosal side down over the levator muscle suture line and attached to the perineal body proximally and to the levator plate laterally. The remnants of Denonvilliers' fascia are identified, and if possible, sutured together in front of the graft to close the defect. The vaginal skin is closed with interrupted absorbable sutures.

The laparoscopy is started in the usual fashion, using four trocars in total, two 10 mm trocars umbilically and suprapubically, and two 5 mm trocars laterally. Anatomical landmarks are identified: rectum, pararectal gutters, vagina, bladder, uterosacral ligaments and ureters. The initial surgical step is to resect the peritoneum of the hernial sac. An incision is made extending along the inside of one uterosacral ligament, across the posterior aspect of the vagina, and down the other. A flap of peritoneum, attached posteriorly to the rectum, is created. The next step is to suture the vaginal skin graft to the uterosacral ligaments on both sides. An effort is made to place the initial sutures as low as possible, thus completing the reinforcement of Denonvilliers' fascia. The vagina is then attached, without tension, to the graft. The peritoneal incision is closed with interrupted sutures to cover the graft.

Following completion of the procedure, the position of the ureters should be checked, as they are invariably displaced medially. Should there be any obstruction to the ureter, the peritoneum can be incised along its medial border to relieve the tension. The incision need not be deep, as the ureter lies immediately below the peritoneum and above the endopelvic fascia at this level. These relief incisions will therefore not weaken the newly created pelvic floor.

16.3.2 Laparoscopic Approach

Laparoscopy is started in the usual manner, using the same trocars as detailed above. Following identification of anatomical landmarks, the enterocele is reduced digitally by the operator under laparoscopic vision. An assessment is made of the degree of vaginal wall elevation and uterosacral displacement likely to result when the defect is closed. It is our experience that wide defects cause excessive displacement of the ureters when sutures are used to occlude the enterocele, and in these circumstances we employ an alternative procedure using Vicryl mesh to bridge the gap between the uterosacral ligaments. The initial surgical step is the same. The peritoneum is divided on the inside along the uterosacral ligaments and across the posterior aspect of the vagina, creating a flap of peritoneum, which is then resected from the rectum. With the aid of sharp and blunt dissection, the rectovaginal septum is entered. The enterocele defect is now visible. Closure of the defect is achieved by opposing the uterosacral ligaments. The first suture is inserted through the right uterosacral ligament, 2–3 cm in front of its dorsal insertion, and into the rectovaginal septum in the midline. The suture is tied, causing the vaginal wall to be elevated and the uterosacral ligament displaced medially. The position of the ureter is checked; if displacement is thought to be excessive, relief incisions can be used as detailed previously, or the suture can be removed and the technique changed to that employing Vicryl mesh. The procedure is repeated on the opposite side such that the posterior aspect of both uterosacral ligaments are opposed in front of the rectum. Further sutures are placed in a similar fashion incorporating the vaginal wall, thus reattaching Denonvilliers' fascia to the uterosacral ligaments, and closing the remaining enterocele defect.

If Vicryl mesh is used to effect repair, the initial surgical step is the same, except that the peritoneum is not resected from the rectum, as this is used to cover the mesh at the end of the procedure.

Following exposure of the rectovaginal septum as previously described, the dissection is continued down to the perineal body. The mesh, having been cut to size, is positioned within the rectovaginal septum. The mesh is first anchored to the most distal ridge of the defect if this can be identified. If remnants of the Denonvilliers' fascia are not identifiable, the dissection is carried further to the zone of fusion of the pelvic organs, which corresponds to the upper aspect of the perineum. At the end of this dissection, the surgeon should be able to identify the anal sphincter and the pubo-rectalis muscles in addition to the posterior vaginal wall and anterior rectal wall. The graft is then anchored to the perineal body. Three to five sutures are required to accomplish this. At least one suture on each side of the graft incorporates the levator muscle (i.e. pubo-rectalis) at the level of the anal sphincter. Then the proximal border of the mesh is attached to the vaginal vault, covering the proximal edge of the fascial defect. The lateral sutures will attach the mesh to the paravaginal tissues along the middle and lower third of the graft, whereas the upper third is attached to the uterosacral ligaments. The peritoneum is then closed, which in effect covers the graft.

Closure of the cul-de-sac will have a tendency to elevate and elongate the vagina. The pressure transfer from the abdomen to the urethra will be reduced, which may exacerbate pre-existing urinary incontinence. As previously discussed, complications involving the ureters can occur during enterocele repair, and in some cases it may be necessary to define the course of the ureter surgically, especially on the left side. Injury to the anterior border of the rectum can occur while dissecting the rectovaginal septum, especially when a previous posterior colporrhaphy has been performed. Injuries below the peritoneal reflection can be repaired as a primary procedure. Injuries above the peritoneal reflection, although less common, are more prone to breakdown if repair is undertaken in the absence of preoperative bowel preparation. The practice of routine residue-free diet with mechanical bowel preparation before operative laparoscopy is highly recommended. It will facilitate primary repair of rectal injuries, and increase the operating space available within the pelvis because the bowel is empty.

16.4 Conclusions

Laparoscopy is an invaluable tool in the treatment and prevention of enterocele, either as a primary mode of access or as a complement to vaginal surgery. Visualisation of the rectovaginal area is significantly better using the laparoscope than the naked eye. The extent of the enterocele defect and the supporting anatomical structures can be defined in greater detail, leading to a reduction in intraoperative blood loss during dissection of the enterocele sac, rectovaginal septum and exposure of the levator hiatus. This technique leads to elongation of the vagina and restoration of its normal upper horizontal axis. By avoiding a vaginal wall incision, the incidence of postoperative dyspareunia may be reduced. The increased surgical skills required to perform these procedures are far outweighed by the benefits to the patient in terms of postoperative morbidity.

References

1. Creighton SM, Pearce MJ, Stanton SL (1992) Perineal video-ultrasonography in the assessment of vaginal prolapse: early observations. Br J Obstet Gynaecol 99:310–313
2. Waters EG (1961) Enterocele: cause, diagnosis and treatment. Clin Obstet Gynecol 4:186–198
3. Nichols DH (1972) Types of enterocele and principles underlying choice of operation for repair. Obstet Gynaecol 40:257–262
4. Vancaillie TG, Butler DJ (1993) Laparoscopic enterocele repair: description of a new technique. Gynaecol Endosc 2:211–216
5. Koninckx PR, Poppe W, Deprest J (1995) Carbon dioxide laser for laparoscopic enterocele repair. J Am Assoc Gynecol Lap 2:181–185
6. Lam A, Rosen D (1997) A new laparoscopic approach for enterocele repair. Gynaecol Endosc 6:211–217
7. Zacharin RF (1992) Use of vaginal skin graft in posterior colporrhaphia. Aust NZ J Obstet Gynecol 32:146

Chapter 17

Endoscopic Needle Suspensions

Dirk De Ridder and Jan Deprest

17.1 Introduction

In this book dealing with minimally invasive endoscopic and laparoscopic techniques in gynaecology and obstetrics, a chapter concerning the vaginal approach for incontinence surgery may seem somewhat strange. However, vaginal surgery for stress incontinence and prolapse still plays a pivotal role in this era of minimally invasive surgery. Besides simple anterior colporrhaphy with Kelly plication, abdominal approaches are most popular for the treatment of urinary incontinence. Needle suspension was introduced by Armand Pereyra, a US Navy gynaecologist, and further popularised, modified and widely implemented by American urologists from 1957 on. The term endoscopic needle suspension refers to vaginal needle suspension techniques under cystoscopic control. In this chapter, the techniques, indications and results of vaginal needle suspension techniques will be discussed.

Diagnosing urinary incontinence and planning for treatment imply a thorough understanding of continence mechanisms and urodynamics. For more detailed descriptions of diagnostic procedures, urodynamics and surgical procedures we refer to other sources, as these are beyond the scope of this book.

17.2 History of Needle Suspension

The history of the different types of needle suspensions helps to explain the shortcomings and discouraging results published earlier. First, these techniques are all referred to as endoscopic needle suspensions, despite the important technical differences between, for instance, a Gittes and Raz suspension. Moreover, some authors are redesigning their approach regularly. For example, the current so-called Raz technique with incorporation of a vaginal wall sling is by no means comparable to the original Pereyra–Raz suspension. These changes in concept and design reflect the problems encountered in patients with combined urethral hypermobility and intrinsic sphincter deficiency, who were not cured by conventional bladder neck suspension alone.

Pereyra was the first to describe needle bladder neck suspension in 1959.[1] Originally, a blind manoeuvre was performed, bringing a trocar-cannula from a small suprapubic wound into the vagina, thus delivering the sutures, which were then tied over the abdominal fascia. To address the problem of suture pull-through, Lebherz and Pereyra proposed modifications.[2] In the final Pereyra technique (the modified Pereyra procedure), a midline vaginal incision gave access to the urethropelvic ligament, allowing more precise suture placement. Moreover, the lateral attachments of these ligaments were perforated to allow finger-controlled passage of the trocar through the retropubic space.[3]

Cystoscopy to control the placement of sutures was introduced by Stamey in 1973.[4] In this modification, the needle is also moved from the suprapubic region to the vagina. Through the cystoscope the close relationship of the suture with the urethra can be visualised. Then the suture is brought up again from the vagina to the suprapubic area through a second pass of the needle, more lateral to the first. To prevent suture pull-through, the bridge of tissue is often buttressed by a Dacron graft. In 1987, Gittes[5] proposed his "no-incision" modification of the technique. A needle is passed from a suprapubic stab wound through the vagina and the suture ends are transferred to the suprapubic area again, where they are tied over the rectus fascia independently. The vaginal sutures are re-epithelialised after a few days. This technique actually relies on the mechanism of suture pull-through to bury the sutures in the subepithelium.

In 1981, Shlomo Raz[6] published his modification of the original Pereyra technique. He preferred an inverted-U vaginal incision to a midline incision, and he incorporated the vaginal wall without its epithelium in the suture suspending the bladder neck.

Raz continued to publish subsequent modifications on his own technique to deal with problems of intrinsic sphincter deficiency and the concurrent or imminent prolapse.

For the correction of concurrent moderate cystoceles, a four-corner suspension was introduced.[7] Later this was changed to the six-corner suspension, which also includes a bilateral suture suspending the mid-urethral complex.[8] To allow better control of sphincter deficiency, a vaginal wall sling was proposed.[8,9]

To improve the repair of concurrent grade four cystoceles, a reduction of the central defect with a dexon mesh was also added where needed.[8] Not only did the vaginal approach undergo several changes, but the fixation of the sutures at the suprapubic site was also redesigned. Leach introduced the concept of bone anchoring of the sutures in an attempt to reduce the suprapubic discomfort experienced by some patients.[10]

Another topic in needle suspension techniques is the use of slings. The concept is based on the Goebell–Stoeckel–Frangenheim procedure, which has been known since 1917. Hadley was the first to combine the principles of needle suspensions with those of sling suspensions, when he used a rectus fascia patch.[11] Since then, several modifications have been described using fascia lata[12] and synthetic material such as Mersilene, Marlex, Silastic, Prolene and Gore-tex. Originally, these techniques were indicated for severe or recurrent stress urinary incontinence. Recently, some authors have published promising results in less severe grades of incontinence.

Sling surgery currently receives a lot of attention as a result of inventive marketing by the medical industry of various sling types with different delivery and fixation systems.

It is clear from this short historical review that there is not one, well-defined technique of endoscopic bladder neck suspension and therefore this common denominator covers a wide area of hardly comparable procedures. The differences in suture placement among the different modifications are demonstrated in Figure 17.1.

It is obvious that comparison of results between the different techniques is difficult. Not only do the techniques vary among authors, but the definitions of cure, the timing and duration of follow-up also differ. For some techniques, like the recent modifications of the Raz technique, one can only rely on the authors' publications to obtain an idea about the efficacy and safety of the procedures, as other authors have not yet gained enough experience with the new techniques. Comparing the results of bladder neck suspension with the retropubic approaches such as the Burch colposuspension or the Marchal–Marcetti–Krantz procedure is even more difficult, as the latter procedures have been tested in large series by several independent authors, while this has not been the case for endoscopic bladder neck suspensions.

In our centre, the different Raz modifications are used, as they can be tailored to the needs of the patient, and sphincter deficiency can be treated from the first procedure.

17.3 Indications and Patient Selection

Optimal selection of patients for anti-incontinence procedures is the clue for success. Clinically, the degree of concomitant prolapse, the degree of urethral hypermobility, obesity, pulmonary disease, age and menopausal status might be influencing factors in the choice of treatment.[13]

Urodynamic investigation is mandatory in the selection process. Genuine stress incontinence is a

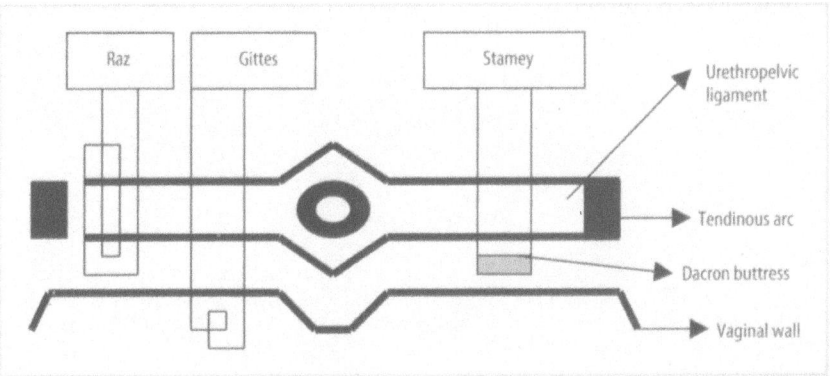

Figure 17.1 The Stamey suspension includes the urethropelvic ligament, with a Dacron graft as buttress for the sutures. The Gittes suspension includes the vaginal wall and the urethropelvic ligaments. The Raz suspension includes the vaginal wall and the pubocervical and medial edges of the urethropelvic ligaments (adapted from Raz[51]).

urodynamic definition, meaning the involuntary loss of urine per urethram in the absence of detrusor contractions.[14] First of all, the presence of stress incontinence has to be demonstrated. Occasional detrusor instability can be detected. Urethral evaluation can be done by measuring the urethral pressure profile or by measuring a Valsalva leak point pressure. Low urethral closing pressure ($< 20\,cm\ H_2O$) or Valsalva leak point pressure ($< 60\,cm\ H_2O$) can suggest the presence of intrinsic sphincter deficiency, which might necessitate a more obstructive sling approach than just a suspension of the bladder neck. Usually, multichannel urodynamics or video-urodynamics are used as standard procedures.

Currently, genuine stress incontinence with urethral hypermobility is considered a good indication for needle suspensions, despite the fact that long-term results are not as good as those of the retropubic suspensions.[15,16]

Obesity of more than 85 kg,[17] prior anti-incontinence surgery,[18] postmenopausal status,[13] age[19] and severe incontinence[20] have been identified as negative prognostic factors.

17.4 Results of Needle Suspension Techniques

Before attempting to summarise any results of needle suspensions, one has to realise the enormous differences in interpretation of definitions of cure and improvement after surgery. Subjective observations and objective measurements are used in a non-systematic way. There is a great need for standardisation for reporting results of this kind. A recent study by Black and Downs (1996)[21] reviewed 11 randomised controlled trials, 20 non-randomised prospective trials and 45 retrospective studies. The methodological quality of the 31 prospective trials was poor, with considerable variation in inclusion criteria, surgical management and assessment of outcome. Besides these remarks there seem to be substantial differences in outcome

between data based on chart review or data based on a third-party questionnaire.[22,23] In an elegant study by Sirls et al.,[23] the cure rate dropped from 72% to 47.1% when the results from a questionnaire were analysed and compared to chart review data.

Currently, recommendations for the best clinical practice cannot be based on scientific evidence, until well-designed clinical trials are available for rigorous statistical analysis.

17.4.1 Gittes Procedure

As with every new procedure, initially excellent results of up to 91% cure were reported.[5,24] Later, however, several authors proved the Gittes procedure to be inferior to other types of suspension. This became clear in comparative efficacy studies[25] as well as in urodynamic and ultrasound studies.[26] The cutting through of the sutures is probably responsible for the recurrent urethral hypermobility and recurrent incontinence.

17.4.2 Stamey Procedure

Initially, Stamey introduced cystoscopy to improve the placement of the suspension sutures.[4] Later publications by these authors mention success rates of 91%, even when the majority of these patients had already had previous surgery.[27] Objective follow-up and outcome analysis by questionnaire showed much lower success rates, as shown in Table 17.1.

Besides lower success rates, comparative studies with Burch colposuspension showed a higher incidence of de novo instability and voiding dysfunction.[28] Compared to the Marshall–Marchetti–Krantz procedure, a higher percentage of patients suffered from urgency following the Stamey procedure, but there was no significant difference concerning the local side-effects.[29] A high incidence of 27% complications other than retention has been reported by Kuczyk et al..[30]

Table 17.1. Success rates of the Stamey bladder neck suspension. N, Number of patients; subjective, follow-up by chart review; objective, follow-up with objective urodynamics; questionnaire, follow-up by questionnaire

Author	N	Follow-up	Type	Cured	Improved
Stamey[27]	203	6 months to 4 years	Subjective	91%	
Hilton[52]	100	27 months	Objective	53%	
Kuczyk[30]	85	44 months	Questionnaire		52%
Mills[53]	30	10 years	Subjective	33%	50%
O'Sullivan[38]	67	5 years	Questionnaire	18%	
Peattie[35]	44	3 months	Objective	39%	
Quentin Clemens[29]	32	15 years	Questionnaire	44%	
Walker[17]	192	2–63 months	Questionnaire	40%	82%

17.4.3 Pereyra–Raz Procedures

The modified Pereyra procedure and the Raz modification[6] are very similar from a technical point of view. The Raz modification introduced the inverted U-shaped incision and the inclusion of vaginal wall in the helical stitches. Therefore the results will be discussed together. Again, interpretation of definitions of cure or improvement varies among authors and has to be considered with care. Another problem is the fact that the Raz technique is still evolving (four-corner, six-corner suspension, incorporation of mesh material) because of the clinical observation of insufficient urethral support in the original suspension technique and because of the continuing search for improvement of the cystocele repair. The results of the Pereyra–Raz procedure are presented in Table 17.2.

17.4.4 Vaginal Sling Procedures

Historically, slings have been used in cases of recurrent stress incontinence or sphincter deficiency with or without urethral hypermobility. The sling principle is increasingly being incorporated in the decision trees of less severe stress incontinence.[31,32] The sling material may be autologous and is then harvested from the abdominal rectus fascia, from the fascia lata, or formed out of the vaginal wall. Artificial slings, like Marlex or Prolene, have been and still are used extensively. There is renewed interest in these foreign materials since several artificial sling delivery systems have been launched by the industry.

The reported results usually show cure or improvement in more than 90%, even with long-term follow-up (up to 17 years). A summary of the results is shown in Table 17.3.

Table 17.3. Results of pubovaginal slings. N, Number of patients; obj, follow-up with objective urodynamics

Author	Sling type	N	Follow-up	Type	Cured
Chaikin[31]	Rectus fascia	251	3.1 (1–15) years	Obj	92%
Raz[20]	Vaginal wall	206	5 years	Obj	90%
Beck[34]	Fascia lata	170	6 weeks to 2 years	Obj	92%

17.5 Complications of Needle Suspensions

Vaginal surgery for stress incontinence has a low morbidity and is minimally invasive. Complications can be related to the surgical technique, such as bleeding and bladder perforation, or may be related to the continence mechanism, such as de novo instability and urinary retention.

In this book on minimally invasive techniques, the surgical complications are of most interest. Most of the published papers, however, focus on the urodynamic effects of needle suspensions and give little information about the surgical complications, although these are usually described as "few". Many series report only on small patient numbers and one could argue that the high incidence of complications in some series is due to the learning curve.

The occurrence of bladder perforation during surgery varies between 0^{33} and 4.8%.[34] None of the reported bladder perforations required additional surgery. The suture, which entered the bladder, was removed and the catheter was left in situ for a longer time.[31] Early detection of this complication is possible when cystoscopy is performed after transferral of the sutures from the vagina to the abdominal site.

Intraoperative bleeding is seldom a problem and is usually controlled by vaginal packing. The incidence in the literature varies between 0 and 6.8%.[35]

Urinary tract infection is more common (3.7–32%). This large variability in the incidence of urinary tract infection is probably due to local factors, like the use of suprapubic or transurethral

Table 17.2. Results of the Pereyra-Raz procedure. N, Number of patients; subjective, follow-up by chart review; objective, follow-up with objective urodynamics; questionnaire, follow-up by questionnaire

Author	N	Follow-up	Type	Cured	Improved
Bergman[16]	98	12 months	Objective	70%	
Bergman[15]	30	5 years	Objective	43%	
Das[32]	10	3 years	Questionnaire	20%	
Holschneider[34]	54	3 years		81.6%	
Korman[19]	151	25 months		47%	64%
Ramon[33]	18	10 months	Subjective	83%	
Raz[20]	206	15 months	Subjective/objective	90%	
Shah[17]	17	2–30 months	Subjective/objective	76%	
Wheelahan[18]	102	5 years	Subjective	69%	

catheters and the eventual use of intraoperative prophylactic antibiotics.

In the Stamey procedure, foreign material (Dacron) is used to buttress the sutures. Infection of these, leading to surgical removal, seems to be common. Bidmead and Cardozo[36] reported a 16% infection rate with consequent excision of the buffers in 9% of cases. Shah[37] reported a 13% infection rate and O'Sullivan[38] had to remove sutures and buffers in 4.8% of his patients.

Besides the above-mentioned complications, low incidences of haematoma,[34] bacteraemia, persisting vaginal discharge,[29] suprapubic pain,[29,38] occult bowel perforation,[17] prolonged ileus, ilioinguinal nerve entrapment[39] and osteomyelitis pubis[40] have been published.

The introduction of bone-anchoring techniques in bladder neck suspensions has led to its own complications. Infection and dislocation of the anchors, as well as formation of soft tissue granuloma, have been described.[41] Removal of the anchors is not always easy, as reported by Bernier and Zimmern,[42] who had to use wedge resection of the os pubis to retrieve the implanted material.

The use of foreign material as slings has also led to complications of infection and erosion. Mersilene was used initially, but has been abandoned because of erosion into the urethra and because of obstruction.[43, 44] Gore-tex, Marlex and Silastic have all been used for the same purpose, with more or less the same complications. Sling removal for infection or obstruction varies among the different series between 3.4[45] and 20%.[46–48] Despite the fact that continence results are comparable to other sling techniques, the risk of infection and sling removal has left these interventions with few supporters, which may be a warning to bear in mind with the new artificial sling types being brought on the market.

A detailed analysis of postoperative voiding dysfunction is beyond the scope of this book.

Four major problems can occur: early and prolonged urinary retention, de novo detrusor instability, recurrent stress incontinence and obstructed voiding.

Recurrent stress incontinence is usually due to secondary sphincter deficiency or to the fact that underlying sphincter deficiency was not properly diagnosed at the time of surgery.

Development of detrusor instability after colposuspension is a well-known risk. However, it is difficult to obtain a good idea about the real incidence, with ranges of 7.6–27% for Burch colposuspension and from 14.6% (objective) up to 70% (subjective) for the Stamey operation.[28,29] The aetiology of the "de novo" instability is unknown. In some cases, obstruction can be the causal factor, in others previously undetected instability or changes in the detrusor behaviour itself could be at the base of this phenomenon.[36] Obstructive voiding can be dealt with by transabdominal or transvaginal urethrolysis. Webster and Kreder[49] described a 93% success rate with a retropubic approach with substitution of the former anti-incontinence procedure by an obturator shelf. McGuire et al.[50] reported a 77% success rate with transvaginal urethrolysis.

17.6 Conclusions

Despite the fact that the literature concerning anti-incontinence procedures in general and needle suspensions in particular is not always clear,[21] there is substantial evidence that needle suspension techniques are successful in correcting stress incontinence. They have a low complication rate and allow correction of intrinsic sphincter deficiency and different pelvic floor disorders in one operation and through one approach. In this way, they can compete easily with laparoscopic approaches or abdominal approaches. In the future, better designed and controlled trials will give an answer about the relative value of the different techniques described above.

References

1. Pereyra AJ (1959) A simplified surgical procedure for the correction of stress incontinence in women. West J Surg 67:223
2. Pereyra AJ, Lebherz TB (1967) Combined urethral vesical suspension vaginal urethroplasty for correction of urinary stress incontinence. Obstet Gynecol 30:537
3. Pereyra AJ, Lebherz TB (1982) The modified Pereyra procedure. In: Buchsbaum HJ, Schmidt JD (eds) Gynecologic and obstetric urology. Saunders, Philadelphia, pp 259–277
4. Stamey TA (1973) Endoscopic suspension of the vesical neck for urinary incontinence. Surg Gynecol Obstet 136:547–554
5. Gittes RF, Loughlin KR (1987) No-incision pubovaginal sling suspension for stress incontinence. J Urol 138:568–570
6. Raz S (1981) Modified bladder neck suspension for female stress incontinence. Urology 17:82–85
7. Raz S, Klutke CG, Golomb J (1989) Four corner bladder and urethral suspension for moderate cystocoele. J Urol 142:712–715
8. Raz S, Stothers L, Chopra A (1996) Raz techniques for anterior vaginal wall repair. In: Raz S (ed) Female urology. WB Saunders, Philadelphia, pp. 344–366
9. Stothers L, Chopra A, Raz S (1995) Vaginal wall sling for anatomic incontinence and intrinsic sphincter damage – efficacy and outcome analysis. J Urol 153:525A
10. Leach GE (1988) Bone fixation technique for transvaginal needle suspension. Urology 31:388–390
11. Hadley RH, Zimmern PE, Staskin DR et al. (1985) Transvaginal needle bladder neck suspension. Urol Clin North Am 12:299–303
12. Karram MM, Bhatia NN (1990) Patch procedure: modified transvaginal fascia lata sling for recurrent or severe stress incontinence. Obstet Gynecol 75:461–463

13. Kursh ED (1992) Factors influencing the outcome of a no incision endoscopic urethropexy. Surg Gynecol Obstet 175:254–258

14. Abrams P, Blaivas JG, Stanton SL et al. (1990) The standardisation of terminology of lower urinary tract function recommended by the International Continence Society. Int Urogynecol J 1:45–48

15. Bergman A, Giovanni E (1995) Three surgical procedures for genuine stress incontinence: five-year follow-up of a prospective randomized study. Am J Obstet Gynecol 173:66–71

16. Bergman A, Koonings PP, Ballard CA (1989) Primary stress urinary incontinence and pelvic relaxation: prospective randomized comparison of three different operations. Am J Obstet Gynecol 161:97–101

17. Walker GT, Texter JH (1992) Success and patient satisfaction following the Stamey procedure for stress urinary incontinence. J Urol 147:1521–1523

18. Wheelahan JB (1990) Long-term results of colposuspension. Br J Urol 65:329–332

19. Korman HJ, Sirls LT, Kirkemo AK (1994) Success rate of modified Pereyra bladder neck suspension determined by outcomes analysis. J Urol 152:1453–1457

20. Raz S, Sussman EM, Erickson DR et al. (1992) The Raz bladder neck suspension: results in 206 patients. J Urol 148:845–850

21. Black NA, Downs ZH (1996) The effectiveness of surgery for stress incontinence in women: a systematic review. Br J Urol 78:497–510

22. Das S (1998) Comparative outcome analysis of laparoscopic colposuspension, abdominal colposuspension and vaginal needle suspension for female urinary incontinence. J Urol 160:368–371

23. Sirls LT, Keoleian CM, Korman HJ et al. (1995) The effect of study methodology on reported success rates of the modified Pereyra bladder neck suspension. J Urol 154:1732–1735

24. Benson JT, Agosta A, McClellan E (1990) Evaluation of a minimal incision pubovaginal suspension as an adjunct to other pelvic floor surgery. Obstet Gynecol 75:844–847

25. Narushima M, Kondo A (1995) Needle suspension of the bladder neck for stress urinary incontinence: surgical results of 3945 patients operated on with quantitative procedures. Jpn J Urol 86:1051–1059

26. Kil PJ, Hoekstra JW, Van der Meijden AP (1991) Transvaginal ultrasonography and urodynamic evaluation after suspension operations: comparison among the Gittes, Stamey and Burch suspensions. J Urol 146:132–136

27. Stamey TA (1980) Endoscopic suspension of the vesical neck for urinary incontinence in females: report on 203 consecutive patients. Ann Surg 192:465–471

28. Wang AC (1996) Burch colposuspension versus Stamey bladder neck suspension. J Reprod Med 41:529–533

29. Quentin Clemens J, Stern JA, Bushman WA (1998) Long-term results of the Stamey bladder neck suspension: direct comparison with the Marshall-Marchetti-Krantz procedure. J Urol 160:372–376

30. Kuczyk MA, Klein S, Grünewald V et al. (1998) A questionnaire based outcome analysis of the Stamey bladder neck suspension procedure for the treatment of urinary stress incontinence: the Hannover experience. Br J Urol 82:174–180

31. Chaikin DC, Rosenthal J, Blaivas ¡G (1998) Pubovaginal fascial sling for all types of stress urinary incontinence: long-term analysis. J Urol 160:1312–1316

32. Cespedes RD, Cross CA, McGuire EJ (1997) Pubovaginal fascial slings. Techniques in Urology 3:195–201

33. Ramon J, Mekras J, Webster GD (1991) Transvaginal needle suspension procedures for recurrent stress incontinence. Urology 38:519–522

34. Holschneider CH, Solh S, Lebherz TB et al. (1994) The modified Pereyra procedure in recurrent stress urinary incontinence: a 15-year review. Obstet Gynecol 83:573–578

35. Peattie AB, Stanton SL (1989) The Stamey operation for correction of genuine stress incontinence in the elderly woman. Br J Obstet Gynaecol 96:983–986

36. Bidmead J, Cardozo L (1998) Four decades of needle bladder neck suspension. Br J Urol 82:171–173

37. Shah PJR, Holder PD (1989) Comparison of Stamey and Pereyra-Raz bladder neck suspensions. Br J Urol 64:481–484

38. O'Sullivan DC, Chilton CP, Munson KW (1995) Should Stamey colposuspension be our primary surgery for stress incontinence? Br J Urol 75:457–460

39. Monga M, Ghoneim GM (1993) Ilioinguinal nerve entrapment following needle bladder suspension procedures. Urology 44:447–450

40. Wheeler JS (1994) Osteomyelitis of the pubis: complication of a Stamey urethropexy. J Urol 151:1638–1640

41. Schultheiss D, Höfner K, Oelke M et al. (1998) Does bone anchor fixation improve the outcome of percutaneous bladder neck suspension in female stress urinary incontinence? Br J Urol 82:192–195

42. Bernier PA, Zimmern PE (1998) Bone anchor removal after bladder neck suspension. Br J Urol 82:302–303

43. Nichols DH (1973) The mersilene mesh gauze hammock for severe stress incontinence. Obstet Gynecol 41:88–93

44. Melnick I, Lee RH (1976) Delayed transection of urethra by Mersilene tape. Urology 8:580–581

45. Staskin DR, Kerr LA (1993) The Gore-Tex patch transvaginal needle suspension: indications, technique, results and follow up of 100 consecutive patients. J Urol 149:291A

46. Stanton SL, Brindley GS, Holmes DM (1985) Silastic sling for urethral sphincter incompetence in women. Br J Obstet Gynaecol 92:747–750

47. Horbach NS, Blanco JS, Ostergard DR et al. (1988) A suburethral sling procedure with PTFE for the treatment of genuine stress incontinence in patients with low urethral closure pressure. Obstet Gynecol 71:648–652

48. Bent AE, Ostergard DR, Zwick-Zaffuto M (1993) Tissue reaction to expanded polytetrafluoroethylene suburethral slings for urinary stress incontinence. Clinical and histological study. Am J Obstet Gynecol 169:1198–1201

49. Webster GD, Kreder KJ (1990) Voiding dysfunction following cystourethropexy: its evaluation and management. J Urol 144:670–673

50. McGuire EJ, Letson W, Wang S (1989) Transvaginal urethrolysis after obstructive urethral suspension procedures. J Urol 142:1037–1039

51. Raz S (1992) The anatomy of pelvic support and stress incontinence. In: Raz S (ed) Atlas of transvaginal surgery. WB Saunders, Philadelphia, pp.1–22.

52. Hilton P, Mayne CJ (1991) The Stamey endoscopic bladder neck suspension: a clinical and urodynamic investigation, including actuarial follow-up over four years. Br J Obstet Gynaecol 98:1141–1149

53. Mills R, Persad R, Handley Asken M (1996) Long term follow up results with the Stamey operation for stress incontinence of urine. Br J Urol 77:86–88

54. Beck RP, McCormick S, Nordstrom L (1988) The fascia lata sling procedure for treating recurrent genuine stress incontinence of urine. Obstet Gynecol 72:699–703

Chapter 18

Laparoscopic Sacral Colpopexy and Sacrospinous Fixation

Thomas L. Lyons, Ted T.M. Lee and Wendy K. Winer

18.1 Introduction

Every honest surgeon of extensive and long experience will have to admit that he is not entirely and absolutely satisfied with his long term results of all his operations for prolapse and allied conditions.
Richard TeLinde

Uterovaginal prolapse is undoubtedly one of the most debilitating and distressing gynaecological conditions for the women who are inflicted with it. It is also a challenging if not frustrating clinical entity for the gynaecological surgeons who attempt to treat it.

The true incidence of uterine prolapse is unknown. In 1964, Quinlivan et al. found that 25% of 600 women over age 60 had significant "uterovaginal relaxation" while Folsome et al. (1956) noted that 3% of 680 elderly institutionalised women had "uterine protrusion."[2,3] The lack of a standardised evaluation for pelvic prolapse likely contributed to the above discrepancy. Wilcox et al. found that 16.2% of all hysterectomies done in the USA between 1988 and 1990 had prolapse as the primary diagnosis. Prolapse is the most common diagnosis for hysterectomy in postmenopausal women, accounting for approximately one-third of all hysterectomies in women over 55 years of age. The true incidence of uterine prolapse is likely to be much higher than these reports suggest, as many symptomatic women are afraid to undergo surgery and in addition many women have asymptomatic prolapse.

The incidence of vaginal vault prolapse is even more difficult to determine. Women who had hysterectomies for uterine prolapse are at higher risk for developing vaginal vault prolapse than those who had hysterectomy for other indications. The risk of prolapse after vaginal hysterectomy has been reported to be as high as 43%, as reported by Backer and Kristoffersen. The lack of attention to correction of various pelvic floor defects and patient selection bias are likely to have contributed to the high incidence in this study. Risk of vaginal vault prolapse after hysterectomies for various indications ranges from 0.2% to 1% in the literature available for review.[7] However, by best estimates, more than 1000 women in the USA will develop vaginal vault prolapse annually.

As uterovaginal prolapse is a common condition suffered by many women, various procedures have been described to treat it. Currently, sacral colpopexy and sacrospinous ligament fixation are the two most accepted vault suspension procedures. Both procedures have success rates exceeding 90% in terms of correction of upper vaginal support.[10] Traditionally, sacral colpopexy is done via a transabdominal approach, whereas sacrospinous ligament fixation is accomplished via a transvaginal approach. With advances in both laparoscopy technology and the skills of endoscopic surgeons, both procedures can now be accomplished via the laparoscopic approach. By providing superior exposure, the laparoscopic approach can be associated with less morbidity than the traditional approach. The following is a relevant discussion on the pathophysiology of uterovaginal prolapse and a description of the technical aspects of accomplishing sacral colpopexy and sacrospinous ligament fixation for the correction of this disorder via laparoscopy. Relevant data and a discussion of complications and morbidity associated with these procedures are also included.

18.2 Pathophysiology and Evaluation of Uterine and Vaginal Vault Prolapse

Uterine and vaginal vault prolapse both share the same pathophysiology. The chief aetiology of uterine and vaginal vault prolapse is breakage or weakening of the attachments of the cardinal–uterosacral ligament complex to the pericervical ring or vaginal vault. Frequently multiple pelvic support defects, i.e. paravaginal defect, cystocele, rectocele and enterocele co-exist. In fact, for significant vault prolapse to exist, paravaginal defects must be present.

Enterocele and vaginal vault prolapse co-exist in the same patients so frequently that at times they are almost considered synonymous. However, enterocele is caused by a distinct pelvic support defect, which requires a separate reparative procedure from that for uterovaginal prolapse. Enterocele is caused by a break in the endopelvic fascia anywhere along the distal pubocervical fascia to the whole length of the rectovaginal septum (Denonvilliers' fascia) including that portion in the cul-de-sac. By definition, histological examination of enterocele defects demonstrates only vaginal mucosa and peritoneum without the intervening endopelvic fascia. When enterocele and uterovaginal prolapse co-exist, defect-oriented enterocele repair must be done prior to a vault suspension procedure in order to prevent "recurrence" of the enterocele defect.

Identification of the edges of the fascial break is the most challenging aspect of any of the reconstructive pelvic procedures. The ability to identify the defect completely allows one to repair it with greater precision. However, even with the aid of laparoscopy, it is not possible to identify these defects precisely in every patient. This difficulty provides fuel for the debate regarding the possibility of stretching the endopelvic fascia instead of specific breakage in these tissues. This inadequacy in identifying the precise defect may have provoked the compensatory-type repairs, including the Halban and the Moschowitz repairs. Sacrospinous fixation, sacral colpopexy and the use of graft material are also methods of correction of diffuse defects.

As uterovaginal prolapse is frequently associated with multiple pelvic support defects, each must be corrected for a better long-term result. In the traditional literature,[1] uterovaginal prolapses were classified into pulsion-type and traction-type prolapse. Pulsion-type prolapse results from an apical defect (detachment or attenuation of cardinal–uterosacral ligament). This type of prolapse is equivalent to the isolated level I defect, as described by Delancey.[2] Classically, the cervix or vaginal vault is the leading point of the prolapse. This is equivalent to the so-called "cervix first" prolapse.[3] Eventually, lower vaginal support became attenuated over time. In a patient with a predominantly pulsion-type prolapse, replacement of the cervix or vaginal vault to its proper position will simultaneously reduce the secondary cystocele or rectocele.

If this manoeuvre does not reduce the cystocele and/or rectocele, a primary level II or level III defect is also present.

Traction-type prolapse, on the other hand, results from initial paravaginal defects (anterior and posterior). The resultant cystocele or rectocele pulls down the cervix or vaginal vault with it. This is the so-called "cervix last" prolapse.[3] In this condition, correction of the paravaginal defects will also normalise the position of the cervix or vaginal vault. Failure to fully correct the vaginal vault position with this manoeuvre suggests the co-existence of a primary apical level I defect.

Distinction of these two main types of uterovaginal prolapse is helpful in directing the necessary extent of the surgical repair in patients with partial prolapse. However, one must note that, regardless of the location of the primary defect, over time the neighbouring support structure will decompensate and total prolapse is the eventual outcome. Obviously, in women with total prolapse, distinction of pulsion and traction prolapse becomes a matter of semantics. In the case of total prolapse, all three levels of pelvic support are compromised. All three levels of support must be reconstructed to assure long-term success.

18.3 Indications

The indications for laparoscopic sacrospinous ligament fixation and laparoscopic sacral colpopexy are not different from those for traditional sacrospinous ligament fixation and abdominal sacral colpopexy. Ideally, if the uterosacral ligament is strong and intact, a McCall's-type culdeplasty should be performed as the primary vault suspension procedure, as it is more anatomical and physiological.[4] Frequently, however, in patients with total prolapse, the uterosacral ligaments are tenuous as a result of multiple pregnancies, hypo-oestrogenism, or genetically poor fascial integrity. These factors can make the uterosacral ligaments unsuitable as the point of anchor for vault suspension.

Compensatory procedures such as sacral colpopexy and sacrospinous ligament fixation are indicated in this situation. Sacral colpopexy and sacrospinous ligament fixation should also be considered in women who failed previous McCall's-type culdeplasty. Sacral colpopexy and sacrospinous ligament fixation are not necessary in women with traction prolapse with intact apical support. A solid paravaginal defect repair and reinforcement sutures of vaginal vault to the uterosacral ligament are more appropriate procedures.

18.4 Procedures

18.4.1 Laparoscopic Sacral Colpopexy

Bilateral ureterolysis from the pelvic brim to the level of the uterosacral ligament insertion is performed to expose the ureters. This can be done with various energy sources, i.e. the contact Nd:YAG laser, electrocautery or the harmonic scalpel. A peritoneal incision is made medial to the ureters to allow visualisation of the ureters and to allow the ureters to splay out laterally. Using a vaginal probe (Apple Medical Corp, Philadelphia, PA), the vaginal vault or cervical stump is anteverted and pushed gently in a ventral direction. This anteversion of the vaginal vault will usually allow for excellent visualisation of the uterosacral ligament. The uterosacral ligament is examined for strength and integrity using a Babcock clamp. If the uterosacral ligaments are attenuated, a decision is usually made to proceed with sacral colpopexy.

The vaginal vault is tented and placed under gentle tension. The peritoneal covering is then stripped off the underlying pubocervical fascia and rectovaginal septum using both sharp and blunt dissection. Dissection of the rectovaginal space is then carried toward the perineal body (Figure 18.1). This dissection of the rectovaginal space is predominantly blunt except for the scarred area of previous episiotomy or repair. If enterocele is suspected preoperatively, effort is made to identify the edges of the enterocele defect. With the aid of improved visualisation of the laparoscope, the edges of the enterocele defect can usually be identified without much difficulty. Frequently, the operator's finger may be used to further delineate these fascial breaks. The edges of the enterocele defect are reapproximated in an anterior–posterior or side-to-side fashion using no. 0 Ethibon sutures. If vaginal length is compromised from prior repair, the side-to-side closure may prevent further shortening of the vagina. On the other hand, side-to-side closure may potentially narrow the upper vagina. Similarly, if a deep transverse defect cystocele is present, it should be repaired at this time. This deep transverse defect can be the source of the "anterior enterocele" defect and is very important to the repair.

A strip of Prolene mesh approximately 22 × 4 cm is introduced into the peritoneal cavity. The mesh is then sutured to the perineal body and the lower perirectal fascia with three Ethibond 0 sutures. The mesh is also sutured to the lateral condensation of the uterosacral ligament on each side of the posterior vaginal wall. The mesh is then wrapped around anteriorly over the vaginal vault and sutured around the vault in a confluent fashion using multiple Ethibond 0 sutures (Figure 18.2). At this time, a McCall's-type Ethibond 0

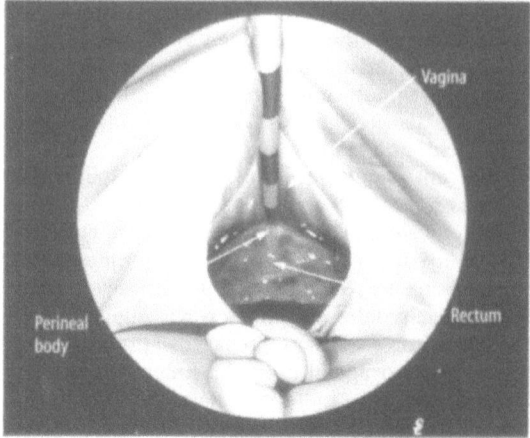

Figure 18.1 Dissection of rectovaginal space is performed to allow for attachment of the mesh to the perineal body.

suture is placed to occlude the cul-de-sac and to remove tension from the mesh at attachment.

The right perirectal gutter peritoneum is opened cephalad toward the sacral promontory and the overlying tissue is dissected using a Kittner. The patient may also be placed in a left tilt position in addition to the 30 of Trendelenburg. This manoeuvre may obviate the constant need to retract the rectosigmoid leftward during this dissection. The patient will have undergone an oral bowel preparation preoperatively, further facilitating this exposure. Vascular structures, including branches of middle sacral artery and vein, are visualised and controlled with bipolar cautery. The anterior longitudinal sacral ligament is isolated directly below the promontory. The mesh is brought over the sacrum and sutured to the anterior longitudinal ligament of the sacrum with two to three Ethibond 0 sutures in a

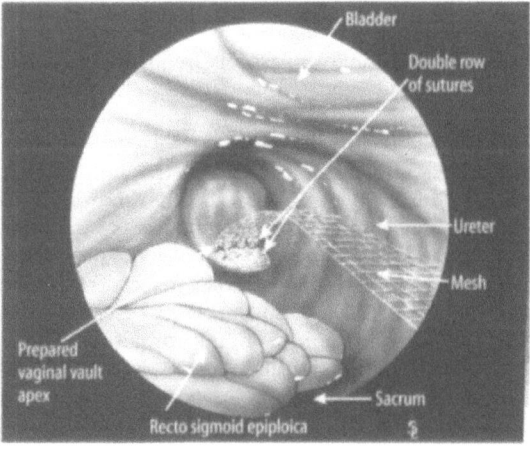

Figure 18.2 After anchoring the mesh to the perineal body, posterior vaginal wall, the mesh is then wrapped anteriorly and sutured to the vaginal vault in a confluent fashion.

tension-free manner. Alternatively, an EMS (Ethicon EndoSurgery, Cincinnati, OH) hernia stapler can be used to anchor the mesh to the sacrum. The excess mesh is then trimmed off. The peritoneum is closed over the mesh using Vicryl 2-0 sutures.

18.4.2 Laparoscopic Sacrospinous Ligament Fixation

The preparation of the vaginal vault and concomitant enterocele and transverse cystocele repair is the same as that for sacral colpopexy as described above. The ischial spine and sacrospinous ligament is first palpated vaginally and the peritoneum of the right perirectal gutter is opened over the underlying sacrospinous ligament. Blunt dissection with an endoscopic Kittner is carried out medially and superiorly toward the coccyx. A rectal probe is placed in the rectum and retracted leftward so the surgeon can dissect this area safely without injuring the rectum. An Ethibond 0 suture on a CT-2 needle is used to suture through the sacrospinous ligament at least 2–3 cm medial to the ischial spine to avoid injuring the pudendal neurovascular bundle. The suture is then passed twice through the posterior vaginal wall including the rectovaginal septum. The suture is left untied until a second suture is placed in a similar fashion. Both sutures are tied snugly to the ligament.

18.4.3 Paravaginal Repair

All patients undergoing a vault suspension procedure undergo a laparoscopic paravaginal repair and, when indicated, a Burch procedure. After development of the space of Retzius and identification of the arcus tendineus of the pelvis, the paravaginal defects are closed with interrupted Ethibond 2-0 sutures, plicating the endopelvic fascia to the arcus. Burch Ethibond 0 sutures may be added if the patient is at risk for urinary stress incontinence. Cystoscopy is performed at the completion of this segment of the procedure in order to document good ureteral performance and to assure that no sutures are present within the lumen of the bladder.

18.5 Complications and Morbidity

The high success rate of sacral colpopexy and sacrospinous ligament fixation accomplished

through the traditional approach comes with the price of substantial morbidity. For abdominal sacral colpopexy, pain and discomfort from the large midline incision is the most obvious morbidity, in addition to the common morbidity associated with midline laparotomy, such as significant blood loss, wound infection, atelectasis and paralytic ileus. Other specific complications distinct to sacral colpopexy include massive haemorrhage from the presacral vessels, ureteral injury, infected mesh and mesh erosion.

Vaginal sacrospinous ligament fixation, though void of the usual morbidity of a laparotomy, carries a substantial risk of bleeding and infection. Significant bleeding can occur in the rectal pillar region during the dissection of the sacrospinous ligament, as well as bleeding from other parts of vaginal repair. The inadequate haemostasis as a result of poor exposure can be a perfect setup for infection. Other complications intrinsic to sacrospinous ligament fixation include pudendal nerve and vessel injury, ureteral injury and rectal perforation.

With the superior exposure provided by the laparoscope, both the morbidity associated with the traditional approaches, as well as morbidity distinct to the specific procedures, can be reduced to a minimum. In our series of cases, this morbidity has not been observed. Operative times have remained in the range of 120 minutes, despite taking a global approach to defect repair. To date, bleeding has been negligible and no mesh complications have been experienced. A consistent morbidity has been that of transient neuralgia in a sciatic distribution on the right side. This problem has been present from 2 to 42 days in patients undergoing sacral colpopexy using permanent mesh (Prolene) and has responded well to non-steroidal anti-inflammatory medications. The neuralgia was rarely disturbing to the patient and resolved completely in all patients.

Because of the fear of mesh complications, Vicryl mesh was used in our initial series. We had hoped that significant scarring from the Vicryl mesh would be enough to suspend the vaginal vault. To our surprise, recurrent prolapse occurred within 3–6 months of the repair in the initial seven patients in whom absorbable mesh was used for the suspension. We have since then used Prolene mesh in our sacral colpopexies. No recurrent vault prolapse was observed in the subsequent series of women in whom permanent graft material was used (Table 18.1).

All procedures were performed as outpatient or 23-hour stays and all patients were capable of voiding by postoperative day 1. Patients were able to resume normal activities in 7–10 days but were restricted from heavy lifting or straining for 6 weeks.

Table 18.1. Laparoscopic sacral colpopexy with Prolene mesh (1994–1997). LSH, Laparoscopic supracervical hysterectomy; LAP, laparoscopic; MMK, Marshall-Marchetti-Krantz; BSO, bilateral salpingo-oophorectomy

Patient	Previous procedures	Concomitant procedures	Follow-up
NF	LSH, LAP rectocele, enterocele, paravaginal defect repair, LAP Burch, high McCall culdeplasty	McCall culdeplasty incorporated into the mesh	16 months, no recurrence
IL	LAP rectocele, enterocele, paravaginal defect repair, LAP Burch, sacral colpopexy with Vicryl mesh	LAP rectocele, enterocele repair. Perineorrhaphy	20 months, no recurrence
PB	LSH, BSO, LAP rectocele, enterocele repair, Burch	McCall culdeplasty incorporated into the mesh	20 months, no recurrence
LR	Abdominal hysterectomy, MMK	LAP rectocele, enterocele, paravaginal defect repair	15 months, no recurrence
OB	Abdominal hysterectomy, MMK	LAP enterocele repair	9 months, no recurrence
MC	LAP Burch, high McCall culdeplasty	LAP enterocele repair	14 months, no recurrence
MH	LSH, LAP Burch, high McCall culdeplasty, perineorrhaphy	LAP enterocele repair	12 months, recurrent enterocele with intact apical support
MA	Vaginal hysterectomy, anterior and posterior colporrhaphy	LAP enterocele, paravaginal defect repair	14 months, no recurrence

This postoperative regimen was significantly less cumbersome for the patients than the reported postoperative course for traditional surgery patients.

18.6 Conclusions

A good reconstructive pelvic surgeon should possess the skills to both identify and repair the specific defects. In our opinion, failure in reconstructive pelvic surgery frequently results from the inability to identify the specific defects rather than from the lack of skills to repair the defects.

Enterocele repair is frequently missing in the treatment of women with uterovaginal prolapse, despite the fact that enterocele defect often co-exists with uterovaginal prolapse. Some of the so-called recurrent vault prolapses were actually unrecognised and unrepaired enteroceles. To repair the enterocele defect adequately, it must be fully dissected and identified. It is not uncommon for a skilled reconstructive pelvic surgeon to confuse an isolated enterocele with intact vault support for vault prolapse. In this case, a simple vault suspension would leave the enterocele unrepaired. One must pay close attention in identifying and repairing the co-existing enterocele when treating women with uterovaginal prolapse. Failure to do so not only leaves the patient with an unrepaired enterocele, but also puts her at risk for suture avulsion from the vaginal vault and potential mesh erosion when an unrepaired enterocele is incorporated into the vault suspension.

Similarly, failure to repair the co-existent paravaginal and transverse defects may leave the patient with urinary stress incontinence and/or cystocele. Previously, both sacral colpopexy and sacrospinous ligament fixation were believed to be associated with postoperative urinary incontinence and recurrent cystocele.[15] Few of these patients actually developed cystocele and urinary incontinence de novo after the vault suspension procedure. Numerous authors have described the paradoxical continence phenomenon seen in women with large cystocele and uterovaginal prolapse.[1,16] In these cases, correction of the prolapse frequently results in incontinence. The defect that caused the incontinence did not develop as a result of the repair, but it was simply unrecognised preoperatively. Brubaker and Varner have reported that underlying urinary stress incontinence exists in 60–80% of women with significant uterovaginal prolapse when urodynamics were done with the prolapse reduced.[7,18] This is not surprising, as we know that most women with significant prolapse have co-existing paravaginal defects, the main aetiology of urinary stress incontinence. In addition, neuromuscular deficits are quite common in women with significant uterovaginal prolapse, and unkinking of the urethra with the correction of the prolapse may unmask underlying intrinsic sphincter deficiency. In addition to correcting most of the cystoceles and treating the underlying stress incontinence, repairing the paravaginal defects also anchors the vagina to the pelvic side walls, assuring long-term success of the reconstruction.

Despite the judicious preoperative clinical assessment, urodynamic evaluations and intraoperative attempts to correct all the defects, anterior vaginal wall support has continued to be a problem for some patients after sacrospinous ligament fixation or sacral colpopexy. Retroversion of the vaginal axis probably plays a part in the pathogenesis of this problem. More importantly, the faulty initial diagnosis of the anterior vaginal wall defect is likely to be responsible for the "recurrence". The current methodology on the diagnosis of the anterior compartment defect is not perfect. This point was voiced by Brubaker in her article "Sacrocolpopexy and anterior compartment: support and function".[7] It is possible that the excellent visualisation with laparoscopy will enhance our ability in identifying the specific defects, thus reducing the possibility of loss of anterior wall support after vaginal vault suspension.

As we approach the 21st century, women are living longer and enjoying an active lifestyle in their golden years. As the number of postmenopausal women increases, so will the numbers of women who suffer from pelvic floor dysfunction, such as urinary incontinence and prolapse. The recent interest in urogynaecology and reconstructive pelvic surgery reflects this trend. With the advance of technology in laparoscopy and refinement in the skills of the endoscopic surgeons, laparoscopy offers the gynaecologist a legitimate approach to the treatment of pelvic floor disorders. With the excellent visualisation of the pelvic support anatomy, laparoscopy allows the gynaecologist to perform a more precise repair with less morbidity. Laparoscopic approaches, while facilitating the repair of the defects of the pelvic floor, have focused attention on the evaluation of these problems and the surgical methods that have been used to correct them. This may revolutionise our understanding of urinary incontinence and pelvic floor prolapse conditions. It is important to note that laparoscopy cannot and should not replace sound vaginal surgical skills, but it is meant to complement one's ability and understanding as a reconstructive pelvic surgeon.

References

1. TeLinde RW (1966) Prolapse of the uterus and allied conditions. Am J Obstet Gynecol 94:444–463
2. Quinlivan LG (1964) The gynecological findings in the elderly women. Geriatrics 19:654–657
3. Folsome CE, Napp EE, Tanz A (1956) Pelvic findings in the elderly institutionalized patient. JAMA 161:1447–1454
4. Wilcox LS, Koonin LM, Pokras R et al. (1994) Hysterectomy in the United States, 1988–1990. Obstet Gynecol 83:549–555
5. Backer OG, Kristoffersen K (1957) Vaginal and abdominal total hysterectomy. Primary and late results. Acta Chir Scand 114:67
6. Symmonds RE, Williams TJ, Lee RA et al. (1981) Post-hysterectomy enterocele and vaginal vault prolapse. Am J Obstet Gynecol 140:852–859
7. Kaser O, Ikle FA, Hirsch HA (1985) Atlas of gynecological surgery, 2nd edn. Thieme-Stratton, New York
8. Dunton JD, Mikuta J (1988) Posthysterectomy and vaginal vault prolapse. Postgrad Obstet Gynecol 8:1
9. Timmons MC, Addison WA, Addison WB et al. (1992) Abdominal sacral colpopexy in 163 women with posthysterectomy vaginal vault prolapse and enterocele. Evolution of operative techniques. J Reprod Med 37:323–327
10. Morley GW, Delancey JOL (1988) Sacrospinous ligament fixation for eversion of the vagina. Am J Obstet Gynecol 158:872–881
11. Nichols DH, Randall CL (1989) Vaginal surgery, 3rd edn. Williams & Wilkins, Baltimore
12. Delancey JOL (1992) Anatomic causes of vaginal prolapse after hysterectomy. Am J Obstet Gynecol 166:1717–1728
13. Porges RF, Smilen SW (1994) Long-term analysis of the surgical management of pelvic support defects. Am J Obstet Gynecol 171:1518–1528
14. Liu CY (1996) Laparoscopic hysterectomy and pelvic floor reconstruction. Blackwell Science, Cambridge
15. Holley RL, Varner RE, Gleason BP et al. (1995) Recurrent pelvic support defects after sacrospinous ligament fixation for vaginal vault prolapse. J Am Coll Surg 180:444–448
16. Grody MHT (1995) Benign postreproductive gynecologic surgery. McGraw-Hill, New York
17. Brubaker L (1995) Sacrocolpopexy and the anterior compartment: support and function. Am J Obstet Gynecol 173:1690–1696
18. Varner RE, Kirby J, Holley R (1995) Effects of sacrosuspension on the lower urinary tract. Am J Obstet Gynecol 173:1684–1689

Chapter 19

Laparoscopic Colposuspension

Jan Deprest, Hans Brölmann, Dirk De Ridder, Michel Degueldre, Jean Vandromme and Pino G. Cusumano

19.1 Introduction

Stress urinary incontinence refers to a symptom or sign. The International Continence Society has adopted the term "genuine stress incontinence" for the involuntary loss of urine when the intravesical pressure exceeds the maximum urethral pressure, in the absence of detrusor activity. The exact diagnosis can therefore be made only by a urodynamic study.

The most likely causes of genuine stress incontinence are:

- abnormal descent of the bladder neck and proximal urethra, leading to a failure of equal transmission of intra-abdominal pressure to the proximal urethra;
- laxity of suburethral support, normally provided by the different pelvic floor structures having a close and delicate inter-relationship. This may lead to ineffective compression during stress.

Another cause is a low spontaneous intraurethral pressure, e.g. as a result of former surgery and radiation.

19.1.1 Rationale for Colposuspension

There are over 160 different operative procedures for patients with genuine stress incontinence.[1] The number of prospective, comparative and particularly randomised trials evaluating these operations is limited. In general, they demonstrate the superiority of retropubic colposuspension (86–92% cure rates) in most surgeon's hands, particularly when compared with vaginal repair combined with the buttress procedure.[2,3] A few years ago, Stanton et al. from St George's Hospital in London published the first long-term results on their colposuspension patients, with an overall cure rate of 69% over 20 years. For primary procedures, the cure rate was about 78% at 15 years.[4] Negative predictive factors could be identified, such as secondary surgery, preoperative weight of over 80 kg, detrusor instability or intraoperative haemorrhage of over 1000 ml. In many countries, colposuspension is therefore considered to be the gold standard in therapy in cases of genuine stress incontinence.

The procedure is believed to be effective because it restores the urethrovesical angle and brings the proximal urethra within the intra-abdominal pressure zone, without affecting the intrinsic urethral sphincter mechanism.[5] This supports to a certain extent the failure of pressure transmission as the theoretical pathophysiological mechanism behind genuine stress incontinence. Surgical elevation and suspension of the bladder neck was first described by Marshall, Marchetti and Krantz for incontinence in men undergoing radical prostatectomy.[6] Sutures were placed in the para-urethral tissues and urethral wall, to be attached to the periosteum of the pubic ramus. Osteitis pubis was a major drawback and Burch therefore proposed suspension of the paravaginal tissue to the ipsilateral ileopectineal ligament.[5] The numerous modifications of this so-called standard procedure may be the most biasing factor when evaluating this operation for incontinence. Many surgeons classify their own technique as a "Burch" colposuspension, although there are considerable differences between individual techniques, and some may be unrelated to what has been described by Burch. For instance, in open surgery we use the modification described by Tanagho,[7] and therefore have mimicked that procedure in our laparoscopic operations.

19.1.2 Laparoscopic Approach to Colposuspension

The advantage of endoscopy over laparotomy is that it offers a magnified and much more bloodless exposure, allowing identification of essential landmarks and eventually specific anatomical defects. This should be of particular interest for pelvic floor reconstruction. The number of procedures that can be handled by laparoscopy has been increasing over the years. It was some time before laparoscopic colposuspension found widespread use, as it requires advanced endoscopic suturing skills. Once a surgeon masters the art of endoscopic suturing, in theory any pelvic floor reconstruction technique is feasible.[8] Vancaillie described the first laparoscopic colposuspension in 1991 and soon after Underwood reported a strictly preperitoneal technique.[9,10] Over the following 10 years, many procedures have been reported, even more than for open surgery during the same period. However, there remains doubt whether the laparoscopic procedure is as effective as its open counterpart, known as the gold standard in incontinence surgery.

In this chapter, we describe our technique, using sutures in a way that mimics the conventional, abdominal operation. We also describe an alternative technique used by the team of one of the co-authors (PC), using synthetic grafts and endoscopic anchoring devices.[11] In Belgium, this technique has found widespread application among endoscopic surgeons. It reduces the need for time-consuming and cumbersome suturing, which may significantly shorten the operation. The modification described here also allows a precise evaluation of the degree of bladder neck elevation. It is obviously yet another modification with its own rationale.

19.2 Technique

19.2.1 Anatomical Considerations

The space of Retzius is a virtual space with an anterior and two lateral compartments. The anterior compartment is bounded by the pubic bone anteriorly, and the endopelvic fascia, surrounding the bladder, posteriorly. There is a rich perivesical venous sinusal network within deposits of fatty tissue. Over the urethra lies the deep dorsal vein of the clitoris, which feeds into these venous channels. The lateral compartments are bounded sideways by the obturator internus fascia and obturator nerve, artery and vein, just beneath the bony arcuate ridge of the ileum. The posterior border of that space is the endopelvic fascia around the internal iliac artery and its branches as they course towards the ischial spine.

The floor of the lateral compartment is formed by the arcus tendineus levator ani, a thickening of the obturator internus fascia. Important landmarks are the ileopectineal or Cooper's ligaments (conjoined tendon). Any suture should be placed relatively medially into this structure to avoid inadvertent laceration of vessels or the ilioinguinal nerve, located on the anterior abdominal wall as it exits the external inguinal ring.

More inferiorly, the space extends to the anterior vaginal wall, becoming visible during dissection because of its "white" endopelvic fascial capsule. Many names have been given to this fascia, according to which part of it is involved. For instance, the area of interest here may be called the pubocervical fascia. Part of it, the area near to the urethrovesical angle, will be the focus of the suspension procedure, at least when doing the colposuspension as originally described. Multiple veins are present on the vaginal vault and should either be avoided or coagulated during the dissection. In principle, the operation is carried out extraperitoneally, but associated procedures may be transperitoneal. For a variety of reasons, some surgeons carry out the laparoscopic procedure via the transperitoneal approach.

19.2.2 Technique of Laparoscopic Colposuspension

Three days prior to the procedure, the patient is put on a soft diet to reduce bowel distension, as for any laparoscopy (this is obviously important for the transperitoneal approach). In our country, the patient provides written consent for a colposuspension, primarily by laparoscopy, but with possible conversion to laparotomy. Cefazolin (2 g) is administered intravenously 1 hour prior to incision. The patient is positioned in the modified lithotomy position, disinfected and draped as for an open Burch colposuspension (which is also performed by the combined abdomino-vaginal approach). The patient's arms are placed alongside the body so the surgeon and assistant can move freely along the sides. A Foley catheter is introduced, and the balloon is filled, usually with more than 15 ml. The balloon catheter will not only keep the bladder empty but will also help to identify the bladder neck (Figure 19.1). This is helpful, as any tactile feedback is lacking in laparoscopy. One can use a three-way catheter so the bladder can be filled with dyed sterile water at any time during the operation. This can be helpful in identifying the border of the bladder or to detect any bladder perforation whenever suspected.

We usually use four trocars: one umbilical 10 mm port, two lateral 5 mm ports, and one port halfway

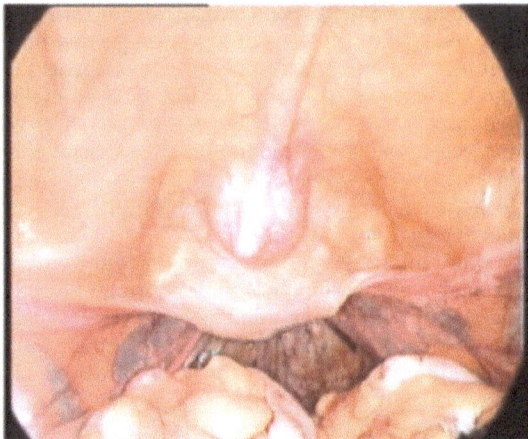

Figure 19.1 Laparoscopic view of the pelvis at the beginning of the procedure, transperitoneal approach. The bladder catheter can be seen bulging.

between the symphysis and the umbilicus. The diameter of the latter port depends on the exact technique used. When doing the procedure with sutures, a diameter of 7 mm or more allows the introduction of needles. It is possible to adapt the curve of the needle for introduction through a 5 mm cannula, or to remove the cannula while introducing the needle. Cannulas with adequate reducers are essential to prevent gas leak. For the mesh technique, a 12 mm port is required for the endostapler. With growing experience, the procedure can be done with three ports (no midline port). Instrumentation is limited to 5 mm rotating monopolar scissors, anatomic and large atraumatic forceps needle holder and knot pusher. A suction–irrigation device is not always necessary, but should be available. We try to avoid irrigation as much as possible, however, as it may pool in the most posterior parts, it dissolves extraperitoneal fat and it does not enhance identification of correct dissection planes. Instead, we use swabs to clean the operative field and – as in open surgery – as a dissecting and presentation device. For large veins, we occasionally need bipolar coagulation forceps.

19.2.2.1 Preperitoneal Approach

If colposuspension is the only procedure to be performed, we prefer to work preperitoneally. Initially, we used a dissection balloon, which is comfortable but expensive. Both rectus muscles are identified and split via open laparoscopy, and a tunnel is prepared under the posterior abdominal muscle sheath, in the direction of the symphysis pubis. Alternatively, an optical trocar has been suggested to control the intentional "fausse route"

into the preperitoneal space. However, nowadays we dissect the space of Retzius digitally, insufflate CO_2 and finalise the dissection under laparoscopic control.

19.2.2.2 Transperitoneal Approach

When the preperitoneal approach fails, a transperitoneal approach may be needed. The procedure can also be primarily transperitoneal, or concomitant surgery may be required. An advantage of the transperitoneal technique is the possibility of inspecting the pelvis for associated pathology or pelvic floor descent, which may also be managed by the laparoscopic approach. The anterior peritoneum is incised about 3 cm above the symphysis (Figures 19.1 and 19.2). We first coagulate the urachus and make an incision from the left to the right obliterated umbilical artery. A large incision may facilitate the manipulation into the space of Retzius, but obviously will take longer to close at the end of the procedure. The dissection must first be oriented to the symphysis, and not laterally. A thin fascial layer must be pierced to reach the posterior aspect of the rectus muscles, to avoid entering the dome of the bladder. In cases of previous lower abdominal surgery, the top of the bladder may be attached to the abdominal wall and peritoneal scar. In that case, filling the bladder may help to identify the upper margin of the bladder and locate the best place for peritoneal incision.

19.2.2.3 Dissection of the Operative Field

Once again, the first landmark is the symphysis pubis. The dissection then extends laterally to the ileopectineal ligaments, and downwards along the

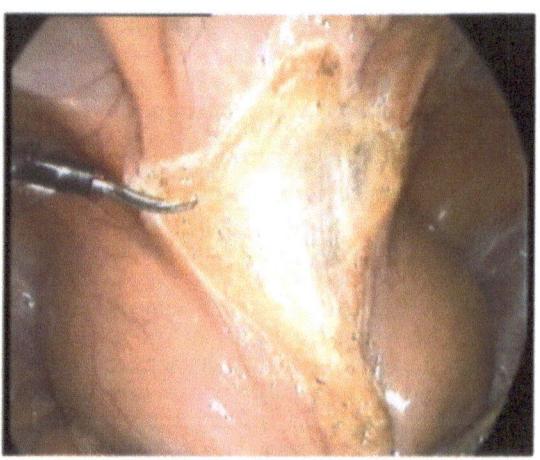

Figure 19.2 Incision of the peritoneum.

midline into the retropubic area. The Cooper's ligaments should not be dissected any further laterally than needed: this will not contribute to the suspension, and can only cause trauma to the veins that course from the inferior epigastric vessels to the obturator vessels (sometimes called the "corona mortis"). The bladder neck and the vaginal vault are the following landmarks. The dissection of the Retzius space is done by blunt dissection, with meticulous haemostasis of small vessels. There is a high potential for bleeding and even limited haemorrhage may mask the visualisation of landmarks, particularly the inferior and lateral bladder border. As visibility is crucial in laparoscopy, we try to avoid any bleeding by prophylactic haemostasis. When dissecting the vagina, one needs to expose a large, conspicuous pale area, with the typical white shining of fascial structures. Fatty tissue must be partly removed for visualisation and this may also enhance postoperative fibrosis (Figure 19.3). We do not transsect the midline structures above the urethra, as they may contain vessels; in any case, these structures do not contribute to continence.

19.2.2.4 Suture Suspension Technique

Any conventional surgical technique can be simulated laparoscopically. We place two to three sutures bilaterally, as in our open technique. We place these midurethral, one about 1.5–2.5 cm beside the bladder neck and one higher up (localisation of sutures according to the Tanagho modification). Obviously, the exact location of the sutures is dependent on the technique used by the surgeon in the open approach, but any of these techniques can be mimicked in laparoscopy. The most distal right-side

stitch is placed first, then the most distal left-side one, returning to the right side. So the operative field closes progressively in a cephalad direction. For each suture, the operator now puts on an extra thin plastic glove over his left latex glove, which will be removed once returning to the abdominal operative field.

The hand is placed into the vagina, pushing the urethra sideways, and exposing the fascia on the vagina to the laparoscopic hand (Figure 19.4). An Ethibond 0 suture with a 3/8 or reverted ski needle, measuring 120 cm (for comfortable extracorporeal knot tying) is introduced. First, a firm vaginal bite is taken, avoiding piercing through the vaginal mucosa (Figure 19.5). To be able to force the needle through the Cooper's ligament, the needle should be oriented perpendicularly to the ligament (Figure 19.6). The introduction of the needle holder through the iplisateral port may enable this. When the suture has been placed (Figure 19.7), the material is pulled out, while elevating the vagina and/or supporting the suture at the vaginal insertion to prepare two symmetrical ends, allowing an extracorporeal "Weston clinch knot" to be made.[12] This knot is a slipping knot that can be locked at any time by traction on the suture ends in opposite directions, even without complete approximation of the sutured tissues, allowing elevation of the vaginal vault as high as desired.

Until now, there have been no objective ways of measuring the degree of bladder neck elevation, but an effort to do so is described below. In theory, the vaginal fornices should be approximated to the ileopectineal ligament, but this may cause "bowstringing", and therefore many surgeons leave the suspension relatively loose, which may not change the outcome.[7] Two additional sutures are placed at each side, alternating left and right.

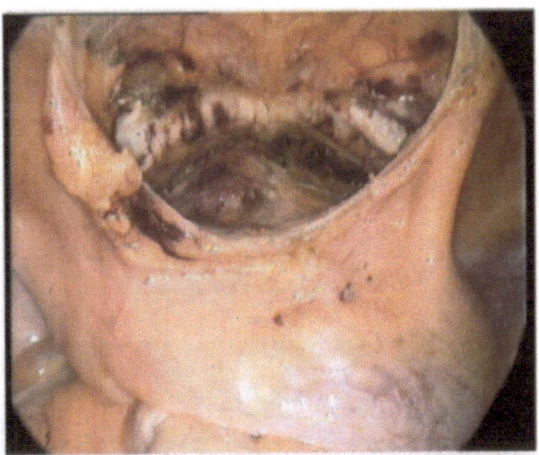

Figure 19.3 View after preperitoneal dissection to expose the landmarks: bladder, urethra, bladder neck, ileopectineal ligaments (Cooper).

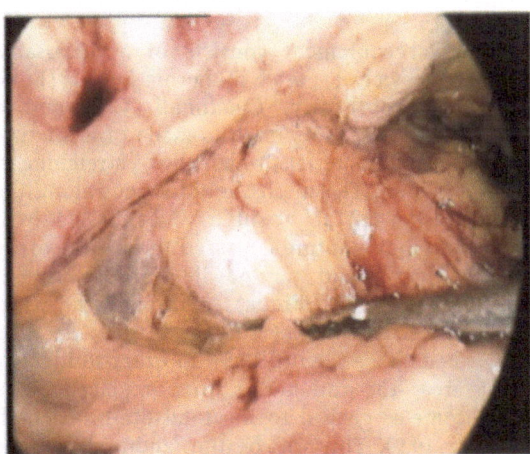

Figure 19.4 The operator's finger is in the vagina, to make insertion of the first stitch in the vagina easier. The whitish shining of the vagina can be seen. All other structures were dissected away.

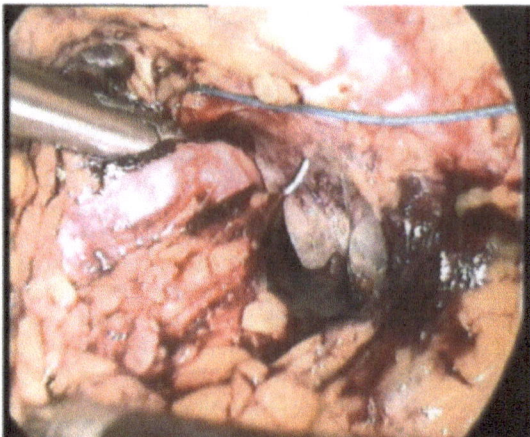

Figure 19.5 First bite by the needle through the vaginal vault.

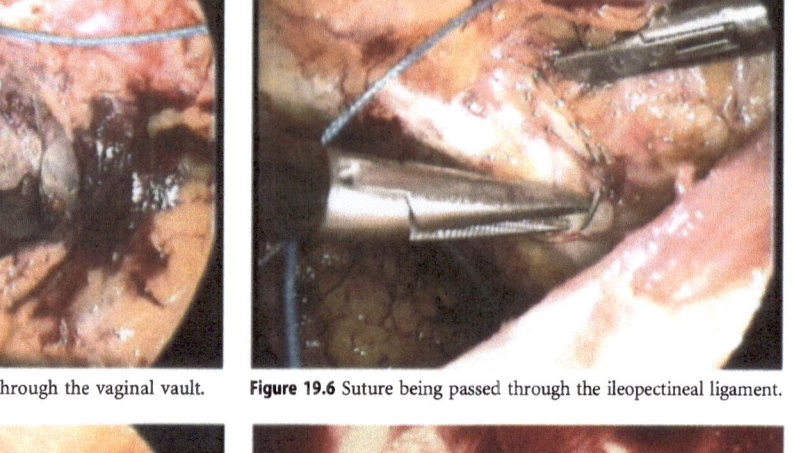

Figure 19.6 Suture being passed through the ileopectineal ligament.

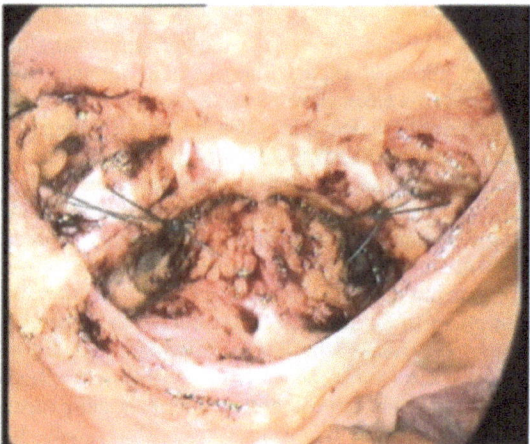

Figure 19.7 Retropubic view after one suture each side; at least one or ideally two sutures will be placed on each side.

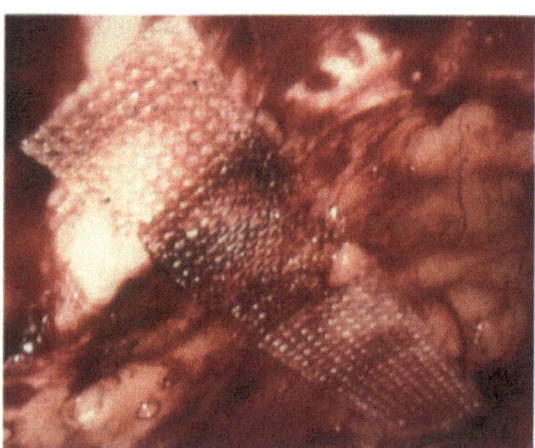

Figure 19.8 Laparoscopic colposuspension using the mesh technique, view at one side, prior to fixation of the mesh.

19.2.2.5 Mesh Technique (Sutures)

Additional equipment consists of a disposable stapling device, as used in hernia repair (EMS, Ethicon Endosurgery, Cincinnati, OH) and a propylene mesh. This mesh is made of a mixture of permanent materials, which allows stretching in one direction. The mesh should be cut along the long elastic axis to about 5×1 cm. A 120 cm Ethibond 0 or 1 suture is passed through a corner of the mesh, and the needle end is brought intraperitoneally to be passed through the paravaginal fascia at the level of the bladder neck, as described above (Figure 19.8). In order to identify that area, the catheter is then replaced by a urethrometer gauged to the total urethral length (Figure 19.9). This will be the landmark for the exact anatomical urethrovesical junction. Once two firm vaginal bites have been taken and a knot has been tied, the mesh is pushed over the free end

of the suture into the Retzius space. In cases of moderate cystocele, one or more additional stitches can be placed more cephalad, obviously well laterally.

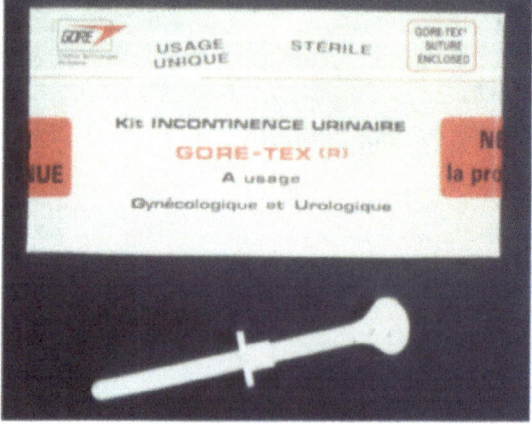

Figure 19.9 Urethrometer.

The mesh is then fixed to the ileopectineal (Cooper's) ligaments. For the right-sided mesh, the forceps are placed through the right port and the endostapler through the midline. The degree of elevation of the bladder neck can also be gauged with the urethrometer. The mesh is put under traction, and when the first downward movement of the external, visible part of the urethrometer is observed, further elevation is avoided. The mesh is anchored to the Cooper's ligament with several staples. Some simply staple the mesh both to the vagina and to the Cooper's ligaments (Figure 19.10).[13–16]

19.2.2.6 End of Operation and Postoperative Regimen

After checking the haemostasis under lower insufflation pressure, and if necessary the integrity of the bladder, the peritoneum is closed with a running suture or stapler (Figure 19.11). We also advocate the closure of any fascial incision of 7 mm or larger to prevent incisional hernia. We normally use a drain in the suprapubic space. We use a transurethral catheter for 24–48 hours, though suprapubic catheterisation is equally good. Most of these instructions vary from place to place, without real scientific background. We usually admit patients for more than 2 days, but shorter admissions are possible, dependent on the incentive for them to be discharged early, which differs between countries. Before discharge, the patient is checked for voiding and residual volumes. When the preoperative bladder volume was normal, we allow a maximal residual of 125 ml. We encourage the patient not to do sport or lift heavy weights for 6 weeks.

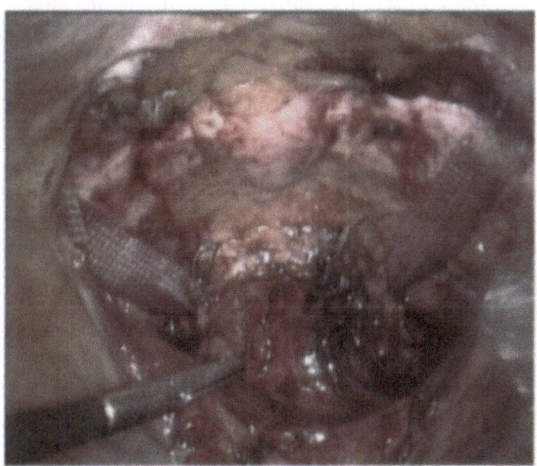

Figure 19.10 Retropubic view of the end of the procedure with the mesh technique.

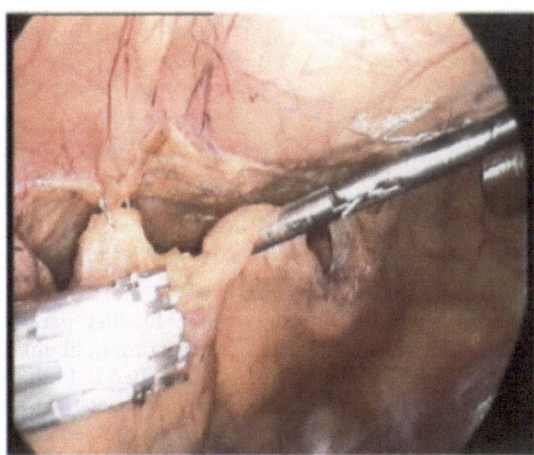

Figure 19.11 Peritoneal closure at the end of the procedure.

19.3 Results

We have compiled the available data comparing open and laparoscopic surgery, and divided it into three categories: observational series (A), non-randomised (B) and randomised controlled studies (C). Characteristics of the different studies are presented in Table 19.1. After the first report in 1991 by Vancaillie, we classified 16 papers in group A,[13–30] eight in group B[28,31–37] and three in group C.[38–41] In the latter group, one study randomised laparoscopically treated patients to either one double-bite or two single-bite sutures; because of its design this study is included in group C.[41] In the (uncontrolled) case series (group A), there were 889 patients; in groups B and C, there were 607 patients.

19.3.1 Intraoperative Parameters and Complications

The operating time for the suture technique is usually longer than when using staples and meshes (123 versus 41 minutes in the case series discussed below). The number of conversions in most case series is lower than 2%, even if additional surgery is required. Blood loss during laparoscopic access is very limited (usually < 50 ml), probably because of meticulous haemostasis and preventive coagulation during the dissection, and the positive pressure, which arrests capillary bleeding. Occasional significant haemorrhage may occur, as in open surgery, and may even be the cause for abandoning the endoscopic approach. When significant haemorrhage occurs (about 2% of procedures), it may be controlled by bipolar coagulation, or by temporary mechanical tamponade with a swab.

Table 19.1. Success rates (%) after laparoscopic Burch colposuspension, using sutures, sutures and staples, staples and mesh, and follow-up period, as reported in 25 published papers

Technique	No. of publications	Success rate (%; range)	Mean follow-up period (months)
Sutures	16	87 (60–100)	18.1
Sutures and staples	3	92 (89–94)	16
Staples and mesh	4	98 (96–100)	12.3
Not specified	2	93 (90–97)	36

Lower urinary tract injury is the most common complication of colposuspension. Bladder perforation is a typical complication, occurring in about 3–5% of cases. Lesions have been described in both the transperitoneal and preperitoneal approach. In our experience, most lesions have occurred in secondary cases. Although the overall incidence is probably decreasing with experience, it is about 3.7%, higher than for the open approach.[42] However, studies have evaluated the value of intraoperative cystoscopy in open Burch colposuspension, quoting a higher rate of bladder injury in open surgery.[43] It is possible that bladder injury is underestimated (or under-reported) in open surgery, as the consequences are not dramatic. Perforation may lead to prolonged catheterisation, as most perforations occur at the dome of the bladder and are not prone to fistulation. They can be easily sutured endoscopically or may not need any treatment except for prolonged catheterisation.

19.3.2 Failure and Success

As this is a functional operation, results are evaluated by cure of the symptoms of incontinence. Success rates differ widely and depend on the definition of success, such as subjective (by questionnaire), objective (urodynamic measurement or pad test), self-reported or by (telephone) interview,

and duration of follow-up. Most authors report success rates but on closer inspection they do not define criteria for success clearly or uniformly. An additional shortcoming is that the majority of studies are not (properly) controlled. All these limitations make a meaningful comparison and analysis impossible.

The range of success rates varied from 60% to 100% after 3–36 months. The mean success rate after 18 (3–36) months was 90%. Hospital stay varied from 1 to 6.3 days (mean 2.1 days). Results did not differ between the different techniques described in those reports, which was confirmed in the study by Ross, randomising different laparoscopic techniques.[28] In the studies where staples were used, the operation was successful in 93% of cases; it was successful in 95% of the suture group, although with a short follow-up period of 6 months.

The studies of groups B and C, comparing results of open and laparoscopic surgery, are presented in Table 19.2. In the ten comparative studies, laparoscopic colposuspension was inferior in three,[41,44,45] superior in three[33,34,40] and not different in four studies.[28,32,36,39] The initial data from randomised trials are indeed discouraging. Burton randomised 60 patients over an open and an endoscopic arm; within months the inferiority of laparoscopic colposuspension became clear.[44] Burton's poor results may be related to unfamiliarity with endoscopic surgery: he embarked on the study after an extremely short learning curve of only ten cases.

Table 19.2. Results of comparative studies on open and laparoscopic colposuspension (open/laparoscopy)

Author	Year	Randomised design (Y/N)	No. of patients	Follow-up period (months)	Operation time (min)	Hospital stay (days)	Resumption of activity (days)	Objective cure assessment (Y/N)	Cure rate (%)
McKinney[36]	1994	N	25/56	> 12		> 1/1			87/96
Ross[28]	1995	N	31/31	24/12		> 1/1			90/93
Polascik[33]	1995	N	10/12	36/21		4.9/1.9			70/83
Das[34]	1998	N	10/10	36					60/90
Miannay[32]	1998	N	72/72	24		6.7/3.0			75/80
Burton[44]	1997	Y	30/30	36				Y	93/60
Su[45]	1997	N	46/46	Not specified					95/80
Ramsay[39]	2001	Y	35/35		41/67	5.1/2.9	33/25	Y	88/92
Carey[40]	2000	Y	100/100	6	85/44	3.7/3.9	17/22	Y + VAS-score	69/80 89/84
Persson[41]	2000	Y	78/83	12	60/77			Y + pad tests	83/58

Su et al compared objective cure rates after 1 year and also demonstrated a significant difference at the expense of laparoscopic colposuspension.[45] More recent studies, however, showed similar or even better results in terms of success and complications. Results of properly conducted studies will eventually be published. The lack of good data is certainly one reason why traditional urogynaecologists have hesitated to embark on laparoscopic colposuspension. This is an important task for endoscopic surgeons in the near future. The true challenge of any study is to find a urogynaecology unit that can assure proper patient selection, correct and objective follow-up, as well as surgical skills, both endoscopic and for open surgery.

19.3.3 Postoperative Complications

As the laparoscopic operation is carried out in a similar fashion to the open Burch colposuspension, it will lead to similar postoperative complications. These include retention and voiding dysfunction, lower urinary tract injury, infections and various less common complications (Table 19.3).

Bladder injury was discussed above, but more worrying is the number of ureteric ligations being reported. This is probably extremely uncommon in open colposuspension.[42,46,47] Over-elevation of the bladder neck, as sometimes done in an effort to correct for cystocele, may kink the ureter(s). When diagnosed in time, the problem may be solved by section of one or more sutures.

Urinary tract infections are extremely common in this surgery, but retropubic abscesses are an uncommon infectious complication. The laparoscopic approach, and the use of extensive irrigation at the end of the procedure may reduce the risk of infection. We are not aware of clinically threatening infectious complications in the literature so far. The general use of prophylactic antibiotics may have helped in reducing wound and urinary tract infections.

Other uncommon complications are deep venous thrombosis, nerve damage and postoperative prolapse.

Table 19.3. Conversions, peroperative complications and delayed effects of open and laparoscopic colposuspension

Nature of complication	Open (%)	Laparoscopic (%)
Conversion to laparotomy		< 2
Haemorrhage	< 1	0.5
Bladder injury	< 1	3.71
Ureteral obstruction	< 0.1	< 0.1
Voiding dysfunction	2–25	5
Detrusor instability	3–25	5
Prolapse	5–27	3
Wound/incisional hernia	Not known	< 0.1

Numbers are difficult to estimate. Groin pain is usually attributed to entrapment of the ilioinguinal nerve as it exits the superficial inguinal ring. Subsequent pain is localised in the medial portion of the groin, labia or thigh. Local injection of steroids may help.

Functional complications may be early or remote. Patients with high residual volumes or hypocontractile bladders are obviously more prone to (transient) retention. They may temporarily require self-catheterisation, or use a suprapubic catheter for a longer time. De novo or recurrent detrusor instability may occur in 3–25% of cases, its course being unpredictable. The numbers for laparoscopic colposuspension are not known yet, but range from 2.8 to 8.0%, with an average of 5%.[48] There have been few reports of enterocele or related prolapse problems, but follow-up is usually too short and more reports are likely, as this is a well-known feature of open Burch colposuspension.

19.4 Conclusions

Theoretically, laparoscopic colposuspension can be a perfect mimic of the original "open" surgery. There should therefore not be much difference in outcome and complications. Reality may be different: not many surgeons have a lot of experience and meticulous follow-up in open colposuspension, and individuals combining this with extensive experience in laparoscopic suturing techniques are even scarcer. In our opinion, this uncommon combination is the main reason for the lack of evidence that laparoscopic colposuspension can indeed substitute open surgery. Initial discouraging randomised studies may have had poor outcomes because the surgeons were still in the learning curve[44] or unusual instruments were used.[45] New studies are underway that may show at least equal outcomes.

In terms of complications, inadvertent cystotomy may be more frequent. Advantages of laparoscopy are reduced postoperative pain and discomfort, a theoretical lower risk of infection, and quicker mobilisation and recovery. This implies a faster return to economical activity, but the costs related to this operation are largely dependent on the health system of the country and/or the individual patient. The more recent vaginal techniques, such as the tension-free vaginal sling operation, discussed in Chapter 20, also have these advantages, while offering similar outcomes. The wide introduction of these alternative minimally invasive techniques have skewed the discussion in recent years.

Obvious disadvantages of laparoscopy are the need for expensive equipment, lengthy operation times and a steep learning curve, which is estimated to be longer than for an open Burch colposuspension.[49]

This emphasises the need for proper training in laparoscopic surgery. If the surgeon fully masters suturing and knot-tying skills, laparoscopic colposuspension may be equivalent to the conventional "open" procedure.

References

1. Horbach NS (1992) Genuine stress urinary incontinence: best surgical approach. Contemp Obstet Gynecol 37:53
2. Jarvis GJ (1994) Surgery for genuine stress incontinence. Br J Obstet Gynaecol 101:371–374
3. Black NA, Downs SH (1996) The effectiveness of surgery for stress incontinence in women: a systematic review. Br J Urol 78:497–510
4. Alcalay M, Monga AK, Stanton SL (1995) The Burch colposuspension: a 10–20 year follow up. Br J Obstet Gynaecol 102:740–745
5. Burch JC (1961) Urethrovaginal fixation to Cooper's ligament for correction of stress incontinence, cystocele and prolapse. Am J Obstet Gynecol 81:281–290
6. Marshall VF, Marchetti AA, Krantz KE (1949) The correction of stress incontinence by simple vesicourethral suspension. Surg Gynecol Obstet 88:509–518
7. Tanagho EA (1976) Colpocystourethropexy: the way we do it. J Urol 116:751–753
8. Vancaillie TG (1997) The role of laparoscopy in the management of pelvic floor relaxation. J Am Assoc Gynecol Laparosc 4:147–148
9. Vancaillie TG, Schuessler W (1991) Laparoscopic bladder neck suspension. J Laparoendosc Surg 1:169–173
10. Underwood L, Smith M (1996) Preperitoneal laparoscopic Burch procedure. In: Cusumano PG, Deprest J (eds) Advanced gynaecological laparoscopy. Parthenon Publishers, London, pp. 143–158
11. Cusumano PG, Beco J (1996) Laparoscopic bladder neck suspension: the mesh technique. In: Cusumano PG, Deprest J (eds) Advanced gynaecological laparoscopy. Parthenon Publishers, London, pp. 159–173
12. Weston PV (1991) A new clinch knot. Obstet Gynecol 78:144–147
13. Liu CY (1994) Laparoscopic treatment of genuine urinary stress incontinence. Baill Clin Obstet Gynecol 8:789–798
14. Lyons TL (1995) Minimally invasive retropubic colposuspension. Gynaecol Endosc 4:189–194
15. Birken RA, Leggett PL (1997) Laparoscopic colposuspension using mesh reinforcement. Surg Endosc 11:1111–1114
16. Ou CS, Presthus J, Beadle E (1993) Laparoscopic bladder neck suspension using hernia mesh and surgical staples. J Laparoendosc Surg 3:563–566
17. Ross JW (1998) Multichannel urodynamic evaluation of laparoscopic Burch colposuspension for genuine stress incontinence. Obstet Gynecol 91:55–59
18. Nieves A (1996) Long-term results of laparoscopic Burch. J Am Assoc Gynecol Laparosc 3:S35
19. O'Shea RT, Seman E, Taylor J (1996) Laparoscopic Burch colposuspension for urinary stress incontinence. J Am Assoc Gynecol Laparosc 3:S36
20. Cooper MJ, Cario G, Lam A et al. (1996) A review of results in a series of 113 laparoscopic colposuspensions. Aust NZ J Obstet Gynaecol 36:44–48
21. Flax S (1996) The gasless laparoscopic Burch bladder neck suspension: early experience. J Urol 156:1105–1107
22. Hannah SL, Chin A (1996) Laparoscopic retropubic urethropexy. J Am Assoc Gynecol Laparosc 4:47–52
23. Lam AM, Jenkins GJ, Hyslop RS (1995) Laparoscopic Burch colposuspension for stress incontinence: preliminary results. Med J Aust 162:18–21
24. Liu CY, Paek W (1993) Laparoscopic retropubic colposuspension (Burch procedure). J Am Assoc Gynecol Laparosc 1:31–35
25. Lobel RW, Davis GD (1996) Long-term results of laparoscopic Burch urethropexy. J Am Assoc Gynecol Laparosc 3: S26–S27
26. Papasakelariou C, Papasakelariou B (1997) Laparoscopic bladder neck suspension. J Am Assoc Gynecol Laparosc 4:185–189
27. Radomski SB, Herschorn S (1996) Laparoscopic Burch bladder neck suspension: early results [see comments]. J Urol 155:515–518
28. Ross JW (1995) Comparison of two techniques of laparoscopic Burch repair for stress incontinence. J Am Assoc Gynecol Laparosc 2:S47
29. Saidi MH, Sadler RK, Saidi JA (1998) Extraperitoneal laparoscopic colposuspension for genuine urinary stress incontinence. J Am Assoc Gynecol Laparosc 5:247–252
30. Tay KP, Lim PH, Ravintharan T (1996) Laparoscopic bladder-neck suspension for urinary stress incontinence in women: our first twenty patients. Int J Urol 3:278–281
31. Kohli N, Jacobs PA, Sze EH et al. (1997) Open compared with laparoscopic approach to Burch colposuspension: a cost analysis. Obstet Gynecol 90:411–415
32. Miannay E, Cosson M, Lanvin D et al. (1998) Comparison of open retropubic and laparoscopic colposuspension for treatment of stress urinary incontinence. Eur J Obstet Gynecol Reprod Biol 79:159–166
33. Polascik TJ, Moore RG, Rosenberg MT et al. (1995) Comparison of laparoscopic and open retropubic urethropexy for treatment of stress urinary incontinence. Urology 45:647–652
34. Das S (1998) Comparative outcome analysis of laparoscopic colposuspension, abdominal colposuspension and vaginal needle suspension for female urinary incontinence [see comments]. J Urol 160:368–371
35. Kung R, Lie KI, Drutz HP (1995) Cost-effectiveness analysis of laparoscopic and abdominal Burch procedures. J Am Assoc Gynecol Laparosc 2:S23–S24
36. McKinney TB (1994) Comparative study of laparoscopic retropubic urethropexy with Prolene mesh and classic Burch suspension. J Am Assoc Gynecol Laparosc 1:S21
37. Su TH, Wang KG, Hsu CY et al. (1997) Prospective comparison of laparoscopic and traditional colposuspensions in the treatment of genuine stress incontinence. Acta Obstet Gynecol Scand 76:576–582
38. Burton G (1997) A three year prospective randomised urodynamic study comparing open and laparoscopic colposuspension. Neurourol Urodyn 16:353–354 (Abstract)
39. Ramsay IN, Morris AR, Reilly ETC, Hassan A, Hawthorn RJ (2001) 5–7 year follow up of a randomised trial comparing laparoscopic and open colposuspension in the treatment of genuine stress incontinence. Presented at International Urogynaecological Association, Melbourne, December 5–8, 2001
40. Carey MP, Maher PJ, Hill DJ (2000) Laparoscopic colpopsuspension. Presented at International Society of Gynaecological Endoscopy (ISGE), Gold Coast, Australia, April 16–19, 2000
41. Persson J, Wolner-Hanssen P (2000) Laparoscopic Burch colposuspension for stress urinary incontinence: a randomized comparison of one or two sutures on each side of the urethra. Obstet Gynecol 95:151–155
42. Demirci F, Petri E (2000) Perioperative complications of Burch colposuspension. Int Urogynecol J 11:170–175

43. Speights S, Moore RD, Miklos RJ (2000) Frequency of lower urinary tract injury at laparoscopic Burch and paravaginal repair. J Am Assoc Gynecol Laparosc 4:515–518
44. Burton G (1994) A randomised comparison of laparoscopic and open colposuspension. Neurourol Urodyn 13:497–498
45. Su T, Wang K, Hsu C et al. (1997) Prospective comparison of laparoscopic and traditional colposuspension in the treatment of GSI. Acta Obstet Gynecol Scand 76:576–582
46. Dwyer PL, Carey MP, Rosamilia A (1999) Suture injury to the urinary tract in urethral suspension procedures for stress incontinence. Int Urogynecol J Pelvic Floor Dysfunct 10(1):15–21
47. Virtanen HS (1995) Ureteric injury following laparoscopic colposuspension. Int Urogynecol J 6:114–118
48. Carter JE (1996) Laparoscopic Burch procedure: avoiding complications. Min Invas Ther Allied Technol 5:372–377
49. Smith A (1995) Laparoscopic pelvic floor surgery. Curr Opin Obstet Gynecol 7:397

Chapter 20

Laparoscopic Suburethral Sling Procedure

Peter von Theobald

20.1 Introduction

Since the sling operation for treatment of genuine stress incontinence was first introduced by von Giordano in 1907 (see Chin and Stanton[1]), many modifications of the operative technique and the material used for the sling have been reported. The original method, as described by Goebbel, Stoekel and Frangenheim, used strips of muscle and fascia, and was performed with laparotomy. Indications for the suburethral sling procedure are recurrent stress incontinence after previous incontinence surgery, low urethral closure pressure (30 cm H_2O or less ; type III), urethral hypermobility (type II), and patients with severe urinary incontinence having an unfavourable prognosis, such as those with severe bronchitis and/or obesity.[2-4] Fascia lata strips, rectus abdominis flaps, lyophilised dura mater, Mersilene, Silastic and polytetrafluoroethylene (PTFE) mesh bands have been tried to replace the original rectus fascia sling, in order to make the procedure easier, quicker to do, and to avoid complications such as herniation at the site of fascial harvesting.

Since the early 1990s, laparoscopy has largely proved its continuing role in the treatment of pelvic floor relaxation, mainly because of the surgeons' ability to identify anatomical structures with far greater precision than with laparotomy, as a result of barohaemostasis and improved exposure and optical magnification of the tissues. Thus, operative endoscopy for women requiring a sling procedure will enhance the quality of the dissection, make the procedure easier to perform and avoid parietal complications. The technique described in this chapter is a laparoscopic preperitoneal suburethral sling procedure using Prolene mesh bands.

20.2 Preoperative Evaluation

Preoperatively, all patients had physiotherapy with electrical stimulation of pelvic diaphragm muscles, and all menopausal women received at least 3 months of oestrogen replacement therapy. Preoperative evaluation included history taking and physical, gynaecological and neurological examination. All patients underwent multichannel urodynamic evaluation, including a waterfill cystometrogram with continuous urethral pressure monitoring and subtracted rectal and abdominal pressures and a static urethral pressure profilometry. The laparoscopic preperitoneal sling procedure was indicated for women without genital prolapse, without unstable detrusor, with normal voiding, having a type II or type III incontinence, and patients with severe urinary incontinence having an unfavourable prognosis, such as those with severe bronchitis and/or obesity.

All the patients gave informed consent to the procedure, being told that laparotomy might be performed in case of technical difficulties or peroperative complications.

20.3 Operative Technique

The patient is placed in the supine position, thighs spread, under general anaesthesia. Intravenous prophylactic antibiotics (ampicillin–sulbactam) are administered immediately before surgery. Pneumoretzius is obtained by two suprapubic incisions and an optic trocar (Visiport, 12 mm). It is then enlarged up to the umbilicus, and a third trocar (10 mm) is placed (Figure 20.1).

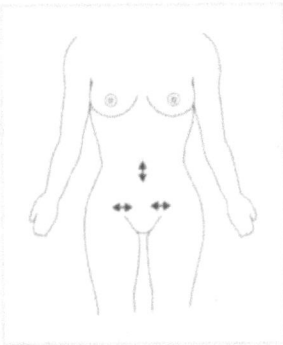

Figure 20.1 Position of the trocars for the laparoscopic suburethral sling procedure.

The optic fibre is placed into the umbilical trocar, and the bladder neck (pointed out by a Foley catheter) is dissected. The pelvic fascia is totally freed from the bladder and the surrounding fat tissue with blunt grasping forceps and two fingers in the vagina. Haemostasis is performed with bipolar cauterisation. The upper sheet of the pelvic fascia (Figure 20.2) is incised 1 cm away from the proximal urethra on each side. A right-angle dissector is used to open the space between the urethrovesical fascia above and the genital fascia (Halban fascia) below, in order to join the contralateral incision of the pelvic fascia. This dissection is performed under vaginal control with two fingers, and with step-by-step haemostasis of the perivaginal vessels with bipolar cautery.

A Prolene mesh band (15 mm wide and 20 cm long) is pulled underneath the urethra through this dissected space with the right-angle dissector. Both ends of the mesh band are grasped with a grasping forceps, and a cystoscopy is perfomed to check the integrity of the urethra and bladder walls, as well as

the correct position of the sling, by pulling the grasping forceps gently upwards, holding the ends of the mesh band. Two or three staples (Endohernia 4.8) on each side of the bladder neck fix the mesh band to the pelvic fascia and close the fascial incisions. The ends of the sling are then sutured to the rectus abdominis fascia with absorbable stitches, closing at the same time the suprapubic 12 mm fascial incisions (Endoclose needle). The tension of the sling must be low: the urethra is pulled only 1 or 2 cm upwards, in order to balance the 8 mmHg CO_2 pressure usually required for this procedure. The Foley catheter is removed on the second or third postoperative day, and the patient is discharged as soon as normal voiding occurs with postvoid residuals less than 20 ml.

20.4 Outcome

The results presented here summarise a prospective study of 31 patients who were scheduled to undergo a preperitoneal suburethral sling procedure by the same surgeon, for stress incontinence, between 1993 and 1998. All women were evaluated pre- and postoperatively at intervals of 6 months. The follow-up period ranged from 1 to 58 months (average 27); no patients were lost to follow-up. The patient population ranged from 35 to 66 years of age (average 47). The population characteristics and operative risk factors are presented in Table 20.1. Concomitant procedures, duration of the procedure and day of discharge are presented in Table 20.2. In six patients, laparotomy had to be performed because of technical difficulties or peroperative complications (Figure 20.4). Complications are presented in Figure 20.5. Six of the main complications occurred in the first nine patients, corresponding to our learning curve; most of these patients had operative risk factors. By the tenth patient, use of the right-angle dissector had been fully mastered, the anatomy of the two sheets of the pelvic fascia was

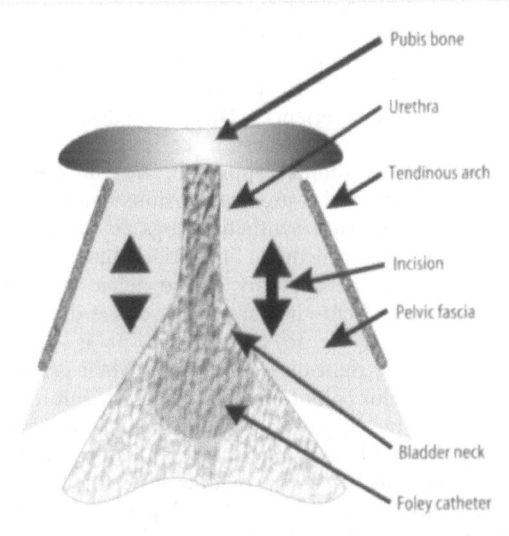

Figure 20.2 The pelvic fascia.

Table 20.1. Population characteristics and operative risk factors. PTFE, Polytetrafluoroethylene

Parity	0–8 (average 3)
Obesity	9 patients (29%)
Previous suprapubic laparotomy	10 patients (32%)
Previous incontinence surgery	4 patients: 2 vaginal PTFE slings (Mouchel) 1 Burch colposuspension (laparotomy) 1 promontofixation + Burch
Preoperative closure pressure	15–70 (average 34) cm H_2O

Table 20.2. Concomitant procedures, duration of procedure and day of discharge

No. of patients	Procedure	Duration (min)	Discharge on day
22	Sling only (incl. laparotomies)	40–130 (average 77)	2–10 (average 5)
16	Sling only (excl. laparotomies)	40–120 (average 74)	2–7 (average 4)
6	Tubal ligation	40–120 (average 72)	2–5 (average 3)
1	Ovarian cystectomy	60	3
1	Myomectomy	90	5
1	Vaginal hysterectomy	100	7

more familiar, the accurate tension of the sling had been evaluated, and minor complications such as bladder injury could be treated without performing laparotomy. The overall success rate of the slings was 84%, with an average follow-up of 27 months.

20.5 Conclusions

Knowledge of the surgical anatomy of the pelvic fascia is essential to avoid secondary erosion of the urethra or the bladder neck. The Prolene mesh band has to be set underneath the urethrovesical fascia, as shown in Figure 20.3. This dissection plane is identical to the one opened by vaginal anterior colpotomy. Starting the suburethral dissection too close to the urethra involves the risk of injury to the bladder or urethra, or of passing the sling between the urethra and the urethrovesical fascia. In this case, secondary erosion of the urinary tissue will occur during the months following the procedure.

The main advantages of laparoscopy applied to the sling procedure are: bloodless dissection, perfect exposure of the tissues and optical magnification, allowing easy recognition of the fascial dissection plane. Operation time is approximately the same as

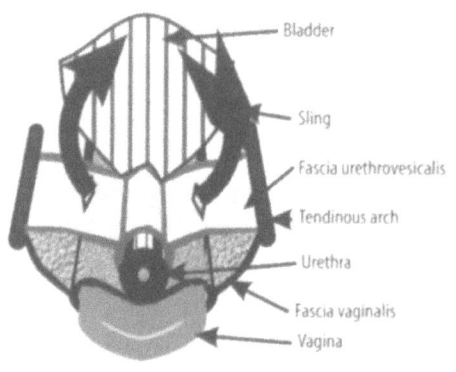

Figure 20.3 Position of the sling.

in classical procedures, and patient discharge is possibly earlier. No parietal complications occur.

Three authors have described their experience of using laparoscopy to perform a sling cystourethropexy. Pelosi[5] performed one transperitoneal sling procedure using a polypropylene mesh; his technique was similar to ours, and the outcome was excellent. Narepalem[6] and Madelenat[7] performed one and 23 sling procedures, using fascia lata and polygalactin strips, respectively. Both authors had good results. All these papers report primary procedures. In our series, four patients had had previous incontinence surgery, and three of these underwent conversion to laparotomy. This emphasises the limits of the laparoscopic sling procedure: secondary surgery is difficult with laparoscopy, requiring more experience and improved dissection devices. We do not believe that secondary surgery is a contraindication to laparoscopic surgery, but the patient should be informed preoperatively of the high risk of laparotomy.

Another discussion concerns the use of slings made of indigenous (fascia lata) or allogenic material. Prosthetic slings are thought to be associated with a higher incidence of urethral erosion,[4,8,9] but also with better long-term results.[9,10] We believe that there is no conclusive evidence in recent literature.

Comparison between different series is impossible, because of the variability of the synthetic (PTFE, Mersilene, Prolene, Marlex, Silastic, Polygalactin) or the allogenic (Lyodura) material used, and particularly the differences in surgical technique, which are sometimes purely abdominal and sometimes abdomino-vaginal. Table 20.3 shows that abdomino-vaginal procedures rarely involve urethral erosions (0.2%), but more frequently sling infection, rejection, granulomas and abscesses (11.2%). Exclusive abdominal procedures involve 4% of erosions with synthetic material. There are no data concerning the incidence of herniation at the site of fascial harvesting (almost 10% after 5 years in our experience). There is no description of the fascial sling procedure carried out by an exclusively abdominal approach. In our opinion, the high incidence of urethral erosions in abdominal procedures (always synthetic slings) is caused not only by the prosthetic material, but also by ignorance of the anatomy of the pelvic fascia (as in the first patients in our series), and a dissection starting too close to the urethra. It is easy to recognise the right dissection plane when performing an anterior colpotomy, but more difficult to find abdominally. Laparoscopy facilitates abdominal recognition of anatomical structures, magnifying the operation site and providing a perfect haemostasis. We believe that the laparoscopic sling procedure is feasible, with good results when performed by experienced endoscopists.

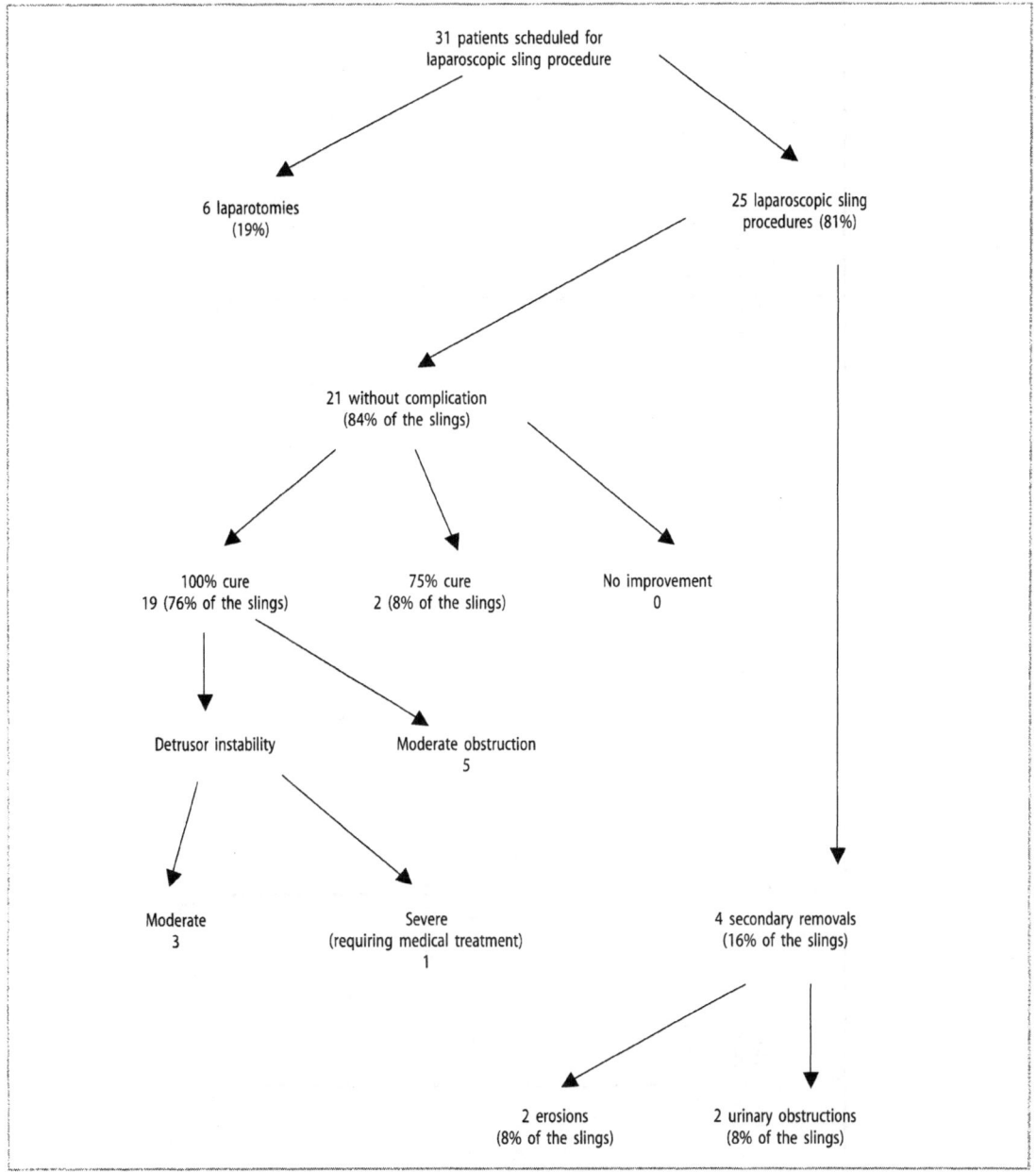

Figure 20.4 Results of the study

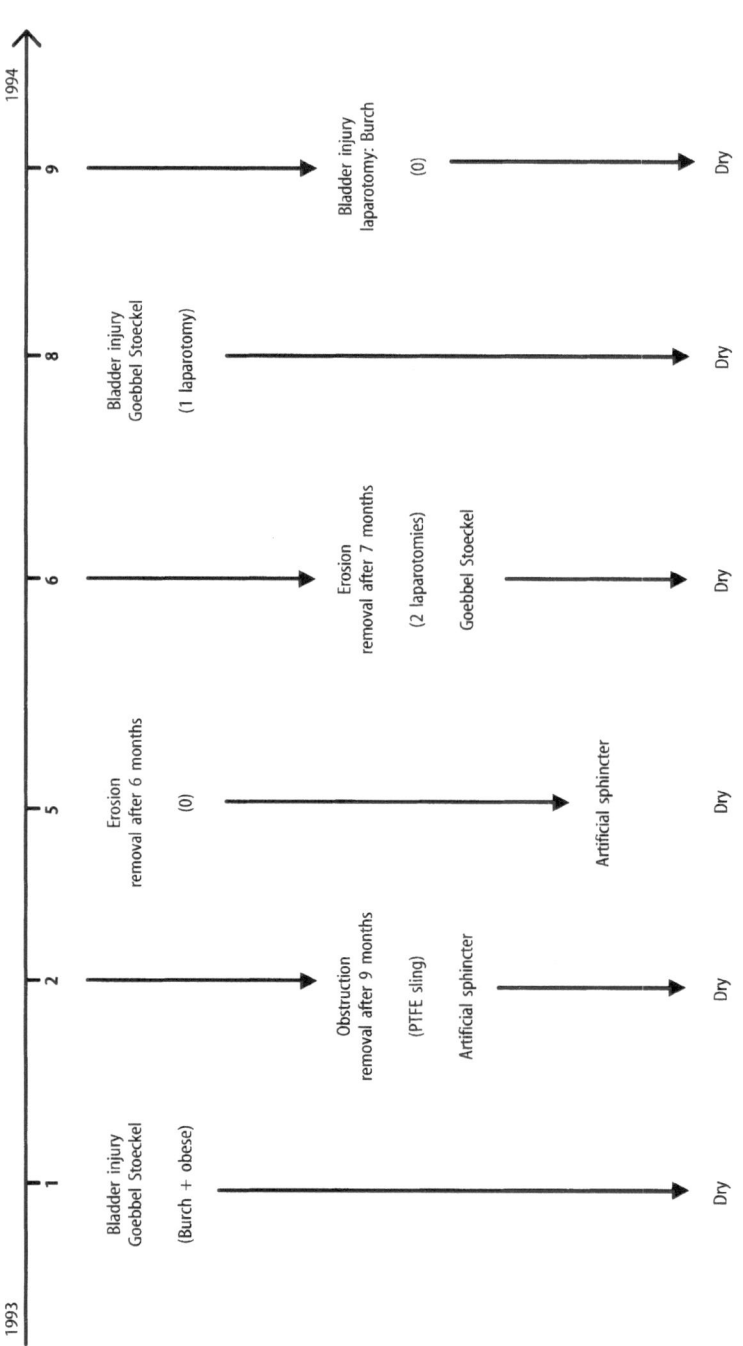

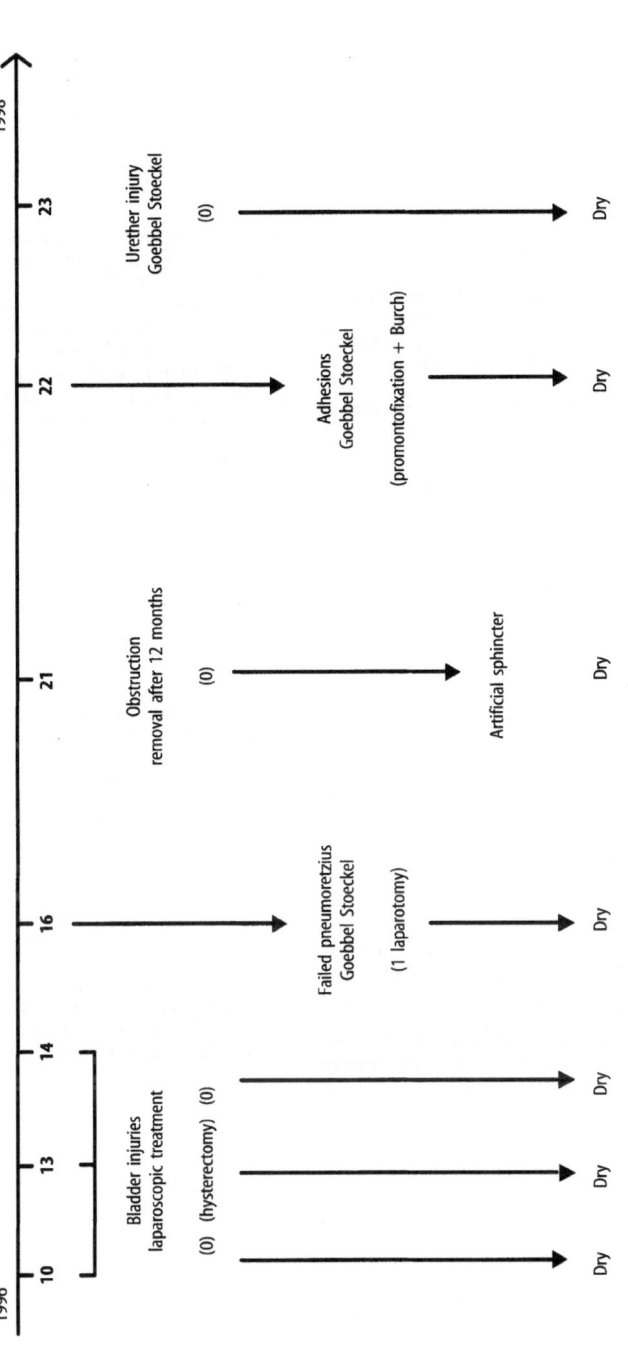

Figure 20.5. Complications: patient chronological number is in bold, with complications, treatment, operative risk factors (in brackets) and outcome below. PTFE, Polytetrafluoroethylene

Table 20.3. Review of the recent literature about sling procedures and their complications. PTFE, Polytetrafluoroethylene

Sling	Technique	Material	Complications
Allogenic	Abdominal	218 Marlex[11]	2 urethral erosions
		74 Silastic[1]	10 urethral erosions
	Abdomino-vaginal	194 Lyodura[12-14]	15 vaginal complications
		290 PTFE[3,7,10,15-17]	66 vaginal complications
			2 urethral erosions
		209 Mersilene[18-20]	4 vaginal complications
		12 Polygalactin[7]	No complications
Indigenous	Abdomino-vaginal	100 rectal fascia[2,10,15]	No complications
		32 muscle flap[21]	1 abscess

References

1. Chin YK, Stanton SL (1995) A follow up of silastic sling for genuine stress incontinence. Br J Obstet Gynaecol 102:143–147
2. Zagora MR (1996) Expanded indications for the pubovaginal sling: treatment of type 2 or 3 stress incontinence. J Urol 156:1620–1622
3. Weinberger MW, Ostergard DR (1995) Long term clinical and urodynamical evaluation of the polytetrafluoroethylene suburethral sling for treatment of genuine stress incontinence. Obstet Gynecol 86:92–96
4. Haab F, Zimmern PE, Leach GE (1996) Female stress urinary incontinence due to intrinsic sphincteric deficiency: recognition and management. J Urol 156:3–17
5. Pelosi MA III, Pelosi MA (1996) Laparoscopic assisted pubovaginal sling procedure for the treatment of stress urinary incontinence. J Am Assoc Gynecol Laparosc 3:593–600
6. Narepalem N, Kreder KJ, Winfield HN (1995) Laparoscopic urethral sling for the treatment of intrinsic urethral weakness (type III stress urinary incontinence). Tech Urol 1:102–105
7. Darai E, Theillier A, Fauconnier A et al. (1998) Suburethral sling procedure by combined laparoscopic-vaginal approach for treatment of stress incontinence. Gynecol Endosc 7:13–18
8. Cholhan HJ, Stevenson KR (1996) Sling transection of urethra: a rare complication. Int Urogynecol 7:331–334
9. Leach GE, Dmochowski RR, Appell RA et al. (1997) Female stress incontinence clinical guidelines panel summary report on surgical management of female stress urinary incontinence. J Urol 158:875–880
10. Barbalias G, Liatsikos E, Barbalias D (1997) Use of slings made of indigenous and allogenic material (Goretex) in type III urinary incontinence and comparison between them. Eur Urol 31:394–400
11. Morgan JE, Farrow GA, Stewart FE (1985) The Marlex sling operation for the treatment of recurrent stress urinary incontinence: a 16 year review. Am J Obstet Gynecol 151:224–226

12. Hägele D, Frühwirth O, Kriesche H et al. (1983) Ergebnisse nach Schlingenoperation mit Tutoplast-Dura. Geburtsh u Frauenheilk 43:762–765
13. Enzelsberger H, Kurz C, Seifert M et al. (1993) Zur operativen Behandlung der Rezidvstressinkontinenz: Burch versus Lyoduraschlingenoperation - eine prospektive Studie. Geburtsh u Frauenheilk 53:467–471
14. Enzelsberger H, Helmer H, Schatten C (1996) Comparison of Burch and Lyodura sling procedures for repair of unsuccessful incontinence surgery. Obstet Gynecol 88:251–256
15. Ogundipe A, Rosenzweig BA, Karram MM (1992) Modified suburethral sling procedure for treatment of recurrent or severe stress urinary incontinence. Surg Gynecol Obstet 175:173–176
16. Horbach NS, Blanco JS, Ostergard DR et al. (1988) A suburethral sling procedure with polytetrafluoroethylene for the treatment of genuine stress incontinence in patients with low closure pressure. Obstet Gynecol 71:648–652
17. Bent AE, Ostergard DR, Zwick-Zaffuto M (1993) Tissue reaction to expanded polytetrafluoroethylene suburethral sling for urinary incontinence: clinical and histologic study. Am J Obstet Gynecol 169:1198–1204
18. Falconer C, Ekman-Ordeberg G, Malström A et al. (1996) Clinical outcome and changes in connective tissue metabolism after intravaginal slingplasty in stress incontinent women. Int Urogynecol 7:133–137
19. Young SB, Rosenblatt PL, Pingeton DM et al. (1995) The Mersilene mesh suburethral sling: a clinical and urodynamic evaluation. Am J Obstet Gynecol 173:1719–1726
20. Guner H, Yildiz A, Erdem A et al. (1994) Surgical treatment of urinary stress incontinence by a suburethral sling procedure using a Mersilene mesh graft. Gynecol Obstet Invest 37:52–55
21. Wall L, Phil D, Galloway NTM (1996) Use of a pedicled rectus abdominis muscle flap sling in the treatment of complicated stress urinary incontinence. Am J Obstet Gynecol 175:1460–1466

Part V

Ovarian Masses

Contents

Summary

Transvaginal ultrasonography can be used to characterise accurately the majority of ovarian masses. An ultrasound report should now not only report the presence of a mass but provide an assessment of the likely pathology. Physiological ovarian cysts are common and repeat scans must be performed to avoid unnecessary surgery on these lesions. Morphological assessment is the mainstay of the evaluation of persistent ovarian masses. Solid papillary projections into the cyst are often associated with malignancy. The size of a lesion is an issue, as beyond 5.0 cm it becomes difficult to examine the entire cyst wall. Subjective impression of the likely nature of a mass by an experienced operator is highly accurate. Statistical models show promise but have yet to perform better than subjective impression, and care must be taken regarding the application of these models outside the populations from whom they are derived. A surgeon should expect to know the nature of an ovarian mass before starting a procedure and plan surgery accordingly.

The introduction of laparoscopy has transformed the management of ovarian masses, but made preoperative evaluation more important. Most benign ovarian masses can be treated by laparoscopy. The surgical approach for these tumours is discussed. When malignancy is suspected, laparotomy remains the standard, although a suspicious lesion may be treated by laparoscopic oophorectomy as long as the lesion is removed intact from the abdomen in an endobag. The role of laparoscopy in the management of patients with ovarian cancer remains controversial; however, it may be a feasible alternative to second-look laparotomy in some cases.

Key points

- The presence of a cyst on the ovary must be related to the patient's age and menstrual cycle. Repeat scans must be performed to allow resolution of a cyst in order to avoid unnecessary surgery
- Even in postmenopausal women, unilocular simple cysts of less than 20 mm diameter do not merit removal
- A conservative management strategy should be considered for unilocular simple cysts that measure between 20 and 50 mm. All tumours that are complex and suspicious of malignancy should be removed
- The majority of ovarian masses can be characterised on the basis of subjective impression. Complex mathematical models do not perform as well as an expert operator
- Dermoid cysts and endometriomas can be reliably identified with ultrasound
- Solid papillary projections into the cyst cavity are a sinister morphological feature and are associated with malignancy
- Surgery should be considered for masses of over 5.0 as small solid projections may be missed by the vaginal probe
- The data relating to colour Doppler are conflicting. Doppler plays a limited role in the evaluation of ovarian masses in clinical practice
- Care must be taken when evaluating data from statistical models because of the problems that arise when applying these models to different populations
- Most benign ovarian masses can be treated by laparoscopy
- Cyst puncture and drainage facilitates cystectomy in most cases
- Ovarian tissue should be removed from the abdomen in an endobag
- Laparoscopy should not be considered as a primary procedure when there is a significant risk of malignancy
- Second-look laparoscopy may be a viable alternative to laparotomy in some cases, although its role in the oncology patient is controversial

Chapter 21

The Use of Ultrasound to Assess the Morphology of Ovarian Tumours

Seth Granberg, Erling Ekerhovd, Dirk Timmerman and Tom Bourne

21.1 Introduction

The rapid development of ultrasound technology has led to an increase in the detection rate of ovarian cysts. Such cysts can be diagnosed at any age or stage of a woman's life, from as early as the fetal stage to as late as the postmenopause. A high number of cystic structures are seen in the ovaries, even in post-menopausal women. Many of these regress spontaneously or remain unchanged. The clinical dilemma that these cystic structures cause for the clinician is well documented. Furthermore, it is also well known that transvaginal sonography plays an important role, not only in the detection of ovarian cysts, but also in the characterisation of these lesions. The problem for the clinician remains the same. Which cystic structures on the ovaries can be managed conservatively, and which need to be removed? Advances in surgery have now led to a further issue. If there is an ovarian cyst, is it suitable for minimal access surgery or are the services of a gynaecological oncologist required?

This chapter will discuss some of the problems that appear at a clinical practice when using B-mode ultrasound and will also try to explain the significance of certain morphological features of ovarian tumours.

21.2 Transvaginal Ultrasound

By placing the ultrasound probe closer to the area of interest, it is possible to use higher frequency ultrasound transducers; this in turn leads to the production of higher resolution images. As a result, applications have been found for transvaginal ultrasonography in many areas of gynaecological practice.[1-4] Its ability to reveal details of ovarian structure and volume has been clearly demonstrated in the field of infertility.[5,6] The technique of transvaginal ultrasonography has been described before.[7] In the context of ovarian cancer screening, transvaginal ultrasonography has the practical advantage of not requiring a full bladder.[8] This is particularly relevant as the target population may well have problems in maintaining urinary continence.

A close correlation has been found between ovarian volume and morphology as described using transvaginal ultrasonography and subsequent operative findings at laparotomy.[9] In this study, 52 patients were examined before laparotomy, and the correlation coefficient between ultrasound and surgical measurement was 0.78 in normal and 0.99 in abnormal ovaries. Out of 104 ovaries, 85 were visualised at ultrasonography (82%). Those not seen were confirmed as being small and atrophic at the time of surgery. Ninety per cent of ovarian abnormalities were detected, and there were no false-positive findings. In this series, only one case of carcinoma was found – it had a complex structure. Other workers have assessed the interobserver variation in the measurement of ovarian volume. Based on independent measurements of 86 ovaries, the correlation coefficient between the ovarian volume measurements of each observer was 0.96.[10] Comparisons with transabdominal ultrasonography support the view that transvaginal ultrasonography provides improved diagnostic information in the majority of cases. Mendelson et al.[11] studied 59 patients with adnexal or ovarian pathology using transvaginal and transabdominal ultrasound; transvaginal ultrasound was thought to be better in 78% of cases. Therefore, the use of transvaginal ultrasonography seems accurately to reflect ovarian morphology and volume, as well as offering an advantage over the transabdominal route.

Preliminary data were initially reported on the use of this technique in a screening programme for ovarian carcinoma by Higgins et al..[12] An abnormal postmenopausal ovary was defined in this study as having a volume of over $8.0\,cm^3$ or any complex or solid areas. In premenopausal ovaries, the maximal permissible volume was $18\,cm^3$. Cystic changes compatible with the stage of the patient's menstrual cycle were classified as normal. Twelve ovarian lesions were found in a sample of 506 asymptomatic women. Ten of these women agreed to surgery: nine had a benign lesion and there was one case of metastatic carcinoma from the colon. The authors claim that 86% of the ovaries in the study were visualised, although there is no reference method to validate this. The same group subsequently published their data on the first 1000 women in their programme who had undergone both a prevalence screen and one follow-up screen.[13] All the women were asymptomatic. It is of interest to note that, while 9.2% of premenopausal women had some sort of ovarian abnormality on their initial scan, in only 3.8% was the lesion persistent when the scan was repeated. This emphasises the need to reassess carefully any ovarian abnormality found on a screening examination. Twenty-four women underwent surgery in the course of this study, and one metastatic ovarian carcinoma was found. However, it must be remembered that no attempt was made in this study to reduce the false-positive rate using any kind of second-stage tests.

In another study, 442 women were scanned, 13 underwent surgery, and one stage I serous cystadenocarcinoma was found.[14] The impressive number of 13 operations being performed on women with a positive test result to find one cancer is to some extent due to the fact that about 30% of this group of patients had a positive family history of ovarian cancer. In four of the 13 patients who underwent surgery, the authors did not recommend an operative intervention. This demonstrates an important practical point. Once a woman has been told she has an ovarian cyst, no matter what advice is given to her, a proportion will insist on surgery. What is more, she will inevitably find a doctor who will carry out that surgery. In some of these cases at least, the use of laparoscopic surgery could reduce both operative morbidity and unnecessary bed occupancy. Therefore an important issue needs to be addressed, i.e. what criteria can be used to decide which persistent lesions need to be removed and which can safely be left in situ?

Two ultrasound-based approaches have been proposed with respect to this problem: morphological assessment using B-mode imaging alone, and vascular assessment with transvaginal colour Doppler. Only morphological assessment will be discussed in this chapter.

21.3 Morphology Assessment

Using the morphological appearances of ovarian tumours in order to predict the likelihood of malignancy has been described with a variable degree of success. It must be emphasised that attempts to characterise tumours morphologically are applicable only to high-resolution transvaginal ultrasonography. Transabdominal ultrasonography may be useful for the evaluation of large tumours extending beyond the range of a vaginal probe, but it is not suitable for making a detailed morphological assessment.

The appearance of any adnexal mass can be described in terms of several criteria, including the size or volume of the lesion, the number of cysts (monocystic or multicystic), number of locules for a given cyst (unilocular or multilocular), echogenicity (cystic, solid or mixed), cyst outline (regular or irregular), papillary projections (presence or absence), wall thickness, septal thickness, echodense foci (presence or absence), acoustic shadowing, mobility of the lesion, and finally ascites (presence or absence). Each of these factors will be reviewed in turn.

21.4 The Size of a Lesion

The size of an ovary is usually measured in three perpendicular planes and the volume calculated according to the formula for a prolate ellipsoid: $\pi/6 \times D1 \times D2 \times D3$ (where D1, 2, and 3 represent the three diameters of the ovary).

In clinical practice, the largest diameter is usually used as the most convenient index; furthermore, this measurement is associated with little subjective bias or interobserver variability.

In general, the risk of malignancy rises with increasing tumour size. In a major study, Granberg et al.[15] reported the macroscopic appearances of a series of ovarian tumours that had been removed from both pre- and postmenopausal women. They described 1017 tumours, of which 789 (77.6%) were benign, 25 (2.5%) were borderline, and 203 (20.0%) were malignant. The tumours were arbitrarily divided into three size categories based on their maximum diameters: < 5 cm, 5–10 cm and > 10 cm. Ninety-four per cent of tumours less than 5 cm were benign, eight were borderline and 14 malignant (6%). When lesions are measured using ultrasonography, similar results are obtained. Granberg et al.[16] performed preoperative transvaginal ultrasonography on 180 masses in both pre- and postmenopausal women. One hundred and forty-one (78%) were benign and 39 (21%) were malignant. Of the 54 tumours that measured less than 5 cm, only one was malignant. Other workers have reported similar findings. Sassone et al.[17] found 97 % of masses less than 5 cm were benign, irrespective of menopausal status.

The survey of ovarian cyst histology by Granberg et al.[15] also demonstrates how the risk of malignancy rises with increasing cyst size. This study shows a positive predictive value for malignancy of 5.9% for cysts < 5.0 cm, 21.3% for 5–10 cm and 43.6% for > 10 cm. On the basis of these data, it would seem unwise to apply morphological or indeed Doppler criteria for malignancy for lesions greater than 10 cm in diameter, and possibly also for those between 5 and 10 cm. However, the data derived from ultrasonography are more variable. Granberg et al.[16] reported that the risk of malignancy for lesions > 10 cm was as high as 71.8%, whereas in contrast, the data of Sassone et al.[17] suggested the risk may be of the order of 12.5%. This discrepancy can be largely explained by the different prevalence of malignancy in the two series: 21.7% in the former and 5% in the latter.

In a series of 300 consecutive patients presenting with persistent adnexal masses, Timmerman et al.[18] found no significant correlation between size of the tumour and the risk of malignancy. In this study, performed in a referral centre, very few functional cysts were present and 27.7% of the masses were malignant, including many (30%) stage I cancers. Of all lesions < 5.0 cm, 28.1% proved to be malignant, whereas 42.5% of those > 10 cm were malignant.

Other workers have stratified their data according to menopausal status. Their findings merely reflect the greater prevalence of malignancy seen in the post-menopausal population. Notwithstanding these limitations, the probability of malignancy associated with tumours > 10 cm is too high for a conservative management strategy to be adopted irrespective of either the morphological or colour Doppler appearances of the lesion. Furthermore, tumours of this size are sometimes unsuitable for morphological evaluation as they extend beyond the depth of penetration of most vaginal ultrasound probes. Hence, in a paper by Bourne et al.,[19] only lesions of less than 5.0 cm were considered suitable for evaluation by second-stage tests. When the lesion is less than 5.0 cm, the risk of malignancy is relatively low, and morphological information may be of interest to clarify the situation further. Between 5 and 10 cm is a grey area. If the entire cyst structure can be visualised by transvaginal ultrasonography, a morphological evaluation may be a reasonable strategy. If not, the risk of malignancy must be of concern.

For the reasons discussed above, the morphological and Doppler assessment of ovarian lesions is probably of relevance only to lesions < 5.0 cm. For lesions larger than this, more detailed ultrasound findings are unlikely to alter the decision whether to operate or not, but they may alter the surgical approach (laparoscopy or laparotomy with or without preoperative staging examinations).

21.5 Locularity and Septations

A loculated cyst is one that is divided into compartments by septations, and should not be confused with a multicystic ovary, which contains a number of separate cysts. This distinction can, however, be difficult in some cases. The commonly used term of "simple cyst" refers to a monocystic, unilocular lesion with no irregular features (Figure 21.1). In contrast, the term "complex cyst". refers to any cyst, which may have all or any

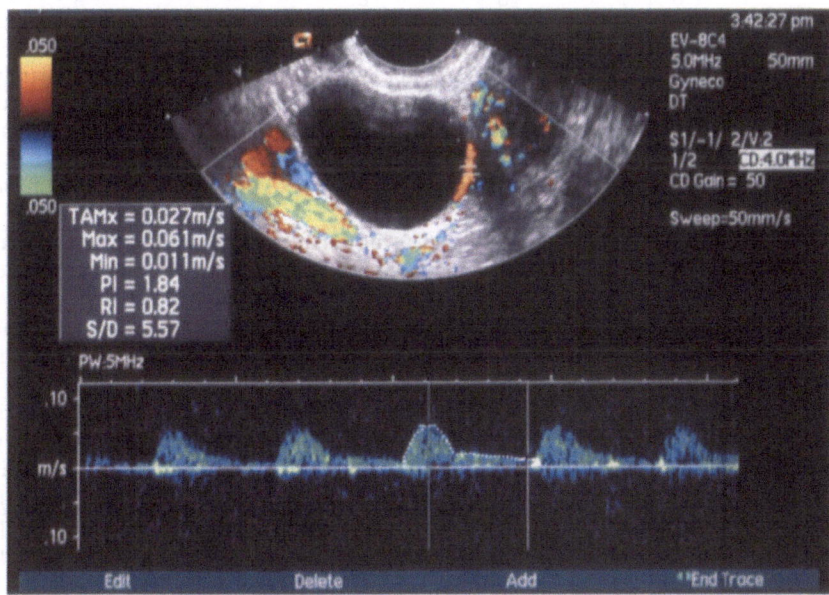

Figure 21.1. Simple cyst with anechoic contents (benign serous cystadenoma).

combination of features such as multicysts, multiloculations and/or the presence of papillary projections.

Published data show that a multilocular lesion is more likely to be malignant. To test the idea that complex cysts are more likely to be malignant, it is instructive to return once more to the histology review carried out by Granberg et al..[15] This study included 499 (49%) unilocular, 438 (43%) multilocular and 80 (8%) solid tumours. Only five of the unilocular cysts harboured malignant or borderline pathology (1%), compared to 191 (44%) of the lesions described as multilocular. Of the 80 solid tumours, 32 (39%) were malignant or borderline. These data represent the most convincing argument relating to morphology and ovarian pathology. It shows clearly the tendency towards more serious pathology with increasing morphological complexity. Simple unilocular cysts are unlikely to represent a malignancy; once septae or solid areas are present, the risk of malignancy increases. Attempts to produce weighted morphology scoring systems must therefore carry an inherent risk of missing cancer, a point made clear from the results by Bourne et al..[19] The further study by Granberg et al.[16] of 180 tumours examined by transvaginal ultrasonography confirmed these findings. This is hardly a radically new observation. Two earlier studies using transabdominal ultrasonography, which categorised lesions into either unilocular or complex cysts, also showed the relatively low risk of malignancy associated with unilocular cysts (1.8–2.6%).[20,21] With complex cysts, however, 24.2% were malignant in one study[20] and 72.7% in another.[21]

If the size of a lesion is included as a variable, as well as the presence or absence of solid papillary projections, more useful information can be extracted. In both the histology- and ultrasonography-based studies by Granberg et al.,[15,16] which have already been discussed, none of the unilocular lesions less than 5 cm was malignant. In this study, it was shown that, while the overall positive predictive value for malignancy for a multilocular lesion is 37.4%, when 10 cm, the risk of malignancy exceeds 90%.

In postmenopausal women, unilocular cysts and their risk for malignancy have been studied by ultrasound for more than two decades. It is known that the percentage of postmenopausal women in the whole population (including both sexes) is increasing to 18%. It is also known that unilocular cysts (including paraovarian cysts) will be found in 12–20% of postmenopausal women. This means that about 600 000 out of 21 million people in the Nordic countries are women who are postmenopausal and have a unilocular ovarian cyst measuring 20–50 mm in diameter (Granberg et al., unpublished data). Data show that the mortality from a laparoscopic surgical operation is 3/100 000.[22] This means that if

all these women in the Nordic countries undergo laparoscopic surgery, 18 will die as a result of the operation. The question is: "Is the risk for malignancy in unilocular ovarian cysts so high that this can be accepted?"

The first study suggesting that unilocular cysts found in postmenopausal women did not need to be removed was by Goldstein and colleagues in 1988.[23] Since that time, several studies have been published.[24–31] Kroon and Andolf published a study in which they had followed 83 postmenopausal women with a unilocular cyst between 1983 and 1992.[32] No malignant ovarian tumour was reported during this follow-up. They concluded that non-palpable ovarian cysts are commonly detected by ultrasound in asymptomatic women, but the risk of malignancy appears to be very low. They recommended ultrasound follow-up of static lesions and that surgery should be confined to symptomatic cases or those in which there is a family history of ovarian, breast or colon cancer. Several studies have been published that make the same suggestions and recommendations.[23–32]

One study by Osmers et al.[33] found that 9.6% (13/135) of unilocular ovarian cysts in postmenopausal women contained either a borderline or invasive carcinoma. The corresponding figure for premenopausal women was 0.8% (5/641). These figures should be compared to a study in which borderline or invasive lesions were found in 1.6% (4/247) of postmenopausal and 0.73% (3/413) of premenopausal women.[34] In this study, no borderline or malignant cyst measured < 75 mm. However, when unilocular cysts were complicated by papillary projections, malignant or borderline lesions were present in tumours in 10% (13/130) of postmenopausal women and 2.1% (11/514) of premenopausal women. These figures are in agreement with those of Osmers et al.. These data suggest that some of the unilocular cysts described by Osmers in fact had papillary projections that were missed. The fact that in the German study the scans were performed by general gynaecologists with no particular expertise in vaginal ultrasonography tends to support this view.

During the past few years, several studies have shown a very low risk of malignancy in unilocular cysts measuring less than 50 mm.[26–29] In these four studies, a total of 577 unilocular cysts were evaluated by ultrasound and only four were found to be borderline or invasive malignancies. However, these four cysts measured over 50, 70, 110 and 180 mm respectively.

In a study by Ekerhovd et al.,[34] in which more than 1300 unilocular cysts were classified by transvaginal sonography prior to surgery as unilocular simple without papillary formations (group I) and unilocular with papillary formations (group II), a very low risk for malignancy was reported in group I. In this group, three of 413 cysts (0.73%) in premenopausal women and four of 247 cysts (1.6%) in postmenopausal women proved to be borderline or malignant. However, all the borderline and malignant cysts measured more than 70 mm and turned out to have papillary formations on the internal wall of the cyst, which had been missed by transvaginal sonography. The corresponding figures for cysts in group II were 11 of 514 cysts (2.1%) and 13 of 130 cysts (10%), respectively. The authors concluded that locularity is not sufficient to discriminate between a benign, borderline or malignant unilocular cyst when solid parts/papillary formations are present, and that if the cysts measure more than 50 mm, papillary formations on the internal cyst wall can easily be missed by transvaginal sonography.[34]

In summary, the data suggest that the only lesion that is associated with a very low risk of malignancy is one that is simple, unilocular and less than 5.0 cm in size. Any morphological deviation from this is associated with a variable increased risk of malignancy. Similarly, any lesion greater than 10 cm has a definite increased risk of harbouring a cancer. Any morphological score that introduces variations from the simple unilocular cyst will reduce the detection rate for cancer. It is important that this is appreciated. The precise risk of malignancy associated with any particular feature is difficult to ascertain because of the prevalence effect inherent in many of the studies quoted above. However, the low risk of malignancy in relatively small unilocular cysts is now generally accepted. Accordingly, we should consider the operative risks involved in removing ovarian cysts and consider avoiding surgery completely in many cases.

21.6 Papillary Projections

These project from the inner surface of cysts, and are the result of localised overgrowth of epithelium. Histological examination usually reveals stroma of variable density covered by tall columnar epithelium. Large papillary projections can be seen relatively easily using transvaginal ultrasonography (Figure 21.2). However, to exclude them, the entire cyst wall must be visible and carefully examined. More subtle irregularities of the wall of a cyst may be more difficult to identify, nor is it known when an irregular cyst wall becomes a papillary projection.

The significance of papillary projections has been recognised for some time, even with the rudimentary ultrasound equipment available in the early 1970s. It is the one ultrasound feature most strongly associated with malignancy. Few, if any, clinicians are happy to manage such lesions conservatively, a policy supported by the literature. Returning yet again to the data of Granberg et al.,[15,16] 152 out of 1017 tumours showed macroscopic evidence of the presence of papillary projections. Of these, 81 (53%) were either malignant or borderline lesions. In their subsequent ultrasound-based study, ultrasonography tended to overdiagnose the presence of papillary projections; these were reported in 51 tumours by ultrasonography compared to 43 on macroscopic examination of removed tissues. However, the associated risk of malignancy in these 43 cases was 67%. Even with transabdominal ultrasound, Meire et al.[35] found that 83% of the tumours in his series with solid projections were cancers. More recently, Sladkevicius et al.[36] also found a high risk of malignancy associated with

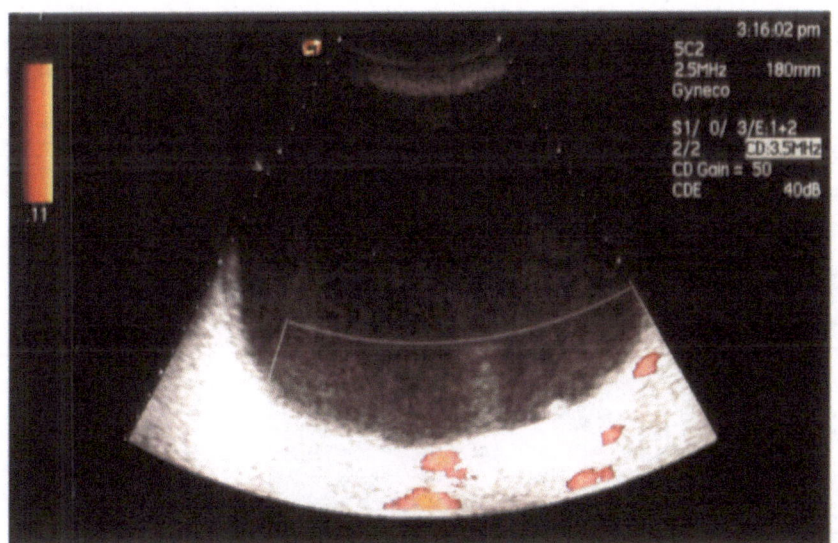

Figure 21.2. Unilocular-solid cyst with small papillary projections and low-level internal echoes (borderline malignant endometroid adenocarcinoma).

papillary projections. In their series of 300 patients examined with transvaginal ultrasound, Timmerman et al. visualised papillary projections (> 3 mm) in 26% of all adnexal masses.[18] They found cancer in 71% of these masses.

It is clear that papillary projections within an ovarian cyst are an ominous sign. There is evidence that the likelihood of malignancy increases proportionately with the number of such irregularities present.[16] However, the use of a quantitative analysis in this context will do little to change the management of the patient. A persistent cyst with solid papillary projections needs to be removed surgically as it is associated with a risk of malignancy that makes conservative management unsuitable.

21.7 Wall and Septal Thickness

As the names imply, both these refer to the thickness of the septae in multilocular lesions or of the cyst wall. However, difficulties exist in standardising the measurements of these structures, or, in some cases, recognising the structures at all. Furthermore, the concept of quantifying wall thickness, in common with other morphological criteria, suffers from the huge assumption that cancer develops in a linear fashion. It seems unlikely that the biology of ovarian cancer is so convenient as to reveal itself by a gradual increase in septations, wall thickness or the number of papillary projections. By concentrating on these factors, it may be that the earliest "simplest looking" cancers will be missed when they are most curable.

The importance of wall or septal thickness for the prediction of malignancy is uncertain. However, there has been a consensus view that benign ovarian cysts are more likely to have thin and smooth septae compared to the thick irregular septae associated with malignancy.[37] A thick septum has been

arbitrarily defined as one greater than 3.0 mm. Using this cut-off, Meire and colleagues[35] found that out of their 27 multilocular lesions, 19 had thin septae and eight had thick septae. Nine (47%) of those with thin septae and seven (88%) with thick septae were malignant. Sassone et al.[17] incorporated these features into a morphological scoring system, but with limited success. Problems arise with benign teratomas and endometriomas. Of the 24 benign teratomas, over 50% had thick walls. This led the same group to utilise an alternative scoring system,[38] which retained a score for septal thickness but excluded wall thickness altogether. With univariate and multivariate logistic regression analysis, septal thickness was no significant parameter to distinguish between benign and malignant masses.[39]

Overall the current data do not support the use of septal thickness as a continuous variable. The presence of septae increases the risk of malignancy; trying to quantify this risk further will lead to cancers being missed.

21.8 Echodense Foci and Acoustic Shadowing

Echodense foci are areas within the lesion that appear almost white on the grey-scale image because they are highly reflective to sound waves.

When scanning adnexal masses, dystrophic calcification near necrotic areas or structures with calcified densities such as teeth will be seen as echodense foci. These foci are usually accompanied by acoustic shadowing and the latter is generally taken as a favorable sign in that it is usually indicative of benign teratomas (Figure 21.3).

However, this generalisation is not without its hazards. Lerner et al.[40] introduced this feature in their new morphology scoring system, weighting it

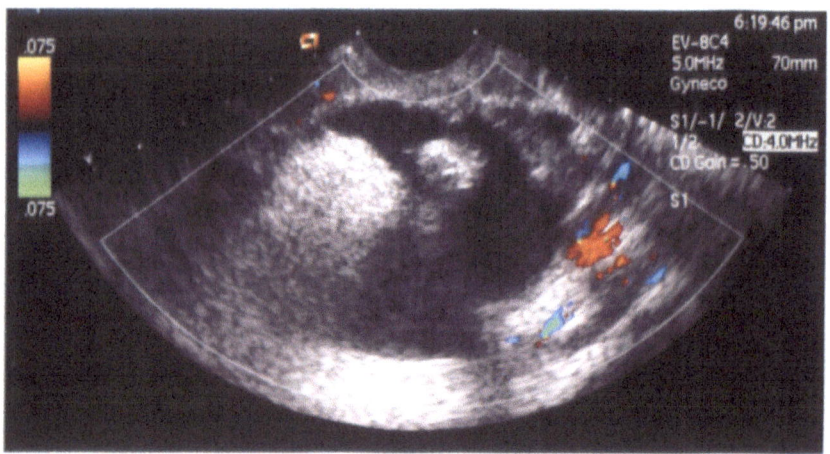

Figure 21.3. Echodense foci in benign cystic teratoma.

so that lesions scored lower if they had shadowing. This was meant to reduce the scores of benign teratomas, which often have high scores as a result of having other high-scoring features such as mixed echogenicity, irregular cyst outline and increased wall thickness.[17] Their results showed that although 86.2% of the teratomas had shadowing, 28.6% of malignant and borderline tumours also shared this feature. In 29 out of 300 adnexal masses, Timmerman et al. found shadowing and five of them (17.2%) were malignant.[18]

In summary, echodense foci and acoustic shadowing are useful give-away signs of teratomas but they are not exclusive to these lesions. The use of these features in characterising adnexal masses must be applied cautiously. Perhaps they should be used only to strengthen the diagnosis of teratoma when a suspicion of this already exists, rather than using these features to exclude the presence of malignancy. Once again, this shows the difficulty of rigidly adhering to morphological scoring systems. Most experienced ultrasound users would characterise a teratoma correctly in the majority of cases on the basis of a subjective assessment of the overall appearance; to a lesser extent the same may be said of endometriotic cysts. It seems more logical to exclude from morphological second-stage assessment those lesions that can be confidently classified subjectively. Having said that, we did not include such subjective assessments in any of our ovarian cancer screening trials. The aim of these protocols was to make things as simple as possible, rather than to introduce subjective bias.

21.9 Echogenicity of Cyst Contents

Serous fluid within an ovarian cyst is virtually anechoic (or sonolucent) and so appears black on the ultrasound screen. In contrast, cysts containing mucinous fluid may have a homogeneous grey appearance due to low-level echoes and yet still appear darker than the surrounding stromal element of the ovary. These areas, which reflect some echoes but not sufficiently to acquire the same grey-scale colour of the surrounding stroma, are referred to as hypoechoic. Lesions containing old blood tend to have this characteristic, and are often described as having a "ground glass" appearance, a feature common to endometriomas (Figure 21.4). Solid elements in an enlarged ovary will tend to have a heterogeneous appearance (Figure 21.5).

The relative echogenicity of an ovarian lesion features in almost all scoring systems, with completely anechoic lesions scoring low and heterogeneously hyperechoic lesions scoring high. Indeed, in 57 out of 300 adnexal masses, "ground glass" appearance was noted and most of them proved to be endometriotic cysts.[18] However, 10 (17.5%) were malignant (e.g. endometrioid cystadenocarcinoma). Echogenicity is a helpful indicator for predicting malignancy, but like many of the other morphological characteristics described above, it cannot be used in isolation.

21.10 Morphology Scoring Systems

Of all the characteristics listed above, it should be possible to decide whether a lesion is simple, unilocular or anechoic and thus lacking either septae or papillary projections. Providing the whole lesion has been examined and is within the focal range of the vaginal probe, such an evaluation should be possible by most if not all ultrasound users. Such a lesion would be most unlikely to be malignant. Once the different morphological features discussed above are introduced into the equation, the risk of a particular lesion that contains any of them being a cancer increases. The issue

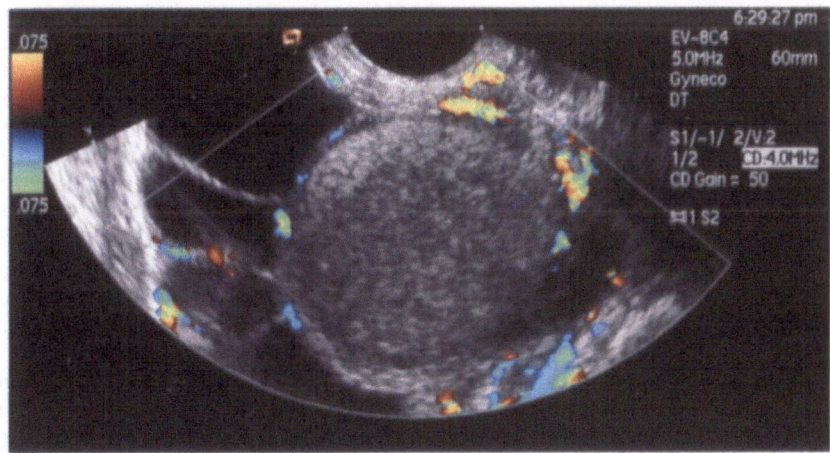

Figure 21.4. Endometrioma with "ground glass" appearance of old blood surrounded by adhesions and anechoic fluid.

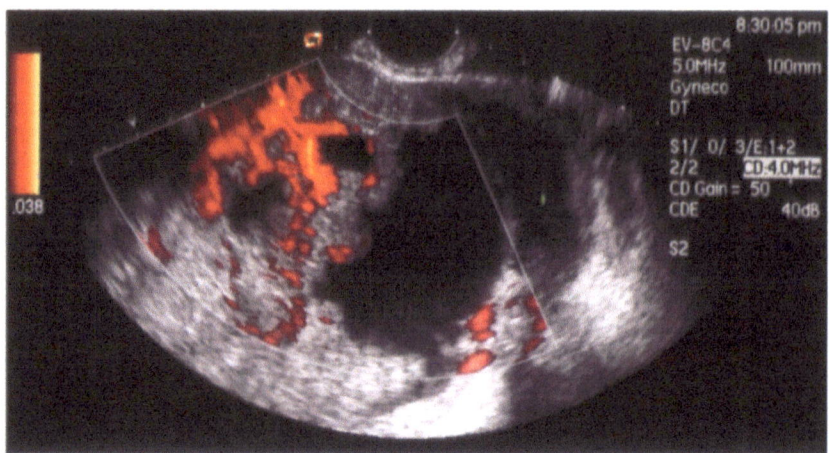

Figure 21.5. Multilocular-solid mass with papillary structures and a strong and irregular vascularisation at power Doppler imaging (serous papillary adenocarcinoma).

therefore is deciding what risk, if any, is acceptable in clinical practice. This is a point that is addressed prospectively in a paper by Bourne et al.[19] Not surprisingly, attempts have been made to give individual elements of the morphological appearances of a cyst a numerical value, in order to arrive at a quantitative description of the risk of malignancy of any lesion. Such an approach must be of concern, given our relative lack of understanding of the natural history of ovarian pathology. Does a thin septum grow thick, does an irregular wall become a papillary projection, and what is the time scale involved? This approach merits detailed evaluation.

A score is derived by giving each morphological feature a range of values dependent on the appearance. The index is then calculated by a simple summation of the individual scores of the different features. Designing a scoring system based on categorical variables is relatively straightforward, i.e. the presence or absence of a feature. Including continuous variables such as wall thickness makes things more complicated, as ranges of values then have to be assigned scores on the assumption that the progression from benign to malignant disease is continuous for that variable.

One of the first attempts to give ultrasound appearances a numerical score was reported by Finkler and colleagues.[41] It was not a true scoring system in that the numerical index was not calculated by a summation of individual scores of the characteristics, but more on the basis of "pattern recognition". A specified score was given to a pre-defined combination of characteristics, for example a clear cyst with slightly irregular outline was given a score of 2 and a multilocular or irregular cystic mass with papillary projections was given a score of 8. Finkler et al. chose 7 as a cut-off to indicate malignancy. Out of their 37 malignant tumours in 102 patients, this scoring system correctly identified only 23 (62%) of the malignant and 62 (95%) of the benign

tumours in the series. However, as the adnexal masses could have alternatively been labelled as either malignant or benign according to the same pre-defined characteristics, instead of giving them a score greater than or less than 7, the object of giving a numerical score seems almost irrelevant.

Sassone and colleagues suggested a true scoring system, which incorporated four variables, namely: inner wall structure, wall thickness, septal thickness and echogenicity.[17] After a retrospective analysis on 143 patients with adnexal masses, a cut-off value of 9 was selected in order to achieve 100% sensitivity for the detection of malignancy. However, this was associated with a relatively high false-positive rate of 17%; the study also has limited value because of its retrospective design. Many of the false-positive diagnoses arose from benign teratomas. This scoring system was then applied prospectively to 94 adnexal masses, which included 16 malignancies.[38] The detection rate for cancer was 94%, the specificity 87%, and positive predictive value 60%. This system was applied to a further series of 36 benign and 27 malignant tumours.[42] Four cancers were missed (a detection rate of 85.2%) and there were 11 false-positive test results for cancer, which reduced the specificity to 69.4% and positive predictive value to 67.6%.

A further version of this same scoring system was proposed by Lerner et al..[40] There were three important differences, namely: the variable called wall thickness was replaced by another described as acoustic shadowing, the number of categories for each variable was reduced to a maximum of three, and the individual score for each category was reduced. A lesion with acoustic shadowing was given a lower score to indicate a reduced probability of malignancy. This was designed to reduce the index score of benign teratomas. They evaluated their new system on 350 masses, of which 31 were malignant. Using a numerical cut-off value of 3, the detection rate for malignancy was 97%. However, the false-positive rate was 23% and positive predictive value 29.4%. Despite refining the system, the overall performance of the test still had serious limitations. Furthermore, as is the case with many studies, the relatively low prevalence of malignant disease in both this and other study populations suggests that the data should be interpreted with caution. The surgical stage of the cancers evaluated is a further important variable. Most cancers assessed by scoring systems (and as discussed in Chapter 22, with colour Doppler) in the literature are either of a late stage, or the stages are not stated. The morphological differences between a stage III ovarian cancer and simple cyst are of course dramatic, but we know little about the morphological appearances of very early cancers. It must be remembered that by applying second-stage tests we may miss the earliest, and possibly most treatable cancers.

Of most interest in the paper of Lerner et al.[40] was the inclusion of age as a variable. Using the elaborate artifice of incorporating the age of the patient as a variable into the scoring system by adding a tenth of the age to the overall score, they were able to reduce the number of false-positive test results and improve the specificity and positive predictive values to 81% and 33.3% respectively. In this study, the mean ages of patients with benign and malignant lesions were approximately 43 and 60 years respectively. This is in accordance with the expected distribution of the disease in the population. The prevalence of ovarian cancer is lower in younger age groups, and any ovarian mass is less likely to be malignant in such women.

The last morphological system we will mention here is the scoring system by Ferrazzi and co-workers, who reported a modified older scoring system compared with four others from the literature.[43] The aim of this work was to compare the accuracy of five different morphological scoring systems to identify malignant ovarian masses in a prospective multicentre study. Four of the systems had previously been reported by Granberg,[16] Sassone,[17] De Priest[26] and Lerner[40] and the fifth is newly developed. A total of 330 ovarian neoplasms were collected in three different centres, which adopted the same diagnostic procedures. Of these, 261 masses were benign (mean diameter 50 ± 26 mm) and 69 were malignant (mean diameter 69 ± 33 mm) (prevalence 21%). The area under the receiver operating characteristic (ROC) curve for the multicentre score was 0.84. This was significantly better than the areas of the other four scores, which ranged from 0.72 to 0.75. The cut-off levels derived from the five ROC curves achieved a sensitivity that ranged from 74% (Sassone score[17]) to 88% (De Priest score = 5), and a specificity from 40% (De Priest[26]) to 67% (multicentre); the highest positive predictive value was 41% (multicentre). With a cut-off level of 9, the accuracy of the multicentre score was significantly better than the scores of Granberg[16] and De Priest[26] (McNemar's test p < 0.0001).

Similar results were obtained in 207 ovarian masses of 5 cm mean diameter, and also for the 19 borderline and 11 stage I cancers. For the clinical purposes of a screening test, a possible cut-off level of 8 was also used, which increased the sensitivity to 93%, with a drop of specificity to 56%. With the use of the same criteria for the scores of the different authors, the following values were obtained for sensitivity: 96%, 81%, 93% and 90%; and for specificity: 23%, 56%, 28% and 49%. The multicentre score performed well at distinguishing malignant from benign lesions, and was better than the other four traditional scores, for both large and small masses. This was mainly due to the introduction of two criteria that allowed correction for typical dermoids and endohaemorrhagic corpora lutea. A completely reliable differentiation of benign from malignant masses cannot be obtained by ultrasonographic imaging alone. This model seems to be easy to use in clinical practice compared with many others.

The menopausal status of the patient is an important consideration at the time of any scan. The data of Granberg et al.[15] relating to histology support this view. In this study, the median age of patients with benign and malignant lesions was approximately 43 and 64 years respectively.

A clear illustration of the prospective application of morphological assessment of persistent ovarian masses can be derived from the familial ovarian cancer screening study by Bourne et al..[19] These data also allow a direct comparison of morphological assessment and colour Doppler, as well as the outcome of morphological outcomes based on either a simple or complex evaluation.

21.11 Risk of Malignancy Index

Jacobs et al.[44] were the first to combine morphology, serum CA 125 levels and menopausal status. In a retrospective study using transabdominal ultrasonography, the following features suggestive of malignancy have been assessed: multiloculated cysts, evidence of solid areas, evidence of metastases, presence of ascites and bilateral lesions. An ultrasound score (U) of 0 was given when none of these features was recorded, a score of 1 was given when one feature was present and a score of 3 was given when two or more of the above features were noted. A score (M) of 1 or 3 was given to pre- and postmenopausal patients, respectively.

The following equation was proposed: risk of malignancy index = $U \times M \times$ serum CA 125, where U and M are the ultrasound and menopausal scores, as defined above.

The main advantage of this rather simple test is that it can be applied easily in less specialised departments and several groups have confirmed that the results are reproducible.

21.12 Mathematical Models

In a natural progression from the use of simple scoring systems, a further interesting model to predict the risk for malignancy in ovarian tumours was reported by Tailor et al..[45] They tested a multivariate logistic regression analysis to predict the risk for malignancy in adnexal masses. Ten different parameters were used and when cross-validating the model, 100% sensitivity and specificity was found. However, for the entire data set, the best sensitivity and specificity were 93.3% and 90.4% respectively, at a cut-off value of 25% probability of malignancy. They concluded that the accuracy of this prediction appears to be better than that of morphological or Doppler criteria when the latter are used independently. Furthermore, they concluded that the value of this model needs to be tested prospectively.[45]

A comparison of methods for the preoperative discrimination between benign and malignant adnexal masses using a new logistic regression model was described in a prospective study by Timmerman and colleagues.[39] This model also confirmed the low risk for malignancy in unilocular ovarian cysts. The same group recently reported on the use of artificial neural networks to help discriminate between malignant and benign adnexal masses.[46] The aim was to generate and evaluate artificial neural network (ANN) models from simple clinical and ultrasound-derived criteria in order to predict whether or not an adnexal mass will have histological signs of malignancy. In this study the data were collected prospectively from 173 consecutive patients who were scheduled to undergo surgical investigations. The outcome measure was the histological classification of excised tissues as malignant (including borderline tumours) or benign. The ANN models were trained on a randomly selected set of 116 patient records and tested on the remainder (n = 57). The performance of each model was evaluated using ROC curves and compared with corresponding data from an established risk of malignancy index[44] and a logistic regression model.[39] The authors concluded that an ANN can be trained to provide clinically useful information in most cases. The input variables used were: the patient's menopausal status, serum CA 125 levels, and some simple ultrasonographic criteria. None of the simple unilocular cysts was malignant.

In a further study, the subjective impression of the ultrasound appearances of an ovarian mass was used to characterise a set of 300 ovarian lesions.[47] They concluded that the subjective evaluation of an ovarian mass by an experienced ultrasonographer is an accurate method for discriminating between benign and malignant ovarian masses. Therefore, any analysis using mathematical approaches such as logistic regression or neural networks would have to obtain very high levels of test performance to be comparable to an expert. Where such models are likely to be of value is to help those operators with less experience to mimic a more experienced operator and so obtain a better overall diagnostic accuracy.

21.13 Conclusions

It is clear that the presence or absence of certain morphological features may be useful when trying to discriminate between benign and malignant ovarian masses. However, it seems wise to be cautious. The use of second-stage tests such as morphological assessment is associated with a reduction in the detection rate for cancer, and so this approach must be considered carefully in relation to high-risk groups, such as women with a family history of ovarian cancer. The fact that so few early cancers have been scrutinised using these scoring systems means that those using them must be aware of this limitation. A simple description of a cyst as being simple or complex will reduce the false-positive rate for cancer, and be more likely to maintain the detection rate. The chances of a simple unilocular cyst of less than 5.0 cm representing a malignancy, particularly in a younger woman, appear to be very low indeed (< 1.0%). It seems reasonable to use this as a criterion on which to make clinical decisions; however, for scoring systems, prolonged use will be associated with missed opportunities to diagnose cancers. There are some lesions with morphological features that are specific enough for the lesion to be characterised on the basis of "pattern recognition". Some teratomas and endometriomas would fall into this category. Morphological assessment will be able to characterise a number of lesions correctly. However, only unilocular echo-free ovarian cysts < 50 mm without papillary formations can be classified as benign by ultrasound with almost 100% accuracy. Cyst rupture is associated with a worse prognosis in patients treated for stage I ovarian cancer.[48] Preoperative ultrasound could help in selecting patients for laparoscopic treatment. Cyst rupture should be avoided if malignancy is suspected.

References

1. Wikland M, Enk L, Hamberger L et al. (1987) Use of a vaginal transducer for oocyte retrieval in an IVF/ET programme. J Clin Ultrasound 15:245–250
2. Quinn MJ, Beynon NJ, McC Mortenseon NJ et al. (1988) Transvaginal endosonography: a new method to study the anatomy of the lower urinary tract in urinary stress incontinence. Br J Urol 62:414–418
3. Timor-Tritsch IE, Farine D, Rosen MG (1989) A close look at early embryonic development with the high frequency vaginal transducer. Am J Obstet Gynecol 159:676–681
4. Khullar V, Salvatore S, Cardozo LC et al. (1994) A novel technique for measuring bladder wall thickness in women using transvaginal ultrasonography. Ultrasound Obstet Gynecol 4:220–223
5. Gonzalez CJ, Curson R, Parsons J (1988) Transabdominal versus transvaginal ultrasound scanning of ovarian follicles: are they comparable? Fertil Steril 50:657–659
6. Bonilla-Musoles F, Pardo G, Perez-Gil M et al. (1989) Abdominal ultrasonography versus transvaginal scanning: accuracy in follicular development evaluation and prediction for oocyte retrieval in stimulated cycles. J Clin Ultrasound 17:49–91
7. Timor-Tritsch IE, Bar-Yam Y, Elgali S et al. (1988) The technique of transvaginal sonography with the use of the 6.5 MHz probe. Am J Obstet Gynecol 158:1019–1024
8. Goldstein SR (1990) Incorporating endovaginal ultrasonography into the overall gynecologic examination. Am J Obstet Gynecol 162:625–632
9. Rodriguez MH, Platt LD, Medearis AL et al. (1988) The use of transvaginal ultrasonography for evaluation of postmenopausal ovarian size and morphology. Am J Obstet Gynecol 159:810–814
10. Higgins RV, van Nagell JR, Woods CH et al. (1990) Interobserver variation in ovarian measurements using transvaginal sonography. Gynecol Oncol 39:69–71
11. Mendelson EB, Bohm-Velez M, Joseph N et al. (1988) Endometrial abnormalities: evaluation with transvaginal sonography. Am J Radiol 150:139–142
12. Higgins RV, van Nagell Jr JR, Donaldson ES et al. (1989) Transvaginal sonography as a screening method for ovarian cancer. Gynecol Oncol 34:402–406
13. Van Nagell Jr JR, De Priest PD, Puls LE et al. (1991) Ovarian cancer screening in asymptomatic women by transvaginal ultrasonography. Cancer 68:458–462
14. Crade M, Crade K (1995) Preliminary ovarian screening data from Long Beach Memorial Hospital. Personal communication
15. Granberg S, Wikland M, Jansson I (1989) Macroscopic characterisation of ovarian tumors and the relation to the histological diagnosis: criteria to be used for ultrasound evaluation. Gynecol Oncol 35:139–144
16. Granberg S, Norström A, Wikland M (1990) Tumors in the lower pelvis as imaged by transvaginal sonography. Gynecol Oncol 37:224–229
17. Sassone AM, Timor-Tritsch IE, Artner A et al. (1991) Transvaginal sonographic characterisation of ovarian disease: evaluation of a new scoring system to predict ovarian malignancy. Obstet Gynecol 78:70–76
18. Timmerman D (1997) Ultrasonography in the assessment of ovarian and tamoxifen-associated endometrial pathology. Thesis, University of Leuven, Belgium (ISBN 906186 857 2)
19. Bourne TH, Campbell S, Reynolds K et al (1993) Screening for early familial ovarian cancer with transvaginal ultrasonography and colour blood flow imaging. Br Med J 306: 1025–1029
20. Hermann UJ, Locher GW, Goldhirsch A (1987) Sonographic patterns of ovarian tumors: prediction of malignancy. Obstet Gynecol 69:777–781
21. DeLand M, Fried A, van Nagell JR et al. (1979) Ultrasonography in the diagnosis of tumors of the ovary. Surg Gynecol Obstet 148:346–348
22. Champault G, Cazacu F, Taffiner N (1996) Serious trocar accidents in laparoscopic surgery – a French survey of 103 852 operations. Surg Lap Endosc 6:367–370
23. Goldstein S, Subramanyam B, Snyder J et al. (1988) The postmenopausal cystic adnexal mass: the potential role of ultrasound in conservative management. Obstet Gynecol 73:8–10
24. Valentin L, Sladkevicius P, Marsal K (1994) Limited contribution of Doppler velocimetry to the differential diagnosis of extrauterine pelvic tumors. Obstet Gynecol 83:425–433
25. Morley P, Barnett E (1970) The use of ultrasound in the diagnosis of pelvic masses. Br J Radiol 43:602–616
26. De Priest P, Gallion H, Pavlik E et al. (1997) Transvaginal sonography as a screening method for the detection of early ovarian cancer. Gynecol Oncol 65:408–414
27. Gerber B, Muller H, Kulz T et al. (1997) Simple ovarian cysts in premenopausal patients. Int J Gynaecol Obstet 57:49–55
28. Bailey C, Ueland F, DePriest P et al. (1998) The malignant potential of small cystic ovarian tumors in women over 50 years of age. Gynecol Oncol 69:3–7
29. Obwegeser R, Deutinger J, Bernascheck G (1993) The risk of malignancy with an apparently simple adnexal cyst on ultrasound. Arch Gynecol Obstet 253:117–120
30. Auslender R, Atlas I, Lissak A et al. (1996) Follow-up of small postmenopausal ovarian cysts using vaginal ultrasound and CA-125 antigen. J Clin Ultrasound 24:175–178
31. Conway C, Zalud I, Dilena M et al. (1998) Simple cyst in the postmenopausal patient: detection and management. J Ultrasound Med 17:369–372
32. Kroon E, Andolf E (1995) Diagnosis and follow-up of simple ovarian cysts detected by ultrasound in postmenopausal women. Obstet Gynecol 85:211–214
33. Osmers R, Osmers M, von Maydell B et al. (1998) Evaluation of ovarian tumors in postmenopausal women by transvaginal sonography. Eur J Obstet Gynecol 77:81–88
34. Ekerhovd E, Wienerroith H, Staudach A et al. (2001) Preoperative assessment of unilocular adnexal cysts by transvaginal sonography: a comparison between sonographic morphological imaging and histolopathologic diagnosis. Am J Obstet Gynecol 184:48–54
35. Meire HB, Farrant P, Guha T (1978) Distinction of benign from malignant ovarian cysts by ultrasound. Br J Obstet Gynaecol 85:893–899
36. Sladkevicius P (1994) Doppler ultrasound studies in gynaecology. Thesis, Lund University, Malmö, Sweden
37. Bourne T (1995) Screening for early familial ovarian cancer and the diagnosis of endometrial and ovarian pathology using transvaginal ultrasonography with and without color Doppler. Thesis, University of Göteborg, Sweden
38. Timor-Tritsch LE, Lerner JP, Monteagudo A et al. (1993) Transvaginal ultrasonographic characterization of ovarian masses by means of color flow-directed Doppler measurements and a morphologic scoring system. Am J Obstet Gynecol 168:909–913
39. Timmerman D, Bourne TH, Tailor A et al. (1999) A comparison of methods for the pre-operative discrimination between benign and malignant adnexal masses: the development of a new logistic regression model. Am J Obstet Gynecol 181:57–65
40. Lerner JP, Timor-Tritsch IE, Federman A et al. (1994) Transvaginal ultrasonographic characterisation of ovarian masses with an improved, weighted scoring system. Am J Obstet Gynecol 170:81–85
41. Finkler NJ, Benacerraf B, Lavin PT et al. (1988) Comparison of serum CA 125, clinical impression, and ultrasound in the preoperative evaluation of ovarian masses. Obstet Gynecol 72:659–664

42. Hata K, Hata H, Manabe A et al. (1992) A critical evaluation of transvaginal Doppler studies, transvaginal ultrasonography, magnetic resonance imaging, and CA 125 in detecting ovarian cancer. Obstet Gynecol 80:922-926

43. Ferrazzi E, Zanetta G, Dordoni D et al. (1997) Transvaginal ultrasonographic characterization of ovarian masses: comparison of five scoring systems in a multicenter study. Ultrasound Obstet Gynecol 10:192-197

44. Jacobs I, Oram D, Fairbanks J et al. (1990) A risk of malignancy index incorporating CA 125, ultrasound and menopausal status for the accurate preoperative diagnosis of ovarian cancer. Br J Obstet Gynaecol 97:922-929

45. Tailor A, Jurkovic D, Bourne T et al. (1997) Sonographic prediction of malignancy in adnexal masses using multivariate logistic regression analysis. Ultrasound Obstet Gynecol 10:41-47

46. Timmerman D, Verrelst H, Bourne T et al. (1999) Artificial neural network models for the pre-operative discrimination between malignant and benign adnexal masses. Ultrasound Obstet Gynaecol 13:17-25

47. Timmerman D, Schwärzler P, Collins WP et al. (1999) Subjective assessment of adnexal masses using ultrasonography: an analysis of interobserver variability and experience. Ultrasound Obstet Gynecol 13:11-16

48. Vergote I, De Bralanter J, Fyles A et al. (2001) Prognostic importance of degree of differentiation and cyst rupture in stage I invasive epithelial ovarian cancinoma. Lancet 357: 176-182

Chapter 22

Colour Doppler

Lil Valentin

22.1 Introduction

Two reports published in 1989 suggested Doppler ultrasonography to be an excellent tool for discriminating between benign and malignant adnexal masses with virtually no overlap in Doppler results between the two categories.[1,2] Malignant masses were found to yield colour Doppler signals and arterial Doppler shift spectra almost always, whereas benign tumours often yielded no colour Doppler signals and seldom yielded arterial Doppler shift spectra.[1] Moreover, much lower resistance index (RI) and pulsatility index (PI) values were recorded from malignant than from benign masses.[1,2] A few years later, however, benign and malignant adnexal masses were reported to be characterised by considerable overlap in Doppler results,[3,4] and the value of Doppler ultrasound examination in the differential diagnosis of pelvic tumours was questioned in several publications.[5-12]

In the following, I shall systematically review published literature on the use of Doppler ultrasound examination in the differential diagnosis of adnexal masses, and report the experience of the Malmö group. I have deliberately chosen to discuss adnexal masses – not only ovarian masses – because it is not always possible to determine whether an adnexal mass is of ovarian or extraovarian origin at grey-scale ultrasound examination. To compare the properties of different diagnostic tests, I have plotted the sensitivity of each test against its false-positive rate (false-positive rate being defined as 1 – specificity). I have defined the best test as that detecting most malignancies with the lowest false-positive rate.[13] Some of the sensitivities and false-positive rates presented in this chapter have not been published but have been calculated by myself on the basis of the raw data reported in the publications cited.

22.2 Which Doppler Variable is Best for Discriminating Between Benign and Malignant Adnexal Masses?

22.2.1 Resistance Index and Pulsatility Index

No Doppler variables have been more extensively tested regarding their ability to discriminate between benign and malignant adnexal masses than PI and RI. Various malignancy-specific cut-off values have been suggested, the most commonly cited being PI < 1.0 and RI < 0.4 to indicate malignancy.[8] Figures reported for the sensitivity of PI and RI range from 26 to 100%, and those for false-positive rate from 0 to 54%.[8] Most studies showed benign and malignant adnexal masses to manifest considerable overlap in PI and RI values, and the use of these variables in making clinical decisions was strongly discouraged in a recent review.[8]

22.2.2 Localisation of Blood Vessels

Benign tumours are said to be characterised by peripheral vascularisation and malignant tumours by central vascularisation,[8,12,14-21] the reported sensitivity of central vascularisation varying from 64 to 97%, and the reported false-positive rate from 5 to 41%.[8,12,14-17,21] At least to some extent, vessel localisation depends on tumour morphology. Only tumours with septa or solid components, which are often malignant, can have central vascularisation, whereas cysts without septa or solid components, which are usually benign, can only be peripherally vascularised. The Malmö group found the solid components of malignant multilocular solid tumours (i.e., tumours with one or more septa and solid parts or papillary excrescences) to be more vascularised than those of benign multilocular solid tumours[22] (and Valentin et al. 1994, unpublished data), and PI values to be significantly lower and time-averaged maximum velocity to be significantly higher in the septa of malignant multilocular solid tumours than in those of benign multilocular solid tumours (Valentin et al. 1994, unpublished data). However, we found no difference in the localisation of blood flow between benign and malignant solid tumours, i.e., tumours where the solid components comprised 80% or more of the tumour[22] (and Valentin et al. 1994, unpublished data).

22.2.3 "Notch"

Doppler shift spectra with a notch have been reported to be recorded from 11 to 89% of benign adnexal tumours, but from very few malignant pelvic tumours.[7,8,14,17,20,23] Thus, a notch in the spectrum is suggestive of benignity. The Malmö group found Doppler shift spectra with a notch to be recorded more often from extraovarian masses than from ovarian masses (39 versus 19%; Valentin et al. 1994, unpublished data). In my own experience, a spectrum with a notch is very rarely recorded from an ovarian mass. A notch in the spectrum suggests that the mass is extraovarian (e.g., hydrosalpinx, peritoneal cyst or paraovarian cyst), or that the spectrum was obtained from a vessel outside the mass.

22.2.4 Blood Flow Velocity (Peak Systolic Velocity, Time-averaged Maximum Velocity, End-diastolic Velocity)

The ability of PI and/or RI and blood flow velocity to discriminate between benign and malignant adnexal masses has been compared in 15 studies.[5,7,16,17,21,22,24–32] Blood flow velocity was a better discriminator between benign and malignant tumours than PI or RI in eight of these studies.[7,22,24,26,27,29,30,32] Eight studies compared the diagnostic properties of different blood flow velocities.[7,21,22,26,27,29,30,32] In six of these studies, time-averaged maximum velocity was a better predictor of malignancy than peak systolic velocity[7,26,27,29,30,32] or end-diastolic velocity;[26] in one study, peak systolic velocity and time-averaged maximum velocity had similar diagnostic properties,[22] and in one study the end-diastolic velocity was superior to both peak systolic velocity and time-averaged maximum velocity.[21] Prömpeler and

co-workers, who compared a large number of Doppler variables, found the sum of all time-averaged maximum velocities (calculated by summation of the time-averaged maximum velocity of each vessel in a tumour) to be the best Doppler variable for discrimination between benign and malignant tumours.[26] Only the highest time-averaged maximum velocity and the highest peak systolic velocity recorded from a tumour have been cross-validated prospectively, a time-averaged maximum velocity ≥ 7.2 cm/s being found to detect all malignancies with a false-positive rate of 51%,[30] a peak systolic velocity ≥ 14.4 cm/s to detect 79% of malignancies with a false-positive rate of 36%,[30] and a peak systolic velocity ≥ 15 cm/s to detect 47% of malignancies with a false-positive rate of 19%.[25]

22.2.5 Evaluation of the Colour Doppler Image

In the pioneer study, colour Doppler signals were almost always seen in malignancies but almost never detected in benign pelvic tumours.[1] With modern and more sensitive Doppler equipment, vascularity can be detected in most adnexal tumours irrespective of whether they are benign or malignant, and in normal ovaries.[7,8,10,12,14,22,25,26,29,33–36] Therefore, the elicitation of colour Doppler signals within an ovary or adnexal mass is no longer taken to indicate malignancy. On the other hand, failure to elicit colour Doppler signals speaks in favour of benignity. According to literature published after 1992, 0–25% of malignant adnexal masses lack detectable flow at colour Doppler ultrasound examination, whereas colour Doppler signals are undetectable in between 0 and 47% of benign adnexal masses.[7,8,10,12,14,16,21,22,25,26,29,33,34,37–42]

According to findings in several studies, more vessels are visible at colour Doppler ultrasound examination and more arterial Doppler shift spectra can be recorded from malignant than from benign tumours.[7,15,19,26,43,44] Possibly, this difference may be explained – at least partly – by differences in tumour morphology, as it is probably easier to detect flow and to record arterial Doppler shift spectra from complex tumours containing much tissue, which are likely to be malignant, than from simple tumours containing little tissue, which are likely to be benign. Prömpeler and coworkers suggested five or more detectable vessels in a tumour, or at least one detectable vessel in the centre of a tumour, to indicate malignancy.[26] To the best of my knowledge, these cut-off values have not been tested prospectively.

The Malmö group found the total colour content of the tumour scan as rated subjectively by the ultrasound examiner on a visual analogue scale (tumour colour score) to be a better variable than PI or blood flow velocity for discriminating between benign and malignant pelvic masses (Figures 22.1 and 22.2), and Carter and colleagues found subjective evaluation of the colour Doppler image to be a better test than PI or RI for distinguishing benign and malignant gynaecological tumours.[5,22] Carter and coworkers defined abnormal colour flow as "colour aliasing, dilated and prominent tumour vessels appearing to start and go nowhere and seen as hot spots".[5] It is not surprising that evaluation of the colour Doppler image has been found by some research teams to be a good method for distinguishing benign and malignant tumours. The colour Doppler image might be said to give an overall impression of tumour vascularisation in that it probably reflects both the number and size of tumour vessels and their functional capacity. Kurjak and Predanic suggested that randomly dispersed vessels, as opposed to regularly separated vessels, indicate malignancy,[45] and Jain proposed continuously fluctuating colour rather than pulsatile colour at colour Doppler ultrasound examination to be suggestive of malignancy.[46] I know of no published studies in which the latter two criteria of malignancy have been tested prospectively.

22.2.6 Prospective Cross-validation of Different Doppler Criteria of Malignancy/Benignity

The diagnostic properties of previously defined Doppler criteria of malignancy/benignity were cross-validated and compared prospectively in four studies. Carter and coworkers compared PI, RI, peak systolic velocity, time-averaged maximum velocity, end-diastolic velocity and subjective evaluation of the colour Doppler image. They found subjective evaluation of the colour Doppler image to be the best Doppler variable for discrimination between benign and malignant gynaecological conditions (sensitivity 57%, false-positive rate 9%). However, their study comprised not only adnexal masses but also other kinds of pelvic tumour and normal findings.[5] The Malmö group compared PI, RI, time-averaged maximum velocity, peak systolic velocity and tumour colour score. We found time-averaged maximum velocity to be the best discriminator between benign and malignant adnexal masses, values ≥ 7.2 cm/s indicating malignancy (sensitivity 100%, false-positive rate 51%).[30] The presence of internal colour Doppler signals was found to be the best Doppler variable in a study by Stein and coworkers, who compared PI, RI, detectable colour

Doppler signals, and the presence of internal colour Doppler signals (sensitivity 77%, false-positive rate 31%).[12] Buy and colleagues, who compared PI, RI and peak systolic velocity, found PI to be the best Doppler variable for distinguishing benign and malignant masses, values ≤ 1.0 indicating malignancy (sensitivity 71% and false-positive rate 33%).[25] Plotting the sensitivity of the best test found in each of the four studies against its false-positive rate, shows time-averaged maximum velocity and evaluation of the colour Doppler image to detect most malignancies with the lowest false-positive rate. Thus, these Doppler variables seem to be better than PI for discriminating between benign and malignant pelvic tumours.

22.2.7 Multivariate Analyses to Select the Doppler Variable Most Predictive of Malignancy

It is reasonable to suppose many Doppler variables to be related. It is also reasonable to expect a relationship to exist between some Doppler findings and the ultrasound morphology of a tumour: the localisation of vessels, the number of vessels detectable in a tumour, the number of Doppler shift spectra that it is possible to record from a tumour, and the total colour content of a tumour scan should – at least to some extent – depend on tumour morphology. Multivariate analyses, taking into account both grey-scale findings and Doppler findings, are needed to determine which grey-scale findings and which Doppler variables independently predict malignancy.

Carter and colleagues, who included subjective evaluation of the colour Doppler image, PI, RI, peak systolic velocity and time-averaged maximum velocity as independent variables, and benignity and malignancy as dependent variables in multivariate analysis, found only abnormal colour Doppler imaging results to be independently related to malignancy.[5] This is in agreement with the results of the Malmö group.[22] Using multiple logistic regression analysis with menopausal status, tumour volume, colour content of the tumour scan (tumour colour score), time-averaged maximum velocity, peak systolic velocity and the presence of "colour lakes" in the colour Doppler image as independent variables, and benignity and malignancy as dependent variables, we found the tumour colour score to be the only Doppler variable independently predicting malignancy and benignity.[22] Using a regression model including the woman's age, five grey-scale variables and four Doppler variables (peak systolic velocity, time-averaged maximum velocity, PI, RI),

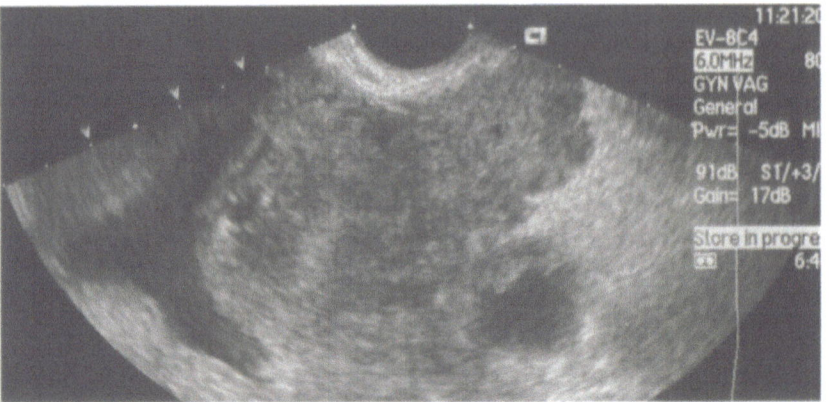

a

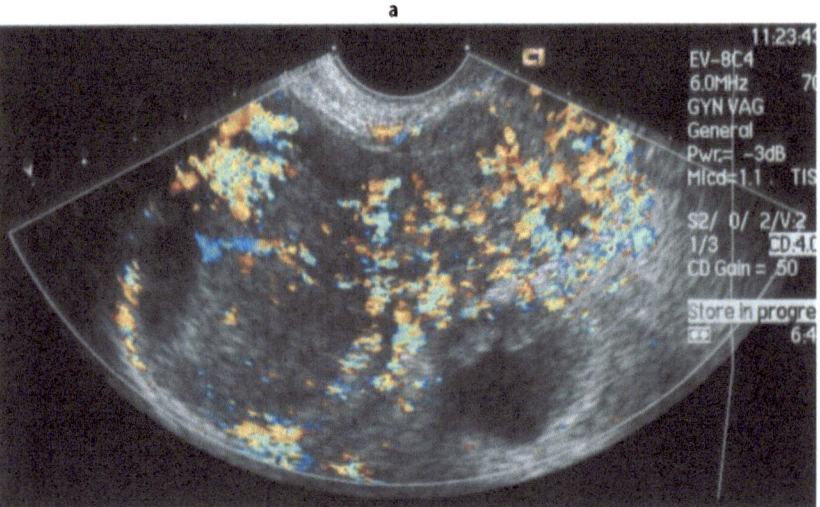

b

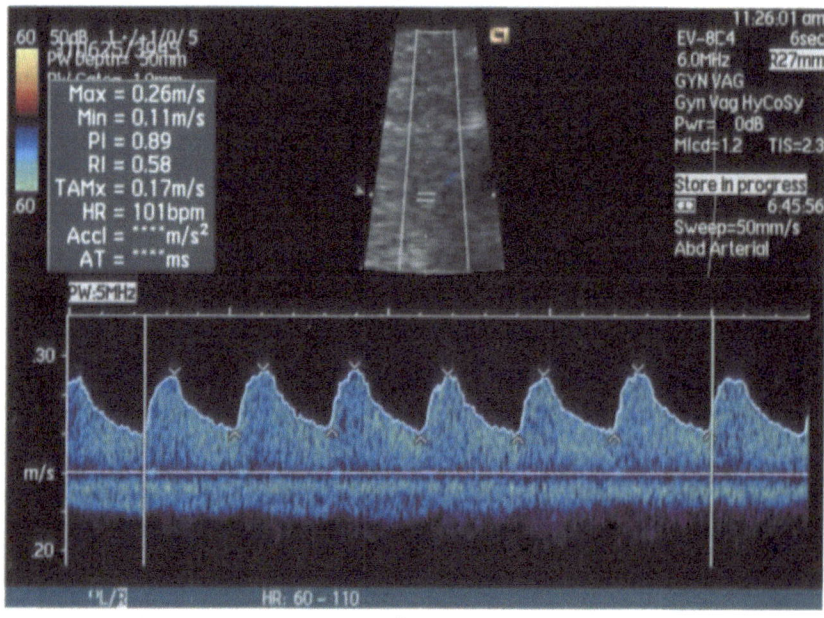

c

Figure 22.1 **a** Grey-scale, **b** colour Doppler and **c** spectral Doppler ultrasound images from a case of ovarian cancer.

Tailor and colleagues found the age, "papillary projection score" and time-averaged maximum velocity to be independent predictors of the presence or absence of malignancy.[27] Most other research teams who have later used multivariate logistic regression analysis to test the ability of clinical variables, grey-scale ultrasound variables, Doppler variables and biochemical variables to predict malignancy in adnexal masses[21,38,39,47–49]

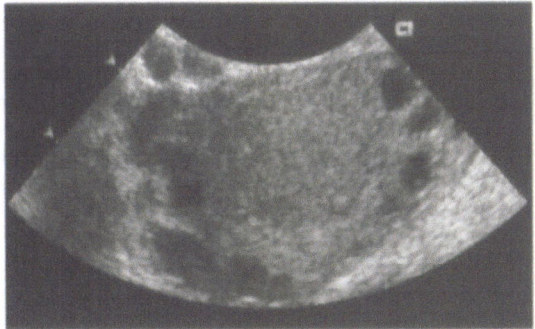

a

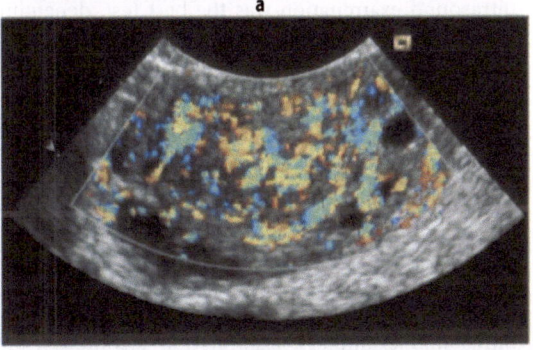

b

found both Doppler variables and grey-scale variables to independently predict malignancy.[21,38,39,47,48] However, the Doppler variables included in the final models vary: centrally located flow,[21,48] the colour content of the tumour scan,[47] peak systolic velocity and RI,[39] or only RI[38] were selected to be included. Nonetheless, the results of multivariate logistic regression analyses indicate that Doppler results do contain diagnostic information in addition to that obtained from grey-scale ultrasound examination. The discrepant results with regard to the Doppler variables included in the models may be explained by differences in tumour populations, examination technique, and the model-building process itself.

22.2.8 Summary and Comments

In most studies comparing the diagnostic properties of different Doppler variables, subjective evaluation of the colour Doppler image and blood flow velocity were better than PI or RI for discriminating between benign and malignant adnexal masses. The colour Doppler image probably reflects tumour vascularity better than any other Doppler variable, but because evaluation of the colour Doppler image has the disadvantage of being entirely subjective, it is difficult to obtain reproducible results.[50] It seems desirable to develop an objective method of quantifying the number and/or intensity of colour Doppler signals detectable in a tumour. However, even an objective method of quantifying the colour content of a tumour scan would almost certainly

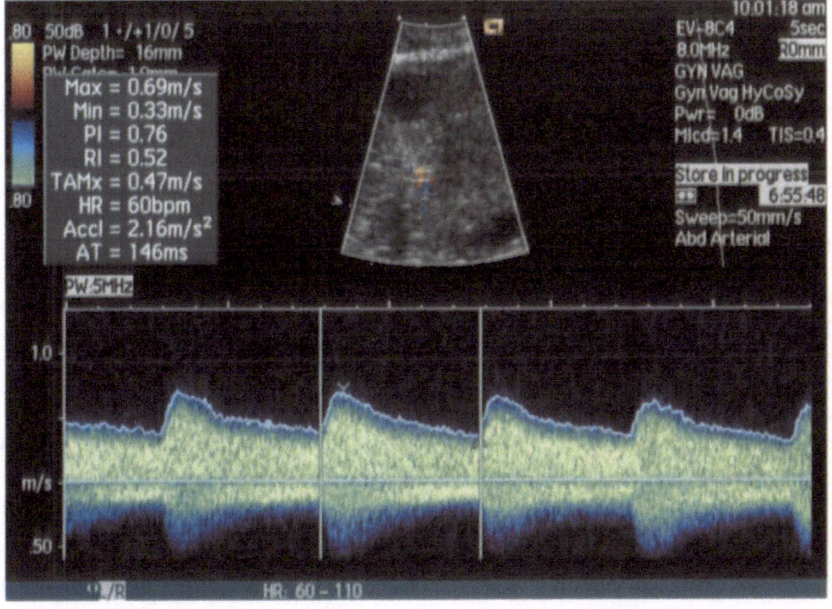

Figure 22.2 a Grey-scale, b colour Doppler and c spectral Doppler ultrasound images of a case of benign intraovarian Leydig cell tumour.

have the disadvantage of yielding results applicable to only one type of ultrasound system, i.e., the results of an objective method would probably be "equipment-dependent". Meanwhile, however, the time-averaged maximum velocity seems to be a useful Doppler variable for discriminating between benign and malignant adnexal masses. There is no consensus in published literature as to the reproducibility of Doppler measurements of blood flow velocity, PI or RI in tumour vessels.[29,50,51]

22.3 The Clinical Role of Colour Doppler Ultrasound Examination for Discrimination Between Benign and Malignant Adnexal Masses: Literature Review and the Experience of the Malmö Group

Gray-scale imaging is quite a good method for discriminating between benign and malignant masses, with a sensitivity of 70–100% and a false-positive rate of 4–63% (Tables 22.1 and 22.2). Is colour Doppler ultrasonography better for this purpose? Is it possible to achieve higher sensitivity and a lower false-positive rate by defining criteria of malignancy based on both grey-scale and Doppler findings?

Of 15 studies in which the diagnostic properties of grey-scale imaging and those of Doppler ultrasonography were compared, Doppler examination was superior in eight[15,18,24,33,41–43,58] (Table 22.1). Seventeen studies compared the diagnostic properties of grey-scale imaging, Doppler ultrasonography, and a combination of the two, and five studies compared a combination of the two methods with either grey-scale imaging alone or Doppler examination alone (Table 22.2). The combined method was the best method in 11 of 22 studies,[7,12,21,22,25,27,34,37,47,60,62] but in three of these the results of the combined method were only marginally better than those obtained with grey-scale imaging alone.[12,21,60] Doppler examination was the best method in four studies,[6,32,45,61] and grey-scale imaging was the best method in five studies.[28,30,63–65] Gray-scale imaging and the combined method yielded equally good results in two studies.[10,11] In some of the studies cited, the combined method is the use of a multivariate logistic regression model or of an artificial neural network including results of both grey-scale and Doppler ultrasound examination.[27,32,47,64,65]

In several studies shown in Tables 22.1 and 22.2, the comparison of methods was unsatisfactory, as grey-scale imaging was cross-validated prospectively, whereas Doppler ultrasonography or the combined method was not (i.e., previously defined grey-scale criteria of benignity and malignancy were used to classify the tumours, whereas Doppler criteria or combined criteria of benignity and malignancy were established on the basis of the results of the study itself).[4,6,10,11,24,28,34,41,43,57,59,60–63] Such an approach favours the method not tested prospectively, in this case the Doppler method or the combined method. In eight studies where both grey-scale imaging and Doppler examination were cross-validated prospectively,[9,15,18,33,42,46,58,60] grey-scale imaging was much better than Doppler ultrasonography in three studies,[9,46,60] whereas Doppler examination was much better than grey-scale imaging in three studies[18,42,58] and marginally better in two studies[15,33] (Table 22.1). All three methods (grey-scale imaging, Doppler ultrasonography, and a combination of the two) were cross-validated prospectively in four studies.[12,25,30,37] In three of them, the combination of the two methods was the best alternative,[12,25,37] though the improvement achieved by combining the two methods was minimal in one of the studies.[12] In the fourth study, either grey-scale imaging or Doppler ultrasound examination was the best test, depending on which grey-scale imaging method was used[30] (Table 22.2). Two studies prospectively cross-validating grey-scale imaging versus combined methods (multiple logistic regression analysis, artificial neural networks) showed grey-scale imaging to be superior to the mathematical models.[64,65]

The discrepant results shown in Tables 22.1 and 22.2 are probably to be explained by differences in study design (prospective versus non-prospective), study populations, grey-scale ultrasound and Doppler criteria of malignancy, experience and skill of the ultrasound examiners, examination techniques, and quality of ultrasound systems. However, if we limit our comparisons of methods to only those studies where all methods were cross-validated prospectively (which is probably most appropriate), we find that adding Doppler ultrasound examination to grey-scale imaging contributed nothing or little to the diagnostic performance in five[12,21,30,64,65] of seven studies.[12,21,25,30,37,64,65] The experience of the Malmö group is that the role of Doppler ultrasound examination in the differential diagnosis of benignity and malignancy in adnexal masses depends on which grey-scale imaging method is used. If the grey-scale imaging method used is a very simple classification system, whereby tumours without any solid components are classified as benign and tumours with solid components as malignant, Doppler ultrasound examination (using time-averaged maximum velocity ≥ 7.2 cm/s to indicate malignancy) is superior to grey-scale imaging for discriminating between benign and malignant masses.[30] If the grey-scale imaging method used is the Lerner score, the role of adding Doppler examination to grey-scale imaging is to decrease the

Table 22.1. Ability of grey-scale imaging and colour Doppler examination to predict malignancy in adnexal masses. GS, Gray-scale imaging; D, Doppler; Sens, sensitivity; FP, false-positive rate; P, prospective cross-validation of previously defined criteria of malignancy; NP, not prospective, i.e., criteria of malignancy were defined on the basis of the results of the study itself; PSV, peak systolic velocity; subj, subjective; PI, pulsatility index; RI, resistance index. Figures in bold denote the best test in each study

Study	Prospective testing?		GS method	D method	GS		D		Best method[a]
	GS	D			Sens (%)	FP (%)	Sens (%)	FP (%)	
Sassone[32]	NP		Sassone score		100	17			
Ferrazzi[53]	P		Sassone score		74	35			
Lerner[54]	NP		Lerner score		97	23			
Ferrazzi[53]	P		Lerner score		90	51			
Clayton[55]	P		Lerner score		86	39			
De Priest[56]	NP		De Priest score		100	26			
Ferrazzi[53]	P		De Priest score		88	60			
Hata[24]	P	NP(?)	Sassone score	PSV $\geq$ 16cm/s	87	31	83	8	D
Hata[24]	P	NP(?)	Sassone score	RI $\leq$ 0.72	87	31	93	32	D
Kawai[63]	P	NP	Classification	1/PI $\geq$ 0.8	89	40	89	0	D
Hata[4]	P	NP(?)	Sassone score	RI $\leq$ 0.72	85	31	93	47	GS
Franchi[57]	P	NP	Subj evaluation? Classification? Score?	RI $\leq$ 0.65	84	16	76	28	GS
Weiner[58]	P	P(?)	Subj evaluation? Weiner classification?	PI $\leq$ 1.0	94	31	94	3	D
Zanetta[33]	P	P	Sassone score	PI < 1.0	97	21	97	13	D
Zanetta[33]	P	P	Sassone score	RI < 0.60	97	21	91	15	GS = D
Zanetta[33]	P	P	Sassone score	RI < 0.56	97	21	85	9	GS = D
Zanetta[33]	P	P	Sassone score	RI < 0.50	97	21	67	4	GS
Jain[46]	P	P	Subj evaluation	RI $\leq$ 0.4	100	5	70	18	GS
Levine[9]	P	P	Subj evaluation	RI < 0.4	100	39	25	14	GS
Kawai[15]	P	P	Classification	1/PI $\geq$ 0.8	90	35	70	12	D
Alcazar[31]	NP	NP	Sassone score	RI $\leq$ 0.45	100	7	100	11	GS
Caruso[41]	P(?)	NP	Sassone score De Priest score Classification	Own vascular score	100 100 100	25 31 39	100	8	D
Sawicki[42]	P	P	Vera/Rottem score	RI < 0.4	100	39	100	6	D
Mercé[18]	P	P	Own score	Utero-ovarian RI $\leq$ 0.55	96	18	91	1	D
[b]Reles[59]	P	NP	Classification	PI $\leq$ 1.1	91	16	90	26	GS
[c]Strigini[60]	P	P	Own criteria	PI < 1	84	5	84	26	GS

[a] Best method defined as that detecting most malignancies with the lowest false-positive rate.[13]
[b] Reles also tested a combination of GS and D, but it is not possible to understand from their publication what kind of combined criteria they used.
[c] Strigini also tested combined criteria but only in postmenopausal women, the results being shown in Table 22.2.

false-positive rate without decreasing the sensitivity.[62] If the grey-scale imaging method used is subjective evaluation of the grey-scale ultrasound image by an experienced examiner, the role of adding Doppler examination to grey-scale imaging is to increase the confidence with which a correct diagnosis is made.[30]

The use of multivariate logistic regression models or artificial neural networks incorporating grey-scale and Doppler ultrasound variables to calculate the risk of malignancy in an adnexal mass merits comment. These mathematical models performed extremely well in the studies where they were created.[27,38,39,47,48,66,67] Some of them[27,38,47,67] have been externally cross-validated prospectively,[64,65,68] whereby they manifested much poorer performance than in the original studies. Other models have not been cross-validated prospectively.[39,48,66] It is im-

portant to emphasise that in those studies where grey-scale sonography was prospectively compared to a multivariate logistic regression model or an artificial neural network, grey-scale imaging (subjective evaluation of the grey-scale ultrasound image or the Lerner score) was superior to the more complicated mathematical models.[64,65]

22.4 The Role of Colour Doppler Ultrasound Examination when Making a Specific Diagnosis in an Adnexal Mass

Only little has been published on colour Doppler findings characteristic of specific types of tumour

Table 22.2. Ability of grey-scale imaging, colour Doppler examination, and the combination of the two to predict malignancy in adnexal masses. GS, Gray-scale imaging; D, Doppler; Sens, sensitivity; FP, false-positive rate; P, prospective; NP, not prospective; PSV, peak systolic velocity; subj, subjective; PI, pulsatility index; RI, resistance index; TAMXV, time-averaged maximum velocity; S-score, Saasone score; K-score, Kurjak score; B-score, Benacerraf score; MLR, multiple logistic regression model; ANN, artificial neural networks. Figures in bold denote the best test in each study

Study	Prospective testing?		GS method	D method	GS		D		GS+D		Best method[a]
	GS	GS+D			Sens (%)	FP (%)	Sens (%)	FP (%)	Sens (%)	FP (%)	
		D									
Timor-Tritsch[54]	P	NP	NP	S-score	RI < 0.46	94	13	94	1	**100**	**0**	Combined use
Timor-Tritsch[54]	P	NP	NP	S-score	PI < 0.62	94	13	88	3	**100**	**0**	Combined use
Kurjak[45]	NP?	NP?	NP?	K-score	D-score	92	5	**97**	**0**	97	5	D
Salem[10]	P	P	NP	Subj evaluation	PI < 1.0	**100**	40	77	21	77	16	Combined use = GS
Bromley[6]	P	NP	NP	B-score	RI < 0.6	92	48	67	19	**92**	**48**	D
Schneider[11]	P	NP	NP	Subj evaluation	RI < 0.8	88	15	**94**	**44**	82	8	Combined use = GS
Valentin[7]	NP	NP	NP	S-score	RI < 0.8	88	25	94	44	**82**	**15**	Combined use
Valentin[22]	NP	NP	NP	Classification	PI, PSV, TAMXV	**100**	27	93	28	**100**	**17**	Combined use
Sengoku[61]	P	NP	NP	Classification	Colour content	**100**	61	85	20	**100**	**32**	Combined use
Leenen[28]	P	NP	NP	S-score	PI < 1.5	81	33	**81**	**8**	**100**	33	D
Stein[12]	P	P	P	S-score	RI < 0.45	70	15	71	39	**74**	**26**	GS
				Subj evaluation	PI < 1.0	98	38	67	34	**66**	**20**	GS
				Subj evaluation	RI < 0.4	98	38	24	10	**23**	**7**	GS
				Subj evaluation	Internal flow	98	38	77	31	**74**	**20**	GS
Buy[25]		P	P	Subj evaluation	Colour seen	98	38	98	87	**96**	**34**	Combined use
				Subj evaluation	Colour D findings	88	18	71	33[b]	**88**	**3**	Combined use
					PI ≤ 1.0			18	2[b]			
					RI ≤ 0.4			47	19[b]			
					PSV ≥ 15cm/s							
Valentin[30]	P	P		Subj evaluation	Subj evaluation	87	4			**83**	**3**	GS
Valentin[30]	P	P		Classification	TAMXV, PSV	96	63	**100**	**51**	79	31	D
Valentin[62]	P	P	NP	Lerner score	TAMXV	92	37	**100**	**51**	92	23	Combined use
Guerreiro[57]	P	P	P	Subj evaluation	Colour D findings	100	17			**100**	**8**	Combined use
					PI ≤ 0.8				85	33		
					RI ≤ 0.4				58	23		

Table 22.2. Ability of grey-scale imaging, colour Doppler examination, and the combination of the two to predict malignancy in adnexal masses. GS, Gray-scale imaging; D, Doppler; Sens, sensitivity; FP, false-positive rate; P, prospective; NP, not prospective; PSV, peak systolic velocity; subj, subjective; PI, pulsatility index; RI, resistance index; TAMXV, time-averaged maximum velocity; S-score, Sassone score; K-score, Kurjak score; B-score, Benacerraf score; MLR, multiple logistic regression model; ANN, artificial neural networks. Figures in bold denote the best test in each study (*continued*)

Study	Prospective testing?		GS method	D method	GS Sens (%)	FP (%)	D Sens (%)	FP (%)	GS+D Sens (%)	FP (%)	Best method[a]
	GS	GS+D									
Rehn[63]	P	NP	S-score	PI $\leq$ 1.0	**84**	27	67	47	92	60	GS
	D: P		Classification		90	35			98	64	
Strigini[60]	P	NP	Own criteria	PI < 1	77	10	85	19	92	24	Combined
	D: P								69	5	criteria (postmenopausal women only)
Schelling[21]	P	P	Solid area present	Colour present in solid area	97	19			92	6	Combined use
Timmerman[47]	GS: NP(?)	NP	Lerner score	Colour score	96	39	80	37	88	8	Combined method (i.e. MLR)
	D: NP			TAMXV							
Tailor[27]	NP	NP		TAMXV			87	27	93	10	Combined method (i.e. MLR)
Aslam[22]	NP(?)	P		PSV			74	21	43*	8*	D
				TAMXV			78	21			* = MLR of Tailor[27]
				PI			61	24			
				RI			65	26			
Valentin[64]	P	P	Subj evaluation		83	9			71*	18*	GS * = MLR of Tailor[27]
					86	13			62**	21**	** = MLR of Timmerman[47]
Mol[65]	P	P	S-score		90	66			90*	55*	GS
	P	P	Lerner score		77	11			90**	54**	* = MLR of Tailor[27]
	P	P	De Priest score		90	31			90#	40#	** = ANN of Timmerman[67]
	P	P	Ferrazzi score		93	49					# = ANN of Timmerman[67]

[a] Best method defined as that detecting most malignancies with the lowest false-positive rate.[13]
[b] Combination with GS findings not tested.

(e.g. dermoid cyst, endometrioma, haemorrhagic corpus luteum cyst, etc.) in the female pelvis.[69-72] The role of Doppler ultrasound examination when trying to make a specific diagnosis in an adnexal mass seems to be very limited.[73]

22.5 Conclusions

A problem with Doppler ultrasound examinations of adnexal tumours is the dependence of results on the examination technique and the equipment used. Results obtained with one type of equipment or examination technique will almost certainly differ from those obtained with other equipment or another examination technique.

Pulsatility index and RI seem to be the least suitable Doppler variables for discrimination between benign and malignant adnexal masses. Evaluation of the colour Doppler image or measurement of time-averaged maximum velocity are probably better. A high level of colour content in the tumour scan and high blood flow velocity support the presence of malignancy.

The extent to which Doppler examination will contribute to the correct diagnosis of an adnexal mass will depend on which grey-scale imaging method is used. If a good grey-scale imaging method is used (such as subjective evaluation of the grey-scale ultrasound image by an experienced examiner using a good ultrasound system), the contribution of Doppler examination to a correct diagnosis is much smaller (if it contributes at all) than if a poorer grey-scale imaging method is used (such as a rough classification of tumours). Based on the results of prospective studies, there is little to support an important role of Doppler examination in the differential diagnosis of adnexal masses. In most cases a correct diagnosis can be made on the basis of the grey-scale ultrasound image alone.

References

1. Kurjak A, Zalud I, Jurkovic D et al. (1989) Transvaginal color Doppler for the assessment of pelvic circulation. Acta Obstet Gynecol Scand 68:131-135
2. Bourne T, Campbell S, Steer C et al. (1989) Transvaginal colour flow imaging: a possible new screening technique for ovarian cancer. Br Med J 299:1367-1370
3. Tekay A, Jouppila P (1992) Validity of pulsatility and resistance indices in classification of adnexal tumours with transvaginal color Doppler ultrasound. Ultrasound Obstet Gynecol 2:338-344
4. Hata K, Hata T, Manabe A et al. (1992) A critical evaluation of transvaginal Doppler studies, transvaginal sonography, magnetic resonance imaging, and Ca 125 in detecting ovarian cancer. Obstet Gynecol 80:922-926
5. Carter J, Saltzman A, Hartenbach E et al. (1994) Flow characteristics in benign and malignant gynecologic tumors using transvaginal color flow Doppler. Obstet Gynecol 83:125-130
6. Bromley B, Goodman H, Benacerrraf BR (1994) Comparison between sonographic morphology and Doppler waveform analysis for the diagnosis of ovarian malignancy. Obstet Gynecol 83:434-437
7. Valentin L, Sladkevicius P, Marsál K (1994) Limited contribution of Doppler velocimetry to the differential diagnosis of extrauterine pelvic tumors. Obstet Gynecol 83:425-433
8. Tekay A, Jouppila P (1996) Controversies in assessment of ovarian tumors with transvaginal color Doppler ultrasound. Acta Obstet Gynecol Scand 75:316-329
9. Levine D, Feldstein VA, Babcook CJ et al. (1994) Sonography of ovarian masses: poor sensitivity of resistive index for identifying malignant lesions. Am J Roentgenol 162:1355-1359
10. Salem S, White LM, Lai J (1994) Doppler sonography of adnexal masses: the predictive value of the pulsatility index in benign and malignant disease. Am J Roentgenol 163:1147-1150
11. Schneider VL, Schneider A, Reed KL et al. (1993) Comparison of Doppler with two-dimensional sonography and CA 125 for prediction of malignancy of pelvic masses. Obstet Gynecol 81:983-988
12. Stein SM, Leifer-Narin S, Johnson MB et al. (1995) Differentiation of benign and malignant adnexal masses: relative value of gray-scale, color Doppler, and spectral Doppler sonography. Am J Roentgenol 164:381-386
13. Richardson DK, Schwartz JS, Weinbaum PJ et al. (1985) Diagnostic tests in obstetrics: a method for improved evaluation. Am J Obstet Gynecol 152:613-618
14. Maly Z, Riss P, Deutinger J (1995) Localization of blood vessels and qualitative assessment of blood flow in ovarian tumors. Obstet Gynecol 85:33-36
15. Kawai M, Kikkawa F, Ishikawa H et al. (1994) Differential diagnosis of ovarian tumors by transvaginal color-pulse Doppler sonography. Gynecol Oncol 54:209-214
16. Kurjak A, Predanik M, Kupesic-Urek S et al. (1993) Transvaginal color and pulsed Doppler assessment of adnexal tumor vascularity. Gynecol Oncol 50:3-9
17. Fleischer AC, Rodgers WH, Kepple DM et al. (1993) Color Doppler sonography of ovarian masses: a multiparameter analysis. J Ultrasound Med 12:41-48
18. Mercé LT, Caballero RA, Barco MJ et al. (1998) B-mode, utero-ovarian and intratumoral transvaginal color Doppler ultrasonography for differential diagnosis of ovarian tumors. Eur J Obstet Gynecol Reprod Biol 76:97-107
19. Takac I (1998) Analysis of blood flow in adnexal tumors by using color Doppler imaging and pulsed spectral analysis. Ultrasound Med Biol 24:1137-1141
20. Twickler DM, Forte TB, Santos-Ramos R et al. (1999) The Ovarian Tumor Index predicts risk for malignancy. Cancer 86:2280-2290
21. Schelling M, Braun M, Kuhn W et al. (2000) Combined transvaginal B-mode and color Doppler sonography for differential diagnosis of ovarian tumors: results of a multivariate logistic regression analysis. Gynecol Oncol 77:78-86
22. Valentin L (1997) Gray scale sonography, subjective evaluation of the color Doppler image and measurement of blood flow velocity for distinguishing benign and malignant tumors of suspected adnexal origin. Eur J Obstet Gynecol Reprod Biol 72:63-72
23. Fleischer AC, Rodgers WH, Rao BK et al. (1991) Assessment of ovarian tumor vascularity with transvaginal color Doppler sonography. J Ultrasound Med 10:563-568
24. Hata K, Hata T, Kitao M (1995) Intratumoral peak systolic velocity as a new possible predictor for detection of adnexal malignancy. Am J Obstet Gynecol 172:1496-1500
25. Buy J-N, Ghossain MA, Hugol D et al. (1996) Characterization of adnexal masses: combination of color Doppler and

conventional sonography compared with spectral Doppler analysis alone and conventional sonography alone. Am J Roentgenol 166:385–393

26. Prömpeler HJ, Madjar H, Sauerbrei W et al. (1994) Quantitative flow measurements for classification of ovarian tumors by transvaginal color Doppler sonography in postmenopausal patients. Ultrasound Obstet Gynecol 4:406–413

27. Tailor A, Jurkovic D, Bourne TH et al. (1997) Sonographic prediction of malignancy in adnexal masses using multivariate logistic regression analysis. Ultrasound Obstet Gynecol 10:41–47

28. Leeners B, Schild RL, Funk A et al. (1996) Color Doppler sonography improves the pre-operative diagnosis of ovarian tumors made using conventional transvaginal sonography. Eur J Obstet Gynecol Reprod Biol 64:79–85

29. Tailor A, Jurkovic D, Bourne TH et al. (1996) A comparison of intratumoral indices of blood flow velocity and impedance for the diagnosis of ovarian cancer. Ultrasound Med Biol 22:837–843

30. Valentin L (1999) Prospective cross-validation of Doppler ultrasound examination and gray scale ultrasound imaging for discrimination of benign and malignant pelvic masses. Ultrasound Obstet Gynecol 14:273–283

31. Alcazar JL, Ruiz-Perez ML, Errasti T (1996) Transvaginal color Doppler sonography in adnexal masses: which parameter performs best? Ultrasound Obstet Gynecol 8:114–119

32. Aslam N, Tailor A, Lawton F et al. (2000) Prospective evaluation of three different models for the pre-operative diagnosis of ovarian cancer. Br J Obstet Gynaecol 107:1345–1353

33. Zanetta G, Vergani P, Lissoni A (1994) Color Doppler ultrasound in the preoperative assessment of adnexal masses. Acta Obstet Gynecol Scand 73:637–641

34. Timor-Tritsch IE, Lerner JP, Monteagudo A et al. (1993) Transvaginal ultrasonographic characterization of ovarian masses by means of color flow-directed Doppler measurements and a morphologic scoring system. Am J Obstet Gynecol 168:909–913

35. Sladkevicius P, Valentin L, Marsál K (1993) Blood flow velocity in the uterine and ovarian arteries during the normal menstrual cycle. Ultrasound Obstet Gynecol 3:199–208

36. Sladkevicius P, Valentin L, Marsal K (1995) Transvaginal gray-scale and Doppler ultrasound examinations of the uterus and ovaries in healthy postmenopausal women. Ultrasound Obstet Gynecol 6:81–90

37. Guerriero S, Ajossa S, Risalvato A et al. (1998) Diagnosis of adnexal malignancies by using color Doppler energy imaging as a secondary test in persistent masses. Ultrasound Obstet Gynecol 11:277–282

38. Alcazar JL, Jurado M (1998) Using a logistic model to predict malignancy of adnexal masses based on menopausal status, ultrasound morphology, and color Doppler findings. Gynecol Oncol 69:146–150

39. Biagiotti R, Desii C, Vanzi E et al. (1999) Predicting ovarian malignancy: application of artificial neural networks to transvaginal and color Doppler flow US. Radiology 210:399–403

40. Roman LD, Muderspach LI, Stein SM et al. (1997) Pelvic examination, tumor marker level, and gray-scale and Doppler sonography in the prediction of pelvic cancer. Obstet Gynecol 89:493–500

41. Caruso A, Caforio L, Testa AC et al. (1996) Transvaginal color Doppler ultrasonography in the presurgical characterization of adnexal masses. Gynecol Oncol 63:184–191

42. Sawicki W, Spiewankiewicz B, Cendrowski K et al. (1997) Transvaginal color flow imaging in assessment of ovarian tumor neovascularization. Eur J Gynaecol Oncol 18:407–409

43. Kawai M, Kano T, Kikkawa F et al. (1992) Transvaginal Doppler ultrasound with color flow imaging in the diagnosis of ovarian cancer. Obstet Gynecol 79:163–167

44. Wu CC, Lee CN, Chen TM et al. (1994) Incremental angiogenesis assessed by color Doppler ultrasound in the tumorigenesis of ovarian neoplasms. Cancer 73:1251–1256

45. Kurjak A, Predanic M (1992) New scoring system for prediction of ovarian malignancy based on transvaginal color Doppler sonography. J Ultrasound Med 11:631–638

46. Jain KA (1994) Prospective evaluation of adnexal masses with endovaginal gray-scale and duplex and color Doppler US: correlation with pathologic findings. Radiology 191:63–67

47. Timmerman D, Bourne TH, Tailor A et al. (1999) A comparison of methods for preoperative discrimination between benign and malignant adnexal masses: the development of a new logistic regression model. Am J Obstet Gynecol 181:57–65

48. Brown DL, Doubilet PM, Miller FH et al. (1998) Benign and malignant ovarian masses: selection of the most discriminating gray-scale and Doppler sonographic features. Radiology 208:103–110

49. Hata K, Akiba S, Hata T et al. (1998) A multivariate logistic regression analysis in predicting malignancy for patients with ovarian tumors. Gynecol Oncol 68:256–262

50. Sladkevicius P, Valentin L (1995) Inter-observer agreement in the results of Doppler examinations of extrauterine pelvic tumors. Ultrasound Obstet Gynecol 6:91–96

51. Tekay A, Jouppila P (1997) Intraobserver variation in transvaginal Doppler blood flow measurements in benign ovarian tumors. Ultrasound Obstet Gynecol 9:120–124

52. Sassone AM, Timor-Tritsch IE, Artner A et al. (1991). Transvaginal sonographic characterization of ovarian disease: evaluation of a new scoring system to predict ovarian malignancy. Obstet Gynecol 78:70–76

53. Ferrazzi E, Zannetta DG, Dordoni D et al. (1997) Transvaginal ultrasonographic characterization of ovarian masses: comparison of five scoring systems in a multicenter study. Ultrasound Obstet Gynecol 10:192–197

54. Lerner JP, Timor-Tritsch IE, Federman A et al. (1994) Transvaginal ultrasonographic characterization of ovarian masses with an improved, weighted scoring system. Am J Obstet Gynecol 170:81–85

55. Clayton RD, Snowden S, Weston MJ et al. (1999) Neural networks in the diagnosis of malignant ovarian tumours. Br J Obstet Gynaecol 106:1078–1082

56. De Priest PD, Shenson D, Fried A et al. (1993) A morphology index based on sonographic findings in ovarian cancer. Gynecol Oncol 51:7–11

57. Franchi M, Beretta P, Ghezzi F et al. (1995) Diagnosis of pelvic masses with transabdominal color Doppler, CA 125 and ultrasonography. Acta Obstet Gynecol Scand 74:734–739

58. Weiner Z, Thaler I, Beck D et al. (1992) Differentiating malignant from benign ovarian tumors with transvaginal color flow imaging. Obstet Gynecol 79:159–162

59. Reles A, Wein U, Lichtenegger W (1997) Transvaginal color Doppler sonography and conventional sonography in the preoperative assessment of adnexal masses. J Clin Ultrasound 25:217–225

60. Strigini FA, Gadducci A, Del Bravo B et al. (1996) Differential diagnosis of adnexal masses with transvaginal sonography, color flow imaging, and serum CA 125 assay in pre- and postmenopausal women. Gynecol Oncol 61:68–72

61. Sengoku K, Satoh T, Saitoh S et al. (1994) Evaluation of transvaginal color Doppler sonography, transvaginal sonography and CA 125 for prediction of ovarian malignancy. Int J Gynecol Obstet 46:39–43

62. Valentin L (2000) Comparison of Lernefs score, Doppler ultrasound examination, and their combination for discrimination between benign and malignant adnexal masses. Ultrasound Obstet Gynecol 15:143–147

63. Rehn M, Lohmann K, Rempen A (1996) Transvaginal ultrasonography of pelvic masses: evaluation of B-mode technique and Doppler ultrasonography. Am J Obstet Gynecol 75:97–104

64. Valentin L, Hagen B, Tingulstad S et al. (2001) Comparison of 'pattern recognition' and logistic regression models for discrimination between benign and malignant pelvic masses. A prospective cross-validation. Ultrasound Obstet Gynecol 18:357–365.

65. Mol BW, Boll D, De Kanter M et al. (2001) Distinguishing the benign and malignant adnexal mass: an external validation of prognostic models. Gynecol Oncol 80:162–167

66. Tailor A, Jurkovic D, Bourne TH et al. (1999) Sonographic prediction of malignancy in adnexal masses using an artificial neural network. Br J Obstet Gynaecol 106:21–30

67. Timmerman D, Verrelst H, Bourne TH et al. (1999) Artificial neural network models for the preoperative discrimination between malignant and benign adnexal masses. Ultrasound Obstet Gynecol 13:17–25

68. Aslam N, Banerjee S, Carr JV et al. (2000) Prospective evaluation of logistic regression models for the diagnosis of ovarian cancer. Obstet Gynecol 96:75–80

69. Kurjak A, Kupesic S (1994) Scoring system for prediction of ovarian endometriosis based on transvaginal color Doppler sonography. Fertil Steril 62:81–88

70. Aleem F, Pennisi J, Zeitoun K et al. (1995) The role of color Doppler in diagnosis of endometriosis. Ultrasound Obstet Gynecol 5:51–54

71. Zalel Y, Caspi B, Tepper R (1997) Doppler flow characteristics of dermoid cysts: unique appearance of struma ovarii. J Ultrasound Med 16:355–358

72. Tinkanen H, Kujansuu E (1993) Doppler ultrasound findings in tubo-ovarian infectious complex. J Clin Ultrasound 21:175–178

73. Valentin L (1999) Pattern recognition of pelvic masses by gray scale ultrasound imaging: the contribution of Doppler ultrasound. Ultrasound Obstet Gynecol 15:338–347

Chapter 23

Statistical Models

Anil Tailor

23.1 Introduction

The ultrasound based characterisation of adnexal masses continues to be a challenge. A reliable, objective and reproducible method to predict malignancy in these tumours remains elusive. For the clinician such information on the probability of malignancy would be very helpful in the management of the patient. On the basis of this information, any patients deemed to have a high probability of malignancy could be selected for referral to tertiary centres for surgery to be performed by gynaecological oncologists. At the other end of the spectrum, patients with benign tumours could be operated on by minimally invasive techniques. There may be another subgroup of patients whose tumours appear so benign that the need for surgery could be questioned. In such instances, the information on the probability of malignancy could be utilised to reassure the patient and arrange the appropriate follow-up.

23.2 Current Methods of Managing Adnexal Masses

The exclusion of malignancy is one of the main concerns of the clinician when a patient presents with a suspected pelvic mass. The diagnostic pathway includes a careful history, concentrating on any risk factors that may be present such as age, menopausal status, symptoms, family history and past history of gynaecological tumours. On clinical examination, the size and mobility of the mass and the presence of any ascites are assessed. A serum CA 125 level is usually measured and ultrasound examination of the pelvic mass requested. The sonographer in turn tries to determine the size, locularity and echogenicity. Additional features such as the presence of papillary projections and ascites are sought. If the facilities are

available, the ultrasonographer may go on to investigate the vascularity of the tumour. In particular, the presence of high-velocity, low-impedance blood flow within the tumour will be sought. The referring clinician then has at his disposal all the information from the patient's age to whether her tumour has suspicious blood flow. At some centres a further evaluation with computed tomography or magnetic resonance imaging may be undertaken. On the basis of all this information, the clinician will attempt to make an intellectual guess on the possibility of malignancy and plan the subsequent management. Thus, a tentative diagnosis is reached using a multifactorial approach.

This is in vast contrast to the unifactorial approach that some have unsuccessfully advocated. After serum CA 125 was identified as a tumour marker,[1] it was hoped that, on the basis of this single marker, malignant tumours could be selected. However, a suboptimal diagnostic accuracy has prevented this.[2-4] With the advent of Doppler ultrasound, it was hoped that single impedance parameters such as the pulsatility index (PI) or the resistance index (RI) could usefully discriminate benign and malignant tumours.[5-7] When the initially impressive results with impedance parameters could not be reproduced,[8-10] some investigators experimented with velocity parameters such as the peak systolic velocity (PSV)[11,12] and the time-averaged maximum velocity (TAMXV)[9,11] to determine whether they held any promise. The possibility of using two Doppler parameters instead of one has also been investigated. While this provided marginal improvement, the results were still suboptimal.[11] Concurrently, others abandoned the unifactorial approach and attempted to develop algorithms based on multifactorial parameters. For example, various morphology scoring systems were developed, which incorporated tumour characteristics such as locularity, echogenicity, papillary projec-

165

tions, cyst outline, septal thickness, wall thickness, acoustic shadowing, ascites, etc.[3,13-15] This method, however, still concentrated only on data obtained from sonographic examination.

The main problems with the simple multifactorial approaches (morphology scoring systems) have been on deciding which multiple parameters to combine within an algorithm. Furthermore, how should each chosen parameter be allocated an appropriate weight relative to its importance? Lerner et al[14] attempted to generate an objective morphology scoring system incorporating an optimum set of variables and weights derived by multiple linear regression analysis. This method is different from the techniques of statistical modelling proposed in the following discussion.

23.3 Multiple Logistic Regression Analysis

This is a statistical method that generates an equation describing the relationship between a dichotomous outcome variable (e.g. presence or absence of malignancy) to multiple predictive variables (e.g. age, menopausal status, CA 125, ultrasound appearance and vascularity). This regression equation can be used in two ways: first, to select the best predictive variables and their relative weights and, second, the numerical output of the equation can be interpreted as the probability of the outcome variable being present. Therefore, if the outcome variable happens to be the presence of malignancy, the equation will generate a numerical value for any given patient that will be directly proportional to the probability of malignancy being harboured by that patient.

To generate the regression equation, experimental data need to be collected for many patients. Information regarding their age, menopausal status, CA 125, various grey-scale ultrasound characteristics such as locularity, echogenicity, presence of papillary projections, size, Doppler indices, and finally, the histology of the operative specimen needs to be recorded. Once an adequate number of patients have been recruited, the overall sample should be randomly separated into two sets. These include the training set, which will comprise about 75% of the overall data set on which the logistic regression analysis will be carried out, and the testing set, which will be the remainder and on which the generated model will be tested prospectively. The patients' data contained within the training set are then fed through a dedicated computer program capable of performing multiple logistic regression analysis. A manual analysis without computers is also possible but this is very complex and time-consuming. Various soft-

ware packages have algorithms that will allow the investigator to choose the most predictive variables for the equation rather than generating the latter from all the available variables. The reason for not using too many input variables is that, for a given amount of training data, the greater the number of predictive variables used in the regression equation, the greater the risk of a chance relationship.[16] The resulting model will perform almost perfectly on the retrospective data from which it has been derived, but is likely to cross-validate very poorly on the testing set. It is therefore unlikely to be of any clinical value. Hence, the more variables one wishes to include in the model, the more patients one has to recruit for the training set. As a rule of thumb, the number of patients in the training set with the outcome of interest (malignancy) must be approximately ten times the number of variables used. For example, with four predictive variables such as age, serum CA 125, presence of papillary projections and PI, 40 patients with malignant tumours will be required in the training set. Therefore, if the prevalence of malignancy in the study sample is approximately 30% (i.e. 30% of the patients presenting with a known adnexal mass actually harbouring a malignancy), an additional 95 patients with benign tumours are also required in the training data set. Hence a total of approximately 135 patients need to be recruited for the training set alone. If this set comprised 75% of the whole data set, an additional 45 patients need to be recruited into the testing set. Therefore, approximately 180 patients need to be recruited when a logistic regression analysis with four variables is contemplated. Table 23.1 shows the relationship between the total number of patients that need to be recruited and the desired number of variables for the regression equation.

The derived regression model looks like:

$$\text{Probability of Malignancy} = \frac{1}{1 + e^{-z}}$$

where z = constant + $k_1 var_1$ + $k_2 var_2$ + $k_3 var_3$ +$k_n var_n$, and e is the mathematical constant and base value of natural logarithms.

Table 23.1. Relationship between number of desired variables to be incorporated in a model and the number of patients that need to be recruited based on assumptions that the training and testing sets are divided in a ratio of 75 : 25 and that the prevalence of malignancy in the overall study population is 30%

No. of variables	Size of:		Total no. of patients required
	Training set	Testing set	
2	65	25	90
3	100	35	135
4	135	45	180
5	165	55	220
10	335	110	445

The logistic regression analysis derives the values for the constant and the coefficients k_1, k_2, k_3, k_n. For any given patient, the value for var_1, var_2, var_3, var_n are determined preoperatively. Therefore z is calculated accurately and can range from $-\infty$ to $+\infty$. If z is very large and positive, e^{-z} will be very small and almost zero. Therefore, the probability of outcome will be numerically equal to one. If z is very large but negative, e^{-z} will be very large and almost infinite. In this case the probability of outcome will equal $1/\infty$, which is zero. This illustrates the fact that the probability of outcome can mathematically achieve numerical values only within the range of zero and one. The former would imply the absence of the outcome and the latter, the presence of the outcome. Intermediate values can be interpreted as the probability of the outcome. For example, for a given patient, if the regression equation generates a value of 0.65, the probability of malignancy for that patient is 65%.

In the final stage of deriving the regression model, the probabilities of malignancy for all the patients in the testing set are calculated. These are then compared with the actual histology to check how accurately the model is performing. This is an important exercise as a poor accuracy is almost certainly indicative of excessive shrinkage, i.e. the derived model refers to a chance relationship and is unable to generalise well. A likely cause would be the inclusion of too many input variables.

23.3.1 Advantages and Disadvantages of Multiple Logistic Regression Analysis

The advantages of this statistical method are:

- it chooses the most appropriate and independent variables for predicting the outcome of interest;
- the coefficients for each variable are calculated to reflect the relative importance of each variable;
- the output value of the regression model is conveniently equal to the probability of the outcome of interest. This value can be used for counselling and planning management.

The disadvantages of this statistical method are:

- it requires fast computational power for its derivation. Furthermore, once the model is derived, a computer or at least a programmable calculator would be required to calculate the probability of malignancy for any prospective patient;
- the models may not be portable, i.e. a model generated at one scanning unit may not be usable at another unit unless identical recruitment criteria and methodology for defining patient

characteristics (e.g. presence or absence of papillary projections, random echogenicity, low impedance blood flow, etc.) are present;

- significant interactions may exist between the chosen input variables. While allowances can be made for these interactions, the resulting model becomes very cumbersome. For instance, suppose that among the input variables there are two whose values need to be large simultaneously for the outcome of interest to occur. This implies that the two variables are not completely independent. Under some circumstances, e.g. the value for one variable is very large and the other normal for a given patient, the model may incorrectly predict the outcome of interest. The value for the former would have to be large enough to compensate for the smallness of the other. To make this model more accurate, a correction variable would have to be incorporated into the model, making it cumbersome to use.

23.4 Artificial Neural Networks

These are computer-based decision-making tools, which are modelled on the structure and learning behaviour of biological nervous systems. They are used to generate a numerical probability of an output (e.g. presence of malignancy) from the input of clinical and technical data. Information from examples (retrospective data) is used to develop algorithms (supervised learning) in the same manner as a clinician learns to make a particular diagnosis based on previous experience. The potential of this approach to aid radiological diagnosis has been recognised for some years.[17] In particular, the technique has been applied to texture analysis in ultrasonography,[18] differential diagnosis from chest X-rays,[19] prediction of pulmonary embolism from ventilation/perfusion scans[20] and the prediction of breast cancer from mammography.[21]

The term "neural network" is derived from the close resemblance of its structure with the neuronal interconnections within the brain. Individual neurons in the physiological nervous system receive multiple synaptic inputs from surrounding neurons. The activation level of any given neuron is dependent on the activation of the preceding neuron and the strength of synaptic connections between them and this neuron. Neurophysiologists have long been aware that in simple animal models, learning is accompanied by changes in morphology and neurotransmitter release at synaptic junctions that can be visualised with the electron microscope. It has therefore been proposed that learning takes place by adjusting the strengths of individual synaptic connections.

In the artificial neural network (ANN), the input signals (e.g. age, menopausal status, etc.) are propagated forward through layers of processing nodes to emerge eventually as the output signal (e.g. histopathology of an adnexal mass). The most commonly used structure for an ANN utilises three layers: input layer, hidden layer and output layer (Figure 23.1). The input layer consists of individual processing nodes (analogous to individual sensory neurons) for each parameter that is thought to be important for contributing towards the eventual output. The output layer also contains individual processing nodes for all the desired outputs. The hidden layer is slightly more difficult to conceptualise and also contains processing nodes. These receive signals from the input layer and, after processing, relay them to the output layer. The connectivity of the network is such that each input-processing node is connected to all the nodes within the hidden layer. Each of these nodes in turn is connected to all the nodes in the output layer. All the individual connections are weighted depending on the relative importance of each of the nodes in the preceding layer. Initially, before the training of the network begins, these weights are set at random. During training, when examples are presented to the network, these weights are adjusted at each iteration until, after multiple iterations, these weights have been fine-tuned such that a maximum number of patients in the training data are correctly classified.

The connection weights are adjusted when examples are presented to the network during supervised learning. This process can be achieved with various learning algorithms, but the classical method is called the "back propagation" method. Briefly, the network calculates the error between the projected network output and the actual desired output for all the cases. In this manner the mean square error for all the input–output pairs in the training data is computed with the current set of weights. The information regarding the magnitude of this mean square error is "back propagated" to the individual weights, which are then adjusted for the next iteration. With this new set of weights, the error is again calculated and the adjustment repeated. This process can be carried on ad infinitum to minimise the mean square error or, alternatively, it can be terminated following a set number of iterations, even if maximal reduction in mean square error has not occurred. It must be noted that a high number of iterations during training for thorough fine-tuning of the weights does not necessarily result in a better model than one that had the iterations terminated at the optimum time early on during the training process. This is because, with increasing training time, the model can over-train. This is analogous to memorisation. If the network model memorises each of the input–output pairs in the training data, it may not be able to generalise well with new data that is presented to it in the future. Therefore, the aim of any network-building process is to ensure that it is able to generalise rather than memorise all the different combinations of input–output pairs that are presented to it.

The preceding paragraphs have given a general overview of the structural architecture of neural networks and how certain elements within this network are adjusted to produce the desired output. A basic understanding of the neural networks can perhaps be achieved by considering what happens to input data as it is presented to a network. The

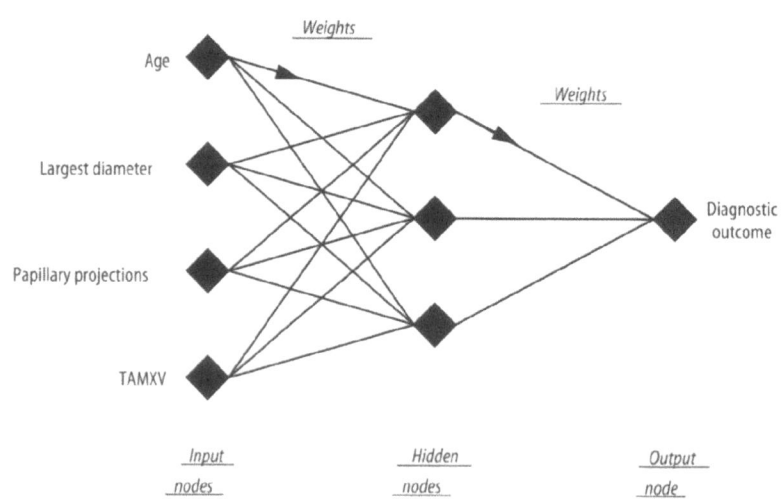

Figure 23.1 Architecture of the neural network for predicting ovarian malignancy from demographic and sonographic data. TAMXV, Time-averaged maximum velocity.

magnitude of each input can be thought of as the activation level of a given neuron in the input layer. The amount of this activation that will be relayed to the neuron in the next layer (hidden layer) will be dependent on the weight or strength of the connection between the two. This neuron in the hidden layer, meanwhile, will also be receiving other stimuli from the other neurons in the input layer, depending on their individual activation levels and the strengths of the connections between them. Therefore, for a given neuron in the hidden layer, its level of activation will depend on the sum of all the stimuli that it receives. This activation is then propagated forward to the neuron in the next layer if it is high enough. This is analogous to a neuron firing if the activation level exceeds the threshold. The decision to propagate its stimulus forward is achieved by processing the overall activation level through a "transfer function". This is usually the sigmoid function and it determines the threshold for the stimulus. The amount of stimulus that the neuron in the next layer receives is also dependent on the connection strength between the two. Assuming that this is an output neuron, it will have a high activation level (indicating a greater possibility of malignancy in our study) if the summation of all the weighted stimuli it receives from other neurons in the hidden layer is high.

23.4.1 Method for Generating Artificial Neural Network Model

The initial process of data collection and separation into training and testing sets is similar to that described for multiple logistic regression analysis. Dedicated computer software capable of generating neural network models is used with the training set as the substrate. Similar rules as described above for logistic regression models apply regarding the number of input variables that should be incorporated. The combination of variables likely to give the best neural network model has to be chosen by the investigator on a trial-and-error basis. This is unlike multiple logistic regression analysis, in which the most independent and predictive variables can be statistically selected. Therefore, with ANNs, numerous models with various combinations of input variables have to be generated individually. Each of these models then has to be compared with the others until the best model with the appropriate input variables emerges. Receiver operating characteristic (ROC) curve analysis using the statistic provided by area under the graph can be used to perform this comparison of different models.[22]

23.4.2 Advantages and Disadvantages of Artificial Neural Networks

The advantages of this technique are:

- the model is more accurate than the one generated by multiple logistic regression analysis because it has inherent mechanisms for adjusting interactions between input variables.[22] When enough patients have been recruited to allow numerous input variables, the chances of interactions increase, making this modelling technique more superior;
- unlike logistic regression analysis, which can predict only two outcomes (e.g. absence or presence of malignancy), ANN can predict any number of outcomes (e.g. benign, borderline, invasive and metastatic). However, this would require a large data set.

The disadvantages of this technique are:

- it cannot inherently choose the best set of independent variables and hence the generation of the best model is cumbersome and time-consuming.[22] This may be overcome in the future with dedicated software that will not only generate the model, but also instantaneously carry out the ROC curve analysis on the generated model. The area under the graph statistic may be stored for subsequent comparisons;
- artificial neural network models use matrix algebra and complex functions to generate the output value, unlike the relatively simpler regression equation derived by logistic regression analysis. The use of these models on prospective patients then requires a dedicated database on a relatively fast computer.

23.5 Experimental Results

Statistical modelling to predict malignancy in ovarian tumours has only recently been investigated with the advent of faster computing power. Our own experience has been based on a sample of 67 patients who were known to have an adnexal mass and were about to undergo surgery.[22,23] All the patients underwent a preoperative scan and had data collected on their age, menopausal status, size of their tumour, echogenicity, locularity, presence of papillary projections and Doppler indices, such the PSV, TAMXV, PI and RI. Unfortunately, complete data on serum CA 125 was not available. This sample of 67 patients was separated randomly into two sets: a training set, which contained 52 patients (41 benign, 11 malignant), and a testing set, which contained 15 patients (11 benign, 4 malignant). The derived regression model retained three independent variables, including "age", "TAMXV" and "papillary projections score (0, 1)".[23] The probability of malignancy was given by:

$$\text{Probability of Malignancy} = \frac{1}{1 + e^{-z}}$$

Where $z = (0.1273 \times \text{age}) + (0.2794 \times \text{TAMXV}) + (4.4136 \times \text{papillary projection score}) - 14.2046$ and e is the mathematical constant and base value of natural logarithms. This model gave a sensitivity and specificity of 90.9% and 87.8% respectively for the training set at a cut-off value for probability of malignancy of 25%. When cross-validated on the testing set, a 100% accuracy was achieved. Therefore, the overall sensitivity and specificity for the whole data set at the cut-off value of 25% probability was 93.3% and 90.4% respectively.[23]

We used the same data set to derive an ANN model.[22] Two hundred and five different models, each with a different combination of four input variables, were designed and compared. The best model contained "age", "largest diameter", "papillary projection score" and "TAMXV" as the input variables. These were modulated through a single hidden layer containing three nodes, as shown in Figure 23.1. Using a lower cut-off value of 5% probability, the sensitivity and specificity for the whole data set using the best ANN model were 100% and 96.2% respectively. Figure 23.2 shows the ROC curves for the ANN and logistic regression models, and TAMXV and PI for comparison. It shows clearly

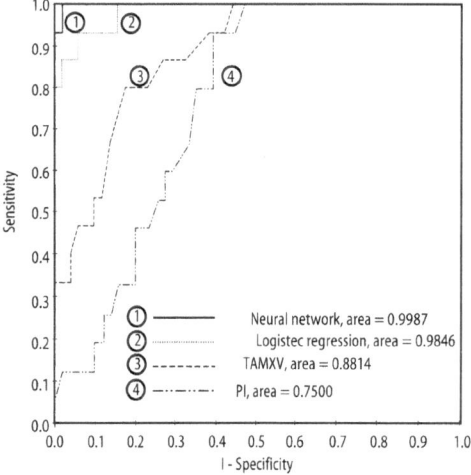

Figure 23.2 Receiver operating characteristic curve comparing the diagnostic accuracy of the neural network model, multiple logistic regression model, time-averaged maximum velocity (TAMXV) and pulsatility index (PI).

that better discrimination is achieved using the statistical models.

Some cases of actual data are shown as examples in Table 23.2 to illustrate the workings of the logistic regression model.[23] The first patient (case A) was only 31 years of age. There were no papillary projections, but the TAMXV was higher than our optimum cut-off value of > 12 cm/s, which would have made this tumour malignant according to Doppler criteria alone. However, the model correctly identified this lesion as benign. Conversely, case B was that of a 65-year-old whose tumour had papillary projections. The TAMXV was lower than the optimum cut-off value of 12 cm/s, which would have made it a benign lesion according to the Doppler criteria alone. Despite the low TAMXV, the model correctly identified this lesion as malignant.

The other two cases in Table 23.2 relate to those who were classified incorrectly by the model. Case C was a young patient of 37 years of age, whose tumour had no papillary projections and the TAMXV was higher than the optimum cut-off value. The tumour in this case was shown to be of borderline malignancy on the basis of histological criteria. We suspect that the model failed because the TAMXV was not high enough to offset the effects of the young age and the absence of papillary projections. A close inspection of case D shows that it was incorrectly classified as positive because of the high TAMXV.

Important data on statistical modelling have also been produced by Timmerman and colleagues.[24] Their sample included 191 patients separated randomly into the training and testing sets at a ratio of two-thirds to one-third. The best logistic regression model retained four variables including "colour score" (a subjective semi-quantitative assessment of blood flow on colour Doppler imaging ranging from zero to four), "serum CA 125", "presence of papillary projections", and "menopausal status".[24] The probability of malignancy was given by $1/1 + e^{-z}$, where z was equal to $(2.6369 \times \text{colour score}) + (0.0225 \times \text{CA 125}) + (7.1062 \times \text{papillary projection score}) + (2.6423 \text{ postmenopausal status score}) - 13.6796$. At a cut-off value of 25% probability of malignancy, this model gave a sensitivity and specificity of 97.1% and 90.8% respectively on the training set. When cross-validated on the testing set, these reduced to 92.9% and 78.4% respectively. Therefore, the overall sensitivity and specificity for the whole data set was 95.9% and 87.1% respectively.[24]

Timmerman and colleagues have also experimented with ANN models.[25] Their best model derived and tested on 173 patients contained seven input variables, including "presence of papillary projection (0, 1)", "presence of smooth outline (0, 1)", "presence of unilocular cyst (0, 1)", "presence of

Table 23.2. Example cases to illustrate derivation of probability and odds from logistic regression model. TAMXV, Time-averaged maximum velocity

	Age (years)	Papillary projection	TAMXV (cm/s)	Probability (%)	Odds[a]	Classification of test result
A	31	No	17	0.4	1 : 247	True negative
B	65	Yes	8	67.2	2 : 1	True positive
C	37	No	26	9.7	1 : 9	False negative
D	48	No	32	70.0	7 : 3	False positive

[a] Odds of patient having ovarian cancer based on test result.

ascites (0, 1)", "presence of bilateral involvement (0, 1)", "postmenopausal status (0, 1)" and "serum CA 125 level". These were modulated through a hidden layer containing two nodes. At a cut-off value of 60% probability of malignancy, their model gave a sensitivity and specificity of 97.0% and 92.8% respectively on the training set and 93.8% and 95.1% respectively on the testing set.

A logistic regression model based on 155 patients has also been produced by Schutter et al.[26] Their input variables were "clinical examination findings (0, 1)", "ultrasound morphology score" (based on Finkler et al[3]), "serum CA 125" and "serum CA72-4". Their z-score for the regression equation was equal to –5.6816 + (2.2677 × ultrasound score) – (2.4928 × clinical examination score) + (1.6057 × CA 125) + (1.5866 × CA72-4). With this regression model they obtained a sensitivity and specificity of 81.3% and 90.2% respectively. The cut-off value for probability of malignancy at which this performance was achieved was not stated. It also appears that no attempt was made to cross-validate the derived model on a testing set.

Alcazar and colleagues derived a logistic regression model on 73 patients and tested it on a further 58 patients.[27] Their input variables included an "ultrasound morphology score" based on Sassone et al[13] and a "colour Doppler score" based on the RI value. The z-score for their regression model was equal to –5.002 + (4.263 × morphology score) + (3.095 × Doppler score). At a cut-off value of 75% probability of malignancy, their model, when tested on the 58 patients, gave a sensitivity of 84.6% and a specificity of 100%.

Clayton and colleagues derived and tested neural network and logistic regression models on 217 cases.[28] Their variables included age, CA 125 level and Lerner ultrasound score.[14] Their neural network model was 95% sensitive and 78% specific and the logistic regression model was 82% sensitive at a specificity of 51%.

More recently, data has emerged on prospective validation of logistic regression models. Aslam and colleagues at King's College Hospital, where our original logistic regression model was produced, failed to obtain any decent accuracy with the original model when tested prospectively on 61 women with adnexal masses.[29] At a cut-off value of 50% probability of malignancy, the sensitivity and specificity were 43% and 92% respectively. It was reported that there was a lack of homogeneity between the cases that had been used to generate the original model and those that were used to test the model prospectively. More specifically, in our original data set, there were no cases of non-epithelial ovarian malignancy. In contrast, the data used to test the model prospectively contained five out of 23 non-epithelial ovarian malignancies. As the original model was developed from a small number of non-diverse cases, it could not have been expected to perform accurately if it was not trained to cater for these odd cases. Indeed, we had stated in our original study that our aim was to report a potentially useful application of multivariate logistic regression analysis on data to predict the presence of malignancy in an adnexal mass. It was not our intention that the model be used definitively to calculate probabilities. This was because it was derived from a small number of cases and the extent to which this form of modelling was sensitive to variation in the scanning technique and interpretation of features was unknown.

Therefore, the study by Aslam and colleagues merely confirms that precise models based on logistic regression have to be generated from a large number of diverse cases. It does not prove that these statistical modelling techniques are ineffective.

23.6 Future Directions

One of our future aims should be to build models on easily collectable data, such as serum CA 125, presence or absence of a relevant family history, locularity, size, etc., instead of complex data such as the Doppler indices. The latter require expertise and are generally less reproducible than the former. Certain aspects of ultrasound morphology and its interpretation are also affected by operator experience and bias. For example, what may represent a papillary projection to one operator may merely be interpreted as an irregular outline by another. Similarly, a suspiciously mixed echogenicity within a tumour may not be perceived as such by another operator. Because these elements play a vital role in most algorithms, we need to find ways of standardising their interpretation. Only then are statistical models likely to become portable. Perhaps, we need to experiment with allowing artificial intelligence to take over this role of interpretation. The use of neural networks for texture analysis in ultrasonography is not new.[18] It should therefore be possible to develop expert systems based on neural networks that will extract the necessary information, such as papillary projections, echogenicity, locularity, etc. in real time while ultrasonography is being performed. This information could be fed directly into resident statistical models programmed into the ultrasound hardware, so that a final result is made available immediately on completion of the examination.

23.7 Conclusions

Statistical modelling to predict ovarian malignancy appears to be a logical way forward in our search for the perfect algorithm to discriminate benign and malignant tumours. It is useful that the numerical outputs of these models can conveniently be interpreted as a probability. These can be usefully applied in terms of counselling patients and planning management. Most experimental evidence on the usefulness of these models is based on retrospective analysis of data. This inherently exaggerates the accuracy of these models. The few data on prospective validation appear to suggest that these precise models will have to be generated from relatively large samples of diverse cases.

References

1. Bast RC Jr, Feeney M, Lazarus H et al (1981) Reactivity of a monoclonal antibody with human ovarian carcinoma. J Clin Invest 68(5):1331–1337
2. Chen DX, Schwartz PE, Li XG et al (1988) Evaluation of CA 125 levels in differentiating malignant from benign tumors in patients with pelvic masses. Obstet Gynecol 72(1):23–27
3. Finkler NJ, Benacerraf B, Lavin PT et al (1988) Comparison of serum CA 125, clinical impression, and ultrasound in the preoperative evaluation of ovarian masses. Obstet Gynecol 72(4):659–664
4. Kawai M, Kikkawa F, Ishikawa H et al (1994) Differential diagnosis of ovarian tumors by transvaginal color-pulse Doppler sonography. Gynecol Oncol 54(2):209–214
5. Bourne TH, Campbell S, Steer C et al (1989) Transvaginal colour flow imaging: a possible new screening technique for ovarian cancer. Br Med J 299:1367–1370
6. Kurjak A, Zalud I, Alfirevic Z (1991) Evaluation of adnexal masses with transvaginal color ultrasound. J Ultrasound Med 10(6):295–297
7. Hata T, Hata K, Yamane Y et al (1988) Real-time two-dimensional and pulsed Doppler ultrasound detection of intrapelvic neoplastic tumors and abnormal pathogenic changes: preliminary report. J Cardiovasc Ultrasonography 7:135–141
8. Bromley B, Goodman H, Benacerraf BR (1994) Comparison between sonographic morphology and Doppler waveform for the diagnosis of ovarian malignancy. Obstet Gynecol 83 (3):434–437
9. Valentin L, Sladkevicius P, Marsal K (1994) Limited contribution of Doppler velocimetry to the differential diagnosis of extrauterine pelvic tumours. Obstet Gynecol 83:425–433
10. Stein SM, Leifer-Narin S, Johnson MB et al (1995) Differentiation of benign and malignant adnexal masses: relative value of gray-scale, color Doppler, and spectral Doppler sonography. Am J Roentgenol 164:381–386
11. Tailor A, Jurkovic D, Bourne TH et al (1996) A comparison of intratumoural indices of blood flow velocity and impedance for the diagnosis of ovarian cancer. Ultrasound Med Biol 22(7):837–843
12. Hata K, Hata T, Kitao M (1995) Intratumoral peak systolic velocity as a new possible predictor for detection of adnexal malignancy. Am J Obstet Gynecol 172:1496–1500
13. Sassone AM, Timor-Tritsch IE, Artner A et al (1991) Transvaginal sonographic characterization of ovarian disease: evaluation of a new scoring system to predict ovarian malignancy. Obstet Gynecol 78(1):70–76
14. Lerner JP, Timor-Tritsch IE, Federman A et al (1994) Transvaginal ultrasonographic characterization of ovarian masses with an improved, weighted scoring system. Am J Obstet Gynecol 170(1 Pt 1):81–85
15. Bourne TH, Campbell S, Reynolds KM et al (1993) Screening for early familial ovarian cancer with transvaginal ultrasonography and colour blood flow imaging. Br Med J 306 (6884):1025–1029
16. Astion ML, Wilding P (1992) The application of back-propagation neural networks to problems in pathology and laboratory medicine. Arch Pathol Lab Med 116:995–1001
17. Boone JM, Gross GW, Greco-Hunt V (1990) Neural networks in radiologic diagnosis: I Introduction and illustration. Invest Radiol 25:1012–1016
18. DaPonte JS, Sherman P (1991) Classification of ultrasonic image texture by statistical discriminant analysis of neutral networks. Comput Med Imaging Graph 15(1):3–9
19. Gross GW, Boone JM, Greco-Hunt V et al (1990) Neural networks in radiologic diagnosis. II Interpretation of neonatal chest radiographs. Invest Radiol 25(9):1017–1023
20. Scott JA, Palmer EL (1993) Neural network analysis of ventilation-perfusion lung scans. Radiology 186(3):661–664
21. Floyd CE Jr, Lo JY, Yun AJ et al (1994) Prediction of breast cancer malignancy using an artificial neural network Cancer 74(11):2944–2948
22. Tailor A, Jurkovic D, Bourne TH et al (1999) Sonographic prediction of malignancy in adnexal masses using an artificial neural network. Br J Obstet Gynaecol 106(1):21–30
23. Tailor A, Jurkovic D, Bourne TH et al (1997) Sonographic prediction of malignancy in adnexal masses using multivariate logistic regression analysis. Ultrasound Obstet Gynecol 10(1):41–47
24. Timmerman D, Bourne TH, Tailor A et al (1999) A comparison of methods for preoperative discrimination between malignant and benign adnexal masses: the development of a new logistic regression model. Am J Obstet Gynecol 181(1):57–65
25. Timmerman D, Verrelst H, Bourne T et al (1999) Artificial neural network models for the preoperative discrimination between benign and malignant adnexal masses. Ultrasound Obstet Gynecol 13:17–25
26. Schutter EM, Sohn C, Kristen P et al (1998) Estimation of probability of malignancy using a logistic model combining physical examination, ultrasound, serum CA 125, and serum CA 72-4 in postmenopausal women with a pelvic mass: an international multicenter study. Gynecol Oncol 69(1):56–63

27. Alcazar JL, Jurado M (1998) Using a logistic model to predict malignancy of adnexal masses based on menopausal status, ultrasound morphology, and color Doppler findings. Gynecol Oncol 69(2):146–150
28. Clayton RD, Snowden S, Weston MJ et al (1999) Neural networks in the diagnosis of malignant ovarian tumours. Br J Obstet Gynaecol 106(10):1078–1082
29. Aslam N, Tailor A, Lawton F et al (2000) Prospective evaluation of three different models for the pre-operative diagnosis of ovarian cancer. Br J Obstet Gynaecol 107 (11):1347–1353

Chapter 24

Treatment of Adnexal Masses and Laparoscopy

Michel Canis, Arnaud Wattiez, Revaz Botchorishvili, Patrice Mille, Marie-Claude Anton, Hubert Manhes, Gérard Mage, Jean-Luc Pouly and Maurice-Antoine Bruhat

24.1 Introduction

The laparoscopic treatment of adnexal masses has become the gold standard within the last few years. However, there are few extensive descriptions of the procedure; it is generally summarised as a "stripping" procedure without any detail. Nevertheless, a good laparoscopic technique and adequate surgical management are required to ensure optimal patient care. In this chapter, we will discuss:

- the treatment technique that should be adapted to each pathological diagnosis;
- postoperative adhesions;
- the limits of the laparoscopic approach, accounting for all the clinical and experimental data recently reported about tumour dissemination.

Obviously, any significant and reliable improvement in preoperative evaluation would be a major step forward in the surgical management of adnexal masses.

24.2 The Surgical Technique

24.2.1 Entering the Abdomen

The initial steps of the laparoscopy procedure have been described elsewhere.[1] However, a specific technique should be used to manage large adnexal cysts, in order to avoid blind punctures with the Veress needle or with the umbilical trocar. To treat a cyst of more than 8 cm, the pneumoperitoneum is created in the left hypochondrium with a Veress needle inserted perpendicularly to the abdominal wall. In very large masses, up to 20 cm, the first trocar may be inserted above the umbilicus or with an open laparoscopy technique.

A very large mass is not a contraindication to the laparoscopic approach as long as a reliable preoperative examination of the internal capsule of the cyst has been carried out. As very large masses are often difficult to examine using ultrasound, we routinely use a second imaging technique, preferably magnetic resonance imaging (MRI), to confirm that the mass is entirely or almost entirely cystic. If there are large solid areas inside, the laparoscopic approach may be considered to inspect the upper abdomen, but not for the treatment.

In adnexal masses, large solid contents should be considered an absolute contraindication for laparoscopic surgery. Ovarian morcellation is always an unacceptable in such cases.

24.2.2 The Ancillary Ports

Ancillary trocars should be inserted perpendicularly to the abdominal wall. This is particularly important when treating an adnexal mass. Indeed, if a cancer is diagnosed or missed during the laparoscopic procedure, a restaging procedure will be required. As trocar site metastases have been reported,[2] excision of the trocar sites is recommended when performing a restaging. However the information obtained from an excision, performed perpendicularly to the abdominal wall, is reliable only if the trocars were inserted in the same way.

24.2.3 Laparoscopic Treatment

The cyst wall should be removed completely. Ablation of the cyst wall with laser or bipolar coagulation cannot be considered as a valid treatment, except in selected cases, such as endometriomas in young infertile patients. Pathological examination of the entire cyst wall is required to make a reliable diagnosis.

When learning the technique for laparotomy, we were taught the concept that an adequate cystectomy should be performed without puncture or rupture to avoid spillage of malignant ovarian tumours. However, we believe that puncture of a tumour of low malignant potential and of an early invasive cancer has no effect on the prognosis when the tumour is removed immediately by laparotomy.[3-5] A rupture is not the catastrophic event described by Williams in 1973.[6]

In our opinion:

- it is difficult to achieve an ovarian cystectomy without puncture or rupture;
- avoiding puncture is impossible when treating an early ovarian cancer. Indeed, if a tumour is malignant, it invades the cleavage plane and cannot be separated from the surrounding ovarian tissue without rupture. In these cases, cystectomy without rupture is impossible.

The key steps in the management of an ovarian mass are the diagnosis and the choice between salpingo-oophorectomy and ovarian cystectomy.

24.3 The Laparoscopic Diagnosis[7]

First, a peritoneal fluid sample and/or peritoneal washings for cytological examination are aspirated from the posterior cul-de-sac, or from the paracolic gutters and the vesicouterine cul-de-sac, when the pouch of Douglas is obliterated by adhesions or filled by a large adnexal mass. Thereafter, the cystic ovary, pelvic peritoneum, contralateral ovary, paracolic gutters, diaphragm, omentum, liver and bowel are carefully inspected. The value of this inspection has been confirmed by Possover et al, who reported that metastases easily accessible to laparoscopic inspection were always present in patients with metastasis of the small bowel and of the mesentery.[8] If signs of malignancy such as ascites, peritoneal metastases or extracystic ovarian vegetations are found, the mass should be treated as suspicious or malignant.

In the remaining cases, an intracystic evaluation is required to rule out malignancy. Several techniques may be used to perform this essential step of the surgical diagnosis (Table 24.1). Adnexal masses are punctured only when assumed to be benign from the initial laparoscopic inspection and from the preoperative work-up. This is simple when managing adnexal masses that are non-suspicious at ultrasound. In this group, the incidence of malignancy is low, and the false negatives are explained by two possibilities:

- a solid tumour is found on the surface of the cystic mass or beside the lesion identified by ultrasound;

Table 24.1. Techniques for intracystic examination.

Preoperative	Abdominal ultrasound
	Vaginal ultrasound
	Computed tomography scan or magnetic resonance imaging
Intraoperative	Laparoscopic inspection without puncture
	Laparoscopic ultrasound
	Ovarioscopy (a second endoscope is required)
	Laparoscopic intracystic inspection (an incision is required)
Postoperative	Macroscopic pathological examination

- very small vegetations (less than 1 mm in diameter) not visible at ultrasound are present inside the cyst and may be identified only at laparoscopy using an endocystic inspection with the magnification provided by the laparoscope.

In contrast, the situation is more difficult when the adnexal mass is suspicious at ultrasound. Indeed, most masses are benign (Table 24.2) and conservative treatment would be possible in most cases, whereas a routine salpingo-oophorectomy is unacceptable. From the results of ultrasound examinations performed preoperatively in our department, we propose the following management of this sometimes difficult clinical situation.

In young patients (< 40 years old) (Figure 24.1), the laparoscopic inspection allows a reliable diagnosis of:

- physiological cysts, which are identified using previously reported macroscopic signs (Table 24.3);
- endometriomas, which are recognised from the ovarian adhesions and the peritoneal implants;
- suspicious paraovarian cysts, whose solid contents may be seen through the cyst wall.

Moreover, teratomas may be diagnosed from the preoperative ultrasonographic examination, computed tomography (CT) scan or MRI.

In the remaining cases, which represent fewer than 10% of patients aged less than 40 years, the management should be adapted to each case. If only one small intracystic papillary formation was found at ultrasound, endocystic examination with frozen section may allow conservative treatment. In contrast, if there were numerous papillary formations, if the tumour was mixed or mainly solid, if numerous vessels with a low resistance index were found or if the tumour is very large, an adnexectomy without puncture is the reasonable treatment.

Puncture is not routine; it should be discussed cautiously as an essential step of the management with potential but unknown prognostic consequences, which cannot justify a routine salpingo-oophorectomy.

In patients aged 40–50 years, laparoscopy remains an important diagnostic tool, given the frequency of physiological and paraovarian cysts and of endome-

Table 24.2. Pathological diagnosis according to age and ultrasonographic appearance. Values are n (%)

| Age (years) | Non-suspicious masses[a] | | | | Suspicious or solid masses[b] | | | |
	< 40	> 40 – < 50	> 50	Total	< 40	> 40 – < 50	> 50	Total
Physiological	94 (22.5)	28 (15.9)	2 (2.0)	124 (17.9)	23 (11.7)	7 (10.8)	3 (4.8)	33 (10.2)
Serous	87 (20.9)	62 (35.2)	70 (70.7)	219 (31.6)	18 (9.2)	6 (9.2)	26 (41.9)	50 (15.5)
Paraovarian	53 (12.7)	17 (9.7)	10 (10.1)	80 (11.6)	3 (1.5)	2 (3.1)	1 (1.6)	6 (1–9)
Mucinous	53 (12.7)	19 (10.8)	9 (9.1)	81 (11.7)	9 (4.6)	5 (7.7)	8 (12.9)	22 (6.8)
Dermoid	20 (4.8)	0 (0.0)	2 (2.0)	22 (3.2)	103 (52.6)	16 (24.6)	9 (14.5)	128 (39.6)
Endometrioma	105 (25.2)	48 (27.3)	5 (5.1)	158 (22.8)	26 (13.3)	25 (38.5)	1 (1.6)	52 (16.1)
Low malignant potential	4 (1.0)	2 (1.1)	1 (1.0)	7 (1.0)	6 (3.1)	1 (1.5)	5 (8.1)	12 (3.7)
Cancer	1 (0.2)	0 (0.0)	0 (0.0)	1 (0.1)	8 (4.1)	3 (4.6)	9 (14.5)	20 (6.2)
Total	417	176	99	692	196	65	62	323

[a] Non-suspicious masses: entirely cystic masses, entirely cystic masses with echogenic fluid, cysts with one or several thin septae.
[b] Suspicious masses at ultrasound: thick septae, vegetations, mixed tumours.

triomas (Table 24.2), but difficult cases are managed by salpingo-oophorectomy.

In postmenopausal patients and patients over 50 years old, where the incidence of malignant tumours is high (22.6%), laparoscopic diagnosis is helpful to inspect the diaphragm and the upper abdomen. All benign masses are treated by bilateral salpingo-oophorectomy. As the incidence of malignancy is high, frozen sections should be available when managing this group of patients.

24.4 Laparoscopic Puncture: The Technique

Care should be taken to minimise spillage when puncturing a cyst. Briefly, the adnexa is grasped and stabilised with an atraumatic forceps placed on the utero-ovarian ligament. The puncture should be performed perpendicularly to the ovarian surface and, as discussed below, it should be located on the

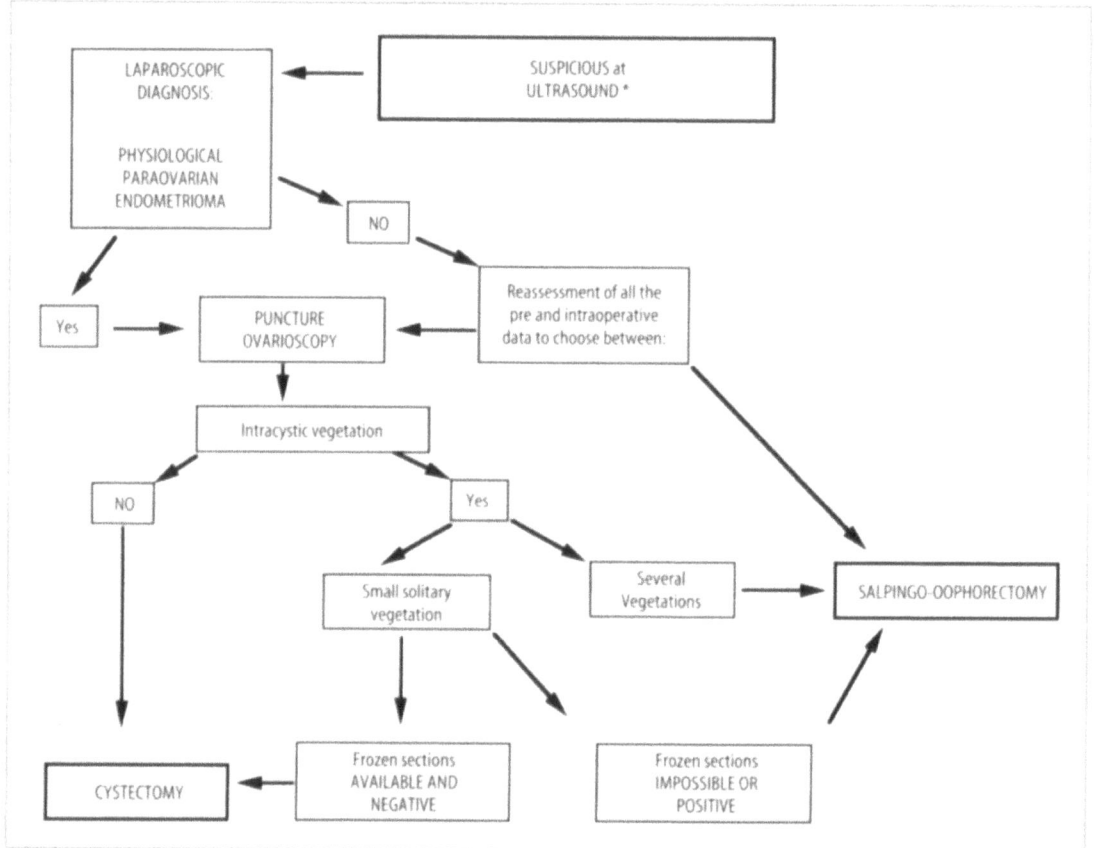

Figure 24.1 Management of patients < 40 years old with adnexal masses.

Table 24.3. Laparoscopic criteria to distinguish benign ovarian neoplasms and physiological cysts

	Benign neoplasm	Functional cyst
Utero-ovarian ligament	Lengthened	Normal
Cyst wall	Thick	Thin
Cyst vessels	Comb-like from the hilum	Scanty, coral-like
Fluid	Clear, chocolate	Saffron yellow
Internal appearance	Smooth	Retinal-like aspect
Cystectomy	Possible	"Impossible"

antimesenteric border of the ovary. Small cysts are aspirated with a needle connected to a 20 or 50 ml syringe. Cysts of more than 5 cm are punctured with a 5 mm conical trocar and emptied with an aspiration lavage device 5 mm in diameter. A 5 mm conical trocar is used to puncture large cysts for the following reasons:

- the penetration of cone-shaped instruments depends on the perforating effect of the instrument and on the elasticity of the cyst wall, so that the puncture is more watertight than when performed with a cutting instrument;
- the 5mm reusable conical trocar can be inserted through a 5.5 mm disposable trocar, so no trocar changes are necessary after the puncture;
- a large and powerful aspirating device is used for aspiration of the cyst contents.

As a puncture performed with currently available instruments cannot be completely watertight; other devices are being developed to decrease the risks associated with a puncture. The first possibility is to introduce a large bag in the abdomen, to put the bag in the pelvis and to place the adnexa in the bag, so that the cyst fluid will be collected in the bag if any leakage occurs. This technique is not particularly effective when managing very large adnexal masses, or in patients with significant pelvic adhesions. Another possibility would be aspiration of the cyst through a watertight membrane stuck on the surface of the ovary. The solution should be simple but the device should be watertight during the puncture and after aspiration to allow a safe endoscystic evaluation of the cyst wall. Any progress in this field would be welcome.

The following arguments may be proposed:

- puncture and endoscopic inspection are the final steps of the surgical diagnosis;
- in our view there is no rationale for avoiding laparoscopic puncture, as the risks of dissemination are minimal when the tumour is removed entirely and immediately;

- laparoscopic cystectomy is much easier and faster after a puncture, than when trying to remove the cyst intact.

Therefore, the classical laparoscopic approach, which includes a puncture, appears to be reasonable and can be used for the management of most cysts, including serous or paraovarian cysts, as well as unilocular or bilocular mucinous cysts.

The cyst fluid is examined macroscopically and sent for cytological examination. The cyst and the pelvic cavity are then washed many times with small volumes of fluid to avoid contamination of the upper abdomen. The cyst is opened with scissors and the internal cyst wall inspected carefully. If signs of malignancy are found, the mass should be diagnosed as suspicious or malignant.

Very large cysts (> 10 cm) are aspirated, inserting the second puncture trocar high enough to allow visual control of the puncture site.

In most cases, endometriomas are fixed to the broad ligament by adhesions located close to the ovarian hilum. As these adhesions generally involve the endometrioma itself, the cyst will often be ruptured while freeing the ovary. The puncture should not be performed before ovariolysis. Indeed, a puncture performed on the posterior surface of the ovary is an unnecessary trauma, as an incision located on the anterior surface is almost always required to treat the cyst. In endometriomas, ovariolysis should be the first step and a puncture is performed only when the cyst has not been ruptured.

In multilocular mucinous cysts with less than 3 mm septae, puncture is often difficult, as several punctures are necessary to empty the mass. When there are more than three different cystic cavities, conservative treatment is rarely possible and probably involves a high risk of early recurrence, as small mucinous cysts may be missed around the main ones. Therefore, in large multilocular cystic masses, salpingo-oophorectomy should be discussed with the patient before surgery.

Laparoscopic puncture and/or rupture of an ovarian teratoma may induce a granulomatous peritonitis. This complication is uncommon (1.1%; two cases out of 178 teratomas punctured in our experience);[9] however, many other unreported cases have occurred. Moreover, from the data collected at incidental and/or routine second-look laparoscopy, we found that adhesion formation is not uncommon after the laparoscopic treatment of ovarian teratoma. In contrast, adhesion formation appeared to be uncommon after the laparoscopic treatment of other types of benign ovarian neoplasm (Table 24.4), suggesting that the cyst contents, rather than the laparoscopic procedure, explained postoperative de novo adhesion formation. Therefore, the spillage of

Table 24.4. Adhesions after laparoscopic cystectomy: 20 patients, 22 treated adnexae, 17 contralateral adnexae. IPC, Intraperitoneal cystectomy; EAC, cystectomy by mini-laparotomy

Group	n	Diameter (mm)	Adhesion score[a]
All	22	70.4 ± 37 (30-180)	2.7 ± 5.9 (0-24)
IPC	15	68.7 ± 42 (30-180)	2.4 ± 6.1 (0-24)
EAC	7	74.3 ± 27 (50-120)	3.3 ± 5.9 (0-16)
Teratomas	13	68.4 ± 33 (30-140)	4.6 ± 7.2 (0-24)
Other pathological diagnoses	9	73.3 ± 45 (30-180)	0.0 ± 0.0
Contralateral adnexae	17		0.0 ± 0.0

[a] This adhesion score at second-look laparoscopy was calculated using the American Fertility Society classification.

teratoma contents should be avoided whenever possible. An accurate preoperative diagnosis is essential to help the surgical management. Although many ovarian teratomas are diagnosed by ultrasonographic examination, it may be worth confirming the diagnosis with a second imaging technique to identify the fatty tissue inside the cyst. Indeed, if fatty tissue is found inside a cyst, the diagnosis of teratoma is probable, malignancy is unlikely and cystectomy without puncture can be performed. Both CT scan and MRI with fat

suppression sequences can be used to identify the fatty tissue. Whether the decrease in complications and adhesions is worth the additional costs will have to be evaluated in prospective clinical trials.

On the other hand, a cystectomy cannot be achieved without rupture in large masses of more than 8 cm, in a pelvic cavity of 10 cm diameter. Therefore teratomas greater than 8cm are emptied with a 10 mm aspiration device. A very large teratoma is not a contraindication for conservative treatment. A laparotomy should be performed if it seems reasonable to preserve the ovary (Figure 24.2).

24.5 Treatment Techniques

24.5.1 Benign Ovarian Neoplasms

After puncture, the pressure in the ovary decreases and the cyst wall and the remaining ovarian stroma, which present different degrees of elasticity, retract differently and open the cleavage plane spontaneously. Careful inspection of the ovarian incision will allow identification of this plane. To achieve a laparoscopic ovarian cystectomy, effective grasping forceps are required. In our group, the

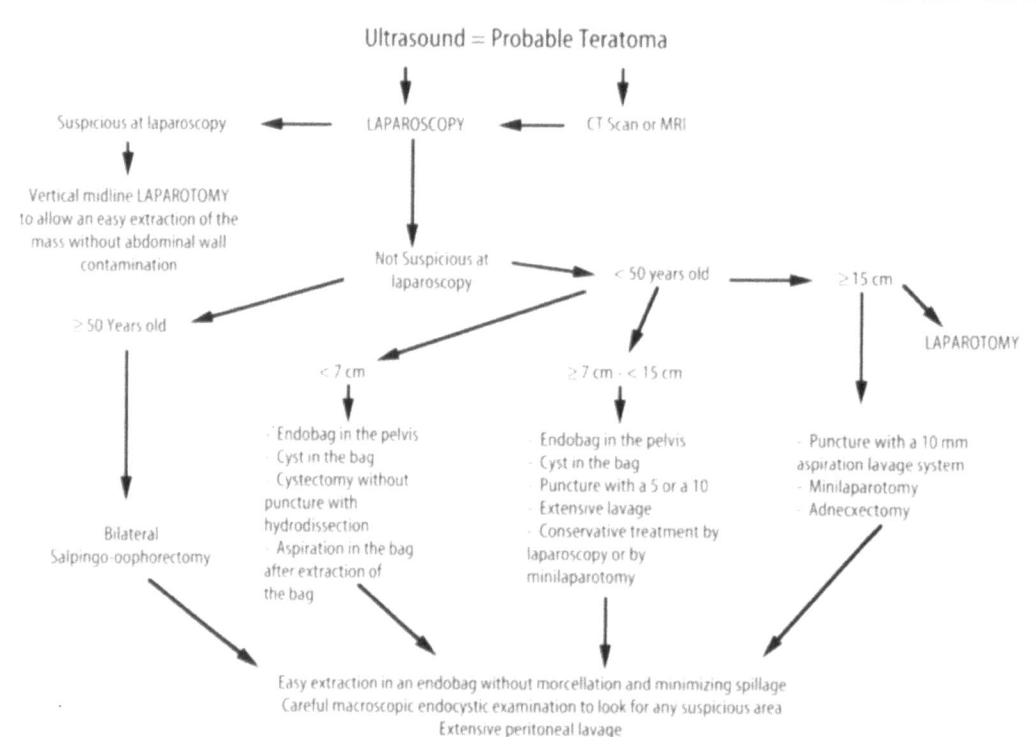

Figure 24.2 Management of patients with teratoma.

number of intraperitoneal laparoscopic ovarian cystectomies performed increased rapidly after the development of the Manhes "grip" forceps. Three effective grasping forceps should be available to treat large cysts. This procedure is simple and is taught to first-year residents as soon as they feel comfortable with the laparoscopic view. However, a strict technique and some rules are required to make it reliable, to ensure that the cyst wall is removed without any tearing.

The procedure should be performed under permanent visual control; therefore, the cleavage plane should always be perfectly exposed, implying that:

- when pulling forceps in opposite directions, one should use short and slow movements and move the forceps on the cyst wall and on the remaining ovarian tissue often enough to obtain a perfect exposure;
- haemostasis should be performed during the dissection, first because bleeding may obscure the cleavage plane and second because the haemostasis is often more difficult at the end of the procedure when the ovarian tissue is retracted.

It is better first to separate the cyst and the ovary on both sides of the ovarian incision. To speed up the procedure, one should avoid allowing the part of the cyst wall, which has just been dissected, to retract. Instead, another forceps should be used and applied on the cyst wall closer to the cleavage plane. When the cyst wall retracts, it is necessary to grasp it two or three times to expose the cleavage plane again.

To avoid ovarian damage, one should follow the "best" cleavage plane. This plane is identified when the outside surface of the cyst wall is white. If there is red tissue on the cyst wall, one is probably removing some healthy ovarian tissue.

24.5.2 Paraovarian Cysts

As the cyst wall is thin and covered only by the peritoneum, the cyst fluid can be seen through the cyst wall and the cyst appears blue. If there are abnormal intracystic areas (vegetations), the cyst wall is thicker and appears white, so that intracystic evaluation can often be achieved without puncture.

When treating these cysts, it is important to open the peritoneum and to identify the cleavage plane before the puncture. For small cysts, if the puncture is performed first, it will be difficult to find the cyst in the retroperitoneal space. Again, the correct cleavage plane is identified only when there is no more red tissue or vessels on the surface of the cyst. If dissection is carried out without choosing the optimal plane, extensive coagulation close to the

ovary is often required, whereas this is rarely needed in optimally dissected paraovarian cysts. Often paraovarian cysts can be removed and treated without puncture. However, large ones should be punctured after identification of the plane.

24.5.3 Endometriomas

Small ovarian endometriomas of less than 3 cm should be treated with a CO_2 laser or with bipolar coagulation. It is generally not possible to identify a cleavage plane in these small cysts.

The treatment of larger endometriomas is controversial. In our department we use a cystectomy technique. In in-vitro fertilisation, we obtained satisfactory pregnancy rates and number of ovocytes in most cases, except in patients who underwent several treatments for ovarian endometriomas. So the impaired ovarian function sometimes reported after ovarian cystectomy may be a consequence of the damage induced by the disease rather than a result of the surgical procedure. In the ovarian cortex biopsied around an endometrioma, Maneschi et al found a fewer follicles and vessels than in the ovarian cortex biopsied around teratoma.[10]

The dissection of an ovarian endometrioma is often difficult and includes several steps. The cleavage plane is difficult to identify along the rupture induced by the adhesiolysis, as if the cyst itself was stuck on the broad ligament. To identify the plane, it is necessary to enlarge the incision. Thereafter, the initial steps of the dissection are easy. When about one-third to one-half of the endometrioma has been dissected, other difficulties are encountered. Red fibrotic tissue is seen on the surface of the cyst, meaning that some ovarian tissue is being removed. If the dissection is continued in this plane, bleeding and possibly damage to the ovarian vessels will occur. To avoid this, one should stay close to the cyst wall. The procedure is guided by the colour of the cyst wall: when it is white, the plane is correct; when it is red, the dissection is too far from the cyst wall. This is achieved by using three instruments: two grasping forceps to expose the plane, and scissors or bipolar coagulation to dissect the cyst. One should be careful at the end of the dissection, as the most difficult part of the cleavage is located close to the ovarian hilum and to the utero-ovarian ligament.

Adhesions are the main problem in the treatment of ovarian endometriomas; we have shown that postoperative adhesion formation is uncommon, but that adhesion reformation occurs in more than 90% of the adnexae (Table 24.5).[11] The number of oocytes was not lower after the laparoscopic treatment of an ovarian endometrioma (Table 24.6).

Table 24.5. Adhesions after laparoscopic treatment of large endometrioma

Group	n	Adnexal adhesion score Laparoscopic treatment	2nd look	p
All cases	53	12.7 ± 10.8	10.4 ± 10	> 0.1
Stage III	15	6.1 ± 5.9	5.8 ± 5.6	> 0.7
Stage IV	38	15.2 ± 11.3	12.1 ± 10.8	> 0.1
Diameter < 6 cm	32	14.9 ± 11.3	11.3 ± 10.9	> 0.07
Diameter > 6 cm	21	9.2 ± 9.3	8.9 ± 8.6	> 0.8
Unilateral	31	12.6 ± 11.4	9.4 ± 9.7	> 0.1
Bilateral	22	12.7 ± 10.2	11.8 ± 10.5	> 0.4
Treated adnexae				
Ovarian adhesion score ≤ 4	19	3 ± 2.4	6.5 ± 7.4	> 0.1
Ovarian adhesion score ≥ 8	34	18.1 ± 9.9	12.5 ± 10.7	< 0.01
Contralateral adnexae				
All cases	21	3.9 ± 8.6	2.6 ± 4.2	> 0.6
Adnexal adhesion score ≤ 4	17	0.5 ± 1.3	1.4 ± 2.7	> 0.08

24.5.4 Teratomas

Two other techniques of laparoscopic ovarian cystectomy may be used for teratomas: "transparietal cystectomy" by mini-laparotomy and cystectomy without puncture.

24.5.4.1 Transparietal Cystectomy

Transparietal cystectomy is a cystectomy performed by mini-laparotomy after a laparoscopic diagnosis. In our group, this technique was used for all cysts before 1985 when the grip forceps was not available. Nowadays it is used only for the treatment of large teratomas. After puncture and drainage of the cyst with a 5 mm and/or a 10 mm aspirating device, a 3 cm low transverse incision is performed. The fascia and the muscles are opened using a classical surgical technique. Then the cyst and the ovary are grasped through the peritoneum, which is incised while pulling the ovary against the abdominal wall, thus facilitating the extraction of the ovary. Thereafter the drainage of the cyst is finished using the 3 cm incision and the ovary is extracted through the abdominal wall. The cystectomy is performed using a classic surgical technique. The ovary is released in the peritoneal cavity without any suture and the abdominal wall is closed.

Table 24.6. Mean number of oocytes obtained during in-vitro fertilisation cycles

Indication	No. of cases	No. of ovocytes
Tubal infertility	253	8.43
Endometriosis		
Without previous endometrioma	83	8.22
After treatment of endometrioma	67	8.49
After treatment of endometrioma by cystectomy	34	7.96

As protection of the abdominal wall is difficult or impossible, this technique should not be used in the treatment of suspicious masses.

24.5.4.2 Cystectomy Without Puncture

The ovary is grasped on the antimesenteric surface with atraumatic forceps. A small superficial incision of the ovarian cortex is performed with scissors. Then an aquadissection is performed through this small incision. The incision should be enlarged carefully. The plane is identified with atraumatic grasping forceps or with scissors. The surface of the cyst is white without any red tissue. Most cases of rupture occur while enlarging the incision, even though the cleavage plane has already been identified. To avoid rupture and/or to minimise its consequences:

- perform the dissection without grasping the cyst and without pushing it;
- always move the instruments away from the cyst;
- be patient and careful, particularly at the end of the procedure;
- put the cyst in a large bag before dissection;
- aspirate the cyst contents immediately and effectively.

In our department this procedure is successful in about 50% of the cases, but it is not used for cysts of more than 7 cm in diameter (Figure 24.2).

24.6 Laparoscopic Adnexectomy

This procedure is simple when the enlarged ovary has stretched the adnexal ligaments, making haemostasis of the adnexal vessels both easy and safe, as the distance between the infundibulopelvic ligament and the ureter is increased.

In contrast, adnexectomy and/or oophorectomy may be very difficult when the ovary is fixed to the broad ligament by dense adhesions. In such cases an excision of the posterior leaf of the broad ligament is required to ensure complete excision of the ovarian tissue and to avoid the risks of recurrences and ovarian remnant syndrome. The ureter should be identified on the pelvic brim and dissected up to the uterine vessels. When the ovary is stuck to the broad ligament, identification of the ureter on the pelvic brim does not imply that the entire ovary may be safely excised without further uereteral dissection. Indeed, complete dissection of the ureter is required. This dissection is particularly important and difficult in patients with endometriosis, as endometriosis frequently invades the retroperitoneal space and the ureter may be involved in the fibrosis induced by the implants.

Haemostasis of the adnexal vessels can be achieved either with bipolar coagulation or with suturing techniques, according to the surgeon's preference. Although much more expensive, the stapling devices present no advantages. In our department, bipolar coagulation is used in more than 95% of the cases. This technique is safe as no postoperative bleeding has been observed over the past 5 years. To make haemostasis of the infundibulopelvic ligament easier, it is important to open the peritoneum between the ovarian vessels and the round ligament and, whenever possible, to open the posterior leaf of the broad ligament. In this way, the ovarian vessels can be stretched much more effectively than when covered by the peritoneum. Moreover, the coagulation is more effective, as it is applied on the ovarian vessels and not on the peritoneum, which would retract, thus decreasing the effects of the electric current on the vessels.

24.7 Extraction of the Cyst Wall and/or the Mass

We have reported one case of abdominal wall endometriosis, which occurred on a trocar site after the laparoscopic treatment of an active endometrioma.[7] As this complication is uncommon, we assumed that this was induced by a part of the cyst wall left in the abdominal wall while extracting it. This complication, which occurred when endobags were not available, showed that the abdominal wall should always be protected when extracting an adnexal mass.

Several techniques can be used. Currently, we use an endobag in most cases. An endobag should be:

- large enough to allow the extraction of masses of 8cm and more; smaller bags should be available to

allow the extraction of small cysts without enlarging the skin incision;

- easy to open in the abdomen; it should remain spontaneously open in the peritoneum;
- long enough to allow easy extraction of the bag in obese patients;
- solid enough to prevent rupture when the surgeon is pulling through the abdominal wall;
- transparent, to allow visual control of punctures performed in the bag.

The bag is extracted either through a 10mm port inserted in an appendectomy scar or through the umbilical trocar. When extracting a cyst without an endobag, the cyst wall may be cut by the trocar sleeve and a part of it may be lost in the abdominal cavity or in the abdominal wall.

Small cysts can also be extracted through a 10 mm trocar, with a 5 mm reducer and a 5 mm forceps.

It is more difficult to extract a mass that has not been punctured. An endobag is required even if the mass is extracted through the vagina.

Large masses should be punctured or drained before extraction. We puncture the mass through the abdominal wall after the extraction of the neck of the bag. Performing a puncture in a bag that is still in the peritoneal cavity increases the risks of spillage. However, when puncturing through the abdominal wall, visual control is required to ensure that the puncture is performed inside the bag and not through it. This is easy in thin patients with a 10 mm incision, whereas a larger incision is required in obese patients. It is sometimes necessary to put a 10mm trocar in the bag to identify the surface of the cyst before the puncture.

One of the port sites or the posterior fornix may be used for extraction of the bag. The colpotomy should be performed by laparoscopy using the Spuller instrument designed by the Lausanne group, which allows the posterior fornix to be opened and the bag grasped without losing the pneumoperitoneum.

When an adnexectomy is associated with a hysterectomy, the adnexectomy is performed first. The mass is placed in a bag, which is closed and placed in a paracolic gutter. Extraction takes place after the hysterectomy.

Whether or not to suture depends on several factors:

- ovarian non-closure is a valuable technique, as shown by several experimental studies. In rabbit models, non-closure of an ovarian surgical incision is less adhesiogenic than a microsurgical closure;[12,13]
- the shape of the ovary needs to be approximated to allow satisfactory healing and to prevent postoperative adhesion. In experimental studies, the ovaries were bivalved so that the shape of the

ovary was spontaneously approximated at the end of the procedure;

- adhesion formation is increased at the surface of the ovary, when compared to the peritoneum;[14]
- ischaemia reduces plasminogen activator concentration and increases adhesion formation, so if sutures are used, they should be placed inside the ovary, not on the ovarian surface.

From these results and our experience, some rules may be proposed to improve laparoscopic cystectomy. As in these experimental models, ovarian puncture and incision should be performed on the antimesenteric surface of the ovary, as far as possible from the fimbria, so that the edges of the incision will be grossly approximated when the ovary falls back in the posterior cul-de-sac. The puncture site should be included in the ovarian incision. The cystectomy should be performed using only one incision, which should be large enough to avoid any additional tear of the ovarian cortex. Meticulous haemostasis should be achieved. Finally, the shape of the ovary may be approximated using a minimal resection of the remaining ovarian tissue or a superficial coagulation of the ovarian stroma to induce an inversion of the ovary, just as coagulation of the serosa is used to obtain eversion of the distal part of the tube. When the incision is adequate, ovarian sutures are not necessary, but when the shape of the ovary is not spontaneously approximated at the end of the procedure, one or two intraovarian sutures should be used to facilitate ovarian healing.

24.8 Conclusions

The following should be kept in mind when deciding on surgical management. The treatment of an ovarian tumour should be complete and immediate.[15] At laparoscopy, one cannot distinguish benign vegetations from malignant ones. When treating macroscopically suspicious adnexal masses by laparoscopy, the consequence is that some ovarian cancers and tumours of low malignant potential are treated laparoscopically.[16]

Frozen sections should not be used to decide the treatment of the ovary or to choose between laparoscopy and laparotomy. The most difficult part of the diagnosis is taking a biopsy for frozen section. Most false negatives of frozen sections are explained by inadequate biopsies.[17,18] The only exception to this rule is a young patient with a small and solitary vegetation. In this situation, a biopsy is reliable, as there is only one suspicious area and the incidence of malignancy is low, below 10%.[19]

In contrast, frozen sections are required to decide staging procedures and the treatment of the contralateral adnexa. Whenever possible, this treatment should be performed during the same anaesthesia, as 20% of the patients may refuse a restaging.

Morcellation of an ovarian tumour is always unacceptable.[16] Most adnexal masses suspicious at ultrasound are benign, even in postmenopausal patients (Table 24.2). A reliable surgical diagnosis is required to decide the treatment of adnexal masses suspicious at ultrasound and to avoid laparotomies using a transverse incision for ovarian cancer.

Most recent experimental studies concerning surgery and tumour growth suggest that tumour growth is greater after laparotomy but that tumour dissemination is worse after laparoscopy.[20–26] There are no long-term follow-up data after the laparoscopic treatment of ovarian cancer.

We propose a simple scheme for management:

- adnexal masses suspicious at ultrasound should be surgically diagnosed by laparoscopy;
- adnexal masses suspicious at surgery should be treated by laparotomy;
- at laparotomy, suspicious masses should be treated by adnexectomy and then managed according to the results of frozen sections. As already discussed, young patients with a solitary vegetation are the only exception to this rule;
- high-risk patients such as postmenopausal patients with adnexal masses suspicious at ultrasound should be managed in oncology departments.

The clinical consequences of these simple rules are summarised in Tables 24.7 and 24.8. The theoretical incidences of laparotomy and of salpingo-oophorectomy were calculated using data obtained in our department. The same methods may be used to evaluate the consequences of this management in each department.

Table 24.7. Calculated incidence of laparotomy: based on data from patients treated in our department between 1992 and 1994

Data used to calculate the theoretical incidence of laparotomy	Total
Total no. of patients	516
Cancer and borderline tumours	28
Benign masses suspicious at surgery	59
Including masses > 6 cm	22
Including masses > 6 cm and/or with external vegetations	36
Benign masses non-suspicious at surgery	429
Laparotomies for technical difficulties	9
Results: No. and rate of laparotomy[a] if indicated for:	
All benign masses suspicious at surgery	97 (18.8%)
Benign masses suspicious at surgery > 6 cm	60 (11.6%)
Benign masses suspicious at surgery > 6 cm and/or with external vegetations	55 (14.3%)

[a] This result includes all the malignant tumours (cancer, borderline) and all the laparotomies for technical reasons.

Table 24.8. Calculated incidence of adnexectomy among benign masses in patients < 40 years old: based on data from patients treated in our department between 1992 and 1994

Data used to calculate the theoretical incidence of adnexectomy	Total
Total no. of patients	248
Benign masses suspicious at surgery	24
Laparotomy in non-suspicious masses	3
Salpingo-oophorectomy for technical problem in non-suspicious masses	10
Results: No. and rate of adnexectomy[a] if indicated for:	
All benign masses suspicious at surgery	37 (14.9%)
Incidence in the department between 1992 and 1994 in the same group of patients	24 (9.6%)

[a] This result includes all the malignant tumours (cancer, borderline) and all the laparotomies for technical reasons.

It can be seen from Table 24.9 that whatever the pathological diagnosis and the diameter, most patients can be treated conservatively. A diameter > 10 cm should not be an indication for oophorectomy. Conservative surgery has always been the main objective of the pioneers of laparoscopic ovarian surgery.

References

1. Bruhat MA, Mage G, Pouly JL et al (1992) Operative laparoscopy. McGraw Hill Inc, Health Professions Division, New York
2. Hsiu JG, Given FT, Kemp GM (1986) Tumor implantation after diagnostic laparoscopic biopsy of serous ovarian tumors of low malignant potential. Obstet Gynecol 68S:90S-93S
3. Hopkins MP, Kumar NB, Morley GW (1987) An assessment of the pathologic features and treatment modalities in ovarian tumors of low malignant potential. Obstet Gynecol 70:923-929
4. Dembo AJ, Davy M, Stenwig AE et al (1990) Prognostic factors in patients with stage I epithelial ovarian cancer. Obstet Gynecol 75:263-273
5. Sevelda P, Vavra N, Schemper M et al (1990) Prognostic factors for survival in stage I epithelial ovarian carcinoma. Cancer 65:2349-2352
6. Williams TJ, Symmonds RE, Litwak O (1973) Management of unilateral and encapsulated ovarian cancer in young women. Gynecol Oncol 1:143-148
7. Canis M, Mage G, Pouly JL et al (1994) Laparoscopic diagnosis of adnexal cystic masses: a 12 year experience with long term follow up. Obstet Gynecol 83:707-712
8. Possover M, Mader M, Zielinski J et al (1995) Is laparotomy for staging early ovarian cancer an absolute necessity? J Am Assoc Gynecol Laparosc 2:285-287
9. Canis M, Candiani M, Giambelli F et al (1997) Laparoscopic management of ovarian teratoma. Int J Gynecol Obstet 2:47-53
10. Maneschi F, Marasa L, Incandela S et al (1993) Ovarian cortex surrounding benign neoplasm: a histologic study. Am J Obstet Gynecol 169:388-393
11. Canis M, Mage G, Wattiez A et al (1992) Second-look laparoscopy after laparoscopic cystectomy of large ovarian endometriomas. Fertil Steril 3:617-619
12. Wiskind AK, Toledo AA, Dudley AG et al (1990) Adhesion formation after ovarian wound repair in New Zealand white rabbits: a comparison of microsurgical closure with ovarian non closure. Am J Obstet Gynecol 163:1674-1678
13. Brumsted JR, Deaton J, Lavigne E et al (1990) Postoperative adhesion formation after wedge resection with and without ovarian reconstruction in the rabbit. Fertil Steril 53:723-726
14. Pittaway DE, Maxson WL, Daniell JF (1983) A comparison of the CO_2 laser and electrocautery on postoperative intraperitoneal adhesion formation in rabbits. Fertil Steril 40:366-368
15. Maiman M, Seltzer V, Boyce J (1991) Laparoscopic excision of ovarian neoplasms subsequently found to be malignant. Obstet Gynecol 77:563-565
16. Canis M, Pouly JL, Wattiez A et al (1997) Laparoscopic management of adnexal masses suspicious at ultrasound. Obstet Gynecol 89:679-683
17. Obiakor I, Maiman M, Mittal K et al (1991) The accuracy of frozen sections in the diagnosis of ovarian neoplasms. Gynecol Oncol 43:61-63
18. Twaalfhoven FCM, Peters AAW, Trimos JB et al (1990) The accuracy of frozen section diagnosis of ovarian tumors. Gynecol Oncol 41:189-192
19. Granberg S, Wikland M, Jansson I (1989) Macroscopic characterisation of ovarian tumors and the relation to the histological diagnosis: criteria to be used for ultrasound evaluation. Gynecol Oncol 35:139-144
20. Volz J, Köster S, Schaeff B (1997) Laparoscopic management of gynaecological malignancies, time to hesitate. Gynaecol Endosc 6:145-146
21. Mathew G, Watson DI, Rofe AM et al (1996) Wound metastases following laparoscopic and open surgery for abdominal cancer in a rat model. Br J Surg 83:1087-1090
22. Bouvy ND, Marquet RL, Jeekel H et al (1996) Impact of gas (less) laparoscopy and laparotomy on peritoneal tumor growth and abdominal wall metastases. Ann Surg 224:694-701
23. Bouvy ND, Marquet RL, Jeekel J et al (1997) Laparoscopic surgery is associated with less tumor growth stimulation than conventional surgery: an experimental study. Br J Surg 84:358-361
24. Jacobi CA, Ordermann J, Böhm B et al (1997) The influence of laparotomy and laparoscopy on tumor growth in a rat model. Surg Endosc 11:618-621
25. Mathew G, Watson DI, Rofe AM et al (1997) Adverse impact of pneumoperitoneum on intraperitoneal implantation and growth of tumor cell suspension in an experimental model. Aust NZ J Surg 67:289-292
26. Canis M, Botchorishvili R, Wattiez A et al (1998) Tumor growth and dissemination after laparotomy and CO_2 pneumoperitoneum: a rat ovarian cancer model. Obstet Gynecol 92:104-108

Table 24.9. Treatment of benign masses in patients < 40 years old. Values are n (%)

Diameter (mm)	Laparotomy	Laparoscopy	Conservative	Radical
< 70	6 (1.4)	409 (98.6)	386 (94.4)	23 (5.6)
≥ 70- < 120	9 (5.9)	142 (94.1)	121 (85.2)	21 (14.8)
≥ 120	6 (18.1)	27 (81.9)	20 (74.1)	7 (25.9)
All	21 (3.5)	578 (96.5)	528 (91.4)	50 (8.6)

Chapter 25

Second-look Laparoscopy in Patients with Ovarian Cancer

Jan Decloedt and Ignace Vergote

25.1 Introduction

The former widely accepted management for patients with epithelial ovarian cancer consisted of three basic components: (1) initial surgery with complete, thorough staging and debulking of advanced disease; (2) combination platinum-based chemotherapy; and (3) surgical reassessment to determine response to initial therapy.[1] The role of primary debulking surgery in some subgroups of patients with advanced ovarian carcinoma has been questioned in recent years.[2-5] Second-look surgery for ovarian carcinoma has been abandoned in most centres, because of the lack of a good second-line therapy that might increase overall survival. Intraperitoneal radioactive phosphorus as consolidating therapy in patients with negative second-look laparotomy was associated with a considerable number of bowel complications, without improving the overall survival.[6]

The second-look laparotomy or surgical second look (SSL) was initially proposed by Wangensteen[7,8] in the setting of gastrointestinal cancers; it was later introduced as a diagnostic tool in ovarian cancer. It is generally accepted that no therapeutic advantages are gained from SSL. Several reports compared computed tomography (CT) scans and SSL findings in terms of diagnostic performance. In a review by Reuter,[9] the false-negative rate in these studies varied between 8 and 64% for CT. The diagnostic value of CT scans is probably higher as patients with palpable disease or high CA 125 serum levels were often excluded from these studies. Many anatomical sites of interest, such as the mesentery, omentum, surface of intestinal loops and parietal peritoneum, possess structural features that are not amenable to exhaustive CT scan examination, especially for just-visible or microscopic deposits. Despite this inaccuracy, the specificity of CT scans was found to be reasonably good, ranging from 88 to 99%.[9]

25.2 Surgical Second Look Versus Second-look Laparoscopy

Second-look laparoscopy following primary surgery and first-line chemotherapy is nowadays a commonly performed investigation, despite the lack of accurate comparisons of SSL and laparoscopic findings. Though most series only report on a small number of second-look laparoscopies, the main limitations are (1) false-negative laparoscopy findings probably ranging from 29.1 to 55%[10-15] and (2) inadequate visualisation in up to 12% of the patients.[16]

A very interesting series was published by the Italian Northeastern Oncology Cooperative Group and the Ovarian Cancer Cooperative Group.[17] They published a series of 102 patients with ovarian cancer who had complete remission (assessed by clinical findings, markers, and visualisation by CT scan and laparosocpy), after initial debulking and first-line chemotherapy (cisplatinum and cyclophosphamide or doxorubicin and cyclophosphamide). Forty-eight patients were randomly assigned to receive follow-up evaluation only, while 54 patients were assigned to receive second surgery (eight patients refused). Of the 46 surgical patients, 35 had negative and 11 positive surgical findings (24% clinically false-negative). Despite the microscopic residua found at open surgery, and the fact that the patients were then treated with second-line chemotherapy (fluorouracil and cisplatinum), SSL did not increase the probability of survival in this setting. They concluded that: (1) second-line treatment is rarely effective; (2) SSL accurately defines complete responders to first-line chemotherapy; (3) SSL per se does not prolong survival; and (4) if confirmed, a less invasive procedure could replace SSL as a valuable method in new first-line regimens in ovarian cancer patients with clinical complete remission confirmed by laparoscopy.

The second-look laparotomy and laparoscopy techniques in patients with epithelial ovarian cancer were compared by Abu-Rustum,[18] who conducted a retrospective review of 109 patients with stage Ib–IV invasive epithelial ovarian cancer who underwent a second-look operation. Thirty-one patients (28.4%) underwent laparoscopy, 70 patients (64.2%) underwent laparotomy and eight patients (7.3%) underwent both procedures during the same operation. The majority of patients (60.6%) presented with stage IIIc disease. Persistent ovarian cancer was found in 65 of the 109 patients (59.6%), being 54.8% of the patients evaluated by laparoscopy, 61.4% of the patients evaluated by laparotomy and 62.5% of the patients who had both techniques. The mean blood loss, operating time and hospital stay were significantly lower in the laparoscopy group. All intraoperative and immediate postoperative complications were noted in patients who underwent laparotomy. Eight of the 39 patients who were initially evaluated by laparoscopy were converted to laparotomy. The indication for conversion to laparotomy in all patients was the inability to identify gross peritoneal disease at laparoscopy. In these patients, cytological washings were obtained. Of these eight patients, four were positive after laparotomy, all of whom had positive washings taken at the time of laparoscopy. Three patients remained negative after conversion to laparotomy and only one patient had a positive biopsy from a tumour nodule in the posterior right diaphragm that was not seen during laparoscopy but was palpated and biopsied at laparotomy. This patient also had negative washings and was the only patient in whom disease would have been missed if laparotomy was not performed.

25.3 Interval Debulking

By performing a laparoscopy to evaluate operability before primary debulking surgery in patients with advanced ovarian carcinoma, one will be able to select patients in whom complete cytoreductive surgery will be unsuccessful, and will thus avoid unnecessary laparotomies. Interval debulking is therefore regarded as a valuable way of treating this subgroup. The concept of interval debulking in patients with advanced ovarian carcinoma has been studied in a prospective, randomised trial.[19] Four hundred and twenty-five patients (stage IIb–IV) were included in the study and entered in one of the two treatment arms. First, patients who had an initial suboptimal debulking attempt were treated with six cycles of cisplatin and cyclophosphamide chemotherapy. The second group of patients received three cycles of the same chemotherapy and

were then reoperated with the intent to bring all remaining residual disease to < 1 cm in diameter (interval debulking), followed by another three cycles of cyclophosphamide–cisplatinum chemotherapy. Patients in both arms were then encouraged to have second-look laparoscopy and full surgical-pathological staging was performed. Patients who were randomised to the interval debulking arm were discovered to have already been chemically cytoreduced (< 1 cm) at the time of interval debulking surgery in 36% of the cases. Interval cytoreductive surgery was successful in 27% but failed in 37% of the patients. Interestingly, considering all patients who underwent interval cytoreductive surgery, 55% had a pathological complete response at the time of second-look surgery, as compared with only 40% in the group receiving standard chemotherapy. Patients who were unsuccessfully debulked at the time of their interval debulking surgery had a similar survival to patients who had no interval debulking surgery. A multivariate analysis performed on these patients showed that interval debulking surgery was an independent, prognostically significant factor, even after controlling for other risk factors, and was associated with an approximately 33% reduction in the risk of death.

Second-look laparoscopy is a valuable technique to select patients for interval debulking who are not good candidates for primary optimal cytoreduction (no macroscopic residual disease after surgery). In a series of open diagnostic laparoscopies to assess the operability of 58 patients with advanced ovarian cancer, we observed that operability could be successfully predicted in the majority (91%) of patients with ovarian carcinoma.[20] Thirty patients received three or four cycles of platinum-based chemotherapy as the laparoscopy suggested it was impossible to achieve an optimal cytoreduction. In 24 of these patients, an interval cytoreductive operation was performed. Six patients had progressive disease after treatment with first-line chemotherapy and received second-line cytotoxic drugs. By using an open laparoscopy prior to debulking surgery, unnecessary laparotomies could be avoided in 26 out of 83 patients with a suspicious ovarian mass.

25.4 Complications of Second-look Laparoscopy

The complications of second-look laparotomy are well known and include wound infection (12%), urinary tract infections (13%), pulmonary complications (5%), bowel injury (4%) and prolonged ileus (13%).[21] Second-look laparoscopy has been associated with a high complication rate, mainly bowel injury, in 2–9% of the patients.[15,16]

In our experience this complication rate can be decreased by using the open laparoscopy technique. In a series of 89 gynaecological oncology patients at risk for closed laparoscopy, we performed 90 open laparoscopies and observed only one complication (1%).[22] Fifty-three laparoscopies were performed in patients with ovarian cancer, 20 of whom had a laparoscopy evaluation before debulking surgery. Thirty-three patients had second-look laparoscopies for recurrent disease or were reassessed for interval debulking surgery. We had no complications due to the laparoscopy technique in any of the procedures for ovarian cancer.

25.5 Conclusions

Open second-look laparoscopy by a well-trained gynaecological-oncological laparoscopist can be a feasible alternative to second-look laparotomy. Its role in evaluating the response to primary chemotherapy and in selecting candidates for interval cytoreductive surgery needs to be examined.

References

1. Rubin SC (1993) Second-look laparotomy in ovarian cancer. In: Markman M, Hoskins WJ (eds) Cancer of the ovary, 1st edn. Raven Press, New York, pp 175-185
2. Hunter RW, Alexander ND, Souffer WP (1992) Meta-analysis of surgery in advanced ovarian carcinoma: is a maximum cytoreductive surgery an independent determinant of prognosis? Am J Obstet Gynecol 166:504-511
3. Potter ME, Partridge EE, Hatch KD et al (1991) Primary surgical therapy of ovarian cancer: how much and when? Gynecol Oncol 40:195-200
4. Hoskins WJ, Buncy BN, Thigpen JT et al (1992) The influence of cytoreductive surgery on recurrence-free interval and survival in small volume Stage III epithelial ovarian cancer: a Gynecologic Oncology Group Study. Gynecol Oncol 47:159-166
5. Vergote IB, De Wever I (1997) Primäre Zytoreduktive Operation bei Ovarialkarzinom im gortgeschittenen Stadium. Ist sie bei alien Patientinnen erforderlich? Gynäkologe 30:102-107
6. Vergote I, Winderen M, De Vos L et al (1993) Intraperitoneal radioactive phosphorus therapy in epithelial ovarian cancer. Analysis of benefits and complications in 313 patients treated primarily or at second-look laparotomy. Cancer 71 (7):2250-2260
7. Wangensteen OH (1949) Cancer of the colon and rectum. Wes Med J 48:591-597
8. Wangensteen OH, Lewis FJ, Tovgen LA (1951) The "second-look" in cancer surgery. Lancet 71:303-307
9. Reuter KL, Griffin T, Richard E (1989) Comparison of abdominal computed tomography results and findings at second-look laparotomy in ovarian carcinoma. Cancer 63:1123-1128
10. Lele S, Piver MS (1986) Interval laparoscopy prior to second-look laparotomy in ovarian cancer. Obstet Gynecol 68:345-349
11. Rosenoff SH, De Vita VT, Hubbard S (1975) Peritoneoscopy in the staging and follow-up of ovarian cancer. Semin Oncol 2:223-228
12. Smith WG, Day TG, Smith JP (1977) The use of laparoscopy to determine the results of chemotherapy for ovarian cancer. J Reprod Med 18:257-260
13. Mangioni C, Bolis G, Molteni P (1979) Indications, advantages and limits of laparoscopy in ovarian cancer. Gynecol Oncol 7:47-55
14. Piver MS, Shashikant BL, Barlow JJ (1980) Second-look laparoscopy prior to proposed second-look laparotomy. Obstet Gynecol 55:571-573
15. Berek JS, Griffith CT, Leventhal JM (1981) Laparoscopy for second-look evaluation in ovarian cancer. Obstet Gynecol 58:192-198
16. Quinn MA, Bishop GJ, Campbell JJ et al (1980) Laparoscopic follow-up of patients with ovarian cancer. Br J Obstet Gynecol 87:1132-1139
17. Nicoletto MO, Tumolo S, Talami R et al (1997) Surgical second-look in ovarian cancer: a randomized study in patients with laparoscopic complete remission – a Northeastern Oncology Cooperative Group–Ovarian Cancer Cooperative Group study. J Clin Oncol 15:994-999
18. Abu-Rustum NR, Barakat RR, Siegel PL et al (1996) Second-look operation for epithelial ovarian cancer: laparoscopy or laparotomy? Obstet Gynecol 88:549-553
19. Fiorentino M, Brigato G, Cima G et al (1993) Randomized study of redebulking in epithelial ovarian cancer (abstract). Proc Am Soc Clin Oncol 12:267
20. Van Dam P, Decloedt J, Tjalma W et al (1997) Diagnostic laparoscopy to assess operability of advanced ovarian cancer: a feasibility study. In: De Oliveira CF, Oliveira HM (eds) Proceedings of the 10th International Meeting of Gynecologic Oncology. Monduzzi Editore, Bologna, pp 259-266
21. Janisch H, Schieder K, Koelbl H (1989) Diagnostic versus therapeutic second-look surgery in patients with ovarian cancer. Baillieres Clin Obstet Gynecol 3:191-200
22. Decloedt J, Berteloot P, Vergote I (1997) The feasibility of open laparoscopy in gynecologic-oncologic patients. Gynecol Oncol 66:138-140

Part VI

Endometriosis

Contents

Summary

Ultrasonography can be used to predict the likelihood of a patient having endometriosis. The characteristic features of endometriomas are described and the positive predictive value of an ultrasound diagnosis of an endometrioma is very high. Other indirect "soft" markers of possible endometriosis include site-specific tenderness at the time of a scan and an assessment of ovarian mobility. The value of ultrasonography for the woman with pelvic pain is to provide reassurance. A normal scan has a high negative predictive value for the presence of significant pelvic disease. For those women with pathology, an ultrasound scan can also be used to estimate the degree of surgical difficulty. Bilateral masses, lack of ovarian mobility, "kissing" ovaries and the presence of a nodule all indicate that referral to a specialist centre may be appropriate.

The pathophysiology of endometriomas is complex but is thought to relate to invagination of the ovarian cortex. This hypothesis is discussed in detail. The surgical approach for an endometrioma may be conservative, but there is debate regarding the optimal approach. Some advocate eversion of the cyst and coagulation of the cyst wall, while others favour excision of the cyst wall in its entirety. Whether it is better to treat patients with gonadotrophin-releasing hormone analogues either before or after surgery is not certain. For extraovarian advanced endometriosis, the optimal management is controversial. Surgery for deep endometriosis is a challenge and there may be significant complications. The surgical approach for these cases is discussed and the pitfalls illustrated.

Key Points

- A normal scan has a high negative predictive value for the presence of significant pelvic pathology
- Endometriomas can be reliably characterised by ultrasonography
- "Soft" markers can help predict which women have endometriosis
- Ultrasound can be used to help predict surgical difficulty
- Endometriomas > 5.0 cm may require a two-stage laparoscopic procedure
- Surgery for deep endometriosis may be hazardous and requires considerable experience
- Full bowel preparation must be given to women suspected of having a deep endometriotic nodule

Chapter 26

Ultrasound Characteristics of Endometriosis

Dirk Timmerman, Jan Deprest, Emeka Okaro and Tom Bourne

26.1 Introduction

Endometriosis is a benign disease characterised by the presence of viable ectopic endometrium outside the uterine cavity. It is commonly found in women of reproductive age. In 1927, Sampson hypothesised that endometriosis develops from retrograde menstruation.[1] However, retrograde menstruation is common among all menstruating women and during the past decades both a genetic predisposition and immunological dysfunction have been found to be associated with the development of endometriotic lesions.[2-5] The actual prevalence of endometriosis in women of reproductive age is difficult to ascertain because the diagnosis requires laparoscopy and the indications used for surgery will influence the proportion of patients diagnosed with endometriosis. Furthermore, the prevalence of endometriosis seems to be geographically different. One possible explanation might be exposure to irradiation, polychlorinated biphenyls or dioxin.[6,7]

The possible role of ultrasound for the diagnosis of endometriosis has been neglected for years, but recent studies have provided more insight into the value of ultrasound to select patients with chronic pain who might benefit from endoscopic treatment. It is clear that superficial endometriosis can be visualised only at the time of surgery. However, ultrasonography can be used to both detect and follow up cystic ovarian endometriosis. The ultrasound-based diagnosis of deep lesions such as rectovaginal or vesicouterine endometriosis is possible, but requires a higher level of operator experience.

26.2 Symptoms

Endometriosis can be asymptomatic in some women but often causes severe pain. It is particularly associated with dysmenorrhoea and deep dyspareunia. There is also an association with subfertility. The pain of endometriosis is most often cyclical, and bowel and bladder symptoms may occur.

26.3 Endometriosis in Infertile Patients

Some authors have found no significant differences in cumulative pregnancy rates between patients with minimal endometriosis (rAFS-1) and patients with unexplained subfertility.[8] On the other hand, one of the largest randomised controlled trials on endometriosis concluded that surgical treatment of minimal and mild endometriosis may cause a modest improvement in fertility, whereas medical treatment had no positive effect.[9]

26.4 Ultrasound Diagnosis

26.4.1 Endometrioma

At ultrasonography, an ovarian endometrioma is a unilocular or multilocular cyst with homogeneous, low-level internal echoes, often described as "ground glass" (Figure 26.1). It is usually surrounded by a thick wall. The wall may contain hyperechoic foci and sometimes the internal wall is irregular and covered with "sludge". If the lesion is bilateral, both ovaries may be adherent in the midline, a feature usually referred to as "kissing ovaries" (Figure 26.2). Kupfer et al. evaluated the spectrum of ultrasound findings in 37 surgically proven endometriomas and demonstrated that transvaginal ultrasound, in contrast with transabdominal ultrasound, is very specific for the

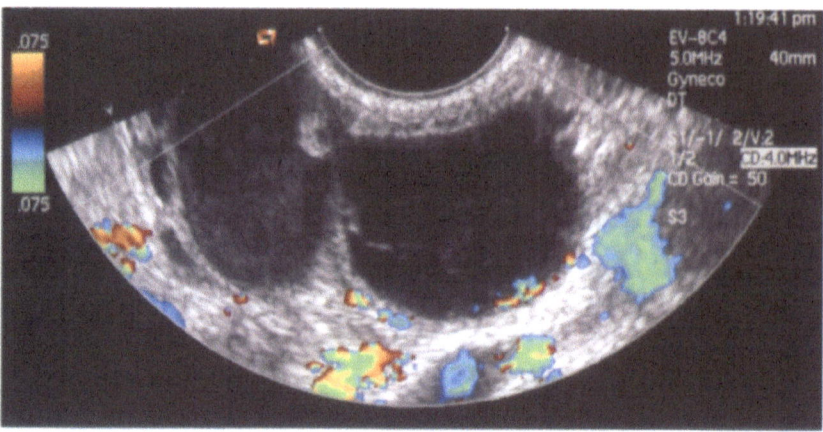

Figure 26.1. Ovarian endometrioma (*left*) with "ground glass" appearance and haemorrhagic cyst (*right*).

preoperative characterisation of an ovarian endometrioma.[10] Subsequently, several studies have confirmed the high specificity of transvaginal ultrasonography for the diagnosis of ovarian endometriomas (Table 26.1). The false-positive test results included cystic teratomas and haemorrhagic cysts, whereas the false negatives included cystic teratomas, haemorrhagic cysts, abscesses and cystadenomas. Persistence of the cyst at the time of a repeat ultrasound scan and measurement of serum CA 125 levels may be helpful in differentiating between endometriomas and physiological cysts (see section 26.5). Common ovarian cysts in young women can usually be characterised accurately. Jermy et al. have shown that the positive predictive value of transvaginal ultrasound for the diagnosis of endometriomas and dermoid cysts is 96.7% and 97.1% respectively, with a false-positive rate of 3.8% and 3.0% respectively.[16]

Whether colour Doppler adds to the diagnostic picture is uncertain. Aleem et al. found no significant differences between Doppler flow indices for endometriomas and other benign cystic lesions.

However, they concluded that scattered vascularity is typical of ovarian endometriomas, and that this finding may help to differentiate them from other lesions of dense vascular distribution, such as corpora lutea or ovarian neoplasms.[17] Guerriero and colleagues also suggested that colour Doppler imaging may be useful to describe the vessel pattern of a lesion and so to distinguish between endometriomas (with "poor" vascularisation) and non-endometriomas exhibiting "rich" vascularisation or the presence of arterial flow in papillary structures or echogenic parts of the cyst.[14] If papillary structures protruding from the internal cyst wall are visualised, ovarian malignancy needs to be excluded.[18] Endometroid adenocarcinoma may develop within ovarian endometriomas (Figure 26.3).

26.4.2 Deep Endometriotic Nodules

Koninckx and Martin consider the endometriotic nodule in the rectovaginal space to be a deep form

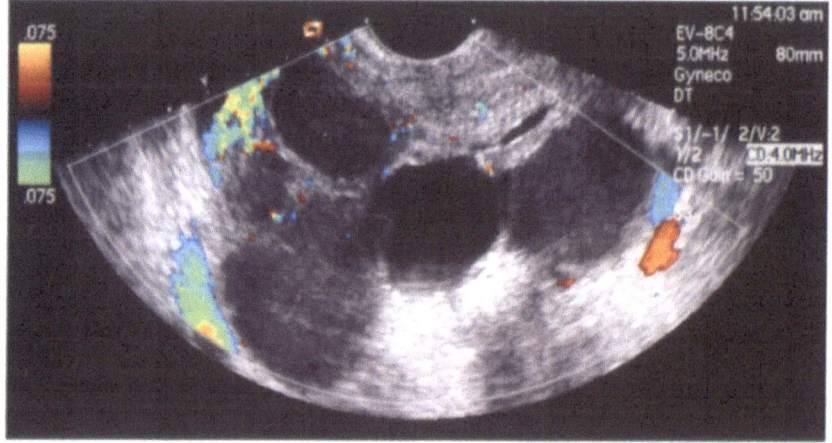

Figure 26.2. Bilateral presence of endometriomas (four locules in right ovary) and centrally located hydrosalpinx.

Table 26.1. The efficiency of transvaginal ultrasound in the diagnosis of ovarian endometrioma

Author	N	Criteria	Sensitivity	Specificity
Mais et al 1993[11]	21	Round-shaped homogeneous hypoechoic "tissue" of low-level echoes within the ovary	84%	90%
Volpi et al 1995[12]	57	Cystic structure with low homogeneous echogenicity and thick regular cyst wall	82%	98%
Dogan et al 1996[13]	107	Typical (group A) or atypical (group B) lesions with irregular margins or septations	86.5%	99%
Guerriero et al 1998[14]	58	B-mode ultrasound alone	81%	96%
		With use of colour Doppler energy	90%	97%
Patel et al 1999[15]	40	B-mode ultrasound alone, Reviewer 1	60%	98%
		B-mode ultrasound alone, Reviewer 2	45%	100%
Jermy et al 2001[16]	80	B-mode ultrasound alone		96%

of infiltrating endometriosis,[19] whereas Donnez and colleagues suggest that this nodule corresponds to an adenomyotic nodule originating from Müllerian remnants by metaplasia.[20] Few ultrasound studies have focused on these nodules. In our experience, deep endometriotic nodules in the rectovaginal space can be visualised as solid lesions with low to moderate vascularity ranging from 0.5 to 4 cm (Figure 26.4), which are often also palpable at vaginal or rectovaginal examination. During menstruation, local pressure with the vaginal probe on the nodule can be very painful. Cancer is usually not painful by pressure with the vaginal probe and often exhibits stronger vascularity (Figure 26.5). On the other hand, vesicouterine endometriotic nodules are not easily palpable at vaginal examination. Vesicouterine endometriotic nodules are usually associated with bladder symptoms such as urinary frequency. Using transvaginal ultrasonography, a solid nodule adherent to the posterior bladder wall may be visualised if the bladder is slightly filled (Figure 26.6). Pressure with the vaginal probe can also elicit local pain.

26.5 Combined Studies using Doppler Ultrasound and CA 125 Values

It is well established that serum CA 125 values are increased in patients with endometriosis, and so it makes sense to take into account the serum CA 125 results in a similar way to that previously described by Jacobs et al. when they proposed a risk of malignancy index to distinguish between malignant and benign adnexal masses.[21] Kurjak and Kupesic[22] improved both the sensitivity and specificity for the diagnosis of an endometrioma by developing a scoring system combining transvaginal ultrasound findings with colour Doppler and serum CA 125 levels. Using their morphological score alone, 16 false-positive test results and 14 false-negative test results were obtained, whereas by using the total score incorporating CA 125 and Doppler data, only two false-positive results and one false-negative result were reported. Using this approach, a sensitivity of 99% and a specificity of 99.6% were obtained. However, these combined data show only a marginal improvement on the data of Jermy et al.[16] based

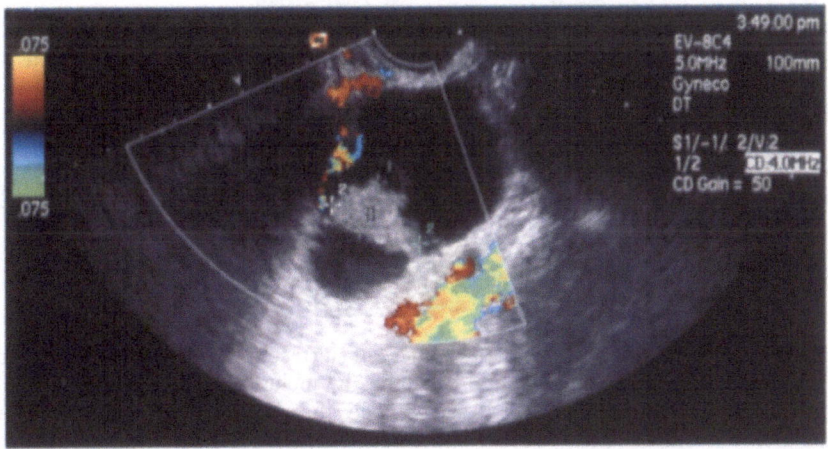

Figure 26.3. Endometroid adenocarcinoma developed in an ovarian endometrioma. Note the centrally located solid structure.

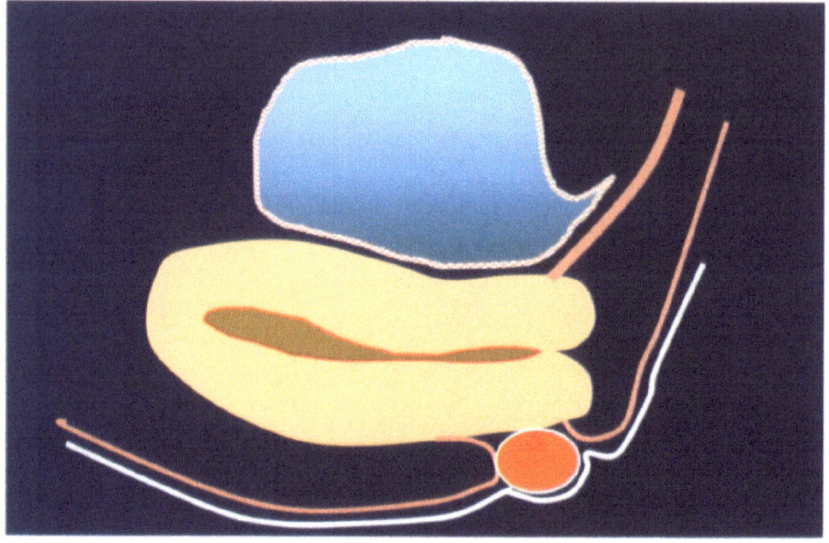

a

Figure 26.4. a Schematic drawing of deep endometriotic nodule in the rectovaginal space.

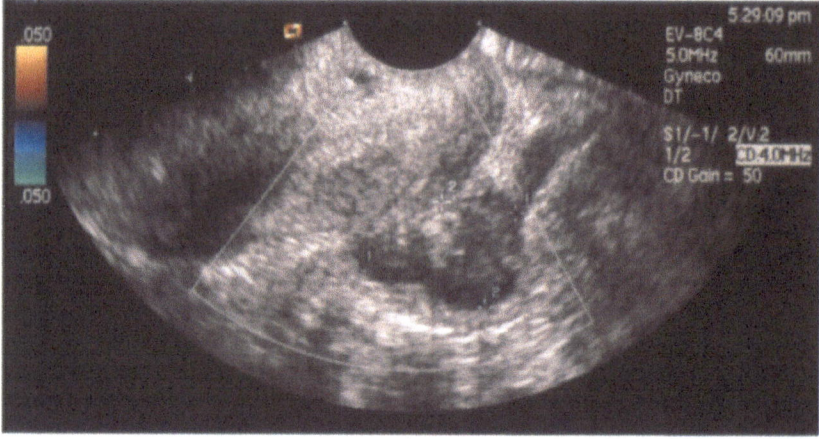

b

Figure 26.4. b Deep endometriotic nodule in the rectovaginal space.

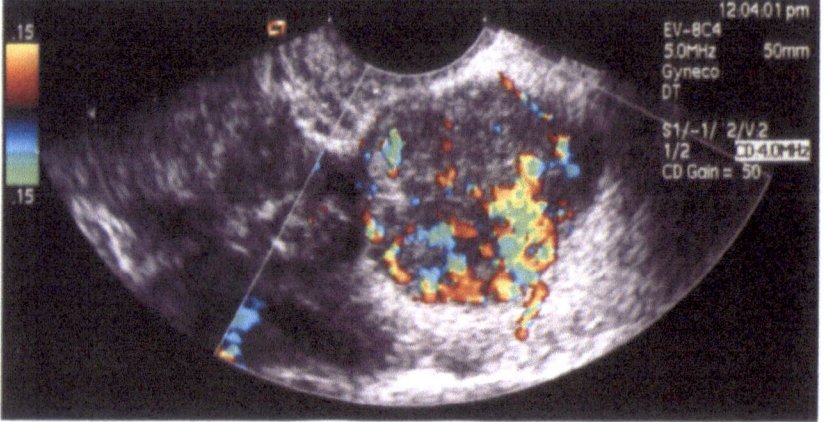

Figure 26.5. Poorly differentiated ovarian adenocarcinoma with metastasis in the rectal wall (*right*) with strong vascularisation.

purely on subjective impression of the morphological appearances of the cysts. Other workers have been unable to replicate the data of Kurjak and Kupesic[22] in relation to the use of colour Doppler.[23] Alcazar et al. found no improvement in the performance of ultrasound for the diagnosis of endometriomas by including colour Doppler.[23]

It seems likely that complicated scoring systems are not useful for the characterisation of these lesions and that most ultrasonographers rely on

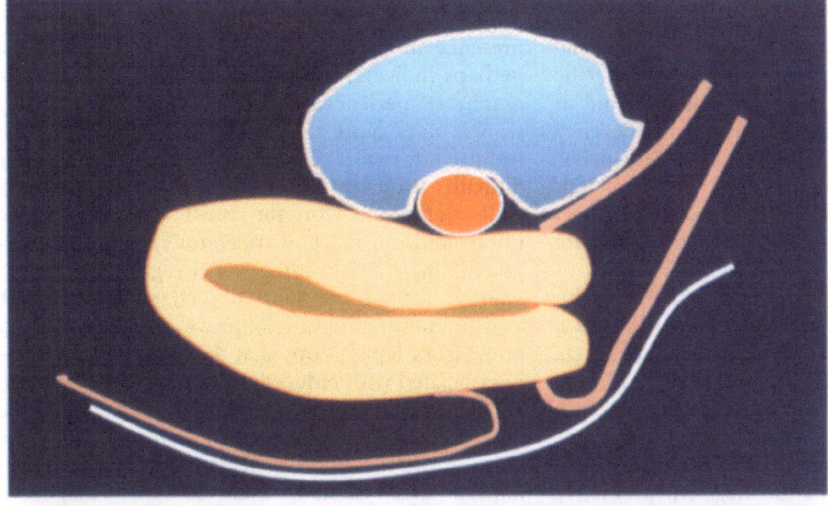

Figure 26.6. a Schematic drawing of a vesicouterine endometriotic nodule.

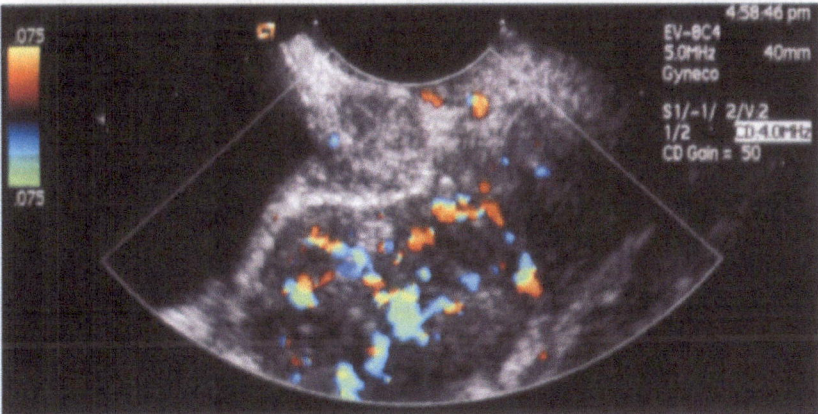

Figure 26.6. b Vesicouterine endometriotic nodules.

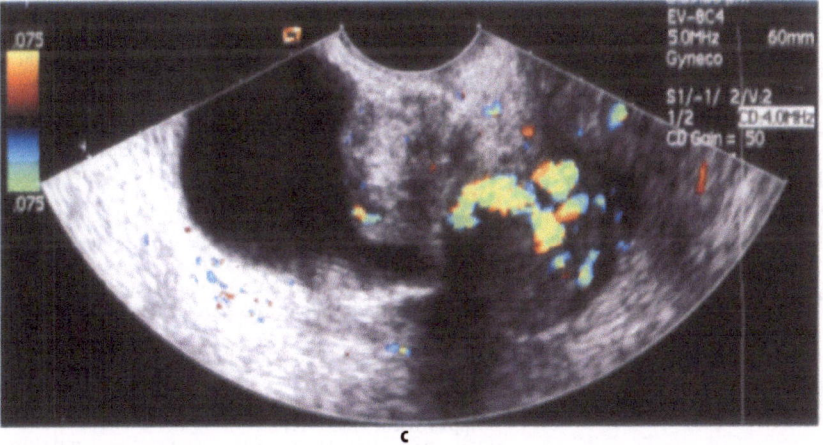

Figure 26.6. c Vesicouterine endometriotic nodules.

their subjective assessment to classify adnexal tumours. Depending on the ultrasonographer's experience, subjective assessment can accurately distinguish between malignant and benign adnexal masses[24] and between endometriomas, cystic teratomas and other common adnexal masses in young women.[16]

Recently, Bourne and colleagues have proposed a different approach to the ultrasound assessment of women with pelvic pain. Conventionally, a scan is performed in these women in order to exclude or detect lesions such as endometriomas or tubal pathology. They have called such lesions "hard markers" for the presence of pelvic pathology.

However, this does not take into account the subtle information that is available to the person performing a scan. This information may include site-specific tenderness, the presence or absence of free fluid in the pelvis, and the degree of ovarian mobility. They have called these findings "soft markers" of pelvic pathology.[25] The inclusion of "soft markers" significantly improved the ability of ultrasound to detect endometriosis or adhesions. Their preliminary data suggest that if "soft" as well as "hard" markers of pelvic pathology are used, 83% of patients with chronic pelvic pain and a normal scan will have a normal pelvis at laparoscopy. Using this approach, in 78% of patients with an abnormal scan, the findings were confirmed at laparoscopy (Table 26.2). If no "hard" or "soft" markers of pathology are found, it is highly unlikely that significant pelvic pathology will be present; the negative predictive value of this new approach to ultrasound seems very high. In such cases it would seem reasonable to avoid laparoscopy and either reassure the patient that significant pathology is unlikely or give a trial of the combined oral contraceptive pill.

26.6 Conclusions

Conventional B-mode ultrasonography can be used confidently to confirm the presence or absence of ovarian cystic endometriosis. Colour Doppler seems to add little to overall diagnostic confidence. However, detecting endometriosis outside the ovaries is a greater challenge. In order to make any progress in this area, it is necessary to use ultrasonography in a different way. Greater emphasis needs to be placed on the more subtle information available at the time of the scan. The images available on the ultrasound screen should be seen in the context of the overall clinical picture and not seen as just "a scan". A fairly reliable prediction of the presence and the severity of endometriosis can be made by taking into account presenting symptoms, clinical examination, ultrasound images and the assessment of the mobility of pelvic organs, as well as the severity and location of any pain induced by pressure with the vaginal probe.

Table 26.2. The efficiency of transvaginal ultrasound for the diagnosis of endometriosis and pelvic adhesions (from Okaro et al,[25] with permission)

	Hard markers alone	Hard and soft markers combined
Sensitivity	24%	85%
Specificity	100%	75%
Negative predictive value	55%	83%
Positive predictive value	100%	78%

The introduction of "soft" markers to indicate the presence of pelvic pathology shows promise, and perhaps indicates the future direction of ultrasonography. Experienced operators often know that a scan is not "quite right"; however, expressing this feeling in a report or in reproducible terms is often difficult. Difficulty arises when obtaining reproducible definitions for the most commonly used ultrasound terms. One operator's solid papillary projection is another's irregular capsule. Standardising more subjective characteristics such as ovarian mobility will not prove easy. However, we know from laparoscopy that the presence of disease is associated with reduced ovarian or tubal mobility, an increase in free or loculated fluid in the pelvis and adhesions. Vaginal examination will often elicit pain. Combining these factors with imaging is logical and should add to the diagnostic performance of ultrasound for the assessment of pelvic pathology. We see ultrasound as a tool to select women who need more invasive management. The negative predictive value of a normal ultrasound scan is high, and may enable the clinician to offer reassurance or a trial of medical therapy. Most patients with positive scan findings will have pathology that would merit laparoscopic intervention.

References

1. Sampson JA (1927) Peritoneal endometriosis due to the menstrual dissemination of endometrial tissue into the peritoneal cavity. Am J Obstet Gynecol 14:422–469
2. Malinak LR, Buttram VC Jr, Elias S et al. (1980) Heritage aspects of endometriosis. II. Clinical characteristics of familial endometriosis. Am J Obstet Gynecol 137:332–337
3. Dmowski WP, Steele RW, Baker GF et al. (1981) Deficient cellular immunity in endometriosis. Am J Obstet Gynecol 141:377–383
4. Oosterlynck D, Cornillie FJ, Waer M et al. (1991) Women with endometriosis show a defect in natural killer cell activity resulting in a decreased cytotoxicity to autologous endometrium. Fertil Steril 56:45–51
5. Vercellini P, Sacerdote P, Panerai AE et al. (1992) Mononuclear cell b-endorphin concentration in women with and without endometriosis. Obstet Gynecol 79:743–746
6. Wood DH, Yochmowitz MG, Salmon YL et al. (1983) Proton irradiation and endometriosis. Aviat Space Environ Med 54:718–724
7. Rier SE, Martin DC, Bowman RE et al. (1993) Endometriosis in rhesus monkeys (macaca mulatta) following chronic exposure to 2,3,7,8-Tetrachlorodibenzo-p-dioxin. Fundam Appl Toxicol 21:433–441
8. Van Rozendaal M, Dunselman GAJ, Evers JLH (1994) Selecting the proper control group in trials of rAFS-1 endometriosis associated subfertility. Hum Reprod 9:161–162
9. Marcoux S, Maheux R, Berube S, the Canadian Collaborative Group on Endometriosis (1997) Laparoscopic surgery in infertile women with minimal or mild endometriosis. N Engl J Med 337:217–222
10. Kupfer MC, Schwimer SR, Lebovic J (1992) Transvaginal sonographic appearance of endometriomata: spectrum of findings. J Ultrasound Med 11:129–133

11. Mais V, Guerriero S, Ajossa S et al. (1993) The efficiency of transvaginal ultrasonography in the diagnosis of endometrioma. Fertil Steril 60:776-780
12. Volpi E, De Grandis T, Zuccaro G et al. (1995) Role of transvaginal sonography in the detection of endometriomata. J Clin Ultrasound 23:163-167
13. Dogan MM, Ugur M, Soysal SK et al. (1996) Transvaginal sonographic diagnosis of ovarian endometrioma. Int J Gyn Obstet 52:145-149
14. Guerriero S, Ajossa S, Mais V et al. (1998) The diagnosis of endometriomas using colour Doppler energy imaging. Hum Reprod 13:1691-1695
15. Patel MD, Feldstein VA, Chen DC et al. (1999) Endometriomas: diagnostic performance of US. Radiology 210:739-745
16. Jermy K, Luise C, Bourne T (2001) The characterization of common ovarian cysts in premenopausal women. Ultrasound Obstet Gynecol 17:140-144
17. Aleem F, Pennisi J, Zeitoun K et al. (1995) The role of color Doppler in diagnosis of endometriomas. Ultrasound Obstet Gynecol 5:51-54
18. Timmerman D, Bourne TH, Tailor A et al. (1999) A comparison of methods for the pre-operative discrimination between benign and malignant adnexal masses: the development of a new logistic regression model. Am J Obstet Gynecol 181:57-65
19. Koninckx PR, Martin D (1992) Deep endometriosis: a consequence of in?ltration or retraction or possible adenomyosis externa? Fertil Steril 58:924-928
20. Donnez J, Nisolle M, Casanas-Roux F et al. (1995) Rectovaginal septum, endometriosis or adenomyosis: laparoscopic management in a series of 231 patients. Hum Reprod 2:630-635
21. Jacobs I, Oram D, Fairbanks J et al. (1990) A risk of malignancy index incorporating CA 125, ultrasound and menopausal status for the accurate preoperative diagnosis of ovarian cancer. Br J Obstet Gynaecol 97:922-929
22. Kurjak A, Kupesic S (1994) Scoring system for prediction of ovarian endometriosis based on transvaginal color and pulsed Doppler sonography. Fertil Steril 62:81-88
23. Alcazar JL, Laparte C, Jurado M et al. (1997) The role of transvaginal ultrasonography combined with color velocity imaging and pulsed Doppler in the diagnosis of endometrioma. Fertil Steril 67:487-491
24. Timmerman D, Schwärzler P, Collins WP et al. (1999) Subjective assessment of adnexal masses using ultrasonography: an analysis of interobserver variability and experience. Ultrasound Obstet Gynecol 13:11-16
25. Okaro E, Condous G, Khalid A et al. (2002) The role of transvaginal ultrasound in the prediction of pelvic pathology in women with chronic pelvic pain. Eur J Ultrasound 15(1): S11.

Chapter 27

The Ovarian Endometrioma: Pathophysiology, Diagnosis and Surgery

Ivo Brosens, Rudi Campo and Stephan Gordts

27.1 Introduction

The ovarian endometrioma represents a severe stage of endometriosis, which, by affecting women in their early reproductive life, can be a major threat to their fertility. It is frequently asymptomatic, but is also a cause of acute and chronic pelvic pain. When initially present on one side, it is likely to affect the other side later. The first surgical procedure is therefore critical for the preservation of the reproductive and endocrine functions of the ovary. In this chapter, we will discuss the pathophysiology, the diagnosis and the techniques of conservative reconstructive surgery.

27.2 Pathophysiology

The ovarian endometrioma is not a simple haemorrhagic cyst of the ovary, but has typical features that make it macroscopically different from other ovarian cysts:

- adhesions;
- spillage during surgery;
- combination with luteal cysts.

The typical endometrioma is adherent on its anterior side to the fossa ovarica, the posterior side of the uterus or the uterosacral ligaments (Table 27.1). Even in the absence of adherence, free-floating adhesions are seen on the ovarian surface and fossa ovarica when

inspected under hydrofloatation (Table 27.2).

It is well known that surgery almost invariably results in so-called "rupture" of the cyst and spillage of the chocolate content. The spillage usually occurs at the site of dense adhesions in the fossa ovarica.

Large endometriomas are frequently associated with luteal cysts, some of which are communicating with the endometrioma (Table 27.3).

The microscopy of the cyst also reveals typical features. The endometrial-like lining is usually without glandular structures and represents a surface epithelium covering a highly vascularised stroma of variable thickness. The lining can extend over the entire wall, but can also occur patchily. In the absence of fibrosis, the endometrial-like lining is loosely attached to the ovarian cortex. In older endometriomas there is extensive fibrotic thickening of the wall with haemosiderin pigmentation.

27.3 Pathogenesis

Sampson[1] discovered endometrial cysts of the ovary by observing that the haemorrhagic cysts of the ovary with some endometrial-like lining showed evidence of typical endometrial shedding when these patients underwent surgery at the time of menstruation. He also described the site of perforation and suggested that chronic spillage was the cause of peritoneal endometriosis. However, in 1927, when he proposed the theory of menstrual regurgitation as the cause of

Table 27.1. Ovarian endometrioma and adhesions

	Size (cm)	n	Adhesions
Sampson[1]	2–10	23	100%*
Nezhat et al[9]	1–2	15	53%
	> 2	144	86%

* 93% with endometrial implants in adhesions.

Table 27.2. Presence of endometriotic adhesions[7]

	No. of ovaries with endometriotic adhesions	
	Present	Absent
Standard laparoscopy	4	17
Transvaginal hydrolaparoscopy	12*	9

* p < .05.

196

Table 27.3. Excision of presumed ovarian endometriomas

	No.	Luteal cyst
Martin and Berry[33]	41	27%
Nezhat et al[8]	216	33%[a]

[a] 8% communicating luteal and endometrial.

endometriosis,[2] he suggested that "endometrial tissue developing on the surface of the ovary caused adhesions which fused the ovary to the uterus and an endometrial cavity developed".

The hypothesis of invagination was later confirmed by serial sectioning of ovaries with the endometrioma in situ (Figure 27.1)[3] and by endoscopic in situ inspection with selective biopsies (Figure 27.2, Table 27.4).[4] In fact, the typical ovarian endometrioma is an ovarian pseudocyst formed by invagination of the ovarian cortex. There is no evidence that the endometrial-like tissue is invading the ovary "like insects eating into an apple". The endometriotic pathology develops on the outside of the ovary. However, follicular activity occurs in the invaginated cortex and, as shown by Sampson[1] on in-situ specimens, the endometrial-like tissue can colonise the surface of a communicating corpus luteum.

The invagination theory is consistent with the specific macroscopic, ovarioscopic and microscopic features of the endometrioma. It is also supported by epidemiological observations: peritoneal endometriosis in reproductive women occurring well before the appearance of ovarian endometrioma;[5] the preferential occurrence of ovarian endometrioma on the left side;[6] and the presence of endometriotic ovarian adhesions in the majority of patients with minimal or mild endometriosis.[7]

Other theories on the pathogenesis of ovarian endometrioma include metaplasia[8] and colonisation of ovulatory follicles.[9] Both mechanisms may occur, but the present evidence is that these are rare.

27.4 Diagnosis

The typical features of the endometrioma make the endoscopic diagnosis very reliable, with a sensitivity, specificity and accuracy of 97, 95 and 96% respectively.[10]

The visual features of a typical endometrioma include:

- size not more than 12 cm in diameter;
- adhesions to the pelvic side wall and/or the posterior broad ligament;
- "powder burns" and minute red spots with adjacent puckering on the surface of the ovary;
- tarry, thick, chocolate-coloured content; however, this is not specific for the endometrioma, as it may be found in lutein cysts and even cystadenomas.

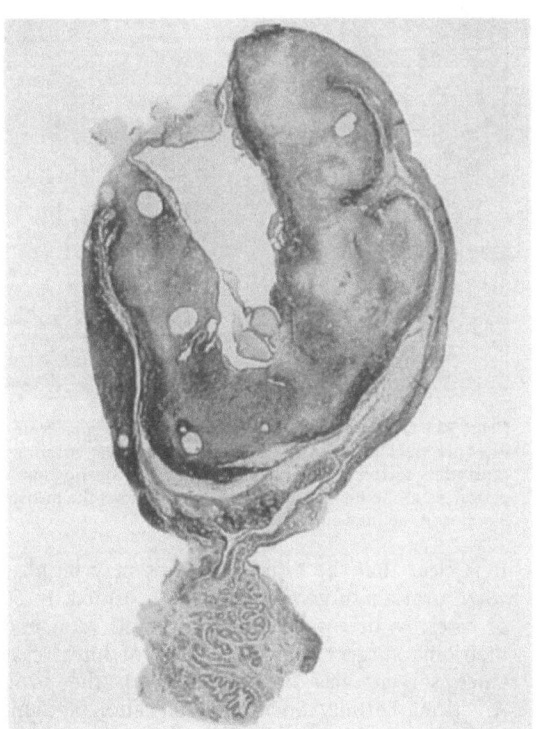

a

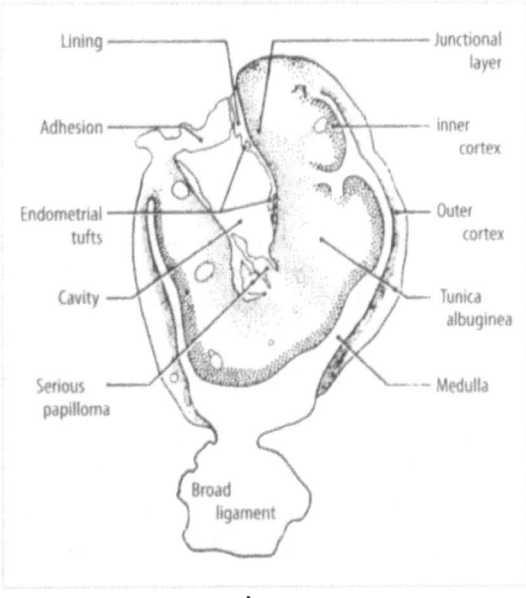

b

Figure 27.1 a Examination of serial sections of the ovary with the endometrial cyst in situ demonstrated that the structure of the vast majority of endometriomas is formed by invagination of the cortex. The specimen shows the adhesion above and the cavity below, surrounded by thickened invaginated cortex. **b** Schematic diagram of **a** showing the various layers and other landmarks. Note the irregular structures like endometrial tufts and the serous papilloma. Reprinted from: Hughesdon (1957) J Obstet Gynaecol Br Empire 64:481–487.[3]

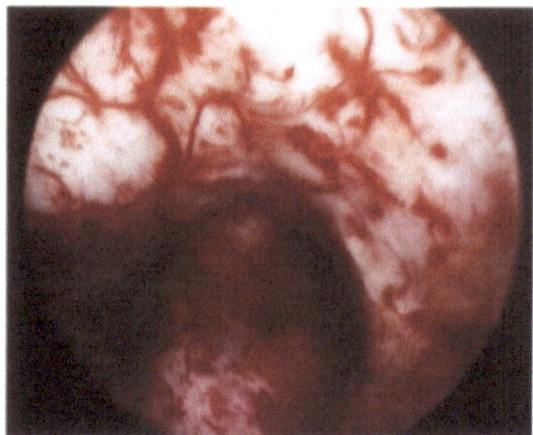

Figure 27.2 Ovarioscopy showing the site of inversion. Note the extensive vascularisation of the endometrial lining covering the pearl-white surface of the inverted cortex. The ovarioscopy was performed at the time of menstruation and shows the menstrual bleeding in the implants.

It is clear that the typical features may be absent when ovarian surgery has been performed. In 50% of cases, recurrent haemorrhagic cysts after endometrioma surgery represent lutein or luteal cysts.[4] Once surgery has been performed, the revised American Fertility Society classification system is no longer applicable, as adhesions can result from the surgical procedure as well as from the disease process.

Ovarian cystoscopy allows optimal visualisation of the wall under hydrofloatation by avoiding collapse of the microvascularisation and filmy structures. It reveals the typical features:

- retraction of the wall and formation of crypts or pockets at the site of invagination;
- old coagulum and fibrosis at the site of retraction;
- complete or partial lining of the wall by a highly vascularised mucosa, which in the non-fibrotic or red endometrioma can be easily dislodged by flushing;
- the colour of the wall varies from the pearl-white, typically cortical colour to yellow and brown-black pigmentation, according to the degree of fibrosis and haemosiderin sedimentation.

Ovarioscopy allows the accurate selection of the site of biopsy by the preservation of neoangiogenesis.

Table 27.4. Selective biopsies of ovarian endometrioma[4]

Site of biopsy	n	Histopathology:		
		Endometrial	Cortical	Fibrous
Random	44	21 (48%)	9 (21%)	14 (32%)
Ovarioscopy-guided red implants	17	14 (83%)	2 (11%)	1 (6%)
Other areas	7	2 (27%)	3 (46%)	2 (27%)

Malignancy does occur occasionally and malignant and atypical changes should be excluded by biopsy.[11] Ultrasound tends to overdiagnose suspected malignant disease, while aspiration cytology may miss malignant cells. It is therefore important that representative biopsies are obtained under direct vision from vascularised or suspected sites.

27.5 Conservative Surgical Techniques

Conservative surgery of ovarian endometrioma has been performed by several techniques. As most endometriomas are characterised by the inversion of the cortex, we will describe the laparoscopic eversion or marsupialisation technique first and then the excision technique. The eversion technique has also been applied successfully using transvaginal hydro-laparoscopy and will be described separately.

27.5.1 Laparoscopic Eversion Technique

The vast majority of endometriomas in young women show the histopathological features of inversion of the ovarian cortex and little fibrosis of the cortical lining. Under these conditions, the technique of eversion or extraovarian surgery can be performed, with selective destruction of the endometriotic tissue and preservation of the ovarian cortex.[12] The first two steps of this technique are fundamentally different from the fenestration technique. However, the coagulation technique is similar to that used for superficial ovarian endometriosis, where there is no invagination.

The eversion technique comprises four steps: first, complete adhesiolysis of the ovary; second, wide opening of the site of inversion for inspection and obtaining representative biopsies; third, superficial coagulation of the endometriotic implants; and finally, coagulation or excision of adenomyotic lesions in adherent tissue.

The adhesiolysis is performed following the plane of cleavage along the ovarian surface to avoid entering the adherent peritoneum. The endometrioma can be densely adherent to the pelvic side wall at the site of inversion, sometimes requiring sharp dissection at this stage. The dissection should be carried out with great care because the ureter is very close and may be adherent. During the adhesiolysis, the endometrioma almost invariably ruptures and the thick haemosiderin-loaden content escapes (Figure 27.3). It is vital to have an efficient suction-irrigator system to remove the chocolate fluid and to irrigate with warm Hartmann solution until the effluent runs clear.

After full mobilisation, the ovary is lifted and the site of inversion is identified by the retraction and pigmentation. The pseudocyst is opened wide by resecting the fibrotic ring. Typically, opening the endometrioma does not cause the walls to collapse, as they represent cortex and remain rigid. Representative biopsies are obtained to exclude malignancy or borderline malignancy.

The vascularised endometriotic implants are destroyed by superficial bipolar coagulation in a similar way as on the outside cortex. The coagulation can be very superficial as the endometrial-like mucosa is thin and the cortex is distended, with the oocytes located within 1 or 2 mm under the surface. Disappearance of the neoangiogenesis is a criterion of adequate coagulation.

Finally, it is important to search for and identify the adenomyotic lesions in the adherent pelvic structures. These lesions may require excision if they are nodular.

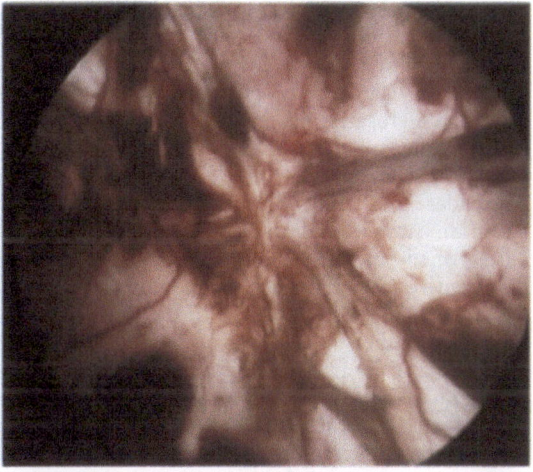

a

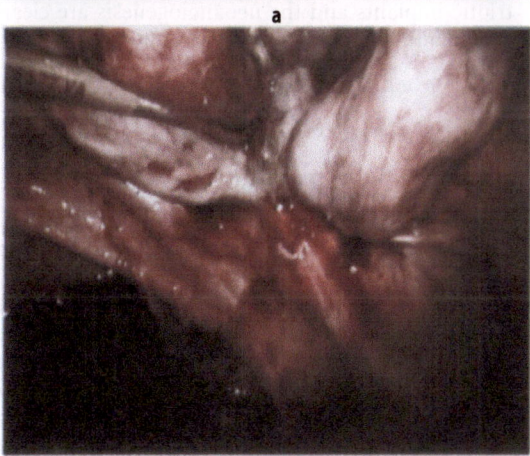

b

Figure 27.3 a Ovarioscopy showing the retraction of the inverted cortex at the site of inversion. **b** The pseudocyst ruptures during ovariolysis at the site of inversion.

27.5.2 The Large Multilocular Endometrioma

The typical endometrioma is not larger than 12cm. However, very large endometriomas are preferably treated by a two-phase procedure for two reasons. First, these large cysts are frequently multilocular and may contain communicating and non-communicating luteal cysts. At the time of surgery it is not possible to distinguish between a luteal and an endometriotic cyst. Second, coagulation of the endometriotic lining in the large and particularly multilocular cyst is difficult, if not impossible.

In the two-phase procedure, the first phase includes the two steps of the eversion technique, with the third step of coagulation remaining unfinished. A 2- to 3-month interval allows for the involution of the cystic structures. During the second-look laparoscopy, the coagulation of vascularised implants is completed and remaining adhesions are removed.

The use of ovarian suppressive therapy during the interval may have the advantage of avoiding the presence of a corpus luteum at the time of surgery and, at least theoretically, of reducing the peritoneal inflammation and the risk of postoperative adhesion formation. However, the primary prevention of postoperative adhesions is achieved by avoiding any unnecessary surgical trauma to normal ovarian cortex or functional structures and by applying strictly microsurgical techniques.

The eversion technique is proposed as the primary approach for conservative reconstructive surgery in young women. The technique is not applicable for old, fibrotic and recurrent endometriomas, where excision is the rule.

27.5.3 Excision Technique

Endometriomas that are adherent to the pelvic wall first need to be teased away by careful ovariolysis in the same way as in the eversion technique.

The endometrioma is entered where it is opposing the fossa ovarica at the site of spontaneous rupture or where the wall shows the inversion stigma or appears thinner. Aspiration and flushing of the tarry, chocolate content is performed as described previously.

The fibrotic capsule is resected and any bleeding is coagulated. It seems illogical to induce ischaemia with surgical knots and therefore the ovarian defect is left open. It is also recommendable to leave 1 litre of warm Hartmann's solution in the peritoneal cavity, to help prevent the initial phase of fibrinous adhesion formation, which occurs in the first 24 hours following surgery.[13]

27.5.4 Eversion Technique by Transvaginal Hydrolaparoscopy

Transvaginal hydrolaparoscopy is a new endoscopic technique, which differs from standard laparoscopy, but also from culdoscopy.[14,15] The technique allows direct exposure and access to the fossa ovarica where the endometrioma is adherent to other pelvic structures. Moreover, the procedure is performed with hydrofloatation of the tubo-ovarian structures, which allows atraumatic manipulation without instruments and bloodless surgery by identification and coagulation of the microvascularisation before cutting.

27.5.4.1 Transvaginal Access and Instrumentation

The transvaginal hydrolaparoscopy is performed as a simple needle puncture technique of the pouch of Douglas, with the patient in a dorsal lithotomy position and using warm saline as distension medium. The specially developed Veress needle is inserted 1.5 cm under the cervix at the midline. A rigid mini-endoscope is used with a 30 optical angle, which is attached to a video-camera system. Once access to the pouch of Douglas is obtained, the Veress needle and the dilating obturator are removed and replaced by the operative endoscope.

Although the view is not panoramic as in transabdominal laparoscopy, the transvaginal approach offers direct access to the ovary and the fossa ovarica, and superior visualisation of the tubo-ovarian structures. The use of an aqueous distension medium keeps the organs afloat, preserves the microvascularisation, allows atraumatic manipulation and provides a remarkable delineation between the tubo-ovarian surface and the adhesions. The technique therefore facilitates the application of atraumatic reconstructive surgery.

The operative channel allows the insertion of 5 Fr scissors and forceps and a thin bipolar coagulating probe (Bicap, Circon ACMI) or a bipolar coagulating and cutting needle (Storz, Tüttlingen, Germany). Before starting the procedure, about 100ml warm saline is instilled in the pouch of Douglas to obtain the necessary distension.

27.5.4.2 Technique

The transvaginal approach includes the same steps as the laparoscopic approach for eversion, but a decision to perform a two-phase procedure is made when the endometrioma is larger than 5cm. Complete coagulation of the endometriotic implants is difficult in cysts larger than 5 cm, but can easily be performed in smaller cysts or after involution of a large cyst.

During the first step, the cyst is dissected and fully mobilised and the site of inversion is identified. The cyst is opened at this site and rinsed.

The site of retraction or inversion is coagulated and opened wide. In a typical endometrioma of less than 5cm, the size and the absence of collapse of the walls allow full inspection of the lining of the wall. Representative biopsies are taken from sites that are suspected or where neoangiogenesis is prominent. The visible vascularised endometriotic implants are coagulated.

27.5.4.3 Advantages of the Technique

In contrast to the transabdominal technique, the transvaginal route offers excellent visualisation of the tubo-ovarian structures, with direct access to the antero-lateral side of the ovaries and the fossa ovarica without instrumental manipulation. The endometrioma is most frequently adherent to the posterior leaf of the broad ligament, the posterior side of the uterus and the uterosacral ligament. All these structures are directly accessible by the transvaginal route.

The use of warm saline as distension medium provides a remarkable delineation between the ovarian surface and the adhesions. As surgery is performed in an aqueous distension medium, preventive haemostasis is mandatory to maintain good visibility. In contrast with the transabdominal access, whether by laparoscopy or laparotomy, the exposure at the transvaginal approach allows for an accurate dissection and in most cases rupture of the endometriotic cyst can be avoided. On close inspection underwater, the vascularised endometriotic implants and the neoangiogenesis are clearly visible and can be biopsied and cauterised.

27.5.4.4 Results

Thirty-three patients have now been followed-up for 6 months to 2 years and no recurrence of endometriosis at ultrasound has been detected. In our series, no conversion to laparoscopy was necessary.

Compared with standard laparoscopy, the recovery after the transvaginal procedures was remarkable. Most patients had no sensation of pain afterwards and at most complained of a light tenderness in the lower abdomen. All patients returned home the same day and resumed their full activities the following day. The 1-day hospitalisation and the low morbidity of the procedure make a second-phase procedure more acceptable for the patient.

27.5.5 Operative Complications

Specific operative complications include:

- profuse bleeding from the ovarian hilus vessels;
- excessive coagulation may lead to ovarian atrophy;
- trauma to the ureter during dissection;
- the most frequent complications are recurrent and de novo postoperative adhesions, which may cause tubo-ovarian infertility, ovarian adhesive disease with chronic pelvic pain and recurrent cyst formation and ultimately, after radical surgery, ovarian remnant syndrome.

When using the transvaginal approach, precautions have to be taken to avoid the risk of rectum perforation. A careful vaginal examination is performed to exclude patients with recto-vaginal indurations.

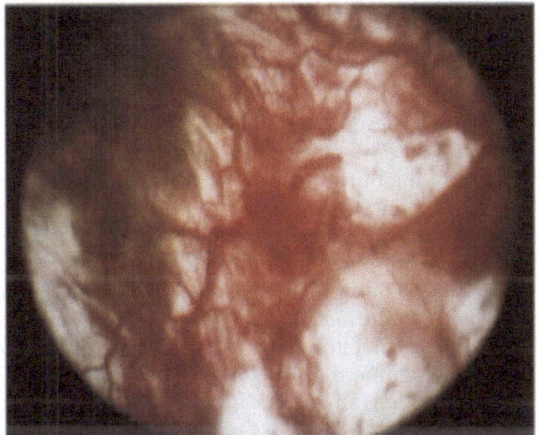

a

27.5.6 Should Spillage be Avoided?

A large retrospective study recently concluded that laparoscopic removal of ovarian cysts should be restricted to patients with preoperative evidence that the cyst is benign.[16]

However, the complex pathology of the ovarian endometrioma renders preoperative exclusion of malignancy practically impossible and ultrasound diagnosis tends to overdiagnose potential malignancy. Laparoscopy remains the gold standard for the diagnosis.

There is no guarantee that surgery via laparotomy will avoid spillage, unless the procedure is performed by retroperitoneal adnexectomy, with the risk of major complications and loss of fertility.

On the other hand, the chocolate cyst of the ovary occurs in young women and is frequently detected when they are attempting their first pregnancy. Therefore, surgery in young women with ovarian endometriomas should be aimed at preserving fertility, excluding malignancy and, in cases of malignancy, achieving accurate diagnosis and localisation.

Laparoscopy with ovarioscopy allows accurate localisation of the endometriotic implants and selection of the representative biopsies (Figure 27.4).[4] The new technique of transvaginal hydrolaparoscopy using hydrofloatation and magnification has been shown to be superior over standard laparoscopy for the detection of subtle ovarian endometriosis, and it preserves the neoangiogenesis.[7]

The preliminary results show that the transvaginal approach also allows dissection of the adhesions of the endometrioma in the fossa ovarica under direct vision and can avoid rupture during the dissection.[17]

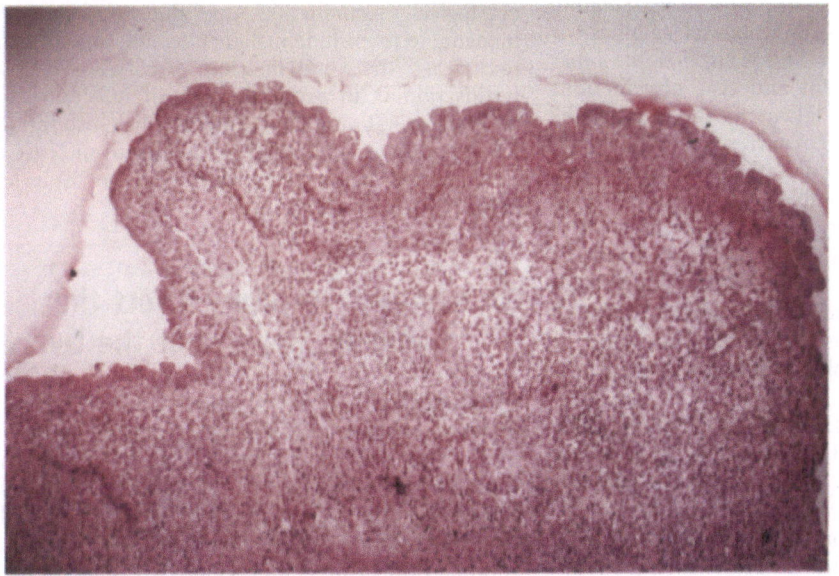

b

Figure 27.4 a Ovarioscopy. The neoangiogenesis of the endometriotic tissue and the old haemorrhagic coagulum lining the cortex allow representative biopsies of endometriotic tissue to be obtained. b The selective biopsy contains the endometrial-like tissue consisting of surface epithelium, vascularised stroma, but no glandular tissue.

Theoretically, it may be questioned whether the conclusions of the Vergote study are applicable to the ovarian endometrioma. Several observations, such as the lateral distribution[18] and anatomo-pathology, suggest that the ovarian endometrioma is different from other non-endometriotic benign ovarian cysts and basically represents an extragonadal tumour. Radical surgery in patients with ovarian endometrioma has not been shown to guarantee that all endometriotic tissue at this site is removed. After radical surgery, these patients are still exposed to reformation of chocolate cysts at this site, as seen after long-term sequential or oestrogen-only hormone replacement therapy.[19]

27.5.7 Comparison of Surgical Techniques

27.5.7.1 Laparoscopy versus Laparotomy

Comparison of laparoscopy with laparotomy has shown that most endometriomas can be treated safely and efficiently by laparoscopic surgery.[20] The recurrence and pregnancy rates are, as expected, comparable. We reported a recurrence rate after microsurgery of 3%[21,22] and after laparoscopic eversion of 6%.[12]

In a case-control study, Hemmings et al[23] found that laparoscopic fenestration and coagulation resulted in faster conception than cystectomy by laparotomy.

27.5.7.2 Comparison of Ovarian-preserving Techniques

Comparison of excision, stripping, laser ablation and drainage by laparoscopy showed significantly more adhesions after excision than after the other techniques, but the extent and type of adhesions before surgery was not taken into account.[24] The same authors found more recurrent endometriomas after the other techniques than after excision. Recurrence due to incomplete surgery is likely to occur when the adhesiolysis is not complete and small endometriotic cysts at the hilus of the ovary or adenomyotic lesions on the adherent pelvic wall are left intact. For the same reasons, the technique of fenestration at the most accessible part is to be avoided and full adhesiolysis and mobilisation of the ovary is the first step.

Recently, Beretta and colleagues[25] presented one of the first randomised trials of two laparoscopic techniques for the treatment of ovarian endometriomas. They found cystectomy to be superior to drainage-coagulation in terms of pain relief, pregnancy rate and, although not

significantly, recurrence. On the other hand, the study is an illustration of the difficulties of a surgical trial that involves a complex pathology and therefore the conclusions need to be interpreted with caution.

It is important to note that the lesions on the outside of the endometrioma may be more important for the outcome factors than the cystic structure. Indeed, the risk of ovarian adhesive disease and consequently recurrent cyst formation, pelvic pain and infertility is largely determined by the type and extent of preoperative adhesions.[26,27] Moreover, the endometriotic lesions outside the ovary rather than the endometriotic cyst may be related to pelvic pain.[28] Drainage or fenestration and coagulation is indeed an inferior technique, which leads to incomplete surgery.

27.6 Management of the Endometrioma before In-vitro Fertilisation

Several studies have addressed the issue of whether the presence of an ovarian endometrioma has an effect on the outcome of in-vitro fertilisation. There is no evidence that, in the absence of extensive adhesions, the ovarian endometrioma has more effect on the outcome of in-vitro fertilisation than superficial endometriosis. Although rare in young women, in principle an ovarian cyst can be malignant. Therefore, reconstructive surgery of the ovarian endometrioma before in-vitro fertilisation is recommended on the basis that the cysts require examination to exclude malignancy. Ultrasound examination combined with aspiration and cytological examination of the aspirate are inadequate to exclude malignancy. A second reason to treat the endometrioma before in-vitro fertilisation is to avoid the risk of infection and abscess formation at the time of follicle aspiration. After endometrioma surgery, the recurrent cyst is frequently a lutein cyst, which can be aspirated before in-vitro fertilisation.

27.7 Does Cystectomy Affect the Follicular Reserve of the Ovary?

Recent studies have raised concern that cystectomy in young women with a suspected endometrioma leads to a loss of follicle reserve.[29-31] El-Sahwi[32] has compared the effect of cystectomy versus fenestration–coagulation in a prospective, randomised-controlled study. Eighty patients with bilateral endometriomas of almost equal size had on one side at random cystectomy by stripping and on the other side drainage–coagulation. Both procedures were performed using CO_2 laser. The recurrence rate at 12 months was similar in both groups (13.8 and 15% respectively). At ultrasound examination, the cystectomy side showed a significantly smaller ovarian volume and at second-look laparoscopy, the cystectomy side had significantly more tubo-ovarian adhesions. During clomiphene citrate stimulation, the cystectomy side also showed less dominance and mature follicles and during in-vitro fertilisation the ovarian dominance, response and number of retrieved oocytes were lower than on the drainage–coagulation side.

References

1. Sampson JA (1921) Perforating hemorrhagic (chocolate) cysts of the ovary. Arch Surg 3:245–323
2. Sampson JA (1927) Peritoneal endometriosis due to the menstrual dissemination of endometrial tissue into the peritoneal cavity. Am J Obstet Gynecol 14:422–469
3. Hughesdon PE (1957) The structure of endometrial cysts of the ovary. J Obstet Gynaecol Br Empire 64:481–487
4. Brosens IA, Puttemans PJ, Deprest J (1994) The endoscopic localisation of endometrial implants in the ovarian chocolate cyst. Fertil Steril 61:1034–1038
5. Redwine DB (1987) The distribution of endometriosis in the pelvis by age groups and fertility. Fertil Steril 47:173–175
6. Vercellini P, Aimi G, De Giorgi O et al (1998) Is cystic ovarian endometriosis an asymmetric disease? Br J Obstet Gynaecol 105:1018–1021
7. Brosens I, Gordts S, Campo R (2001) Transvaginal hydrolaparoscopy, but not standard laparoscopy reveals subtle ovarian endometriosis. Fertil Steril 75:1009–1012
8. Nisolle M, Donnez J (1997) Peritoneal endometriosis, ovarian endometriosis, and adenomyotic nodules of the rectovaginal septum are three different entities. Fertil Steril 68:585–596
9. Nezhat F, Nezhat C, Allan CJ et al (1992) A clinical and histologic classification of endometriomas: implications for a mechanism of pathogenesis. J Reprod Med 37:771–776
10. Vercellini P, Vendola N, Bocciolone I et al (1990) Reliability of the visual diagnosis of ovarian endometriosis. Fertil Steril 53:1198–1200
11. Barbieri RL (1992) Visual diagnosis of endometriosis – reliability? (Letter) Fertil Steril 58:221–222
12. Brosens IA, Van Ballaer P, Puttemans P et al (1996) Reconstruction of the ovary containing large endometriomas by an extraovarian endosurgical technique. Fertil Steril 66:517–521
13. Sutton CJG, MacDonald R (1990) Laser laparoscopic adhesiolysis. J Gynaecol Surg 6:155–160
14. Gordts S, Campo R, Rombauts L et al (1998). Transvaginal salpingoscopy: an office procedure for infertility investigation. Fertil Steril 70:523–526
15. Gordts S, Campo R, Rombauts L et al (1998) Transvaginal hydrolaparoscopy as an outpatient procedure for infertility investigation. Hum Reprod 13:99–103
16. Vergote I, De Brabanter J, Fyles A et al (2001) Prognostic importance of degree of differentiation and cyst rupture in stage I invasive epithelial ovarian carcinoma. Lancet 357:175–182
17. Gordts S, Campo R, Brosens I (2000) Operative transvaginal hydrolaparoscopy of a large ovarian endometrioma. Gynaecol Endosc 9:227–231
18. Vercellini P, Pisacreta A, Vicentini S et al (2000) Lateral distribution of nonendometriotic benign ovarian cysts. Br J Obstet Gynaecol 107:556–558
19. Brosens I (1997) Endometriosis – a disease because it is characterised by bleeding. Am J Obstet Gynecol 176:264–267
20. Adamson GD, Subak LL, Pasta DJ et al (1992) Comparison of CO2 laser laparoscopy with laparotomy for treatment of endometriomata. Fertil Steril 57:965–973
21. Gordts S, Boeckx W, Brosens I (1984) Microsurgery of endometriosis in infertile patients. Fertil Steril 42:520–525
22. Brosens I, Boeckx W, Page G (1988) Microsurgery of ovarian endometriosis. Hum Reprod 3:365–366
23. Hemmings R, Bissonnette F, Bouzayen R (1998) Results of laparoscopic treatments of ovarian endometriomas: laparoscopic ovarian fenestration and coagulation. Fertil Steril 70:527
24. Fayez JA, Vogel MF (1991) Comparison of different treatment methods of endometriomas by laparoscopy. Obstet Gynecol 78:660–665
25. Beretta P, Ghezzi F, Busacca M et al (1998) Randomized trial of two laparoscopic treatments of endometriomas: cystectomy versus drainage and coagulation. Fertil Steril 70:1176–1180
26. Canis M, Mage G, Watiez A et al (1992) Second-look laparoscopy after laparoscopic cystectomy of large ovarian endometriomas (see comments). Fertil Steril 58:617–619
27. Gurgan T, Urman B, Yarali H (1996) Adhesion formation and reformation after laparoscopic removal of ovarian endometriomas. J Am Assoc Gynecol Laparosc 3:389–392
28. Vercellini P, Trespidi L, De Giorgi O et al (1996) Endometriosis and pelvic pain: relation to disease stage and localization. Fertil Steril 65:299–304
29. Nargund G, Cheng WC, Parsons AK (1995) The impact of ovarian cystectomy on ovarian response to stimulation during in-vitro fertilization cycles. Hum Reprod 11:81–83
30. Loh FH, Tan AT, Kumar J et al (1999) Ovarian response after laparoscopic ovarian cystectomy for endometriotic cysts in 132 monitored cycles. Fertil Steril 72:316–321
31. Al-Azmi M, Bernai AL, Gramsbergen I et al (2000) Ovarian response to repeated controlled stimulation in in-vitro fertilization cycles in patients with ovarian endometriosis. Hum Reprod 15:72–75
32. El-Sahwi S (1998) Laparoscopic management of ovarian endometriomas: comparative study incision peeling versus incision coagulation. Abstracts of the 5th Meeting of the Middle East Fertility Society, Amman, Jordan, November 18–20, p 6
33. Martin DC, Berry JD (1990) Histology of chocolate cysts. J Gynecol Surg 6:43–46

Chapter 28

Endometriosis is a Surgical Disease

Philippe R. Koninckx

28.1 Introduction

Our understanding of endometriosis has changed dramatically over the past decade. Introduced clinically at the beginning of this century, as ovarian "chocolate cysts"[1] and as adenomyosis externa,[2-4] it was defined as endometrial glands and stroma outside the uterus. According to this definition, black puckered lesions in the pelvis were soon recognised as endometriosis, making it a frequently observed disease. When, in the 1980s, non-pigmented endometriotic lesions were also described,[5-8] the prevalence of the disease increased from 5–20% to over 60–80% of women with infertility and/or pelvic pain.[9-18] Simultaneously with the increasing awareness of the prevalence of endometriosis, our concepts of aetiology, pathophysiology, natural history and therapy have evolved.

Endometriosis has been considered for decades as the result of the implantation of retrograde menstruated endometrial cells,[19] or metaplasia[20,21] induced by this menstrual debris or lymphatic spread.[22,23] It has been shown that retrograde menstruation occurs in almost all women,[24,25] and that this fluid contains viable cells[26] that can implant on the peritoneum.[27] Progression to cystic ovarian endometriosis and/or deep infiltrating endometriosis was assumed as the natural history of the disease.[28] In recent years this concept of implantation and progression has been challenged by a new concept considering superficial endometriosis to be a physiological condition occurring intermittently in all women, retaining only deep and cystic ovarian endometriosis as a true disease.[29,30]

Treatment of endometriosis consisted of surgical destruction or medical inactivation. As recurrences were considered to be frequent, surgery was often radical. In the last decade, especially since the introduction of endoscopic surgery, concepts such as debulking of deep endometriosis and focal therapy of cystic endometriosis have questioned the concept that surgery should be radical, that endometriotic disease is always progressive, and that recurrence rates are high. Hormone replacement therapy given to women with endometriosis has moreover questioned our concepts of medical therapy and peritoneal fluid.[31]

In order to evaluate critically surgery for endometriosis, we will first discuss the differences in surgical techniques and subsequently describe indications and results of treatment.

28.2 History of Surgical Techniques

To interpret the literature describing the results of surgery for endometriosis, a clear understanding of the evolution and limitations of the various techniques is necessary. Up to the end of the 1970s, minimal and mild endometriosis was destroyed endoscopically by heat application (endothermia) and by unipolar or bipolar coagulation. Treatment of more severe endometriotic disease was mostly radical by hysterectomy, often leaving some rectovaginal endometriosis, whereas in younger women adnexectomies, rarely cystectomies, and anterior resections of the rectum were performed. The literature of this period focuses on infertility and on mild endometriosis and is biased by the fact that deep endometriosis – unless very severe and large – was not recognised. All series of this period are thus "contaminated" by some 5–20% of undiagnosed and thus untreated deep endometriosis.

In the late 1970s and early 1980s, microsurgery was promoted, emphasising careful destruction of superficial endometriosis by bipolar coagulation or resection and removal of cystic ovarian endometriosis followed by reconstruction of the ovary. The underdiagnosing of deep endometriosis continued to be a problem.

From 1986–1987 onwards, the concept of minimal endometriosis and/or non-pigmented endometriosis was introduced.[32] This has caused an important shift in the reported incidence of endometriosis, which depends on recognition and awareness. This increasing recognition of endometriosis has resulted in a progressive shift of women, who would previously have been classified as "normal", to women classified as having minimal endometriosis. This is important in the interpretation of data of this period, such as results of surgery, as the reported groups of "normal" women thus contain variable numbers of unrecognised and untreated women with minimal endometriosis. Simultaneously, the severity of the disease in the groups of women with minimal and mild disease progressively decreases, by dilution with those women with minimal disease. The bias of non-recognition of the majority of deep endometriotic disease still persists.

The increasing use of endoscopic surgery for the treatment of cystic ovarian endometriosis was paralleled by a diversification of techniques with possibly different results. The removal of the cyst wall by stripping followed by suturing or gluing of the ovary is technically similar to microsurgery. Vaporisation of the cyst wall is poorly defined, ranging from focal treatment, to superficial vaporisation, to deeper vaporisation. Besides these differences in techniques, the various studies are biased by the fact that the technique varies with the volume of the endometriotic cyst, but not always to the same extent. In addition, combined endoscopic and microsurgical techniques were proposed.[33]

In the 1990s, deep endometriosis was increasingly recognised during laparoscopic surgery,[18,34] or by clinical examination during menstruation.[35] "Resection of deep endometriosis" comprises techniques ranging from complete resection to debulking and resection–reanastomosis of the rectum, a difference that is rarely stated clearly in the literature. With the recent trend to recognise and to treat deep endometriosis, this "enthusiasm" is already producing and will continue to produce a progressive shift of the severity of the reported series of deep endometriosis, which will include increasing numbers of women with less severe deep endometriosis, which was previously diagnosed as mild disease.

In order to interpret correctly data in the literature on cystic ovarian endometriosis, it is important to consider: (1) the awareness of minimal endometriosis, which is important to judge the "contamination" of the normal group with minimal endometriosis together with the overall severity of endometriosis in the group with minimal endometriosis; (2) the awareness of deep endometriosis will determine the incidence of "unrecognised" deep endometriosis in the minimal–mild groups; whereas (3) only depth of penetration and volume will permit evaluation of the "enthusiasm" of the surgeon to include small spots infiltrating 4–6 mm; (4) the size of cystic ovarian endometriosis, the presence of adhesions, the pathological confirmation of the disease and the technique used, in comparing reported series.

28.3 Minimal and Mild Endometriosis

28.3.1 Methods of Destruction

Ideally, these endometriosis lesions are vaporised or excised with a high-power CO_2 laser. We consider this the method of choice, as this treatment rapidly removes all the endometriosis and not more than the endometriosis, leaving a minimal amount of necrotic tissue. The choice between vaporisation and excision depends on the size of the endometriotic lesion, larger lesions being excised more rapidly. This method takes full advantage of the characteristics of a CO_2 laser as a bloodless and precise cutting instrument, with thermal damage to the surrounding tissue of 100 m or less. However, it requires a high-power CO_2 laser, which is expensive, and a high-flow insufflator of more than 20 l/min,[36] to evacuate smoke and prevent blooming and to maintain a high-power density necessary for minimal thermal damage, at least with a conventional CO_2 laser.

Alternative methods of destruction are bipolar coagulation, endothermia and sharp excision. The two former methods are less adequate than laser vaporisation/excision for typical lesions, since depth of infiltration is difficult to assess by inspection and palpation only. Moreover, the amount of necrotic tissue left behind is more important, which could increase the amount of postoperative adhesions. Sharp excision is theoretically equivalent to CO_2 laser excision. In our experience, however, this method makes it more difficult to find the exact borders between the lesion and the healthy tissue, a process that is more visual than tactile. Sharp dissection, moreover, provides a balance between extensive prophylactic coagulation – which results in tissue damage and difficult planes of cleavage – and no prophylactic coagulation, which is always associated with capillary bleeding and poor visualisation.

28.3.2 Is Destruction Necessary?

If minimal and possibly mild endometriosis is considered a natural condition occurring intermittently in all women,[29,30] it would be logical to postulate that treatment is not necessary as it is not a disease, and it will disappear spontaneously and may reappear later at another localisation.

From a surgical point of view, however, this is an academic discussion. Indeed, the vaporisation of minimal endometriosis, i.e. a few subtle lesions, is so easily performed in a few seconds and generally without risks, that it might be unwise to leave the possibility that some of these lesions would be or become more invasive or aggressive. For slightly larger typical lesions, excision is mandatory to ascertain the depth of infiltration.

28.3.3 Is Destruction Useful?

It is uncertain whether it is useful to treat endometriosis to prevent progression. While most minimal lesions will disappear spontaneously at some stage, it remains extremely likely that at least some of these lesions may have the potential to develop into a more aggressive disease and will eventually do so. To demonstrate this in randomised controlled trials can be argued to be clinically irrelevant, as destruction is so easy, and scientifically it might be practically impossible to achieve. Considering a 60% prevalence of minimal–mild endometriosis with a progression to severe disease in some 10% after 5 years, it would moreover require a randomised trial of hundreds of patients over many years, which is unrealistic.

Whether destruction is useful as a treatment of pain is unknown. Indeed, we favour the hypothesis that subtle and typical endometriosis is rarely painful, except when associated with deeper disease and possibly when larger areas are involved. This view relates to the concept of the activation of spare nociceptors[37,38] with inflammation and the observation that these lesions are specifically painful when stimulated.[39] This discussion, however, is more academic than clinically relevant.

That destruction is useful as an infertility treatment has become increasingly clear. During the late 1970s, an association was shown between endometriosis, luteal-phase insufficiency, unexplained infertility and the luteinised unruptured follicle (LUF) syndrome.[40-42] To understand why this association has been questioned later, it is important to take into account the shift that had taken place in the groups of women reported by the recognition of subtle non-pigmented lesions.[43-46] Studies in the baboon confirmed experimentally that endometriosis was associated with the LUF syndrome, that the LUF syndrome was recurrent and that the LUF syndrome diagnosed by inspection of the ovaries, correlated with the absence of ovulation.[47] Recently, it was shown that treatment improved fertility in women.[48] It should be realised that these observations do not contradict the concept of a natural condition being present intermittently in all women, as subfertility, e.g. a LUF syndrome, might be present predominantly in those months that the lesions are present. If subtle endometriotic lesions are encountered more frequently in women with infertility, this might reduce the overall monthly fecundity rate, e.g. through a LUF syndrome. Again, this discussion might be academic, as surgical destruction can be performed so easily and rapidly.

In conclusion, treatment of minimal and subtle endometriosis can be considered both unnecessary and impossible if it is a recurrent natural condition. The surgical reality of a simple, rapid and harmless destruction, however, favours destruction during laparoscopy, as some of these lesions could have a more aggressive behaviour in the long run, it can be very difficult or impossible to evaluate with certainty the depth of infiltration without excision, and fertility is enhanced in the months following destruction. This argument is based on the assumption that there are facilities for the rapid deployment of the laser, or, if more destructive technology is used, that the surgeon is able to appreciate situations where the position of a lesion may make it unsuitable for destruction.

28.4 Cystic Ovarian Endometriosis

28.4.1 Pitfalls of Diagnosis

The treatment of cystic ovarian endometriosis remains hampered by misdiagnosis of a cystic corpus luteum as a cystic ovarian endometrioma. To the best of our knowledge, this problem has not been addressed specifically in the literature. Even if only women with pathologically confirmed cystic endometriosis were included, these data do not permit a judgment to what extent cystic corpora lutea had been operated on.

A clinical history of the persistence of a cyst is unreliable for diagnosing cystic ovarian endometriosis: over the years we have operated on several women with a "chocolate cyst" on ultrasound, persisting for more than 4 months, even during treatment with luteinising hormone-releasing hormone (LHRH) agonists or when the woman was taking oral contraception. We are fully aware that this clinical observation does not allow any conclusion about frequency, but it is consistent with the observation that ovarian cysts can develop during ovarian down-regulation.[49]

Imaging, such as ultrasound and computed tomography, has a sensitivity of 70–80% and a specificity of 90–95%.[50-54] This is a valuable method of diagnosis to aid the clinical management. It will not, however, prevent errors of judgment during surgery. Ovarian flow measurement does not seem to improve specificity or sensitivity substantially.[50]

Measurement of CA 125 in chocolate fluid has been reported to have a sensitivity and a specificity of nearly 100%.[55,56] Unfortunately, a rapid test, such as a stick assay, is not available to make the diagnosis during surgery.

Our clinical rule of thumb is that, as cystic ovarian endometriosis is so strongly associated with adhesions,[18] a "chocolate cyst" without adhesions has a high probability of being a cystic corpus luteum, whereas the presence of severe adhesions, especially in the fossa ovarica, enhances the suspicion of endometriosis. This, together with inspection of the inside of the cyst by ovarioscopy[57] or inspection with the laparoscope,[58] will help to make a correct judgment in the majority of women. Those with a flattened appearance and red or red and brown mottled ridges are generally endometriosis and those with a dark uniform base, an intracavitary clot, or a yellowish rim are generally corpora lutea or albicans.

In conclusion, however, being aware of the problem, preoperative imaging and CA 125 assays, and peroperative scrutiny did not prevent misdiagnoses in over 10% of women.

28.4.2 Physiopathology

The physiopathology of cystic endometriosis is not entirely understood. It is attractive to consider that many, if not most, cystic ovarian endometrioses originate from invagination of superficial implants.[59] Especially when the ovary becomes adherent to the pelvic wall by endometriotic implants, it seems logic that a "pseudocyst" is formed by the accumulation of old blood and debris, thus stretching the ovarian capsule over this cyst.[60,61] This phenomenon of invagination and stretching of the ovarian capsule explains why the inside of the cyst wall is not always entirely covered by endometriosis, which may be localised as focal endometriotic spots. It thus seems logical to postulate that only these endometriotic spots should be destroyed, and that removing the cyst wall is equivalent to removing the ovarian surface. This mechanism of invagination and stretching of the ovarian capsule does not preclude that some cysts have a different origin, and have a lining covered by endometriosis. Moreover, a careful histology of the cyst wall reveals that endometriotic glands can be present in the so-called cyst wall up to a depth of at least 5–6 mm.

28.4.3 Surgical Pragmatism of Size

From a surgical point of view, the size of the ovarian cyst is most important. For smaller cysts (< 5 cm), the cyst wall can generally be stripped easily from the ovary. This process seems to follow a natural plane of cleavage, confirmed indirectly by the fact that it is associated with little bleeding. For cysts larger than 5 cm diameter, the discussion whether the cyst wall should be removed or destroyed, or whether a focal treatment will be sufficient, is purely academic. Indeed, in these women with a large cyst, the remaining ovarian rim will be so thin that resection becomes either technically impossible or unrealistic in practice, as minimal ovarian tissue will be left. Also the extensive vaporisation of these very large areas is unrealistic.

28.4.4 Methods of Treatment

Aspiration and rinsing of cystic ovarian endometriosis has been attempted, but the recurrence rate is high.[62–64] When we attempted ultrasound-guided aspiration (unpublished data), we noted the presence of chocolate fluid in the pelvis the next day, which might increase adhesion formation,[65] although we have shown that chocolate fluid does not induce adhesions when injected intraperitoneally in mice.[66]

For smaller cysts, i.e. less than 5 cm diameter, the method of stripping the cyst from the ovary, as initially described by the Clermont Ferrand group, seems most attractive.[67–69] It is rapid and technically relatively easy. It is also a complete treatment when invading glands are present. Closure of the ovary by tissucol when necessary results in a "normal ovary" after surgery without denuded areas. The cyst wall could be vaporised. Some report excellent results,[59] but we stopped performing this procedure, as it was too difficult to judge the correct depth of vaporisation. Too superficial destruction will result in an incomplete treatment, whereas too deep destruction often causes bleeding. The cyst wall could be destroyed by unipolar or semi-bipolar coagulation. Although attractive, the reported series are too small to compare this technique with vaporisation. Apart from wall excision and wall destruction, the third option is focal treatment.[70] We feel this is less indicated, as it is difficult in most women to judge which areas are not involved, making focal treatment generally equivalent to vaporisation of the wall.

For larger cysts, the pragmatism of size practically excludes excision and/or vaporisation. The method of making a large window in the cyst wall, followed by rinsing and focal treatment, is attractive and promising. It remains unclear, however, whether during this surgery it is important to do a full adhesiolysis, if necessary, or whether the surgery should be kept to a strict minimum, i.e. marsupialisation to reduce the surgical trauma and possibly adhesion formation. It is also unclear whether medical therapy is helpful postoperatively. This is logical, as it will prevent a corpus luteum from developing and a hypo-oestrogenic milieu could reduce adhesion formation. It also remains unclear whether second-look surgery should always be performed. The number of "large" endometriomata is insufficient in most centres to perform randomised trials, whereas the rapid technical evolution of endoscopic surgery has made a large randomised trial practically impossible.

We favour keeping surgery during the first laparoscopy to a minimum making it a 5- to 10-minute procedure, to vaporise superficially all visible endometriotic spots, and then giving LHRH agonists for 3 months, followed by an ultrasound scan. If a cyst still persists, a second laparoscopy will generally find a small cyst. If no cyst is found, and if there are no complaints of pain or infertility, a second intervention is no longer necessary. This concept has the indirect advantage that the first operation can always be scheduled as a day case, without bowel preparation, whereas the necessity of a bowel preparation for the second intervention will be known in advance.

28.4.5 Results

The results of endoscopic and microsurgical treatment are comparable,[71] ranging between 60 and 80% cure of pain, a cumulative pregnancy rate of 60–70% after 6 months to 1 year and a recurrence rate of some 20%.[72-76] It remains unclear whether preoperative or postoperative medical treatment or ovarian down-regulation significantly affects the results of surgery.[77]

In conclusion, cystic ovarian endometriosis has to be treated, as this condition is associated with pain and infertility and carries the risk of spontaneous rupture. Surgery is the only real treatment, as medical treatment can only inactivate endometriosis and reduce the size of the cyst.[78]

Because of technical and practical surgical considerations, we favour excising smaller cysts by stripping, followed by closure of the remaining flaps if necessary. For larger cysts, we propose a minimal first intervention consisting of marsupialisation, rinsing and focal treatment, followed by LHRH agonists for 3 months and a second intervention when a cyst persists.

28.5 Deep Endometriosis

28.5.1 Diagnosis, Types and Prevalence

Endometriosis can infiltrate the surrounding tissues, resulting in a significant sclerotic and inflammatory reaction, which leads to nodularity, bowel stenosis and ureteral obstruction. The most severe forms, such as rectovaginal endometriosis and endometriosis invading the rectum or the sigmoid, have been known since the beginning of this century. However, these conditions are relatively rare, with an estimated prevalence of less than 1%. This estimation is derived from the observation in Leuven of some 10–20% deep endometriosis in 1988–1991,[79] a period during which endoscopic surgery was not well developed, and in which deep endometriosis was not a well-known entity. Referrals were thus only for infertility and pain, not for deep endometriosis. Assuming that laparoscopies for infertility are performed in some 10–15% of the population, and taking into account the fact that Leuven is a tertiary referral centre, the prevalence of deep endometriosis can be estimated to be between 1% (the prevalence is 10% in younger age groups with infertility, which can be estimated at 15% of the population; in a tertiary centre, the prevalence is probably slightly overestimated) and 3% (prevalence of 20% of the older age group with infertility). Taking into account the observation that deep endometriosis is more frequent on menstrual clinical examination, prevalences between 3 and 10% seem a fair estimate.

The endoscopic excision of endometriosis has revealed that endometriosis invading deeper than 5–6 mm is associated with pain and infertility. Three subtypes have been described.[80]

Type I is characterised by a large pelvic area of typical and sometimes some subtle endometriotic lesions surrounded by white sclerotic tissue. Only during excision does it become obvious that the endometriotic lesion infiltrates deeper than 5 mm. Typically, the endometriotic area becomes progressively smaller as it grows deeper; the lesion is thus cone shaped.

Type II lesions are characterised by retraction of the bowel. Clinically, they are recognised by the obvious bowel retraction around a small typical lesion. In some women, however, no endometriosis can be seen through the laparoscope, and the bowel retraction is the only clinical sign. Diagnosis is generally not too difficult, as the retraction under which an induration is felt is obvious during laparoscopy. In some women, however, it is difficult to see the retraction and to feel the induration. The endometriotic nodule becomes apparent only during excision, emphasising the need for a preoperative diagnosis and training in recognising these lesions.

Type III lesions are spherical endometriotic nodules in the rectovaginal septum. In their most typical manifestation, these lesions are felt as painful nodularities in the rectovaginal septum. At laparoscopy, they generally present as a small typical lesion, and in some women a careful vaginal examination reveals some dark-blue cysts (3–4 mm) in the fornix posterior. Type III lesions are the most severe, and they often spread laterally up and around the uterine artery, sometimes causing sclerosis around the ureter. The spread along the uterine artery can be so obvious that this may be considered an indirect argument for the hypothesis that deep endometriosis has escaped from the inhibitory influence of peritoneal fluid and is mainly under peripheral circulatory control. While being prominent in most women, these lesions are very often missed, as will be discussed later. Sclerosing endometriosis invading the sigmoid is similar to rectal endometriosis, but is situated 10 cm above the rectovaginal septum. This is another form of deep endometriosis, which is fortunately a rare condition and which we could classify as type IV.

Diagnosis of deep endometriosis should be made before surgery. A retrospective analysis showed that only 50% of the larger lesions are diagnosed on routine clinical examination. A menstrual clinical examination is the most powerful tool available to diagnose deep endometriosis types I, II and III. On clinical examination during menstruation,[35] painful nodularities were found in some 30% of women with pain or infertility. In the absence of cystic ovarian endometriosis, these nodularities were caused by deep endometriosis in most of the women. Concentrations of CA 125 are increased in women with deep endometriosis and in those with cystic ovarian endometriosis, and have been proposed as a screening tool. Although specifically increased during menstruation, the variability does not improve the diagnostic accuracy.[81] A late follicular sample has a sensitivity of some 70–90% of endometriotic disease, with a specificity around 95%.[82] Ultrasound and magnetic resonance imaging[83] can be used to diagnose deep endometriosis, but their sensitivity is low, especially for the smaller lesions. For type IV lesions, a contrast enema and/or a rectoscopy are necessary. Although hard data are not available, we presume that this diagnosis is easily missed, making prevalence higher than actually believed.

In conclusion, the most powerful tool to diagnose deep endometriosis is a menstrual clinical examination, whereas a routine clinical examination will reveal mainly the very large lesions. A CA 125 assay is a useful screening aid for deep endometriosis, and it might prove useful as screening for type IV lesions, which, although severe, are easily missed and cannot be diagnosed by clinical examination. The final diagnosis is the estimation of the depth of infiltration during excisional surgery. The prevalence of the disease increases with age and is estimated at 1–10% in the population and at 10–30% in women with pain and/or infertility. A menstrual clinical examination will increase these figures by diagnosing deep endometriosis in women with pain, which is insufficient to perform a laparoscopy.

28.5.2 Surgical Treatment

Surgery for deep endometriosis can be difficult and dangerous. Therefore a preoperative contrast enema and intravenous pyelography should be considered, whereas surgery itself requires a full bowel preparation in order to permit bowel surgery if necessary. This may require the collaboration of a colorectal surgeon, depending on the experience and training of the gynaecologist. If gross distortion of the ureter is present, preoperative ureter stents are recommended. The surgical excision of deep endometriosis relies upon a combination of perfect visual inspection and tactile information.

For type I, II and III lesions, I prefer to use a CO_2 laser (80W, Sharplan), together with a high-flow insufflator (Thermoflator, Storz AG).[36] Guided by visual inspection, together with tactile information about the softness of the tissue, the peritoneum is incised below the lesion at the border between the normal and soft tissue and the harder endometriosis, which glows a yellowish colour under the CO_2 laser beam. First, the lateral edges of the nodule are dissected to free the nodule, if necessary, from the ureter, uterine artery and spinosacral ligament. This is technically the most difficult part of the surgery. Subsequently, the posterior part of the nodule is dissected, thus freeing the rectum. During this dissection, it is important that the nodule remains attached to the uterus and cervix or vagina, thus elevating the nodule, whereas the rectum falls down progressively by gravity. This dissection is continued as far as possible, at least until the rectum is completely liberated from the rectovaginal septum. After completion of the dissection of the posterior part, the anterior side of the nodule is dissected from the cervix, and from the vagina. In some 20% of women, part of the vaginal fornix has to be removed because of endometriotic invasion, whereas we estimate that in 20% of women, the rectum has to be opened to permit a complete resection.[84] It is noteworthy that resection of the rectum has not been necessary in any of the women in the Leuven series.

A careful description of the excisional technique is mandatory to understand the advantages and disadvantages of the reported techniques. The advantages of the technique are the perfect visualisation and the angle of access. Using CO_2 laser excision through the operating laparoscope, excisional surgery is performed with high magnification. Excision can be performed with the laparoscope close in because the laparoscope carries the "knife" and the focal length of the CO_2 laser lens is some 2 cm from the laparoscope. The direction of access of the rectovaginal septum, and especially the posterior side of the nodule, is easier through the laparoscope than through a secondary port. Obviously, this technique requires a high-flow insufflator[85] to maintain a clear picture throughout the excision, and to permit continuous use of the laser.

Three other techniques are used for the resection of deep endometriosis: sharp dissection with electrosurgery through the laparoscope, sharp dissection with electrosurgery through the secondary ports and a partial rectum resection followed by reanastomosis, usually with a circular stapler.

Each surgeon performs best using the techniques with which he is most familiar, and few are familiar with all the techniques. Most have developed the technique they started using for historical reasons, although this should not prevent discussion of the relative advantages of the different approaches, as evaluated by expert surgeons performing surgical procedures often arranged on the basis of friendship.

Sharp dissection with electrosurgery through the laparoscope, as developed by David Redwine,[86–90] is technically almost identical to the CO_2 laser excision, i.e. permitting a very posterior approach and working close in with high magnification in a bloodless operating field. The disadvantage is that this technique is physically demanding, as well as being less suited for video-endoscopic surgery, thus reducing the possibility of help from an assistant. However, it combines the advantage of an improved depth of vision, as a video screen is not used, with enhanced tactile information, as sharp dissection is used.

Sharp dissection with electrosurgery through the secondary ports is the most widely used technique,[68,91–100] for several reasons. It is derived from the other endoscopic procedures; it does not require a CO_2 laser; and possibly even more importantly, a high-flow insufflator was not available during its development. Because the angle of access is much sharper, surgeons using this technique generally start dissection at the anterior site of the nodule, thus freeing nodule and rectum from the rectovaginal septum. Subsequently, the rectum is dissected from the nodule, which has become freely mobile.

Most of these procedures aim at debulking the endometriosis, rather than performing a complete resection. The word "debulking" is chosen when the surgeon prefers not to open the rectum, even if the resection is less complete. It is difficult to estimate whether this debulking attitude is a consequence of the technique used, or of the philosophy often dictated by local and medicolegal considerations. In my experience, resection of endometriosis using this technique is much more difficult than using the CO_2 laser approach, and the best method to avoid bowel lesions is by avoiding traction and using gravity only. These same considerations could explain why some authors, probably in order to perform a complete resection and to avoid recurrences, perform a partial resection and anastomosis in women with larger nodules. It is not known whether those performing a complete resection are overtreating their patients or whether those aiming at debulking the lesion are undertreating the endometriosis.

Type IV endometriosis requires a resection and subsequent reanastomosis. I attempted to perform conservative surgery in three women with type IV endometriosis, but was unsuccessful: the angle of access was too difficult, a third secondary port was necessary to stabilise the sigmoid, and the procedure took more than 2 hours.

28.5.3 Complications, Treatment and Prevention[101–103]

When part of the rectum wall has to be removed, or when the rectum is accidentally opened, the pelvis is rinsed with a 1% hibitane solution and the wall is sutured endoscopically with two layers of 3×0 Vicryl (Ethicon, USA). A defect in the posterior vaginal fornix is sutured either vaginally or endoscopically. Care is taken to ensure that these defects are watertight when sutured. I prefer to suture these defects laparoscopically, for reasons of sterility: during laparoscopic suturing, a continuous flow of CO_2 from the abdominal cavity to the vagina prevents contamination.

Surgical excision of deep endometriosis is thus difficult, as it often necessitates dissection far laterally around the ureter and uterine artery. Also, excision from the bowel wall is difficult, as in 10% of women, part of the bowel wall will have to be resected. In 20% of women, especially those with rectovaginal endometriosis, i.e. type III lesions, excision has to be performed up to and including the posterior vaginal fornix. It is important that neither resection of part of the bowel wall nor of the vaginal fornix should be considered as complications of surgery, as the postoperative follow-up has been uneventful in a series of over 300 women (my series).

Complications of surgery (n = 225) have included transection of the uterine artery in two women, necessitating clipping, a lesion of the ureter in one woman and a late bowel perforation in six women. A ureter lesion is a serious complication, and we therefore advocate a preoperative intravenous pyelogram, careful dissection of the ureter from its landmarks at the pelvic brim and liberal preventive stenting if necessary. This has become even more important since it became evident that a ureter that is only half cut can easily be sutured endoscopically over a double J.[104] A late bowel perforation is an even more serious complication, which has occurred in six women: two women with a type II lesion (1989 and 1991) and one woman with a type III lesion (1992) were readmitted after a week with progressively increasing symptoms of peritonitis; one woman

(1992) with a type I lesion and a history of pouch anastomosis for colitis ulcerosa was observed for 1 week with atypical symptoms, which later proved to be a rectum perforation; two women (1994) with type II lesions had acute pelvic pain 12 hours and 2 days following surgery, respectively. Although symptoms of peritonitis were minimal, an immediate laparoscopy revealed a bowel perforation in both.

It is important to realise that bowel perforations can occur during the early postoperative days, thus necessitating a low-fibre diet and eventually hospitalisation. A perforation generally occurs during straining, with acute pelvic pain as the only symptom. Disturbingly, this pain disappears over the subsequent hours, with slight peritoneal irritation as the only symptom. Liberal use of early second-look laparoscopies is advocated in these women before symptoms of peritonitis develop. In five women, we recently demonstrated that even a bowel perforation can safely be sutured endoscopically, thus avoiding a colostomy.

Prevention of a late perforation is even more important. In January 1996, liberal prophylactic suturing of the rectum was introduced, whenever there is a suspicion of a lesion to the muscularis. Since then, this complication has disappeared.

28.5.4 Medical Treatment

Medical therapy before surgery has been discussed for many years and surgeons have claimed that deep lesions were less vascularised following medical therapy. It was recently demonstrated that pretreatment for 3 months with an LHRH agonist could shrink the volume of deep lesions.[84] Indeed, in this series, decapeptyl (3.75 mg per month) has been given specifically to women with the most severe disease, especially deep lesions. Analysis of data showed that women pretreated with this LHRH agonist had a higher revised American Fertility Society (AFS) score at surgery than those without treatment, confirming the selection bias. Similarly, pretreated women had more and larger cystic ovarian endometriosis, also pointing to the selection bias. As expected, women with pretreatment had a smaller pelvic area of endometriosis. However, pretreated women had a smaller volume of deep endometriosis, notwithstanding the fact that because of the selection bias, they almost certainly had a much higher volume before treatment. For this reason, we advocate pretreating women with severe deep endometriosis medically for 3 months with a gonadotrophin-releasing hormone (GnRH) agonist. Danazol might be equally effective, but our series was too small to prove this statistically. Other medical therapies have not been used frequently enough to be evaluated.

Medical treatment following excision of deep endometriosis has not been evaluated properly. If excision has been performed completely, medical treatment is probably not necessary. Medical therapy, however, should be considered instead of repeat or more radical surgery for recurring symptoms or failures of excision.

Medical treatment alone has not been addressed specifically in any study because of a lack of a clear-cut diagnosis of deep endometriosis without excision. Medical treatment with danazol, GnRH agonists or gestrinone[105-109] does not cure endometriosis. These treatments inactivate the endometriotic lesions, which reappear rapidly after treatment has been stopped.[110] None of these therapies has an important beneficial effect on subsequent fertility.[111] They all improve pelvic pain and the effect persists, often for many months after therapy has been stopped.[112] As deep endometriosis is strongly associated with pelvic pain, and cystic ovarian endometriosis does not respond well to medical therapy, it is suggested that the observations and conclusions concerning severe pelvic pain are probably related to deep endometriosis.

28.5.5 Results

Nehzat[97] reported 25 pregnancies in 67 women following excision of deep endometriosis. We evaluated cumulative pregnancy rates in a consecutive series of 900 women with primary or secondary infertility without severe tubal damage and with a severely subfertile husband. Cumulative pregnancy rates were slightly lower in advanced stages of endometriosis according to the revised AFS classification, being 62 and 44% in classes I and IV respectively. However, when the duration of infertility – the strongest predictor of subsequent conception – was taken into account, the differences in cumulative pregnancy rates between classes I to IV disappeared, suggesting that the differences found between mild and severe endometriosis were mainly a consequence of differences in duration of infertility and possibly in age of the women.[113,114]

The only group with a significantly higher cumulative pregnancy rate following surgery was women with deep endometriosis. By Cox multivariate regression analysis, the following model was established: pregnancy was predicted most strongly by a shorter duration of infertility and by the surgical treatment of cystic ovarian endometriosis and/or of deep endometriosis. From these results, it can be concluded that aggressive and complete excision of deep endometriosis can be advocated, with subsequent spontaneous pregnancy rates up to 60% within 1 year. These results can be considered excellent, taking into account the severity of disease and the large denuded area in the pelvis following excision of deep endometriosis. It remains unclear whether those women who did not conceive after 1 year should be orientated towards in-vitro fertilisation or to a second-look laparoscopy. Indirect evidence indicates that medical treatment alone is probably not the treatment of choice for deep endometriosis and infertility. Medical pretreatment seems to be useful to facilitate surgery, as has been suggested for cystic ovarian endometriosis.[115] Both surgical and medical treatment were reported to be highly successful in treating pelvic pain. Candiani[96] reported absence of dyspareunia and dysmenorrhoea in six and four women out of ten after 40 months. Nezhat[97] reported moderate to complete pain relief in 162 women out of 175, but two or more interventions had been necessary in some women. Preliminary analysis of our results in 250 women, in whom deep endometriosis had been excised with a CO_2 laser, showed a cure rate of pelvic pain in 70%, with a recurrence rate of less than 5% with a follow-up period of up to 5 years. These data should be interpreted carefully, as the completeness of excision has steadily increased. The results of recent years strongly suggest an almost complete cure rate without recurrences; this, however, could be an over-optimistic clinical impression, which will have to be proven by careful analysis of the data. In addition, medical treatment of pelvic pain is highly efficient, and the effect of treatment often persists after treatment has been stopped.[112]

28.6 Conclusions

We advocate a first-line approach to the diagnosis and treatment of endometriosis, which relies on a menstrual clinical examination, an ultrasound scan and eventually an assay of CA 125 (Figure 28.1). Following these examinations, four groups of women can be considered. When the clinical examination during menstruation does not reveal any nodularities, no ovarian cysts are found at ultrasound scan and the CA 125 concentration is normal, women with infertility and/or pain are scheduled for a day-case diagnostic laparoscopy. If an endometrioma larger than 5 cm in diameter is found, these women are also scheduled as a day case for an initial procedure, during which the cyst is opened, rinsed and focally treated. Postoperatively, these women are treated for 3 months with a GnRH analogue, and eventually scheduled for a second intervention. If a small endometrioma is found on scan, these women are also scheduled for day case surgery. They are advised that a bowel preparation may be necessary, but that the probability is less than 5%. If a deep endometriotic nodule is found, preoperative medical treatment, preoperative contrast enema and intravenous pyelography should be considered. These women always receive a bowel preparation and are admitted to hospital for at least 48 hours.

This approach has the advantage that the preoperative clinical examination, together with the ultrasound scan, are used to decide whether the patient will be admitted to hospital or treated in the day clinic, and whether a bowel preparation will be given. From our experience over the past years, the accuracy of this procedure is close to 100%, as unexpected deep endometriosis and unnecessary bowel treatments have virtually disappeared from the department.

Surgery remains the cornerstone of the treatment of endometriosis. Medical treatment seems to be indicated, besides pre- and postoperatively as

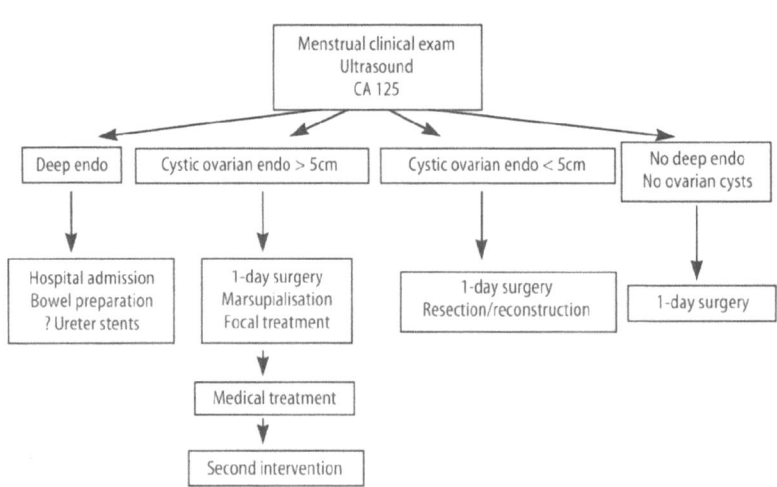

Figure 28.1 Treatment of endometriosis.

discussed, for women with recurrent pelvic endometriosis and pain, or when adequate surgery is not available or is too dangerous.

Acknowledgements

I thank Mr Stephen Kennedy, Nuffield Department of Obstetrics and Gynaecology, Oxford, UK for reviewing this manuscript. I also thank my co-workers and co-authors of the articles that have been reviewed. Stefan Lempereur, Ipsen NV, Belgium and Freddy Cornillie, Director Centocor Europe are thanked for their support and co-operation. This work was supported partially by NFWO research grant no. 9-002090. The manuscript was prepared by Mrs Diane Wolput.

References

1. Sampson JA (1927) Peritoneal endometriosis due to the menstrual dissemination of endometrial tissue into the peritoneal cavity. Am J Obstet Gynecol 14:422–469
2. Cullen TS (1896) Adenoma-myoma uteri diffusum benignum. J Hopkins Hosp Bull 6:133–137
3. Cullen TS (1896) Adeno-myoma of the round ligament. J Hopkins Hosp Bull 7:112–114
4. Cullen TS (1919) The distribution of adenomyomata containing uterine mucosa. Am J Obstet Gynecol 80:130–138
5. Jansen RPS, Russell P (1986) Nonpigmented endometriosis: clinical, laparoscopic, and pathologic definition. Am J Obstet Gynecol 155:1154–1159
6. Stripling MC, Martin DC, Chatman DL et al (1988) Subtle appearance of pelvic endometriosis. Fertil Steril 49:427–431
7. Stripling MC, Martin DC, Poston WM (1988) Does endometriosis have a typical appearance? J Reprod Med Obstet Gynecol 33:879–884
8. Martin DC, Hubert GD, Van der Zwaag R et al (1989) Laparoscopic appearances of peritoneal endometriosis. Fertil Steril 51:63–67
9. Mahmood TA, Templeton A (1991) Prevalence and genesis of endometriosis. Hum Reprod 6:544–549
10. Rawson JMR (1991) Prevalence of endometriosis in asymptomatic women. J Reprod Med Obstet Gynecol 36:513–515
11. Wheeler JM (1989) Epidemiology of endometriosis-associated infertility. J Reprod Med 34:41–46
12. Houston DE, Noller KL, Melton LJ et al (1987) Incidence of pelvic endometriosis in Rochester, Minnesota, 1970–1979. Am J Epidemiol 125:959–969
13. Moen MH (1987) Endometriosis in women at interval sterilization. Acta Obstet Gynecol Scand 66:451–454
14. Hull MGR, Glazener CMA, Kelly NJ et al (1985) Population study of causes, treatment, and outcome of infertility. Br Med J 291:1693–1697
15. Strathy JH, Molgaard CA, Coulam CB et al (1985) Endometriosis and infertility: a laparoscopic study of endometriosis among fertile and infertile women. Fertil Steril 44:83–88
16. Nikanen V, Punnonen R (1984) External endometriosis in 801 operated patients. Acta Obstet Gynecol Scand 63:699–701
17. Bitzer J, Korber HR (1983) Laparoscopy findings in infertile women. Geburtshilfe Frauenheilkd 43:294–298
18. Koninckx PR, Meuleman C, Demeyere S et al (1991) Suggestive evidence that pelvic endometriosis is a progressive disease, whereas deeply infiltrating endometriosis is associated with pelvic pain. Fertil Steril 55:759–765
19. Sampson JA (1927) Peritoneal endometriosis due to the menstrual dissemination of endometrial tissue into the peritoneal cavity. Am J Obstet Gynecol 14:422–469
20. El Mahgoub S, Yaseen S (1980) A positive proof for the theory of coelomic metaplasia. Am J Obstet Gynecol 137:137–140
21. Suginami H (1991) A reappraisal of the coelomic metaplasia theory by reviewing endometriosis occurring in unusual sites and instances. Am J Obstet Gynecol 165:214–218
22. Moore JG, Binstock MA, Growdon WA (1988) The clinical implications of retroperitoneal endometriosis. Am J Obstet Gynecol 158:1291–1298
23. Ueki M (1991) Histologic study of endometriosis and examination of lymphatic drainage in and from the uterus. Am J Obstet Gynecol 165:201–209
24. Koninckx PR, Ide P, Vandenbroucke W et al (1980) New aspects of the pathophysiology of endometriosis and associated infertility. J Reprod Med 24:257–260
25. Halme J, Hammond MG, Hulka JF et al (1984) Retrograde menstruation in healthy women and in patients with endometriosis. Obstet Gynecol 64:151–154
26. Kruitwagen RF (1993) Menstruation as the pelvic aggressor. Baillieres Clin Obstet Gynaecol 7:687–700
27. van der Linden PJQ, de Goeij AFPM, Dunselman GAJ et al (1998) Amniotic membrane as an in vitro model for endometrium–extracellular matrix interactions. Gynecol Obstet Invest 45:7–11
28. Redwine DB, Koninckx PR, D'Hooghe T et al (1991) Endometriosis: will the real natural history please stand up? Fertil Steril 56:590–591
29. Koninckx PR (1994) Is mild endometriosis a condition occurring intermittently in all women? Hum Reprod 9:2202–2205
30. Vercellini P, Bocciolone L, Crosignani PG (1992) Is mild endometriosis always a disease? Hum Reprod 7:627–629
31. Koninckx PR, Kennedy SH, Barlow DH (1998) Endometriotic disease: the role of peritoneal fluid. Hum Reprod Update 4:741–751
32. Jansen RP, Russell P (1986) Nonpigmented endometriosis: clinical, laparoscopic, and pathologic definition. Am J Obstet Gynecol 155:1154–1159
33. Goldenberg M, Oelsner G, Bider D et al (1994) A new approach to ovarian cystectomy – a combined laparoscopic and extra-abdominal microsurgical technique. Gynecol Obstet Invest 37:196–198
34. Cornillie FJ, Oosterlynck D, Lauweryns JM et al (1990) Deeply infiltrating pelvic endometriosis: histology and clinical significance. Fertil Steril 53:978–983
35. Koninckx PR, Meuleman C, Oosterlynck D et al (1996) Diagnosis of deep endometriosis by clinical examination during menstruation and plasma CA-125 concentration. Fertil Steril 65:280–287
36. Koninckx PR, Vandermeersch E (1991) The persufflator: an insufflation device for laparoscopy and especially for CO2-laser-endoscopic surgery. Hum Reprod 6:1288–1290
37. Cervero F (1995) Visceral pain: mechanisms of peripheral and central sensitization. Ann Med 27:235–239
38. Cervero F, Janig W (1992) Visceral nociceptors: a new world order? [see comments] Trends Neurosci 15:374–378
39. Koninckx PR, Renaer M (1997) Pain sensitivity of and pain radiation from the internal female genital organs. Hum Reprod 12:1785–1788
40. Brosens IA, Koninckx PR, Corveleyn PA (1978) A study of plasma progesterone, oestradiol-17ß, prolactin and LH levels, and of the luteal phase appearance of the ovaries in patients with endometriosis and infertility. Br J Obstet Gynaecol 85:246–250
41. Koninckx PR, Brosens IA (1982) Clinical significance of the luteinized unruptured follicle syndrome as a cause of infertility. Eur J Obstet Gynecol Reprod Biol 13:355–368

42. Koninckx PR, Brosens IA (1977) Diagnosis of the luteinized unruptured follicle syndrome. Proc FIGO, Tokyo
43. Schenken RS, Werlin LB, Williams RF et al (1986) Histologic and hormonal documentation of the luteinized unruptured follicle syndrome. Am J Obstet Gynecol 154:839-847
44. Haines CJ (1987) Luteinized unruptured follicle syndrome. Clin Reprod Fertil 5:321-332
45. Scheenjes E, te Velde E R, Kremer J (1990) Inspection of the ovaries and steroids in serum and peritoneal fluid at various time intervals after ovulation in fertile women: implications for the luteinized unruptured follicle syndrome. Fertil Steril 54:38-41
46. Mio Y, Toda T, Harada T et al (1992) Luteinized unruptured follicle in the early stages of endometriosis as a cause of unexplained infertility. Am J Obstet Gynecol 167:271-273
47. D'Hooghe TM, Bambra CS, Raeymaekers BM et al (1996) Increased incidence and recurrence of recent corpus luteum without ovulation stigma (luteinized unruptured follicle syndrome?) in baboons with endometriosis. J Soc Gynecol Investig 3:140-144
48. Marcoux S, Maheux R, Berube S (1997) The Canadian Collaborative Group on Endometriosis. Laparoscopic surgery in infertile women with minimal and mild endometriosis. N Engl J Med 337:217-222
49. Jenkins JM, Anthony FW, Wood P et al (1993) The development of functional ovarian cysts during pituitary down-regulation. Hum Reprod 8:1623-1627
50. Alcazar JL, Laparte C, Jurado M et al (1997) The role of transvaginal ultrasonography combined with color velocity imaging and pulsed Doppler in the diagnosis of endometrioma. Fertil Steril 67:487-491
51. Mais V, Guerriero S, Ajossa S et al (1993) The efficiency of transvaginal ultrasonography in the diagnosis of endometrioma. Fertil Steril 60:776-780
52. Outwater EK, Dunton CJ (1995) Imaging of the ovary and adnexa: clinical issues and applications of MR imaging. Radiology 194:1-18
53. Guerriero S, Ajossa S, Paoletti AM et al (1996) Tumor markers and transvaginal ultrasonography in the diagnosis of endometrioma. Obstet Gynecol 88:403-407
54. Guerriero S, Mais V, Ajossa S et al (1996) Transvaginal ultrasonography combined with CA-125 plasma levels in the diagnosis of endometrioma. Fertil Steril 65:293-298
55. Koninckx PR, Muyldermans M, Moerman P et al (1992) CA 125 concentrations in ovarian 'chocolate' cyst fluid can differentiate an endometriotic cyst from a cystic corpus luteum. Hum Reprod 7:1314-1317
56. Koninckx PR (1993) CA 125 in the management of endometriosis. Eur J Obstet Gynecol Reprod Biol 49:109-113
57. Brosens IA, Puttemans PJ, Deprest J (1994) The endoscopic localization of endometrial implants in the ovarian chocolate cyst. Fertil Steril 61:1034-1038
58. Martin DC, Demos Berry J (1990) Histology of chocolate cysts. J Gynecol Surg 6:43-46
59. Donnez J, Nisolle M, Gillet N et al (1996) Large ovarian endometriomas. Hum Reprod 11:641-646
60. Hughesdon PE (1984) Benign endometrioid tumours of the ovary and the mullerian concept of ovarian epithelial tumours. Histopathology 8:977-990
61. Brosens I, Puttemans P, Deprest J (1993) Appearances of endometriosis. Baillieres Clin Obstet Gynaecol 7:741-757
62. Vercellini P, Vendola N, Bocciolone L et al (1992) Laparoscopic aspiration of ovarian endometriomas. Effect with postoperative gonadotropin releasing hormone agonist treatment. J Reprod Med 37:577-580
63. Giorlandino C, Taramanni C, Muzii L et al (1993) Ultrasound-guided aspiration of ovarian endometriotic cysts. Int J Gynaecol Obstet 43:41-44
64. Aboulghar MA, Mansour RT, Serour GI et al (1991) Ultrasonic transvaginal aspiration of endometriotic cysts: an optional line of treatment in selected cases of endometriosis. Hum Reprod 6:1408-1410
65. Muzii L, Marana R, Caruana P et al (1995) Laparoscopic findings after transvaginal ultrasound-guided aspiration of ovarian endometriomas. Hum Reprod 10:2902-2903
66. Kennedy SH, Cederholm-Williams SA, Barlow DH (1992) The effect of injecting endometriotic 'chocolate' cyst fluid into the peritoneal cavity of mice. Hum Reprod 7:1329
67. Bruhat MA, Mage G, Chapron C et al (1991) Present day endoscopic surgery in gynecology. Eur J Obstet Gynecol Reprod Biol 41:4-13
68. Bruhat MA, Mage G, Pouly JL (1991) Advances in pelviscopic surgery. Ann NY Acad Sci 626:367-371
69. Bruhat MA, Wattiez A, Mage G (1989) CO2 laser laparoscopy. Baillieres Clin Obstet Gynaecol 3:487-497
70. Brosens IA, Van Ballaer P, Puttemans P et al (1996) Reconstruction of the ovary containing large endometriomas by an extraovarian endosurgical technique. Fertil Steril 66:517-521
71. Crosignani PG, Vercellini P (1995) Conservative surgery for severe endometriosis: should laparotomy be abandoned definitively? Hum Reprod 10:2412-2418
72. Adamson GD, Pasta DJ (1994) Surgical treatment of endometriosis-associated infertility: meta-analysis compared with survival analysis. Am J Obstet Gynecol 171:1488-1505
73. Brosens IA (1994) New principles in the management of endometriosis. Acta Obstet Gynecol Scand Suppl 159:18-21
74. Wood C (1994) Endoscopy in the management of endometriosis. Baillieres Clin Obstet Gynaecol 8:735-757
75. Canis M, Mage G, Wattiez A et al (1992) Second-look laparoscopy after laparoscopic cystectomy of large ovarian endometriomas [see comments]. Fertil Steril 58:617-619
76. Fayez JA, Vogel MF (1991) Comparison of different treatment methods of endometriomas by laparoscopy [see comments]. Obstet Gynecol 78:660-665
77. Muzii L, Marana R, Caruana P et al (1996) The impact of preoperative gonadotropin-releasing hormone agonist treatment on laparoscopic excision of ovarian endometriotic cysts. Fertil Steril 65:1235-1237
78. Chang SP, Ng HT (1996) A randomized comparative study of the effect of leuprorelin acetate depot and danazol in the treatment of endometriosis. Chung Hua I Hsueh Tsa Chih Taipei 57:431-437
79. Koninckx PR, Meuleman C, Demeyere S et al (1991) Suggestive evidence that pelvic endometriosis is a progressive disease whereas deeply infiltrating endometriosis is associated with pelvic pain [see comments]. Fertil Steril 55:759-765
80. Koninckx PR, Martin DC (1992) Deep endometriosis: a consequence of infiltration or retraction or possibly adenomyosis externa? Fertil Steril 58:924-928
81. Hompes PG, Koninckx PR, Kennedy SH et al (1996) Serum CA-125 concentrations during midfollicular phase, a clinically useful and reproducible marker in diagnosis of advanced endometriosis. Clin Chem 42:1871-1874
82. Koninckx PR, Meuleman C, Oosterlynck D et al (1996) Diagnosis of deep endometriosis by clinical examination during menstruation and plasma CA-125 concentration. Fertil Steril 65:280-287
83. Deprest J, Marchal G, Koninckx PR (1993) MRI in the diagnosis of deeply infiltrating endometriosis. Abstract AAGL, 22nd annual meeting
84. Koninckx PR, Timmermans B, Meuleman C et al (1996) Complications of CO2-laser endoscopic excision of deep endometriosis. Hum Reprod 11:2263-2268
85. Koninckx PR, Vandermeersch E (1991) The persufflator: an insufflation device for laparoscopy and especially for CO_2-laser-endoscopic surgery. Hum Reprod 6:1288-1290
86. Redwine DB (1991) Conservative laparoscopic excision of endometriosis by sharp dissection: life table analysis of reoperation and persistent or recurrent disease. Fertil Steril 56:628-634
87. Redwine DB (1992) Laparoscopic en bloc resection for treatment of the obliterated cul-de-sac in endometriosis. J Reprod Med 37:695-698

88. Sharpe DR, Redwine DB (1992) Laparoscopic segmental resection of the sigmoid and rectosigmoid colon for endometriosis. Surg Laparoscopy Endosc 2:120–124

89. Redwine DB, Koning M, Sharpe DR (1996) Laparoscopically assisted transvaginal segmental resection of the rectosigmoid colon for endometriosis. Fertil Steril 65:193–197

90. Redwine DB (1997) Severe intestinal (GI) endometriosis (E) and pelvic mapping. Fertil Steril S22

91. Donnez J, Nisolle M, Gillerot S et al (1997) Rectovaginal septum adenomyotic nodules: a series of 500 cases. Br J Obstet Gynaecol 104:1014–1018

92. Crosignani PG, De Cecco L, Gastaldi A et al (1996) Leuprolide in a 3-monthly versus a monthly depot formulation for the treatment of symptomatic endometriosis: a pilot study. Hum Reprod 11:2732–2735

93. Vercellini P, Trespidi L, De Giorgi O et al (1996) Endometriosis and pelvic pain: relation to disease stage and localization. Fertil Steril 65:299–304

94. Donnez J, Nisolle M, Casanasroux F et al (1995) Rectovaginal septum endometriosis or adenomyosis: laparoscopic management in a series of 231 patients. Hum Reprod 10:630–635

95. Martin DC (1995) Pain and infertility – a rationale for different treatment approaches. Br J Obstet Gynaecol 102 (Suppl 12):2–3

96. Candiani GB, Vercellini P, Fedele L et al (1992) Conservative surgical treatment of rectovaginal septum endometriosis. J Gynecol Surg 8:177–182

97. Nezhat C, Nezhat F, Pennington E (1992) Laparoscopic treatment of infiltrative rectosigmoid colon and rectovaginal septum endometriosis by the technique of videolaparoscopy and the CO2 laser. Br J Obstet Gynaecol 99:664–667

98. Reich H, McGlynn F, Salvat J (1991) Laparoscopic treatment of cul-de-sac obliteration secondary to retrocervical deep fibrotic endometriosis. J Reprod Med Obstet Gynecol 36:516–522

99. Ripps BA, Martin DC (1991) Focal pelvic tenderness, pelvic pain and dysmenorrhea in endometriosis. J Reprod Med 36:470–472

100. Martin DC (1988) Laparoscopic and vaginal colpotomy for the excision of infiltrating cul-de-sac endometriosis. J Reprod Med 33:806–808

101. Koninckx PR, Timmerman B, Meuleman C et al (1996) Complications of CO2-laser endoscopic excision of deep endometriosis. Hum Reprod 11:2263–2268

102. Van Rompaey B, Deprest JA, Koninckx PR (1996) Enterocele as a consequence of laparoscopic resection of deeply infiltrating endometriosis. J Am Assoc Gynecol Laparosc 4:73–75

103. Tate JJT, Kwok S, Dawson JW et al (1993) Prospective comparison of laparoscopic and conventional anterior resection. Br J Surg 80:1396–1398

104. Neven P, Vandeursen H, Baert L et al (1993) Ureteric injury at laparoscopic surgery: the endoscopic management. Case review. Gynaecol Endoscop 2:45–46

105. Shaw RW (1993) Endometriosis: current evaluation of management and rationale for medical therapy. In: Brosens IA, Donnez J (eds) The current status of endometriosis. Parthenon Publishing, New York, pp 371–383

106. Fedele L, Bianchi S, Bocciolone L et al (1993) Buserelin acetate in the treatment of pelvic pain associated with minimal and mild endometriosis – a controlled study. Fertil Steril 59:516–521

107. Fedele L, Arcaini L, Bianchi S et al (1989) Comparison of cyproterone acetate and danazol in the treatment of pelvic pain associated with endometriosis. Obstet Gynecol 73:1000–1004

108. Fedele L, Bianchi S, Arcaini L et al (1989) Buserelin versus danazol in the treatment of endometriosis-associated infertility. Am J Obstet Gynecol 161:871–876

109. Redwine DB, Elstein M, Shaw R et al (1992) Nafarelin versus danazol versus surgery. Fertil Steril 58:455–456

110. Evers JLH (1987) The second-look laparoscopy for evaluation of the result of medical treatment of endometriosis should not be performed during ovarian suppression. Fertil Steril 47:502–504

111. Hughes EG, Fedorkow DM, Collins JA (1993) A quantitative overview of controlled trials in endometriosis-associated infertility. Fertil Steril 59:963–970

112. Shaw RW (1990) Nafarelin in the treatment of pelvic pain caused by endometriosis. Am J Obstet Gynecol 162:574–576

113. Koninckx PR, Stukkens K, Meuleman C (1991) Cumulative pregnancy rates following CO2-laser-endoscopic surgery for deeply infiltrating endometriosis. Proc FIGO, Singapore

114. Koninckx PR, Deprest J, Janssen G et al (1993) Cumulative pregnancy rates following CO2-laser endoscopic excision of deeply infiltrating endometriosis. Fertil Steril, Montreal meeting

115. Buttram VC (1993) Rationale for combined medical and surgical treatment of endometriosis. In: Brosens IA, Donnez J (eds) The current status of endometriosis. Parthenon Publishing, New York, pp 32–406

Appendix

The Revised AFS Classification of Endometriosis

AFS Clasification of Endometriosis

Patient's Name _____ Date _____

Stage I (Minimal) - 1–5
Stage II (Mild) - 6–15   Laparoscopy _____ Laparotomy _____ Photography _____
Stage III (Moderate) - 16–40   Recommended Treatment _____
Stage IV (Severe) - > 40   _____

Total _____   Prognosis _____

	ENDOMETRIOSIS	< 1cm	1–3cm	> 3cm
PERITONEUM	Superficial	1	2	4
	Deep	2	4	6
OVARY	R Superficial	1	2	4
	Deep	4	16	20
	L Superficial	1	2	4
	Deep	4	16	20

	POSTERIOR CULDESAC OBLITERATION	Partial		Complete
		4		40

	ADHESIONS	< 1/3 Enclosure	1/3 – 2/3 Enclosure	> 2/3 Enclosure
OVARY	R Filmy	1	2	4
	Dense	4	8	16
	L Filmy	1	2	4
	Dense	4	8	16
TUBE	R Filmy	1	2	4
	Dense	4*	8*	16
	L Filmy	1	2	4
	Dense	4*	8*	16

* If the fimbriated end of the fallopian tube is completely enclosed, change the point assignment to 16.

Additional Endometriosis: _____   Associated Pathology: _____

_____   _____

_____   _____

_____   _____

To Be Used with Normal Tubes and Ovaries	To Be Used with Abnormal Tubes and/or Ovaries

L   R   L   R

EXAMPLES & GUIDELINES

STAGE I (MINIMAL)	STAGE II (MILD)	STAGE III (MODERATE)

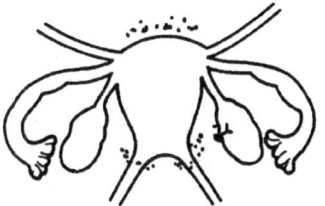 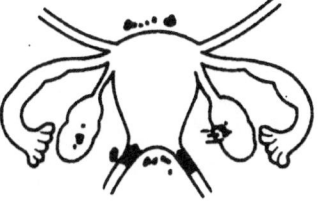 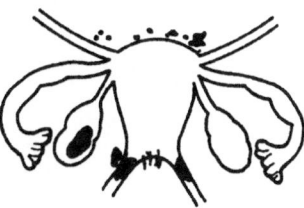

PERITONEUM
  Superficial Endo — 1-3cm - 2
R. OVARY
  Superficial Endo — <1 cm - 1
  Filmy Adhesions — <1/3. - 1
        TOTAL POINTS 4

PERITONEUM
  Deep Endo — >3cm - 6
R. OVARY
  Superficial Endo — <1cm - 1
  Filmy Adhesions — <1/3 - 1
L. OVARY
  Superficial Endo — <1cm - 1
        TOTAL POINTS 9

PERITONEUM
  Deep Endo — >3cm - 6
CULDESAC
  Partial Obliteration - 4
L. OVARY
  Deep Endo — 1-3cm - 16
        TOTAL POINTS 26

STAGE III (MODERATE)	STAGE IV (SEVERE)	STAGE IV (SEVERE)

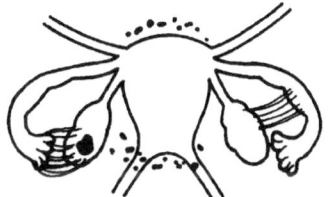 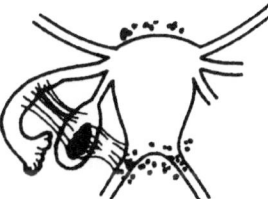 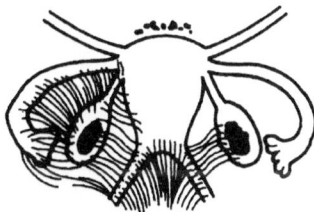

PERITONEUM
  Superficial Endo — >3cm - 4
R. TUBE
  Filmy Adhesions — <1/3 - 1
R. OVARY
  Filmy Adhesions — <1/3 - 1
L. TUBE
  Dense Adhesions — <1/3 - 16 *
L. OVARY
  Deep Endo — <1cm -4
  Dense Adhesions — <1/3 -4
        TOTAL POINTS 30

PERITONEUM
  Superficial Endo — >3cm - 4
L. OVARY
  Deep Endo — 1-3cm - 32 **
  Dense Adhesions — <1-3 - 8 **
L. TUBE
  Dense Adhesions — <1/3 - 8 **
        TOTAL POINTS 52

*Point assignment changed to 16
**Point assignment doubled

PERITONEUM
  Deep Endo — >3cm - 6
CULDESAC
  Complete Obliteration - 40
R. OVARY
  Deep Endo — 1-3cm - 16
  Dense Adhesions — <1/3 - 4
L. TUBE
  Dense Adhesions — >2/3 - 16
L. OVARY
  Deep Endo — 1-3 - 16
  Dense Adhesions — >2/3 -16
        TOTAL POINTS 114

Determination of the stage or degree of endometrial involvement is based on a weighted point sytem. Distribution of points has been arbitrarily determined and may require further revision or refinement as knowledge of the disease increases.

To ensure complete evaluation, inspection of the pelvis in a clockwise or counterclockwise fashion is encouraged. Number, size and location of endometrial implants, plaques, endometriomas and/or adhesions are noted. For example, five separate 0.5cm superficial implants on the peritoneum (2.5 cm total) would be assigned 2 points. (The surface of the uterus should be considered peritoneum.) The severity of the endometriosis or adhesions should be assigned the highest score only for peritoneum, ovary, tube or culdesac. For example, a 4cm superficial and a 2cm deep implant of the peritoneum should be given a score of 6 (not 8). A 4cm

deep endometrioma of the ovary associated with more than 3cm of superficial disease should be scored 20 (not 24).

In those patients with only one adnexa, points applied to disease of the remaining tube and ovary should be multiplied by two. **Points assigned may be circled and totaled. Aggregation of points indicates stage of disease (minimal, mild, moderate, or severe).

The presence of endometriosis of the bowel, urinary tract, fallopian tube, vagina, cervix, skin etc., should be documented under "additional endometriosis." Other pathology such as tubal occlusion, leiomyomata, urine anomaly, etc., should be documented under "associated pathology." All pathology should be depicted as specifically as possible on the sketch of pelvic organs and means of observation (laparoscopy or laparotomy) should be noted.

Part VII

Disorders of Ovarian Function and Subfertility

Contents

Summary

Transvaginal ultrasonography offers an accurate assessment of ovarian morphology. Characteristic patterns such as multifollicular and polycystic ovaries can be recognised. Ultrasound can also assess function: normal follicular and endometrial maturation can be monitored, and indirect evidence of ovulation obtained.

For infertile patients, ultrasound should be part of their initial assessment and can be incorporated into a "one stop" management protocol. A scan at this stage can exclude significant uterine and adnexal pathology. An assessment of tubal patency can be made using an ultrasound contrast agent. Both chronic and acute tubal disease have characteristic patterns that can be recognised.

Most women with pelvic inflammatory disease should have a laparoscopy to confirm the diagnosis, while salpingoscopy might be helpful in some cases.

For every microsurgical technique there is a laparoscopic alternative; the choice is dependent on the clinical state of the woman's pelvis.

Three-dimensional ultrasonography may help to clarify the diagnosis of congenital uterine abnormalities. Operative hysteroscopy can identify these and be used for surgery.

Key Points

- The true prevalence of polycystic ovaries based on ultrasonography is controversial
- The relationship between the morphological appearances of the ovary and function are poorly understood
- Tubal factors account for 25–30% of referrals for infertility
- Hystero-contrast-salpingography can be used as an initial screening test for tubal patency
- An ultrasound scan at an appropriate time of the cycle can exclude most uterine pathology, detect gross tubal pathology and give significant information about ovarion function
- Laparoscopy for pelvic inflammatory disease should be performed as soon as possible, and no longer than 24 hours after admission to hospital. It can be used for both diagnosis and treatment
- Three-dimensional ultrasonography provides all information necessary to classify uterine anomalies
- Subseptate uteri are associated with a higher first-trimester miscarriage rate
- An arcuate uterus appears to carry an elevated risk of second-trimester miscarriage and preterm labour compared with a normal uterus
- Information on reproductive risks associated with congenital uterine anomalies in low-risk women is very limited
- Partial and even complete uterine septa can be treated hysteroscopically

Chapter 29

Amenorrhoea and Polycystic Ovarian Syndrome

Asma Khalid and Tom Bourne

29.1 Introduction

Ultrasound can be used as a marker of ovarian and uterine function in the normal and abnormal menstrual cycle. The ovary and the endometrium have characteristic appearances at certain times and should be evaluated in the context of the patient's menstrual history. The stages of a normal menstrual cycle can be clearly seen on ultrasound using standard grey-scale imaging. Doppler studies give some insight into the pathophysiological changes that are occurring during the cycle and will be discussed later in this chapter, but as yet do not have a practical role in patient management. The most common application of transvaginal ultrasonography to date has been to monitor follicle size and number in women undergoing fertility treatment. Follicle size has been found to be more accurate than serum oestradiol levels in the prediction of ovulation, although a combination of both gives optimum results.

29.2 The Normal Menstrual Cycle

The morphological appearances of both the ovary and uterus show characteristic changes during the cycle. The proliferative-phase endometrium has a non-uniform echogenicity with a thin area of central brightness. The early follicular-phase ovary may mimic the appearance seen in women taking the combined oral contraceptive pill or those women with ovulatory dysfunction.

Ovulation generally occurs when the dominant follicle reaches 20–24 mm in diameter. Morphological changes include a blurring of the edge of the follicle, a reduction in size and the follicle contents becoming more echoic (Figure 29.1). Free fluid is also seen in the Pouch of Douglas.[1] The endometrium shows the classical hypoechoic halo when oestradiol levels reach their peak levels – the "triple line effect".[2] The exact physiology of these changes has yet to be determined. The endometrium then becomes uniformly highly echogenic and increases

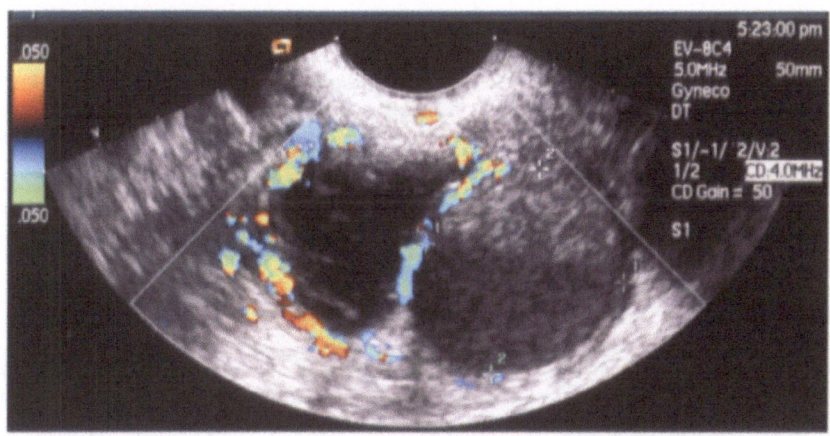

Figure 29.1. Haemorrhagic corpus luteum (*left*) with circular flow and a small endometrioma with "ground glass" appearance (*right*).

221

in thickness up to the time of menstruation. The corpus luteum shrinks in size when fertilisation has not occurred. Its morphology is varied, from an anechoic picture as seen in the dominant follicle to a haemorrhagic "speckled" appearance. Solid corpora lutea, multiloculations and irregular thick walls are not uncommon and it may be necessary to examine the patient in the follicular phase of the next cycle to exclude pathological ovarian cysts.

29.3 Polycystic Ovarian Syndrome

Polycystic ovarian syndrome (PCOS) encompasses a wide spectrum of symptoms and phenotypic variation. For this reason, it has been difficult to establish reproducible diagnostic criteria for this condition. Traditionally, the diagnosis has been made on the basis of ultrasonography. A polycystic ovary is characterised by the presence of a large-volume ovary containing dense hyperechogenic stroma and at least ten peripherally placed follicles (Figure 29.2).[3] Data relating to ovarian volume are difficult to interpret, as they do not seem to include the presence of corpora lutea in a polycystic ovary, which would markedly increase the ovarian volume without increasing the stromal volume. Much of the data relating to PCOS is historical and is based on transabdominal ultrasonography. The introduction of transvaginal ultrasound has provided better resolution of ovarian structures[4] and may provide a suitable alternative to histological examination.[5] Notwithstanding this, there is still debate surrounding the "gold standard" test for PCOS.

Even in early studies, the ovarian stroma of women with PCOS has been noted to be "bright" or hyperechogenic on ultrasonography. This is in keeping with the stromal hypertrophy seen on histological examination of removed ovaries. Attempts to quantify this increase in stroma have been a dominant feature of much of the work relating to

ultrasound and the polycystic ovary. It has been suggested that this ovarian stromal hypertrophy is directly related to androgenic dysfunction. Some data exist which provide objective measurements to directly support this hypothesis. The use of computer-assisted ultrasonography has provided some evidence,[6] although this has been disputed using intensity levels and pixelation technology.[7] The means to measure these multiple parameters in everyday practice are limited and practitioners using traditional definitions of PCOS are dependent on subjective estimations of stromal density. These are unfortunately dependent on machine settings and are therefore unreliable when considered in isolation, as the degree of hypertrophy will often be overestimated.[8] Other workers have tried to measure ovarian area in the maximal longitudinal section to try to provide an indirect method of measuring stromal density.[6,8] Incorporation of the stromal area into a ratio with ovarian area has provided some encouraging results. The stromal to ovarian area ratio has been shown to correlate with circulating levels of serum androgens.[9]

An increase in ovarian volume was noted to be a diagnostic factor in the original observations of PCOS. This has been supported by a series of 104 patients in whom it was found that ovarian volume was significantly greater in women with menstrual irregularity who had PCOS than in normal controls.[10] This has been corroborated in later studies.[9] However, there is no consensus as to the cutoff value for ovarian volume that may be used to define abnormality.

The early definitions of PCOS also incorporated the presence of increased numbers of peripherally distributed follicles. However, the presence of numerous, small, peripheral follicles is not specific to PCOS and can occur in other anovulatory states, multifollicular ovaries or even in the early follicular phase of the menstrual cycle.[5,6,11] Although similar patterns of disease should be observed in both

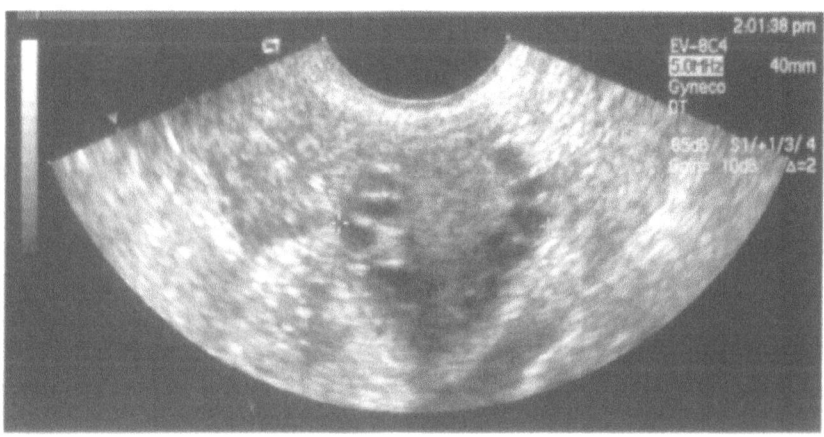

Figure 29.2. A polycystic ovary containing dense stroma and more than ten peripherally placed follicles.

ovaries, this is not always the case, and differences between right and left ovary have been described.[12] These should be borne in mind when making a diagnosis.

PCOS can be described in many cases as a state of chronic anovulation. This results in the endometrium being exposed to the prolonged mitogenic effects of oestrogen. These changes may be detected by the measurement of endometrial thickness, which can be used to select women who are at risk of endometrial hyperplasia. A cutoff value for endometrial thickness of greater than 7 mm has been suggested as an approach to selecting women who are at increased risk of endometrial pathology.[13]

The role of Doppler in the diagnosis of PCOS is limited. The dense stroma is better vacularised but no difference has been shown in the mean uterine artery pulsatility index in women with PCOS and control groups.[14] There have also been attempts to correlate stromal blood flow with the number of subcapsular follicles present;[15] however, these have not proved clinically useful.

29.4 Multifollicular Ovaries

In contrast to the classical polycystic ovary, multifollicular ovaries are normal in size or only slightly enlarged and contain six or more cysts 4–10 mm in diameter (Figure 29.3). They are not associated with hirsutism. Endocrine profiles reveal a normal level of serum luteinising hormone (LH), with a decreased follicle-stimulating hormone level. Ovarian morphology has been shown to revert to normal in women with amenorrhoea associated with weight loss after administration of gonadotrophin-releasing hormone (GnRH). This indicates the possibility that the multifollicular appearance is related to a hypothalamic disturbance of GnRH secretion.[16]

29.5 Ovulatory Dysfunction

The synchrony seen between the endometrium and the ovary in patients with regular menses is not present in anovulatory disorders. The endometrium may be disproportionately thickened with the presence of an inactive ovary. A simple ovarian cyst is not an uncommon finding. This would confirm the existence of an anovulatory cyclical pattern and be a reassuring sign in the presence of abnormal bleeding. The ovary may take the appearance of a classical polycystic ovary or other variants such as a multifollicular ovary. Physiological luteal or follicular cysts are not uncommon. The pathophysiology of anovulation may be explained by changes in the vasculature of the dominant follicle. An anecdotal report of a drug-induced luteinised unruptured follicle has suggested a reduction in vascularisation leading to a failure of blood flow velocity to peak in the immediate periovulatory period.[17] This is consistent with the view that changes in angiogenesis leading to a variation in oxygen tension in the follicle itself are prerequisites for normal ovulation. Subsequent studies have shown that indomethacin administration at the time of ovulation results in the formation of luteinised unruptured follicles. Such changes were associated with altered vascularity.[18] This is discussed in more detail below.

29.6 Blood Flow Studies of Ovarian and Uterine Function

29.6.1 The Ovary

Doppler studies of the normal corpus luteum and endometrium have shown an interesting insight into

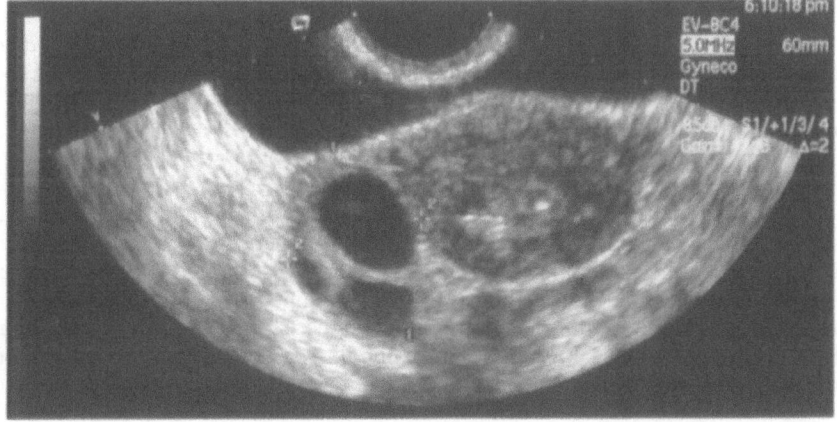

Figure 29.3. A multifollicular ovary next to the uterus.

the physiology of the menstrual cycle, but any role that transvaginal colour Doppler may have in the practical management of infertility problems has yet to be determined. However, preliminary data are of interest. Transvaginal colour Doppler has been used to monitor sequential changes in intrafollicular blood flow in the periovulatory period, and the data obtained related to defined biochemical indices. It is hoped that it will be possible to use information about ovarian blood flow both to predict ovulation, and to investigate ovulatory dysfunction.

Previous studies have shown that it is possible to assess ovarian blood flow during the normal menstrual cycle.[19] This study, using abdominal pulsed Doppler, showed significant changes in ovarian blood flow in the ovarian cycle; in particular there was a marked drop in blood flow impedance within the ovary during the late follicular and luteal phase of the cycle. Although the authors interpret their data as being from the ovarian artery, it is more likely that serial measurements of intraovarian flow have been recorded. Using transvaginal colour Doppler, these areas of vascularity can be clearly visualised on the follicle rim, or within or around the corpus luteum. Transvaginal pulsed Doppler has been subsequently used to record blood flow in the corpus luteum in patients undergoing in-vitro fertilisation following embryo transfer.[20] In the absence of colour flow imaging, the authors had to move the sample volume gate (of 3.5 mm) over the ovarian stroma until suitable waveforms had been obtained. Again, the waveforms are therefore more likely to reflect intraovarian rather than ovarian artery blood flow. Impedance to blood flow was measured on days 3 and 10 following embryo transfer, and significantly higher impedance to flow was observed in the corpora lutea of women who failed to become pregnant.

Kurjak and co-workers have also assessed ovarian and uterine blood flow in the menstrual cycle.[21] Their data suggest a drop in impedance to blood flow within the ovary containing the dominant follicle just prior to ovulation, and with a persistently lower blood flow impedance recorded from vessels within the corpus luteum. In a more detailed study, transvaginal colour Doppler has since been used to monitor intensively vascular events in the periovulatory follicle.[22] Colour Doppler facilitates the detection of small vascular areas in the ovarian stroma and follicle rim that are easy to miss when applying a pulsed Doppler range gate "blind". In this study the aim was to assess each patient every 3–4 hours from the time of the serum LH surge up to the formation of the corpus luteum. Blood flow velocity waveforms from the follicular rim were first seen at the time of the LH surge (or oestradiol peak). There is a sequential increase in vascularity in the

follicle rim from the time of the LH rise, at its peak, and finally just prior to ovulation and the formation of the corpus luteum. These data are supported by studies of ovarian blood flow and volume in laboratory animals,[23] and the fact that red blood cells have been seen in the granulosa cell layer between the time of the LH peak and presumed ovulation.[24] A report of the vascular changes at the time of ovulation shows increased vascularity on the innermost rim of the follicle, and a coincident surge in blood flow velocity just prior to follicular rupture.[25] This may represent the dilatation of new vessels that have developed between the relatively vascular theca cell layer and the normally hypoxic granulosa cell layer of the follicle. Disruption of these vascular changes would have profound effects on the oxygen concentration across the follicular epithelium.[25]

We have reported one case of drug-induced luteinised unruptured follicle, and these preliminary data suggest a reduction in vascularisation and a failure of the blood flow velocity to peak in the immediate preovulatory period.[17] This is consistent with the view that the changes in oxygen tension within the follicle brought about by angiogenesis are necessary for normal ovulation to occur. Transvaginal colour Doppler may be used to monitor hormonal and other methods of increasing or decreasing intrafollicular blood flow. We have subsequently observed eight women with normal ovarian cycles and studied the effect of indomethacin on vascularity around the time of expected ovulation and the formation of such drug-induced luteinised unruptured follicles. These additional data further support the view that changes in vascularity are an important part of the normal ovulatory process, and that its inhibition at a crucial stage may lead to ovulatory dysfunction. Furthermore, steroids that inhibit angiogenesis in the presence of heparin have already been described;[26] if the process of ovulation could be inhibited independently of the main pathways of steroidogenesis, novel methods of contraception might be envisaged. Initial evidence suggests that transvaginal colour flow mapping may be used to monitor progress towards these objectives.

29.6.2 The Uterus

Endometrial thickness can be both measured and characterised in stimulated cycles and has been suggested as a way of predicting successful implantation. Attempts to find markers of endometrial receptivity have led to the investigation of uterine blood flow as a possible factor. It has been shown that transvaginal colour Doppler can be used to obtain reproducible flow velocity waveforms from the uterine arteries at any time during the menstrual cycle.[27] It is apparent that there are complex relationships between the concentration of ovarian hormones in peripheral venous plasma and uterine artery blood flow parameters.

Steer et al.[28] used transvaginal colour Doppler to study uterine artery blood flow in 23 healthy women. The overall trend suggested an increase in perfusion of the uterus during the course of the menstrual cycle. It is particularly interesting that the mean time of lowest blood flow impedance occurs at the time of peak luteal function, which is the time when implantation is most likely. These data are also supported by those of Kurjak et al.[21] In this study of 150 women of proven fertility, the impedance to blood flow in the uterine arteries was at its lowest by day 18 of the cycle. As the authors point out, the differences in the blood flow indices were small between the proliferative and luteal phases of the cycle, and it is uncertain of what use such data will be clinically. It is possible that the differences in flow seen in this study are less convincing than those of Steer et al.[28] because of the use of the resistance index, which tends to be less discriminating between data sets than the pulsatility index.

Having shown these changes in the normal menstrual cycle, it is now possible to hypothesise that suboptimal uterine blood flow at critical times in the menstrual cycle may be associated with infertility. A non-invasive assay of uterine receptivity would enable a clinician to cryopreserve embryos if uterine conditions are adverse, and reduce the number of transferred embryos when conditions are suboptimal. Steer et al. have suggested that studies of uterine artery blood flow may be used to predict a hostile uterine environment prior to embryo transfer.[29] Women who failed to achieve a pregnancy in this study had significantly raised impedance to blood flow in their uterine arteries. There was a zero implantation rate associated with a mean uterine artery pulsatility index of greater than 3.0. According to these data, if this figure was used as the upper limit for the transfer of embryos, the sensitivity of the test for predicting an unreceptive uterus and thus failed implantation would be 35.2%, the specificity 100%, and the positive predictive value of a high impedance blood flow result also 100%.

If substantiated, these data may have important clinical implications, as those women with poor uterine perfusion could be advised that a pregnancy is unlikely in their current treatment cycle, and to have their embryos cryopreserved for transfer at a later date. Colour Doppler may also be used to monitor ways of manipulating the uterine environment. Transvaginal colour Doppler measurement of uterine artery blood flow therefore has the potential for use as a biological assay of uterine receptivity, and may theoretically substantially improve the pregnancy rate per treatment cycle. Prospective controlled clinical trials based on these preliminary data are needed.

29.7 Conclusion

The introduction of ultrasonography truly revolutionised our understanding of the pathophysiology associated with the ovarian cycle. It allows us to recognise normality and assess appropriate functional changes in both the ovary and uterus. It has facilitated the monitoring of ovarian function in both natural and stimulated cycles and can also help to characterise dysfunction. Of interest is the lack of real standardisation available for the diagnosis of common ovarian dysfunction. The diagnosis of polycystic ovaries is often based on the subjective impression of an ultrasound image, and there are few data to establish interobserver variation. There is an overlap between so-called multifollicular ovaries and polycystic ovaries. However, the former reflect hypothalamic–pituitary dysfunction and the latter a primary ovarian problem. Classifying these functional changes in the ovary remains a challenge. Menstrual disturbance may also be associated with ovarian dysfunction and this may be seen with ultrasonography in the form of haemorrhagic or physiological cysts.

Doppler studies of pelvic blood flow reveal interesting insights into ovarian and uterine pathophysiology, but to date the clinical applications of this technique remain limited. However, using Doppler studies of pelvic blood flow as a bioassay of drug effects on the uterus and ovary may yet lead to enhanced approaches to the management of the infertile patient.

References

1. Bourne TH, Jurkovic D, Waterstone J et al. (1991) Intrafollicular blood flow during human ovulation. Ultrasound Obstet Gynecol 1:53–59
2. Greenwald GS, Terranova PF (1988) Follicular secretion and its control. In: Knobel E, Neill JD (eds) Physiology of reproduction. Raven Press, New York, p 387
3. Adams J, Polson DW, Franks S (1986) Prevalence of polycystic ovaries in women with anovulation and idiopathic hirsuitism. Br Med J 293:355–359
4. Takahashi K, Nishigaki A, Eda Y et al. (1990) Transvaginal ultrasound is an effective method for screening in polycystic ovarian disease: preliminary study. Gynecol Obstet Invest 30:34–36
5. Pache TD, Wladimiroff JW, Hop WCJ et al. (1992) How to discriminate between normal and polycystic ovaries: transvaginal ultrasound study. Radiology 183:421–423
6. Dewailly D, Robert Y, Helin I et al. (1994) Ovarian stromal hypertrophy in hyperandrogenic women. Clin Endocrinol 41:557–562

7. Buckett WM, Bouzayen R, Watkin KL et al. (1999) Ovarian stromal echogenicity in women with normal and polycystic ovaries. Hum Reprod 14(3):618-621
8. Robert Y, Dubrulle F, Gaillandre L et al. (1995) Ultrasound assessment of ovarian stroma hypertrophy in hyperandrogenism and ovulation disorders: visual analysis versus computerised quantification. Fert Steril 64:307-312
9. Fulghesu AM, Ciampelli M, Belosi C et al. (2001) A new ultrasound criterion for the diagnosis of polycystic ovary syndrome: the ovarian stroma/total area ratio. Fert Steril 76:326-331
10. Takahashi K, Eda Y, Okada S et al. (1993) Morphological assessment of polycystic ovary using transvaginal ultrasound. Hum Reprod 8(6):844-849
11. Dewailly D (2000) Definition of polycystic ovary syndrome. Hum Fertil 3:73-76
12. Atiomo WU, Pearson S, Shaw S et al. (2000) Ultrasound criteria in the diagnosis of polycystic ovarian syndrome. Ultrasound Med Biol 26(6):977-980
13. Cheung AP (2001) Ultrasound and menstrual history in predicting endometrial hyperplasia in polycystic ovary syndrome. Obstet Gynecol 98:325-331
14. Resende AV, Mendes MC, Dias de Moura M et al. (2001) Doppler study of the uterine arteries and ovarian stroma in patients with polycystic ovary syndrome. Gynecol Obstet Invest 52:153-157
15. Battaglia C, Genazzani AD, Salvatori M et al. (1999) Doppler, ultrasonographic and endocrinological environment with regard to the number of small subcapsular follicles in polycystic ovary syndrome. Gynecol Endocrinol 13:123-129
16. Adams J, Franks S, Polson DW et al. (1985) Multifollicular ovaries: clinical and endocrine features and response to pulsatile gonadotrophin releasing hormone. Lancet 2:1375-1379
17. Bourne TH, Reynolds K, Waterstone J et al. (1991) Paracetamol-associated luteinised unruptured follicle syndrome: effect on intra-follicular blood flow. Ultrasound Obstet Gynecol 1:420-425
18. Athanasiou S, Bourne TH, Khalid A et al. (1996) Effects of indomethacin on follicular structure and function over the peri ovulatory period. Fert Steril 65:556-560
19. Hata K, Hata T, Senoh D et al. (1990) Change in ovarian arterial compliance during the human menstrual cycle by Doppler ultrasound. Br J Obstet Gynaecol 97:163-166
20. Baber RJ, McSweeney MB, Gill RW et al. (1988) Transvaginal pulsed Doppler ultrasound assessment of blood flow to the corpus luteum in IVF patients following embryo transfer. Br J Obstet Gynaecol 95:1226-1230
21. Kurjak A, Kupesik-Urek S, Schulman H et al. (1991) Transvaginal color flow Doppler in the assessment of ovarian and uterine blood flow in infertile women. Fert Steril 56:870-873
22. Collins W, Jurkovic D, Bourne TH et al. (1991) Ovarian morphology, endocrine function and intra-follicular blood flow during the peri-ovulatory period. Hum Reprod 6:319-324
23. Tanaka N, Espey LL, Okamura H (1989) Increase in ovarian blood volume during ovulation in the gonadotrophin-primed immature rat. Biol Reprod 40:762-768
24. Bomsel-Helmreich O, Gougeon A, Thebault A et al. (1979) Healthy and atretic human follicles in the preovulatory phase: differences in evolution of follicular morphology and steroid content of follicular fluid. J Clin Endocrinol Metab 48:686-694
25. Gosden RG, Byatt-Smith JG (1986) Oxygen concentration across the ovarian follicular epithelium: model, predictions and implications. Hum Reprod 1:65-68
26. Ingber DE, Madri JA, Folkman J (1996) A possible mechanism for inhibition of angiogenesis by angiostatic steroids: induction of capillary basement membrane dissolution. Endocrinology 119:1768-1775
27. Scholtes MCW, Wladimiroff JW, van Rijen HJM et al. (1989) Uterine and ovarian flow velocity waveforms in the normal menstrual cycle: a transvaginal Doppler study. Fert Steril 52:981-985
28. Steer CV, Tan SL, Mason BA et al. (1994) Midluteal phase vaginal color Doppler assessment of uterine artery impedance in a subfertile population. Fert Steril 61:53-58
29. Steer CV, Mills CL, Campbell S (1991) Vaginal colour Doppler assessment on the day of embryo transfer (ET) accurately predicts patients in an in-vitro fertilisation programme with suboptimal uterine perfusion who fail to become pregnant. Ultrasound Obstet Gynecol 1(S1): 79

Chapter 30

The Assessment of Tubal Patency: Hystero-Contrast-Salpingography

Karen Jermy and Tom Bourne

30.1 Introduction

Tubal factors are among the most common causes of infertility in women and account for approximately 25–30% of referrals. Demonstration of tubal patency will thus dictate subsequent management; if bilateral tubal occlusion is demonstrated, the patient can be referred for in-vitro fertilisation or tubal surgery. If, however, at least one tube is patent, ovarian stimulation can be recommended, if appropriate.

Established methods of assessing tubal pathology include X-ray hysterosalpingography (HSG) and laparoscopy with dye insufflation.

Laparoscopy allows direct visualisation of peritubal adhesions, endometriosis and pelvic anatomy, and is considered the "gold standard" in the assessment of tubal patency. It is, however, an invasive procedure with the associated risks of general anaesthesia and possible bowel and blood vessel injury. It also provides no information relating to the internal structure of the uterus and ovaries. X-ray HSG provides an assessment of the internal contours of the uterine cavity and fallopian tubes, but offers no information on other pelvic pathology. Although easier, safer and less expensive than laparoscopy, the patient is exposed to ionising radiation and intravenous contrast agents, which have the potential to provoke adverse reactions. The technique also requires the services of the radiology department, and when compared to laparoscopy, concordance rates vary from 57 to 75%.^{1,2}

Transvaginal ultrasonography has an integral role in the investigation and treatment of infertility, providing a non-invasive, cheap, accessible and highly reproducible assessment. B-mode imaging provides highly accurate information regarding not only ovarian volume and morphology, facilitating precise follicular development and guided oocyte retrieval, but also congenital and acquired abnormalities of the uterus. Gross pathology of the fallopian tubes, such as a hydrosalpinx and tubo-ovarian abscess, can be demonstrated easily using the transvaginal probe, as both have characteristic features.^{3} Evaluation of healthy fallopian tubes, using B-mode ultrasonography alone, is difficult as no natural fluid/tissue interfaces exist.

Hystero-contrast-salpingography (HyCoSy) involves the introduction of fluid into the fallopian tubes via the uterine cavity. Sterile saline is an echo-free, or negative, ultrasonographic contrast agent. It has an established role in the sonographic assessment of endometrial and intracavity pathology, such as intrauterine adhesions, polyps, submucous fibroids and congenital uterine abnormalities.^{4,5} A number of studies have evaluated its role in the assessment of tubal patency, with varying results. Intraluminal flow cannot be demonstrated using negative contrast HyCoSy alone, the visualisation of saline in the pouch of Douglas being suggestive of patency of at least one tube, with no scope for localisation of any pathology.^{1,5,6}

The use of positive echocontrast agents such as Echovist (Schering AG, Berlin, Germany) and air/saline mixtures to demonstrate tubal patency has evolved from their use in echocardiography. They both allow consistent visualisation of the fallopian tubes using transvaginal ultrasound and provide a rapid, well-tolerated screening method, which can be performed as part of the initial assessment of the subfertile patient within the outpatient setting. Echovist is the ultrasonographic contrast agent that has been evaluated in the majority of studies, and appears to provide comparable information concerning tubal patency to that achieved by laparoscopy and HSG.

227

Before reviewing its current role alongside laparoscopy with dye insufflation and HSG, we will describe the practical aspects of HyCoSy in more detail.

30.2 Procedure

Hystero-contrast-salpingography is an outpatient procedure, and as such can be carried out in any gynaecology clinic that is equipped with ultrasound equipment. As with any procedure involving instrumentation of the cervix, resuscitation facilities must be available, in case of possible vagal reactions. No analgesia is routinely required. We also recommend antibiotic prophylaxis.

Contraindications to the procedure include concurrent acute genital infections, pregnancy, heavy vaginal bleeding and, when Echovist is the contrast medium, galactosaemia.

The examination should be performed in the preovulatory phase of the cycle; this reduces the chances of disturbing an early pregnancy, and also minimises the possibility of infection.

A Cusco's speculum is passed and after gentle vaginal disinfection with an antiseptic solution, a 2 mm uterine catheter is inserted into the uterine cavity. As the initial part of the examination involves examining the endometrium, better results may be obtained by inserting the catheter only as far as the internal os. The balloon must not be fully inflated within the cervical canal, as this will cause discomfort, but just enough to prevent backflow of contrast. The speculum is removed and the transvaginal probe inserted.

The examination of the premenopausal uterus, tubes and ovaries has been described previously.[7] The diagnostic accuracy of transvaginal ultrasonography has been shown to be similar to hysteroscopy. In a study of 200 patients, assuming hysteroscopy to be the gold standard, the sensitivity of transvaginal ultrasonography for the detection of uterine abnormalities was 98.9% and the false-positive rate 5.5%.[8] A more detailed assessment of the uterine cavity is best achieved using sterile saline rather than a hyperechoic contrast medium such as Echovist.[9] The strong acoustic shadow of contrast media such as Echovist will often obscure details of endometrial pathology.

Having assessed the uterus, the catheter can be pushed fully into the uterine cavity and the balloon fully inflated. Again, care must be taken at this time, as the amount of patient discomfort associated with the procedure seems related to fully inflating the balloon in the cervical canal, or to injecting too great a volume of contrast too quickly.

Echovist is prepared immediately before injection. It consists of a suspension of galactose microparticles in a 20% galactose solution, which, when agitated, produces a suspension of microscopic air bubbles. Having filled the uterine cavity with a few millilitres of contrast media, the tubes should then begin to fill quickly. In the majority of cases, B-mode imaging alone will be sufficient to visualise flow of contrast through the tube (Figures 30.1 and 30.2), with spill into the peritoneal cavity as evidence of patency. The flow in the tube should change easily with the degree of pressure on the syringe. Tubal patency can otherwise be defined as the visualisation of steady tubal flow lasting for more than 10 seconds in one imaged tubal section. Typically, 10 ml contrast media, injected in 1–2 ml aliquots, will be needed up to a maximum possible volume of 30 ml. The whole procedure takes approximately 20 minutes.

30.3 The Role of Doppler

Complete visualisation of the entire tube may not always be possible using B-mode ultrasonography alone. In a study investigating 210 patients for infertility, 404 fallopian tubes were evaluated with B-mode transvaginal ultrasonography and Echovist-200. The additional use of pulsed-wave Doppler improved the results in 31 cases where no flow of contrast media could be demonstrated in the distal portion of the tube using B-mode alone. This led to overall concordance rates with laparoscopy of 92%.[10]

The colour Doppler gate is placed over the presumed mural portion of the tube and will detect the movement of contrast (Figure 30.3). This can be used to direct the positioning of a pulsed Doppler range gate to obtain a flow velocity waveform. The demonstration of a pulsed Doppler waveform from the tube is diagnostic of tubal patency; the amplitude of the waveform will be proportional to the amount of pressure put on the syringe. When a bolus of contrast agent is injected, characteristic Doppler spectra can be generated, representing patent, partially occluded and completely occluded tubes.[11]

30.4 Comparison of Hystero-Contrast-Salpingography with Hysterosalpingography and Laparoscopy

For HyCoSy to have a role in the primary assessment of tubal patency, it must have similar diagnostic capabilities to the established reference methods of laparoscopy and dye and HSG. The majority of studies have evaluated the ability of

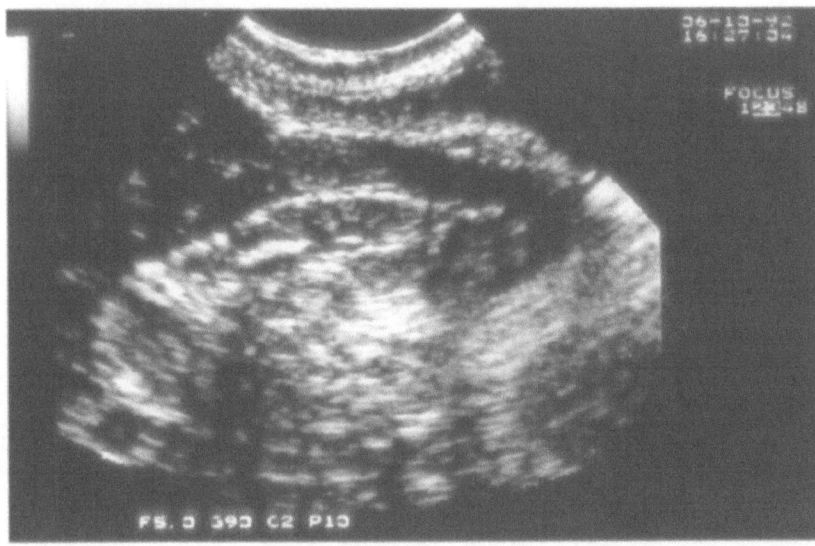

Figure 30.1 Pre-Echovist: this B-mode image demonstrates the intramural portion of the uterus and the proximal fallopian tube.

HyCoSy to demonstrate tubal patency, with Echovist as the ultrasonographic contrast agent. The largest series presented is a meta-analysis from Germany. Almost 1000 patients were assessed, from three clinical studies, comparing Echovist–200 and B-mode transvaginal ultrasonography with HSG or chromolaparoscopy. The findings demonstrated 83% concordance in detecting tubal pathology when HyCoSy was compared to either reference method. Hystero-contrast-salpingography showed "false" occlusion in 10 and 13% of tubes and "false" patency in 7 and 4% of tubes when compared to laparoscopy and dye and HSG respectively. The concordance between laparoscopic and HSG findings for individual tubes was 76%.[12]

Peritubal adhesions, detected by laparoscopy, were found to be the reason for false-positive sonographic tubal findings in 60% of cases; the remainder were possibly due to tubal spasm.[11] Where tubal spasm is suspected, the HyCoSy procedure is safe enough simply to be repeated at a later time.

All studies are based on either HSG or laparoscopy and dye, or both, as the reference methods, despite both having limitations. They all have similar rates of concordance between HyCoSy and

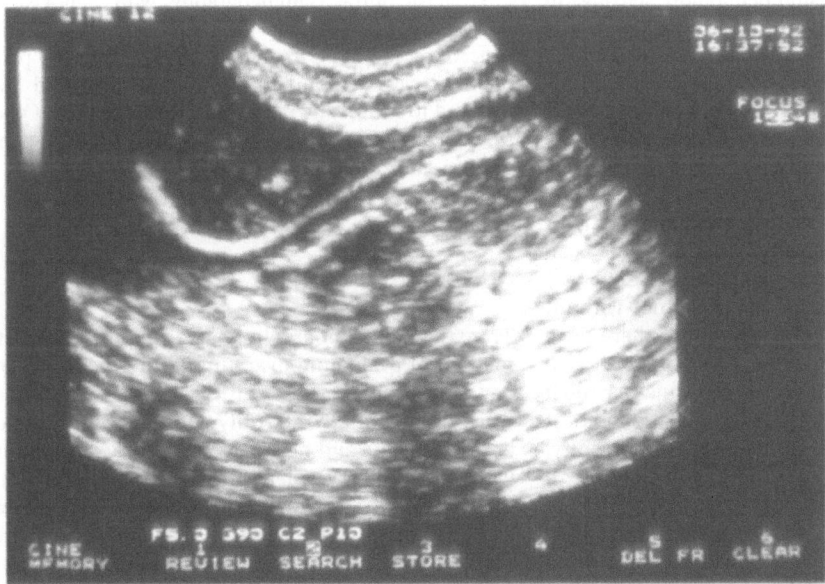

Figure 30.2 Post-Echovist: following the injection of Echovist, the contrast can be seen tracking towards the distal portion of the tube.

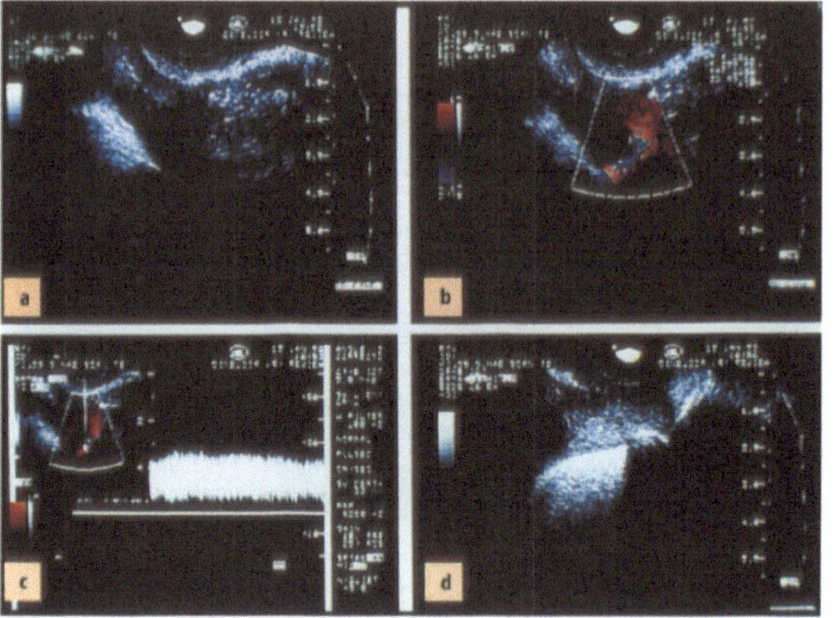

Figure 30.3 View (**a**) shows a suboptimal image where it is uncertain whether contrast is passing through the tube. Colour Doppler can easily demonstrate flow of contrast (**b**) and pulsed Doppler confirms this further in view (**c**). After waiting and adopting a different scanning plane flow can be seen in the mural and ampullary regions of the fallopian tubes (**d**).

the chosen reference method but vary markedly in their sensitivity and specificity.[11–18]

Although Echovist has been the main echogenic contrast agent evaluated, other non-commercial contrast media have been studied. The use of "agitated saline" is a simple technique whereby 10 ml of saline and 10 ml of air are shaken vigorously and then injected into the uterine cavity (keeping the syringe tilted downwards to avoid injection of air). The microbubbles produce bright scintillating echoes on ultrasound, which are easily visible as they pass down the fallopian tube. In a study comparing this technique with HSG, there was 85% concordance in detecting tubal patency, with ultrasound being more sensitive in detecting uterine pathology.[14]

Hystero-contrast-salpingography compares favourably to both established methods, as a reproducible assessment of tubal patency. It is a well-tolerated outpatient procedure, which avoids exposure to ionising radiation and possible allergic contrast agents. There is no general anaesthetic involved, and when combined with colour Doppler and echo-free contrast agents such as saline, can provide detailed information on the uterine cavity and ovarian function. The procedure is not without drawbacks. As with all new methods, there is a learning curve associated with the technique. It also fails to provide information concerning peritubal adhesions or endometriosis. It is this benefit of laparoscopy that makes its increased morbidity, compared to HyCoSy and HSG, tolerable as a primary investigative technique.

A recent study in Oxford questioned the need for routine laparoscopy. Of 140 women who underwent laparoscopy as part of their routine infertility work-up, 71% had normal (minimal or no endometriosis) findings. This would suggest that in comparable populations, non-surgical methods should form the first line of investigation.[17] This study's conclusions were echoed by two others, where a simple ultrasound-based approach, utilising HyCoSy, was used to investigate the infertile couple.[19,20] A degree of information concerning tubal mobility and the presence of periadnexal adhesions can be obtained during HyCoSy, and from the sonographic delineation that is afforded from the presence of saline in the pouch of Douglas.[21]

Hystero-contrast-salpingography with Echovist as the contrast agent is generally a well-tolerated procedure; the most frequent adverse event was pain; rated as severe in up to 10% of women, and was believed to be directly related to tubal occlusion. Other side-effects included vasovagal reactions, flushing and nausea, and occurred in up to 7% of women.[12]

30.5 Conclusions

Transvaginal sonography is a highly accurate method of evaluating ovarian and uterine morphology, and should form an integral part of the initial work-up within the infertility clinic. The addition of both echogenic and negative contrast media, with or without colour Doppler, provides an extension to this basic examination, facilitating a sensitive assessment of the internal morphology of the uterine cavity as well as the patency of the fallopian tubes. The procedure is cheap, quick, well tolerated, safe and reproducible; its ability to demonstrate tubal patency compares favourably with that of HSG and laparoscopy and dye.

Such characteristics lend themselves to establishing HyCoSy as an initial screening tool. It is unlikely ever to replace HSG and laparoscopy and dye completely, but in those patients where tubal patency is demonstrated, early referral for ovulation induction can be facilitated.

The demonstration of tubal, uterine, endometrial or ovarian pathology during this initial assessment will allow appropriate referral for operative laparoscopic interventions, enabling appropriate management strategies to be planned from the outset. This can be enhanced by the investigation taking place solely within the infertility clinic, rather than in several different departments.

Echovist has established itself as more than a research tool in the initial assessment of tubal patency using HyCoSy. The reproducibility of other non-commercial echogenic contrast agents, such as saline and air mixtures, warrants further evaluation. They may provide a more cost-effective, simple alternative to Echovist, while providing comparable information.

References

1. Stern J, Peters A, Coulam C (1992) Colour Doppler ultrasonography assessment of tubal patency: a comparison study with traditional techniques. Fert Steril 58:897–900
2. Kierse M, Vanderwellen R (1973) A comparison of hysterosalpingography and laparoscopy in the investigation of infertility. Obstet Gynecol 41:685–688
3. Timor-Tritsch IE, Lerner JP, Monteagudo A et al (1998) Transvaginal sonographic markers of tubal inflammatory disease. Ultrasound Obstet Gynecol 12(1):56–66
4. Parsons AK, Lense JJ (1993) Sonohysterography for endometrial abnormalities: preliminary results. J Clin Ultrasound 21:87–95
5. Bonilla-Musoles F, Simon C, Serra V (1992) An assessment of hysterosalpingography (HSSG) as a diagnostic tool for uterine cavity defects and tubal patency. J Clin Ultrasound 20:175–181
6. Randolph R, Ying Y, Maier D et al (1986) Comparison of real time ultrasonography, hysterosalpingography and laparoscopy/hysteroscopy in the evaluation of uterine abnormalities and tubal patency. Fert Steril 46:828–832
7. Bourne TH (1991) Transvaginal color Doppler in gynecology. Ultrasound Obstet Gynecol 1:359–373
8. Narayan R, Goswamy R (1993) Transvaginal sonography of the uterine cavity with hysteroscopic correlation in the investigation of infertility. Ultrasound Obstet Gynecol 3:129–133
9. Balen FG, Allen CM, Siddle NC et al (1993) Ultrasound contrast hysterosalpingography – evaluation as an outpatient procedure. Br J Radiol 66:592–599
10. Kalogirou D, Antoniou G, Botsis D et al (1997) Is color Doppler necessary in the evaluation of tubal patency by hysterosalpingo-contrast sonography. Clin Exp Obstet Gynecol 24(2):101–103
11. Kleinkauf-Houcken A, Hüneke B, Lindner CH et al (1997) Combining B-mode ultrasound with pulsed wave Doppler for the assessment of tubal patency. Hum Reprod 12:2457–2460
12. Holz K, Becker R, Schurmann R (1997) Ultrasound in the investigation of tubal patency. A meta-analysis of three comparative studies of Echovist-200 including 1007 women. Zentralblatt fur Gynakologie 119(8):366–373
13. Spalding H, Martikainen H, Tekay A et al (1997) A randomised study comparing air to Echovist as a contrast medium in the assessment of tubal patency in infertile women using transvaginal ultrasonography. Hum Reprod 12:2461–2464
14. Chenia F, Hofmeyr GJ, Moolla S et al (1997) Sonographic hydrotubation using agitated saline: a new technique for improving fallopian tube visualisation. Br J Radiol 70:833–836
15. Campbell S, Bourne TH, Tan SL et al (1994) Hysterosalpingo contrast sonography (HyCoSy) and its future role within the investigation of infertility in Europe. Ultrasound Obstet Gynecol 4:245–253
16. Volpi E, Zuccaro G, Patriarca A et al (1996) Transvaginal sonographic tubal patency testing using air and saline solution as contrast media in a routine infertility clinic setting. Ultrasound Obstet Gynecol 7:43–48
17. Ayida G, Chamberlain P, Barlow D et al (1997) Is routine diagnostic laparoscopy for infertility still justified? A pilot study assessing the use of hysterosalpingo-contrast sonography and magnetic resonance imaging. Hum Reprod 7:1436–1439
18. Dietrich M, Suren A, Hinney B et al (1996) Evaluation of tubal patency by hysterocontrast sonography (HyCoSy Echovist) and its correlation with laparoscopic findings. J Clin Ultrasound 24:523–527
19. Hauge K, Flo K, Riedhart M et al (2000) Can ultrasound-based investigations replace laparoscopy and hysteroscopy in infertility? Eur J Obstet Gynecol Reprod Biol 92(1):167–170
20. Strandell A, Bourne T, Bergh C et al (2000) A simplified ultrasound based infertility investigation protocol and its implications for patient management. J Assist Reprod Genet 17(2):87–92
21. Allhbadia GN (1992) Fallopian tubes and ultrasonography: the Sion experience. Fert Steril 58:901–907

Chapter 31

Laparoscopic Treatment of Tubal Infectious Disease

Filip De Bruyne

31.1 Introduction

When the female genital tract is attacked by infectious organisms, "the acute clinical syndrome associated with ascending spread of micro-organisms from the vagina or cervix to the endometrium, fallopian tubes and/or contiguous structures", defined as pelvic inflammatory disease (PID), occurs. The diagnosis of this entity is difficult because of the wide variation of signs and symptoms. Many episodes of PID are subclinical and not recognised by the patient. Added to this scarcity of clear clinical information, doctors often delay diagnosing the condition, for the same reasons. Acute and silent PID have a certain morbidity. They are responsible for the development of tubo-ovarian abscess as the end stage of acute disease, as well as for the development of chronic pelvic pain, dyspareunia and infertility as long-term sequelae.

31.2 Acute Disease

The role of endoscopy in the management of acute disease can be divided into diagnostic and therapeutic.

Laparoscopy can be used to diagnose the presence of PID. However, laparoscopy cannot diagnose endometritis, so it is useful only in the detection of salpingitis or abscess. In some countries, the laparoscope is used more widely for the diagnosis of PID, but in general, the diagnosis is still made clinically. Initially, one would not expect to perform a laparoscopy whenever there is the slightest suspicion of PID. However, the clinical diagnosis is imprecise, so every extra diagnostic tool to prevent long-term morbidity is welcome, even when it is invasive.

In a recent study to evaluate the reliability of clinical and laboratory data in predicting laparoscopic findings in women with acute salpingitis, Eschenbach et al[1] found no positive association between the severity of clinical and laboratory manifestations and tubal occlusion, suggesting that tubal occlusion with subsequent infertility may be as common in the outpatient with mild clinical findings of salpingitis as in the hospitalised patient with signs of peritonitis. As clinical and laboratory manifestations do not reflect accurately the degree of tubal damage and the nature of the peritoneal response, the authors concluded that these alone were not adequate for classifying the extent and nature of baseline inflammation. Laparoscopy for PID should be performed as soon as possible, and no longer than 24 hours after admission to hospital. It enables the correct diagnosis to be made and immediate therapeutic action to be taken. Hillis[2] evaluated the delayed care of PID as a risk factor for impaired fertility. A 3- to 9-day interval between the onset of pain and treatment doubled the likelihood of later tubal infertility. When the delay increased to ≤ 10 days, a 3.5-fold increase in impaired fertility was reported.

According to the description of various degrees of salpingitis,[3] mild salpingitis consists of tubal erythema and oedema, purulent or fibrinous exudate, no adhesions or only small-diameter "violin-string" adhesions, tubal mobility and grossly open fimbriae. Moderate salpingitis consists of more severe fallopian tube swelling, tubal immobility and inability to see the fimbriae clearly. Severe salpingitis consists of fallopian tubes in which the fimbriae are obviously closed, with or without pelvic peritonitis or abscesses.

Apart from its diagnostic role, endoscopy also plays a role in the therapy of PID. At laparoscopy, a thorough investigation of the pelvis is important and pregnancy must first be ruled out. After tubal microbiological sampling, therapy with antibiotics effective against the most common causative organisms should be started. The end stage of PID is a situation in which a pyosalpinx or tubo-ovarian abscesses can develop. Whenever collections of pus are present or fibrinous exudate causes adhesions, they can be drained or lysed, preferably by blunt or aquadissection, respecting the cleavage plains between tissues. Early in the development of PID, the adhesions between different structures can be separated easily. This is not true when the adhesions are dense and well vascularised, as in longstanding PID. Dissection should be performed with extreme caution, as structures such as the bowel are very fragile at that time and there is a risk of laceration if too much force is exerted. If bleeding occurs during the course of such an adhesiolysis, the creation of a false route must be ruled out. After all pus collections have been opened and drained, the resection of all necrotic tissue and removal of fibrinous material is indicated. The abdomen should be rinsed thoroughly with warm saline. During the cleaning of the pelvis, the patient can be brought alternately in the head-up and head-down position to allow the cleaning of the whole abdominal cavity. The presence of perihepatic adhesions should be looked for. Inspection of the colon descending and the appendix may be informative in the differential diagnosis. The total amount of rinsing fluid often exceeds 3–5 litres. In this kind of surgery, there is no place for extensive use of scissors or electrosurgical devices.

If conservative surgical therapy is not possible or is ineffective, salpingectomy or unilateral adnexectomy, or even total abdominal hysterectomy with bilateral salpingo-oophorectomy may be necessary.

Every physician is concerned about the devastating effects of a PID episode on the reproductive potential of a young woman. In a large cohort study, Weström[4] documented that the visually assessed severity of a PID episode, as well as the total number of PID attacks, were predictors of fertility. Every new episode almost doubled the rate of tubal infertility.

It is advisable to organise a second-look laparoscopy (SLL) when the woman wishes to become pregnant in the future. The exact timing of SLL is a matter of controversy, but can be proposed 3 months after the start of treatment. During the SLL, reparative surgery with meticulous preparation of the female genital tract can be performed when necessary. Raiga[5] presented a group of 39 patients treated laparoscopically for the presence of tubo-ovarian abscess. Four patients were lost to follow-up. Second-look laparoscopy was proposed to the remaining 35 patients, three of whom were also lost. At SLL, all patients had adhesions and corrective surgery was offered. The follow-up consisted of 32 patients after SLL correction. Of the 32 operated patients, 19 wished to have children. Of these 19 patients, 13 had at least one patent oviduct after SLL correction. Of these

13 patients, 12 (63.2%) had a spontaneous intrauterine conception. This reported crude intrauterine pregnancy rate is remarkably high, but could reflect the result of swift and accurate management in the form of combined medical and quick surgical treatment in the case of PID.

31.3 Tubal Infertility

One of the main consequences of a PID episode is the development of tubal infertility. It can create the whole spectrum of tubal alterations, from single peritubal adhesions to the combined presence of proximal and distal tubal occlusion.

In many large fertility surgery centres, the number of microsurgical interventions by laparotomy has decreased in favour of endoscopic operations. This shift is partly a result of the significant technological revolution during the past 5 years. The rise in public awareness and better acceptance have resulted in directed searches for patients suitable for endoscopic operations. Laparoscopy does not represent another technique, it is just another mode of access into the abdominal cavity.

It is not within the scope of this chapter to describe in detail all the microsurgical techniques – adhesiolysis, salpingostomy, tubal anastomosis, cystectomy and so on. The alternative to surgery is assisted reproductive technology (ART). Penzias[6] predicted the decline of fertility surgery, as ART is already superior in terms of monthly fecundity rates. In our opinion, this may become true in the future, but there are currently still indications for surgery. Surgery will always offer the possibility of spontaneous procreation, which is the reason certain infertile couples choose it, given equal success rates with both forms of treatment. Moreover, in many countries, the accessibility of ART is governed by non-medical economic considerations; in Europe, for example, there is a trend to reduce the number of ART centres. This is also true for fertility surgery, but in general, it is more readily available, although substantial microsurgical training and practice is becoming harder to obtain. Reports about cumulative pregnancy rates after multiple ART cycles blur the situation in that they state that fertility surgery is non-competitive.[7] They usually argue that the cost of surgery is too high and the pregnancy rate too low. They forget that real microsurgery, apart from SLL, is offered only once and that the cost of multiple ART cycles is higher than that of a surgical performance.

In daily clinical practice, the two main questions are whether patients should be offered surgery or ART and, once we have decided that surgery is preferable, which method of entry should be used for which indication.

The choice between ART and surgery can be made only after a standard fertility work-up, which also includes diagnostic endoscopy. During the endoscopic evaluation of the genital tract, the combination of hysteroscopy, laparoscopy, chromoperturbation and salpingoscopy offers an almost complete picture of the upper genital tract. Hysteroscopy is informative about the uterine cavity but has limitations in the diagnosis of tubal pathology.[8,9]

There are two points of interest in the diagnosis of tubal pathology, namely: patency and functionality. They are often taken to be the same, but are in fact totally different tubal characteristics. Tubal patency is important, but the demonstration of it is a technical procedure with several limitations. Many variables, such as the delivery systems into the uterus, the degree of occlusion of the cervical canal, the speed with which fluid is injected into the uterine cavity, the physical properties of the injected fluid (viscosity, temperature) and the lack of standardisation can play a determining role in the final interpretation of the test. Special anatomical situations such as congenital infantile tubes can also interfere with the correct diagnosis of patency. These tubes are very long, run very tortuously, have a patchy aplasia of the ampullary muscle and often present a very narrow infundibulum tubae. We regard them as a variation of the normal anatomy. To demonstrate patency at the fimbrial end of these tubes, a sustained and somewhat higher pressure is needed, which is not always easy to perform. Other methods to demonstrate patency are gaseous insufflation, hysterosalpingography, ultrasound with colour Doppler, selective salpingography, tubal catheterisation and chromoperturbation at laparoscopy.

Functional tests differ from the former in that they do not necessarily demonstrate patency, but concentrate more on the functional aspect of the Fallopian tube. They try to link their findings to pregnancy outcome in a prognostic way. Functional testing can be performed by experimental techniques such as laser-scattering spectroscopy. Radionuclide hysterosalpingography is more widely used but does not allow clear delineation of anatomical structures and its general use is hampered by a high rate of equivocal results. Tubal perturbation pressure registration can be performed in an outpatient setting, but clear data on its value are scarce. Direct intraluminal visualisation techniques such as falloposcopy and salpingoscopy are the best-documented procedures.

31.4 Falloposcopy

The unique characteristics of falloposcopy are the ability to visualise the whole tube and the attractive outpatient nature of the procedure. The first attempts at falloposcopy were made transhysteroscopically,[10] but the hysteroscope was later omitted in favour of the freehand tactile technique.[11] In general, there are two systems with which a falloposcopy may be performed. The first is the guide-wire or coaxial system to cannulate the tube and the second is the use of the linear everting balloon catheter system. The balloon has the advantage that there are no shear forces working on the inside of the tube.

In both systems, the falloposcope is introduced under irrigation up to the tip of its protective sheath and a retrograde inspection of the fallopian tube is performed. Irrigation ensures a clean lens and keeps the scope separated from the tubal wall, as failure to do so will compromise the image obtained, causing white-outs. Falloposcopes have an outer diameter of about 0.5 mm and a length of about 1–1.5m. The depth of field is documented from 2 mm up to infinity. However, there are some points of concern. First, the retrograde visualisation reduces the amount of information gained from the procedure. As it is not possible to steer the falloposcope, problems arise when evaluating large hydrosalpinges, as the scope will scrape the ventral tubal wall during the retrograde inspection. It remains to be determined how much of the mucosa has to be evaluated to declare it representative for the whole ampulla. The main problem is the quality of the image produced. Although different authors have repeatedly reported adequate imaging of intratubal pathology, the scopes have an unsatisfactory visual sharpness and definition. The potential for developing better scopes is immense.

Kerin[10] documented the prognostic value of falloposcopy in 71 women. In patients with falloposcopically normal tubes, the pregnancy rate after 1 year follow-up was 21%. Patients with moderate and severe disease had a 9 and 0% pregnancy rate respectively.

31.5 Salpingoscopy

Salpingoscopy is a technique that allows the visualisation of the ampullary part of the fallopian tube. It is therefore more than a simple interpretation of the fimbriated end. Several authors have found discrepancies between fimbrioscopy and salpingoscopy ranging from 23.5 to 49%.[12,13] The link between salpingoscopy and histology has been evaluated by Herschlag[14] and Vasquez.[15,16]

Salpingoscopy can be performed during laparotomy or laparoscopy. We prefer the rigid salpingoscope to the flexible scope, which is far more expensive and has inferior visual quality. A rigid salpingoscope is 40 cm long and has an outer diameter of 2.8 mm. It is protected by an outer sheath of 3.0 mm, which is passed along the operative channel of an endoscope at the umbilicus. The protective sheath is connected to a saline drip to distend the ampulla once the sheath is introduced inside the fallopian tube. The tube is clamped at its infundibulum over the sheath to provide a more or less watertight seal. In this way, the scope can be moved inside the tube without damaging the mucosa. Salpingoscopy can be performed only when the ampullary axis is brought into alignment with the axis of the salpingoscope and when the fimbriated end can be cannulated. This means that hydrosalpinges have to be opened first and that adhesions preventing the mobilisation of the tube have to be lysed.

As with falloposcopy, there are some points of discussion. First, salpingoscopy can only visualise the ampullary part of the fallopian tube, as the diameter of the isthmus is too narrow for the scope to pass. Second, salpingoscopy is used to identify patients who could benefit from a microsurgical operation. However, when adhesiolysis and concomitant salpingostomy have to be performed before a salpingoscopy can take place, one could argue that more than half of the eventual microsurgical intervention has already been carried out. It is not difficult for a well-trained endoscopist to extend a diagnostic 3 mm salpingostomy into a true salpingostomy with eversion of the newly created fimbrial wound edges; nature can then determine later events as far as pregnancy is concerned. This is only true in ideal situations where adhesiolysis is easy. When there are more extensive adhesions to the adjacent organs, the patient can be informed about the increased morbidity and the alternatives can be discussed, given the knowledge about the mucosal involvement. Whenever a salpingostomy remains diagnostic, it is unlikely that the small 3 mm opening will damage the tube irreversibly – it should reocclude spontaneously.

During salpingoscopy, the whole ampullary mucosa can be evaluated. There are major and minor folds in the mucosa. The major folds have secondary folds, which can easily be visualised. We do not know the prognostic value of mucosal alterations inside the tube. Strictures of the wall, vascular alterations and polyps are often reported, but the true meaning of these lesions is not well understood. A recent prospective study of tubal mucosal lesions and fertility outcome in

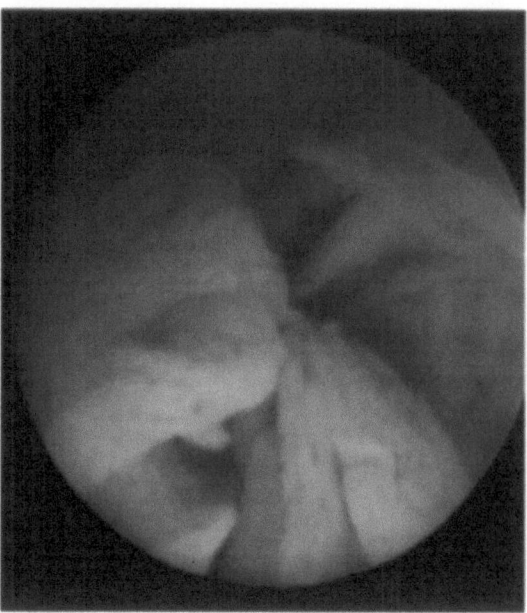

Figure 31.1 Normal tubal mucosa.

hydrosalpinges, evaluating the individual weight of different factors, concluded that adhesions between the folds were the most important feature.[16] Adhesions can present as cobweb-like structures with an irregular form, or as clear strings between different folds. Salpingoscopic findings can be classified as follows:

- class I: normal pattern of folds;
- class II: distended fold pattern;

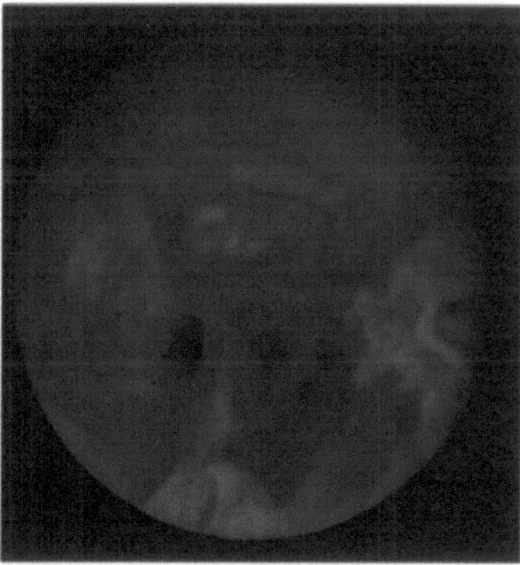

Figure 31.2 Intratubal adhesions.

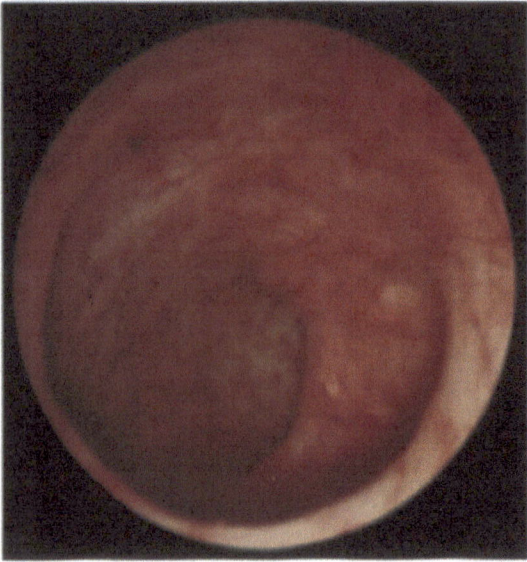

Figure 31.3 Terminally damaged tubal epithelium.

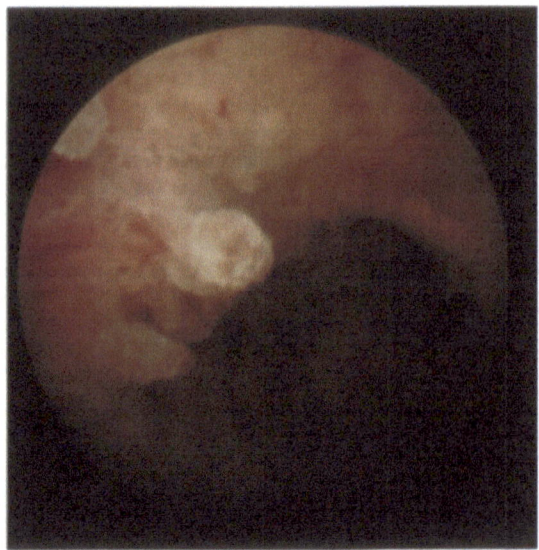

Figure 31.4 Cobweb type of intratubal adhesions.

- class III: focal lesions (adhesions, polyps, strictures, non-specific mucosal deposits);
- class IVa: extensive lesions but preservation of the folds;
- class IVb: extensive lesions with partial disappearance of the mucosa;
- class V: complete loss of the fold pattern.

Classes I–II are regarded as normal and classes III–V represent pathological situations (Figures 31.1–31.5).

The prognostic value of salpingoscopy has been documented in several studies. In a group of 68

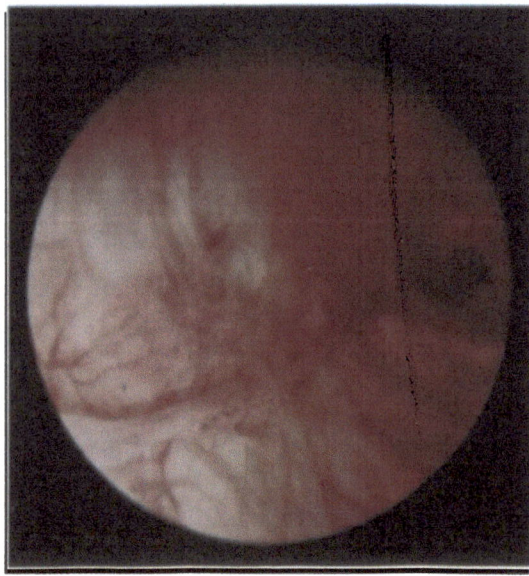

Figure 31.5 Patchy type of intratubal lesions.

patients, Cornier[17] reported 12 intrauterine pregnancies when salpingoscopy revealed normal mucosa. There were no intrauterine pregnancies in patients with severe mucosal damage. On the contrary, four ectopic pregnancies developed in the latter group. No ectopic pregnancies occurred in the group with healthy mucosa. In another study of 42 patients with a follow-up of 13.5 months, a pregnancy rate of 39% was achieved in patients with healthy tubes on salpingoscopy, compared with a 4.1% pregnancy rate in those with intratubal pathology.[18] In a study of 158 patients, Heylen[19] found a pregnancy rate of 71% in salpingoscopy classes I–II versus 34% in class III. There were no pregnancies in patients with more advanced mucosal damage.

Marana[20] reported on 29 patients treated with salpingo-ovariolysis and 23 patients treated with salpingoneostomy. The term pregnancy rates of salpingoscopy class I–II oviducts were 73 and 64% respectively. There were no pregnancies in patients with unhealthy mucosa. Henry-Suchet[13] demonstrated a highly significant correlation between normal ampullary mucosa and pregnancy.

We also evaluated the prognostic value of salpingoscopy in 226 patients with tubal infertility secondary to sequelae of PID. They were all treated by microsurgery and a salpingoscopy was performed prospectively at the end of surgery.[12] The patients were divided into two groups: one with non-obstructive, adhesive disease and one with hydrosalpinx. After a follow-up period of 42 months, the obstetric history of 163 remaining patients was collected and different characteristics were calculated for each salpingoscopic class in the two different groups. The cumulative intrauterine pregnancy rate (CIPR) was calculated using life-table analysis. The CIPR in the non-obstructive group was 51.5% in class I, 90.0% in class II, 38.9% in class III and 36.4% in class IVa. The differences in CIPR for the different salpingoscopic classes were statistically significant. No pregnancies occurred in classes IVb and V. The CIPR in the hydrosalpinx group was 100% in class I, 60% in class II, 57.1% in class III, 16.7% in class IVa and 10% in class IVb. The difference between the salpingoscopy classes was highly significant for the occurrence of intrauterine pregnancies. There were no pregnancies in class V. The CIPR for the salpingoscopy classes I–II versus III–V were 64 and 36.7% in the non-obstructive disease group and 78.6 and 23.5% in the hydrosalpinx group. The differences were statistically significant in both patient groups. As the CIPR in salpingoscopy class III were 38.9 and 57.1% for the non-obstructive and hydrosalpinx group respectively, we propose to offer a surgical form of treatment for those patients with tubal salpingoscopic findings up to class III. Patients with more significant tubal damage, as in salpingoscopy classes IV–V, should be offered ART as the primary form of treatment.

31.6 Conclusions

Salpingoscopy can help in planning treatment for patients with tubal infertility secondary to PID. It avoids unnecessary laparotomies and also gives young patients, with healthy tubes, a chance for natural conception without an increased risk of multiple pregnancy.

Once the decision has been made to offer surgical treatment, the second important question is to choose between laparoscopy and laparotomy as modes of access into the abdomen. For every microsurgical technique, there is a laparoscopic alternative. The main outcome criterion in fertility surgery is the postoperative pregnancy rate. Because of ethical problems, there are very few prospective randomised controlled studies that evaluate laparoscopy versus laparotomy in fertility surgery. However, the available data indicate that the results after laparoscopy are in the range of what microsurgery offers. Trying to solve every situation with only laparoscopy or laparotomy is certainly wrong. The choice between the two modalities is largely dependent upon the abdominal situation and the surgeon. For instance, when a situation is largely dominated by the presence of filmy adhesions, microsurgery would be overtreatment, but if the ovary is stuck to the lateral pelvic wall and the medial part of the mesosalpinx is adherent to the ovarian surface with dense adhesions, microsurgery is more appropriate.

References

1. Eschenbach DA, Wölner-Hanssen P, Hawes S et al (1997) Acute pelvic inflammatory disease: associations of clinical and laboratory findings with laparoscopy findings. Obstet Gynecol 89:184–192
2. Hillis SD, Joesoef R, Marchbanks PA et al (1993) Delayed care of pelvic inflammatory disease as a risk factor for impaired fertility. Am J Obstet Gynecol 168:1503–1509
3. Jacobson L, Weström L (1969) Objectivised diagnosis of acute pelvic inflammatory disease. Diagnostic and prognostic value of routine laparoscopy. Am J Obstet Gynecol 105:1088–1093
4. Weström L, Joesoef R, Reynolds G et al (1992) Pelvic inflammatory disease and fertility. A cohort study of 1844 women with laparoscopically verified disease and 657 control women with normal laparoscopic results. Sex Trans Dis 19:185–192
5. Raiga J, Canis M, Le Bouedec G et al (1996) Laparoscopic management of adnexal abscesses: consequences for fertility. Fertil Steril 66:712–717
6. Penzias AS, DeCherney AH (1996) Is there ever a role for tubal surgery? Am J Obstet Gynecol 174:1218–1221
7. Benadiva CA, Kligman I, Davis O et al (1995) In vitro fertilisation versus tubal surgery: is pelvic reconstructive surgery obsolete? Fertil Steril 64:1051–1061
8. Puttemans P, Brosens I, Dellatin Ph et al (1987) Salpingoscopy versus hysterosalpingography in hydrosalpinges. Hum Reprod 2:535–540
9. Swart P, Mol BWJ, van der Veen F et al (1995) The accuracy of hysterosalpingography in the diagnosis of tubal pathology: a meta-analysis. Fertil Steril 64:486–491
10. Kerin J, Daykhovsky L, Segalowitz J et al (1990) Falloposcopy: a microendoscopic technique for visual exploration of the human fallopian tube from the uterotubal ostium to the fimbria using a transvaginal approach. Fertil Steril 54:390–400
11. Bauer O, Diedrich K, Bacich S et al (1992) Transcervical access and intra-luminal imaging of the Fallopian tube in the non-anaesthetized patient; preliminary results using a new technique for Fallopian access. Hum Reprod 7:7–11
12. De Bruyne F, Hucke J, Willers R (1997) The prognostic value of salpingoscopy. Hum Reprod 12:266–271
13. Henry-Suchet J, Loffredo V, Tesquier L et al (1985) Endoscopy of the tube (= tuboscopy): its prognostic value for tuboplasties. Acta Europea Fertilitatis 16:139–145
14. Herschlag A, Seifer DB, Carcangiu ML et al (1991) Salpingoscopy: light microscopic and electron microscopic correlations. Obstet Gynecol 77:399–405
15. Vasquez G, Winston RML, Boeckx W et al (1983) The epithelium of human hydrosalpinges: a light optical and scanning microscopy study. Br J Obstet Gynaecol 90:764–770
16. Vasquez G, Boeckx W, Brosens I (1995) Prospective study of mucosal lesions and fertility in hydrosalpinges. Hum Reprod 10:1075–1078
17. Cornier E, Feintuch MJ, Bouccara L (1984) La fibrotuboscopie ampullaire. J Gynecol Obstet Biol Reprod 1:49–53
18. Surrey ES, Surrey MW (1996) Correlation between salpingoscopic and laparoscopic staging in the assessment of the distal fallopian tube. Fertil Steril 65:267–271
19. Heylen SM, Brosens IA, Puttemans PJ (1995) Clinical value and cumulative pregnancy rates following rigid salpingoscopy during laparoscopy for infertility. Hum Reprod 10:2913–2916
20. Marana R, Rizzi M, Muzi L et al (1995) Correlation between the American Fertility Society classifications of adnexal adhesions and distal tubal occlusion, salpingoscopy, and reproductive outcome in tubal surgery. Fertil Steril 64:924–929

Chapter 32

Three-dimensional Ultrasound Diagnosis of Congenital Uterine Anomalies

Rehan Salim and Davor Jurkovic

32.1 Introduction

Congenital uterine anomalies are a range of morphological abnormalities of the uterus, which form as a result of aberrant development of the Müllerian ducts at around 8 weeks' gestation.[1] They are associated with a wide range of pregnancy problems, including miscarriage, pre-term delivery, ante-partum bleeding and intrauterine growth restriction.[2] However, our knowledge of congenital uterine anomalies has been limited because of their apparent rarity and the invasive nature of diagnostic tests, which have traditionally been used to assess uterine morphology. Screening for congenital uterine anomalies has therefore been limited to women with poor reproductive histories, such as recurrent first-trimester miscarriage. The prevalence of anomalies in the general population of women, with normal reproductive histories, and their clinical significance have remained largely unknown.

The advent of transvaginal three-dimensional ultrasound has greatly enhanced our ability to assess uterine morphology. The technique is non-invasive and relatively inexpensive, which has enabled the first large-scale screening studies of uterine morphology in low-risk women. In this chapter we will discuss in detail the technique of three-dimensional ultrasound and its impact on the diagnosis and management of congenital uterine anomalies.

32.2 Pathophysiology of Early Pregnancy Failure

The Müllerian ducts form as paired tubes around 5 weeks' gestation. By 8 weeks, the lower portions of the ducts are fused to form the uterus and cervix, while the upper portions remain separate and form the Fallopian tubes. The fusion of the lower parts of the ducts is followed by the resorption of tissue adjoining in a caudo-cranial sequence. The process of fusion and resorption of the Müllerian ducts is a highly ordered process and any deviation from it is likely to result in a congenital uterine anomaly. Developmental abnormalities can occur at any stage, ranging from a complete agenesis of one or both Müllerian ducts to a minor degree of resorption failure after fusion of the ducts.

The most common congenital anomalies of the uterus are duplication anomalies. The arcuate and subseptate uteri form as a result of resorption failure of the adjoining tissue, whereas the bicornuate and didelphys anomalies are mostly the result of fusion failure.[1] This results in a wide range of congenital uterine anomalies, which have different effects on reproductive outcomes.

The mechanism of early pregnancy failure with the subseptate uterus is not clearly understood. As most losses in subseptate uteri occur in the first trimester, it has been proposed that miscarriage is a result of poor decidualisation on a relatively avascular septum. Histological studies of resected uterine septa showed that the septum is relatively avascular in comparison to the myometrium of the lateral uterine wall, which supports this theory.[3-5] In women with an arcuate, bicornuate and unicornuate uterus, pregnancy failure may result from an overall decrease in functional uterine volume, which leads to increased intrauterine pressure causing cervical dilatation.[6] Finally, it has also been suggested that there may be a relative deficiency of oestrogen and progesterone receptors in congenitally malformed uteri, which leads to abnormal uterine contractions.[7]

32.3 Technique of Three-dimensional Ultrasound Examination

Three-dimensional images are generated following the acquisition of a large number of consecutive ultrasound tomograms through the movement of a transducer. The spatial orientation of sonograms is monitored throughout the process of acquisition and these are stored in the computer as a memory set. Mechanical, electromagnetic or acoustic methods can then be utilised to establish the relative position and orientation of the tomograms. The volume dataset obtained can then be examined using three methods: section reconstruction, surface rendering and volume rendering.

Three-dimensional ultrasound images can be reconstructed and any arbitrarily chosen plane can then be displayed. This is an important advantage over two-dimensional ultrasound as it allows visualisation of planes that cannot be seen as a result of restriction on probe movements due to anatomical constraints.

In the assessment of uterine morphology the main advantage of three-dimensional ultrasound is the ability to visualise the uterus in the coronal plane, which is rarely seen with conventional two-dimensional scanning (Figure 32.1). Studies of uterine morphology are performed in a standardised plane,

which is defined by the visualisation of interstitial portions of the Fallopian tubes. This ensures consistency of examination technique and improves the reproducibility of ultrasound diagnosis. Another important advantage of three-dimensional ultrasound, over other methods for the assessment of uterine morphology, it the ability to describe a degree of disruption of uterine morphology in quantitative terms. The depth of fundal indentation, or the length of a uterine septum, can be measured and compared across groups of women with different reproductive outcomes (Figure 32.2).

The differentiation of individual congenital uterine anomalies is important as it has implications for reproductive prognosis and management. Conventional imaging modalities, such as two-dimensional ultrasound, hysterosalpingography and hysteroscopy, are accurate at identifying the presence of an anomaly. However, for a full assessment of uterine morphology, it is necessary to combine methods that examine the uterine cavity (e.g. hysteroscopy or hysterosalpingography) with a laparoscopy, which provides information about the outer uterine contour.[8] Three-dimensional ultrasonography, with its ability to visualise both the endometrial cavity and the serosal contour of the uterus, provides all the information necessary to classify uterine anomalies. Furthermore, it is also possible to identify accurately the presence of

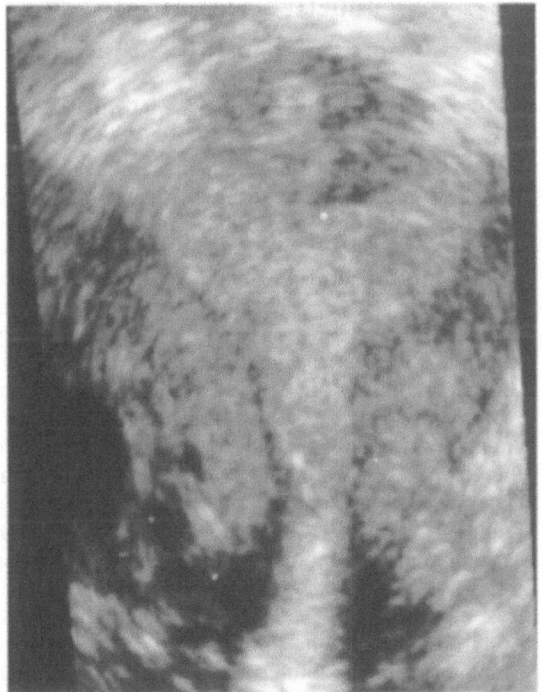

Figure 32.1. A coronal view of an arcuate uterus with the interstitial portions of the Fallopian tubes clearly visible.

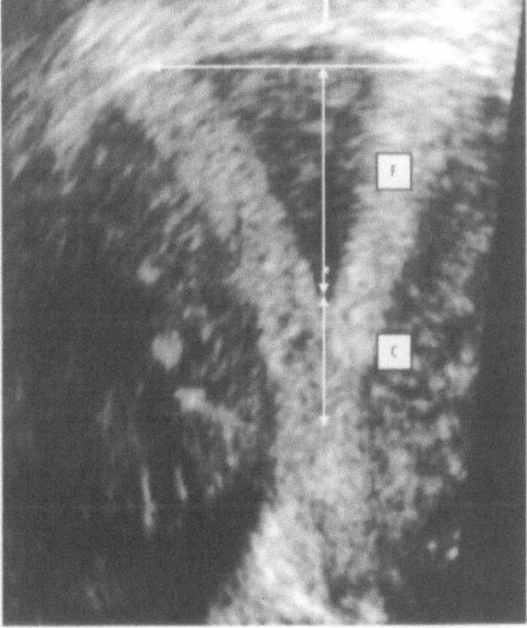

Figure 32.2. An example of a subseptate uterus, which is characterised by the normal outer uterine contour and a uterine cavity that is divided by a septum. The interstitial portions of the Fallopian tubes are used as a reference point to measure the length of the septum (F) and the length of unaffected cavity (C).

rudimentary cornua in women with a unicornuate uterus and demonstrate any connection with the dominant uterine cavity.

32.4 Diagnostic Accuracy of Three-dimensional Ultrasound

There are many classification systems of congenital uterine anomalies. However, the most commonly used system is the American Fertility Society classification for Müllerian anomalies (see Appendix in Part VII).[9] This system divides uterine anomalies into six groups based on their clinical significance, treatment and prognosis. The classification was based on a retrospective analysis of a small group of women.[10] The main problems with this classification are a lack of clearly defined diagnostic criteria, which should be used to classify uterine anomalies. In addition there is no agreement on the most appropriate diagnostic method to assess uterine morphology. As a result, the diagnosis of uterine anomalies in routine clinical practice rests exclusively on the subjective impression of the investigator performing the test. No study has ever been published, which has assessed the accuracy and reproducibility of the diagnosis of uterine anomalies.

Studies of uterine anomalies with three-dimensional ultrasound have adopted the American Fertility Society classification when describing uterine morphology.[11] However, the diagnostic criteria have been more precisely defined and they include the degree of fundal distortion as well (Table 32.1). It is likely that this classification may be further refined once more data on the correlation between the degree of uterine distortion and reproductive outcomes are available.

The accuracy of three-dimensional ultrasound in the diagnosis of congenital uterine anomalies has been investigated in two studies. The initial study included 61 women with infertility or recurrent miscarriage and used hysterosalpingography as the gold standard.[12] Three-dimensional ultrasound was found to be in complete agreement with hysterosalpingography and correctly classified the uterus as normal or abnormal. Furthermore, in the same study, three-dimensional ultrasound was found to be superior to two-dimensional ultrasonography, which detected all cases of anomalies but also gave a high number of false-positive diagnoses. Another study compared three-dimensional ultrasound diagnoses with those found at hysterosalpingography and laparoscopy. There was complete agreement among the three methods, except that in one case the description of the uterine fundus was different at laparoscopy.[13]

32.5 Reproductive Significance of Congenital Uterine Anomalies

32.5.1 General Gynaecological Population

The majority of uterine anomalies are detected in women with a history of adverse pregnancy outcomes. However, they are also found incidentally when women are investigated for indications unrelated to reproductive performance. Little is known about the true prevalence and clinical significance of uterine anomalies in this low-risk population. A recent study has used three-dimensional ultrasound to screen for uterine anomalies in 1022 women with normal reproductive histories. The prevalence of all uterine anomalies was 5.4%, while major anomalies were found in 2.3% of women.[14] The most common anomaly in this study was the arcuate uterus, being found in 3.1%. The subseptate uterus was the most common major anomaly, found in 1.6%. These findings were comparable to previous studies, which used invasive tests such as laparoscopy and hysterosalpingography to investigate the prevalence of major congenital uterine anomalies in women undergoing elective sterilisation procedures. They reported a prevalence of major anomalies of between 1.9% and 3.2%.[15,16]

Table 32.1. Classification of congenital uterine anomalies[9]

Uterine morphology	Fundal contour	External contour
Normal	Straight or convex	Uniformly convex or with indentation < 10 mm
Arcuate	Concave fundal indentation with central point of indentation at obtuse angle (> 90°)	Uniformly convex or with indentation < 10 mm
Subseptate	Presence of septum, which does not extend to cervix, with central point of septum at an acute angle (< 90°)	Uniformly convex or with indentation < 10 mm
Septate	Presence of uterine septum that completely divides cavity from fundus to cervix	Uniformly convex or with indentation < 10 mm
Bicornuate	Two well-formed uterine cornua	Fundal indentation > 10 mm dividing the two cornua
Unicornuate with or without rudimentary horn	Single well-formed uterine cavity with a single interstitial portion of Fallopian tube and concave fundal contour	Fundal indentation > 10 mm dividing the two cornua if rudimentary horn present

A further study from our centre also used three-dimensional ultrasound to compare uterine morphology with previous reproductive outcomes in a large group of low-risk women. This study showed an increased risk of first-trimester loss with subseptate uteri and a higher risk of second-trimester miscarriage with an arcuate uterus (Table 32.2).[11] However, all adverse outcomes were less common than previously reported. A recent meta-analysis of women with subseptate uterus[7] found an overall miscarriage rate of 79%, which was twice as high as our results. Furthermore, contrary to previous reports, our study showed that the risk of miscarriage with a subseptate uterus was confined to the first trimester, with no significant risk of second-trimester miscarriage or pre-term labour.

Only a handful of studies have investigated the reproductive performance of women with an arcuate uterus. All studies have been retrospective and have mostly included women with a history of infertility. Two studies have reported no increase in adverse pregnancy outcomes with live-birth rates of 83–86%.[17,18] A third study, however, reported successful pregnancy outcomes in only 45% of women with an arcuate uterus.[19] In our study, women with an arcuate uterus had a significantly higher number of second-trimester losses and pre-term labours compared to women with a normal uterus. Term deliveries occurred in 64% of pregnancies.

The differences between the results of our study and previous reports almost certainly reflect differences in study designs. While almost all previous studies have investigated women with a history of recurrent pregnancy loss or infertility, we have investigated women who are considered to be at low risk of having an anomalous uterus. The outcomes of previous pregnancies are therefore expected to be better in our study population. However, the results of our study have confirmed that even in a low-risk population there is an association between congenital uterine anomalies and adverse pregnancy outcomes.

32.5.2 Women with a History of Recurrent Miscarriage

A number of studies have investigated the prevalence of congenital uterine anomalies in women with a history of recurrent miscarriage. They have reported a wide range of prevalence figures ranging from 1.8% to 37.8%, depending on the inclusion criteria (two, three or more miscarriages, early and late miscarriages) and the diagnostic method used.[7]

A screening study of 510 women with a history of three consecutive first-trimester miscarriages, using three-dimensional ultrasound as the only diagnostic modality, has found the prevalence of uterine anomalies to be 23.9%. Major anomalies were found in 6.8% of cases.[20] In comparison, in a similar study of low-risk women, the prevalence of all types of anomalies was increased (Figure 32.3). Furthermore, the study also investigated the morphological characteristics of uterine anomalies in women with recurrent first-trimester miscarriage and women with normal reproductive histories. Using three-dimensional ultrasound images, measurements of the fundal indentation in arcuate uteri, septal length in subseptate uteri, and unaffected cavity length were made. The congenital uterine anomalies in women with recurrent first-trimester miscarriage were found to be more severe with a significantly shorter unaffected part of the uterine cavity.

There is a well-recognised association between the subseptate uterus and recurrent first-trimester miscarriage.[7,21] Therefore, women with a subseptate uterus and recurrent first-trimester miscarriage are routinely offered hysteroscopic resection of the septum in an attempt to restore uterine anatomy and thereby improve the prognosis of subsequent pregnancies. Results from retrospective studies have been encouraging. Women with a history of recurrent first-trimester miscarriage had a live birth rate of approximately 80% following hysteroscopic resection of a uterine septum. Only 15% of pregnancies miscarried.[22] However, other studies of pregnancy outcome following septal resection reported no significant change in miscarriage rate.[23] The reasons for such discrepancies may lie in the differing definitions of recurrent miscarriage and differences in diagnostic criteria for congenital uterine anomalies. Our finding of a positive correlation between the severity of a uterine anomaly and the risk of adverse pregnancy outcome may improve the selection of patients for hysteroscopic surgery in the future. There has never been a randomised controlled trial of hysteroscopic metroplasty in women with subseptate uterus and there is urgent need for such a study in order to establish the potential benefits and risks of surgical correction of subseptate uterus.

Table 32.2. Reproductive outcomes in low-risk women[11]

	Uterine morphology		
	Normal	Arcuate	Subseptate
Number of pregnancies per woman (mean and range)	2.0	1.2	2.0
First-trimester miscarriages (%)	235 (12)	14 (15.9)	24 (42.0)
Second-trimester miscarriages (%)	69 (3.5)	7 (7.9)	2 (3.6)
Pre-term labours	114 (6.2)	11 (12.5)	6 (10.5)

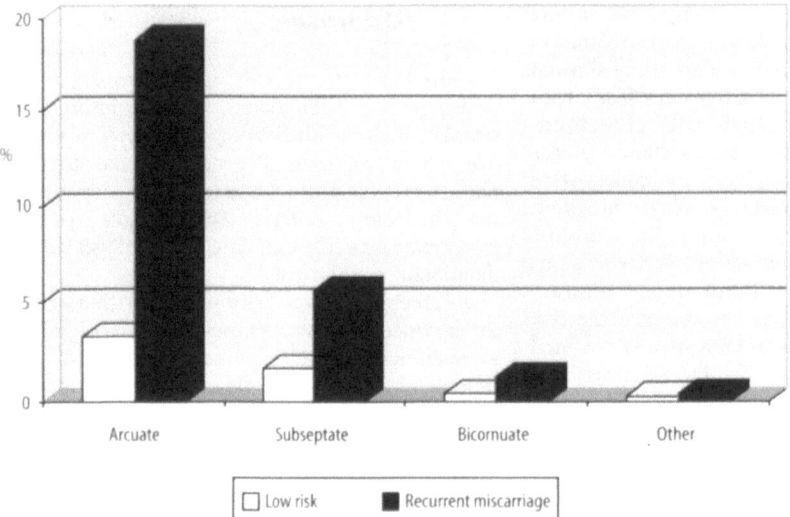

Figure 32.3. Distribution of congenital uterine anomalies in low risk and recurrent miscarriage.

32.6 Conclusions

Three-dimensional ultrasound can be used as an alternative to invasive diagnostic procedures for the diagnosis of congenital uterine anomalies. The test is relatively simple, non-invasive, fast and carries no anaesthetic or surgical risks. However, it is unlikely that three-dimensional ultrasound equipment will be widely available in the immediate future. Therefore, two-dimensional ultrasound should continue to be used as a first-stage screening test. Only those women with suspected anomalies on a two-dimensional scan should be referred for a detailed three-dimensional scan.

In routine clinical practice, screening for uterine anomalies should at present be limited to high-risk women with a history of infertility or recurrent miscarriage. There are several reasons for this. First, using two-dimensional ultrasound as a screening test, a false-positive diagnosis of a uterine anomaly occurs in approximately 6% of women, which is likely to result in a significant increase in workload for tertiary referral centres.[12] In addition, there is very limited information on the reproductive risks associated with congenital uterine anomalies in low-risk women. Furthermore, there is no evidence that surgical correction of an incidentally diagnosed congenital uterine anomaly is of benefit to women.

References

1. Rock J (1997) Surgery for anomalies of the Müllerian ducts. In: Rock J, Thompson J (eds) Te Linole's operative gynaecology. Lippincott-Raven, Philadelphia, pp 687–731
2. Heinonen P, Saarikoski S, Pystynen P (1982) Reproductive performance of women with congenital uterine anomalies. Acta Obstet Gynecol Scand 61:157
3. Candiani G, Fedele L, Zamberletti D et al. (1983) Endometrial patterns in malformed uteri. Acta Eur Fertil 14:35–42
4. Fedele L, Bianchi S, Marchini M et al. (1996) Ultrastructural aspects of endometrium in infertile women with septate uterus. Fertil Steril 65:750–752.
5. Dabirashafi H, Bahadori S, Mohammed K et al. (1995) Septate uterus: new idea on the histological features of the septum in this abnormal uterus. Am J Obstet Gynecol 171:105–107
6. Rock J, Murphy A (1986) Anatomic abnormalities. Clin Obstet Gynecol 29:886–911
7. Homer H, Li T, Cooke I (2000) The septate uterus: a review of management and reproductive outcome. Fertil Steril 73:1–4
8. Reuter K, Daly D, Cohen S (1989) Septate versus bicornuate uteri: errors in imaging diagnosis. Radiology 172:749–752
9. The American Fertility Society (1988) The American Fertility Society classifications of adnexal adhesions, distal tubal occlusion, tubal occlusion secondary to tubal ligation, tubal pregnancies, Müllerian anomalies and intrauterine adhesions. Fertil Steril 49:944–955
10. Buttram V, Gibbons W (1979) Müllerian anomalies: a proposed classification (an analysis of 144 cases). Fertil Steril 32:40–46
11. Woelfer B, Salim R, Banerjee S et al. (2001) Reproductive outcomes in women with congenital uterine anomalies detected by three-dimensional ultrasound screening. Obstet Gynecol 98:1099–1103
12. Jurkovic D, Geipel A, Gruboeck K et al. (1995) Three-dimensional ultrasound for the assessment of uterine anatomy and detection of congenital anomalies: comparison with hysterosalpingography and two-dimensional ultrasonography. Ultrasound Obstet Gynecol 5:233–237
13. Raga F, Bonilla-Muscoles F, Blanes J et al. (1996) Congenital Müllerian anomalies: diagnostic accuracy of three-dimensional ultrasound. Fertil Steril 65:523–528
14. Jurkovic D, Gruboeck K, Tailor A et al. (1997) Ultrasound screening for congenital uterine anomalies. Br J Obstet Gynaecol 104:1320–1321
15. Ashton D, Amin H, Richart R et al. (1988) The incidence of asymptomatic uterine anomalies in women undergoing transcervical tubal sterilisation. Obstet Gynecol 72:28–30

16. Simon C, Martinez L, Prado F et al. (1991) Müllerian defects in women with normal reproductive outcome. Fertil Steril 56:1192–1193
17. Raga F, Bauset C, Remohi J et al. (1997) Reproductive impact of congenital uterine anomalies. Hum Reprod 12:2277–2281
18. Acien P (1993) Reproductive performance in women with congenital uterine malformations. Hum Reprod 8:122–126
19. Tulandi T, Arronet G, McInnes R (1980) Arcuate and bicornuate uterine anomalies and infertility. Fertil Steril 34:362–364
20. Salim R, Woelfer B, Regan L et al. (2001) Three-dimensional ultrasound study of congenital uterine anomalies in women with a history of recurrent miscarriage. Ultrasound Obstet Gynecol 18 (suppl 1):5

21. Grimbizis G, Camus M, Tarlatzis B et al. (2001) Clinical implications of uterine malformations and hysteroscopic results. Hum Reprod Update 7:161–174
22. Fedele L, Bianchi S (1995) Hysteroscopic metroplasty for subseptate uterus. Obstet Gynecol Clin North Am 22:473–489
23. Kirk EP, Choung CJ, Coulam CB et al. (1993) Pregnancy after metroplasty for uterine anomalies. Fertil Steril 59:1164–1168

Chapter 33

The Role of Endoscopy in Congenital Abnormalities: Diagnosis and Treatment

Jacques Donnez, Pascale Jadoul, Michelle Nisolle and Jean Squifflet

33.1 Introduction

The endoscopic technique for the management of uterine septa was first proposed by Eström and Fernström in 1970,[1] but the method has only become widely used in recent years.[2]

In the past, whenever a patient presented with a Müllerian fusion defect that was thought to be the cause of recurrent pregnancy loss, a Jones, Strassman or Tompkins procedure would be performed by laparotomy. These procedures required lengthy anaesthesia. Surgery could be complicated by infection or haemorrhage, necessitating antibiotic treatment and blood transfusions. Also, because the full thickness of the uterine fundus was surgically damaged, the patient would require caesarean section for future deliveries. Some women became infertile as a result of adhesions or tubal occlusion, developing secondary to the procedure itself.

Many Müllerian fusion defects are amenable to hysteroscopic treatment. Several different procedures have been adopted, with more or less similar results. The basic concept involves the transcervical examination of the uterine septum by means of hysteroscopy, followed by its resection.[3-5] The use of an operative hysteroscope permits the passage of surgical instruments.

33.2 Uterine Septum: Partial and Complete

33.2.1 Prevalence and Diagnosis

Uterine septum is the most common Müllerian fusion defect. Its incidence in the general population is estimated to be 1.8%.[5]

Between 1986 and 1998, in our department, 216 patients underwent a hysteroscopic septoplasty with the help of the Nd:YAG laser (Table 33.1). In 85% of cases (183/216), the uterine septum was partial (Figure 33.1) and in 15% of cases (33/216), the uterine septum was complete with cervical duplication. A vaginal septum was noted in 22 cases (10%). The diagnosis of a complete uterine septum may be delayed, particularly if a vaginal septum is associated.[7] Indeed, the vaginal septum can easily be misdiagnosed by gynaecological examination and, at hysterosalpingography, the uterus appears to be unicornuate, unless there is a fistula between the two uterine cavities (Figure 33.2). However, in the absence of a vaginal septum, the diagnosis is simple because two distinct external cervical orifices are clearly visible. The opacification through these two orifices allows the diagnosis of a septate uterus with cervical duplication.

For hysteroscopy the traditional liquid distension medium used to be dextran 70 or a solution of 5% dextrose; however, glycine is now preferred by most authors. This medium is not viscous, permits a clear visual field and is not a conductor of electricity. If electricity is not used, saline or Ringer's lactate can be employed. These are well tolerated when absorbed into the system and represent an advantage of the laser.

Table 33.1. Hysteroscopic septoplasty (1986–1998)

Partial uterine septum	Complete uterine septum
n = 183 (85%)	n = 33 (15%)
	11 (5%) no vaginal septum
	22 (10%) vaginal septum
10 cases (1986–1993)	23 cases (1994–1996)
Nd:YAG laser septoplasty	Nd:YAG laser septoplasty
in two steps	in one step

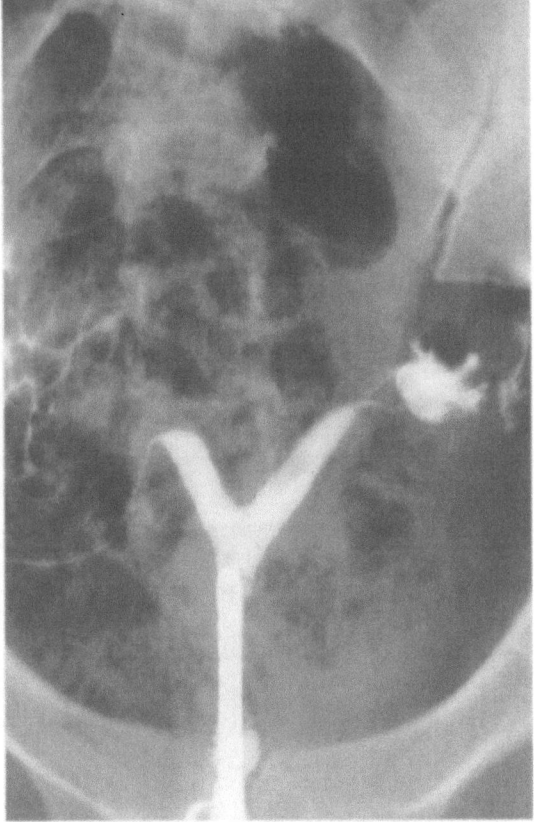

Figure 33.1 Partial uterine septum: hysterography.

33.2.2 Instruments

Various instruments can be used for the resection of the septum: miniature scissors or semi-rigid miniature scissors, which permit the required pressure but are small enough to pass through the hysteroscopic operating sheath and along the cervical canal with no difficulty or risk. The blades can be opened wide enough to allow resection of even thick septa.

Other surgeons[8-10] prefer to use the resectoscope. High-frequency electric sources are advised for safety reasons. The resectoscope has several advantages: it is inexpensive and readily available in most operating rooms, as well as being simple to operate and highly efficient at removing the septum.

Finally, others[11-12] have suggested the use of lasers for this type of hysteroscopic surgery. Argon, krypton, KTP 532 and Nd:YAG lasers have all been used successfully in the resection of uterine septa; however, certain limiting factors must be taken into consideration. First, hyskon should not be used because caramelisation can prove troublesome and may damage the laser fibre, resulting in delay while fibres are replaced or repaired. Second, the surgeon must be thoroughly acquainted with the physics of

the particular laser being used. Third, only bare fibres should be used: CO_2-conducting fibres may cause bubbling of the medium, which may lead to gas embolism, cardiovascular compromise and even death.

The Nd:YAG laser uses a solid-state rig (garnet) in which the neodymium atoms play the active lasing role. The energy is supplied by a flashlight lamp, which illuminates the rod. Both are housed in a container called the resonator. The shape of the resonator is ellipsoidal and its inner surface is coated with a highly reflective material. The lamp and the rod are placed at the two focal points of the ellipsoid. The light emitted by the lamp is reflected by the internal coating of the resonator and is collected, almost in its entirety, by the rod positioned at the opposite focal point.

In contrast to the CO_2 laser, Nd:YAG laser beams propagate well through commercially available glass fibres, very much like visible light. The propagation is effected by a chain of internal reflections occurring at the boundaries of the glass fibre. Hence, the delivery devices used in Nd:YAG lasers are a variety of fibres (see below) equipped with a connector that attaches to the output port of the laser system.

Manufacturers offer Nd:YAG laser units featuring different maximum powers from 40 to 100 W. Nd:YAG laser systems are composed of:

- a laser head or resonator;
- a power supply, which furnishes the flashlight lamp with the necessary electrical energy;
- a closed-circuit water-cooling system, further chilled by a radiator, which removes excess heat from the resonator;
- a control system, based on a microcomputer;
- a He-Ne laser tube;
- an output-port optical assembly, to which the external glass fibre is attached.

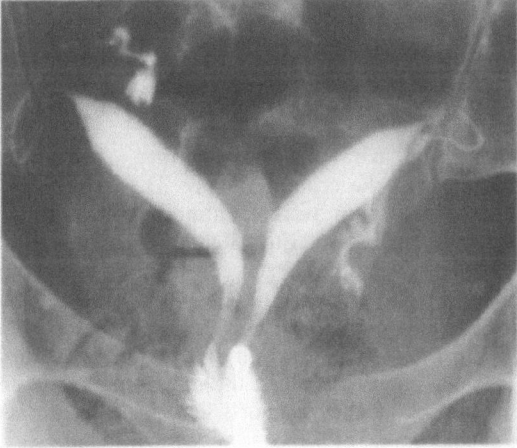

Figure 33.2 Complete uterine septum (uterocervical septum) with a fistula between the two uterine cavities.

The accessories offered with Nd:YAG systems are almost exclusively fibres. They fall into two categories: non-contact fibres and contact fibres.

The distal ends of non-contact fibres are flat and highly polished. They operate at a short distance from the tissue, in order to create deep coagulation. A well-known example of their use is in the treatment of superficial bladder tumours, where the fibres are inserted through a cystoscope. Non-contact fibres have no incision capability. These fibres are usually reusable. However, after a limited number of surgical procedures, they must be repolished with the aid of a special polishing kit.

Contact fibres feature a sharpened sculpted conical tip. The laser radiation is concentrated at the very narrow tip and the fibre functions like a hot knife, capable of performing fine incisions when in contact with the tissue. Moreover, the tapered fibre prevents the rays from progressing forwards, while enabling their exit through the sides of the tip. The end result is that the forward penetration is reduced, much as in the case of the CO_2 laser. The side radiation, on the other hand, produces a haemostatic effect on the lateral surfaces of the wedge created by the incision. Contact fibres are used in a variety of configurations for freehand and endoscopic applications. They feature different shapes (conical, hemispherical) and different diameters (400, 600, 800 and $100\,\mu m$). They are offered as disposable, single-use, sterilised fibres.

Recently, new types of fibres have been introduced onto the market. These fibres possess a polished distal face, which is inclined with respect to the fibre axis. This angle enables the fibre to emit the laser beam at right angles to its long axis. Employed transurethrally, these fibres are used to treat benign prostatic hypertrophy by coagulating the adenoma. Another type of fibre, emanating lateral diffusive radiation from an elongated segment located at its distal end, is used for the interstitial laserthermia of benign and malignant lesions.

33.2.3 Partial Uterine Septum

Using the "bare fibre", the surgeon begins the resection of the septum (Figure 33.3), continuing until it has been resected almost flush with the surrounding endometrium. Regardless of the type of medium employed, the surgeon must be able to see the right and left cornual regions completely and keep the septum in view at all times. Concurrent laparoscopy at the time of hysteroscopic resection is recommended to confirm the diagnosis, but is not mandatory if the diagnosis has been confirmed previously.

The septum is cut using the "touch technique" (Figure 33.3). The hysteroscope with the laser fibre is

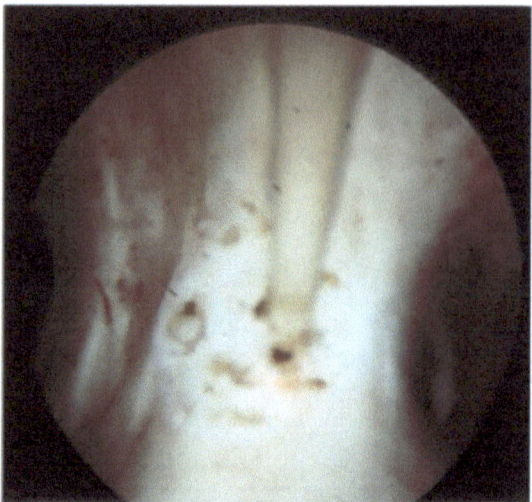

a

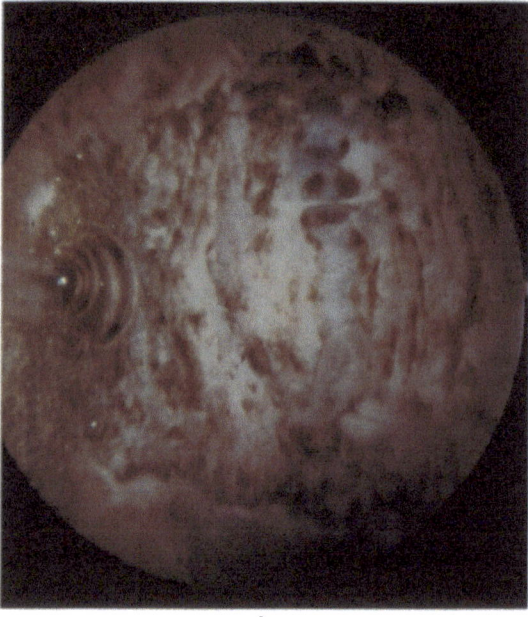

b

Figure 33.3 a Resection of the uterine septum is carried out with the help of the Nd:YAG laser. The septum is cut using the touch technique. The hysteroscope with the laser fibre is advanced. The septum is melted away by a simple advancement of the bare fibre. b Final view.

advanced and melts away the septum, while visual contact is maintained with the right and left uterine ostia. The mean time of hysteroscopic resection is < 15 minutes. The risk of fluid overload is therefore minimal.

The most delicate part of the procedure is probably deciding exactly when the resection is sufficient, and when continuing would cause damage to the myometrium and immediate complications such as perforation, or more delayed complications such as uterine rupture during pregnancy. Almost all surgeons stop resection when the area between the tubal ostia is a line (Figure 33.3). Simultaneous laparoscopic examination is extremely useful for this purpose, especially for beginners. Querleu and associates[13] use echography to distinguish the septum from the myometrium, and thus the decision to stop the resection is easily made.

33.2.4 Complete Uterine Septum

For many years, only partial septal defects were treated hysteroscopically, and wide (>2 cm) or complete septal defects were corrected via an abdominal metroplasty. Donnez and co-workers,[7,12,14] however, described a method that allows even complete septal defects to be managed hysteroscopically. Rock and colleagues[15] proposed the use of the resectoscope for the lysis of a complete uterine septum by means of a new method, which makes it possible to leave the cervical septum intact, thus avoiding any subsequent cervical incompetence. To treat a complete uterine septum, they described a one-stage method where the other cervical os is occluded with the balloon of

a Foley catheter, in order to prevent loss of the distending medium. They believe that it is better not to remove the cervical canal, as this might lead to subsequent cervical incompetence. We do not agree with this hypothesis, and all complete uterine septa are removed using the following surgical procedure, previously done in two steps, but now in one.

In some cases, not only may a double cervical canal be observed, but a vaginal sagittal septum may also be present in the upper vagina or throughout its length (Figure 33.4a). First, the vaginal septum (if present) is resected using a CO_2 laser or unipolar coagulation (Figure 33.4b). The cervical septum is then incised with the scissors or with a CO_2 laser connected to a colposcope, until the lower portion of the uterine septum is seen. In the past, the second step was performed 2 months after the first operation. Now, however, Nd:YAG laser resection of the uterine septum is subsequently carried out (Figure 33.5). The hysteroscope is advanced while visual contact is maintained with the right and left uterine ostia. Because the septum is poorly vascularised, bleeding is usually minimal. When this procedure was carried out in two steps, hysterosalpingography demonstrated the presence of a

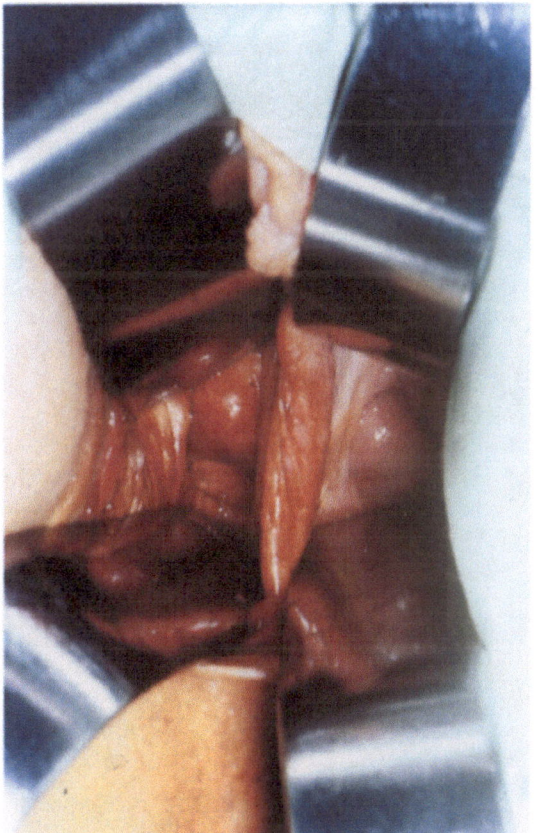
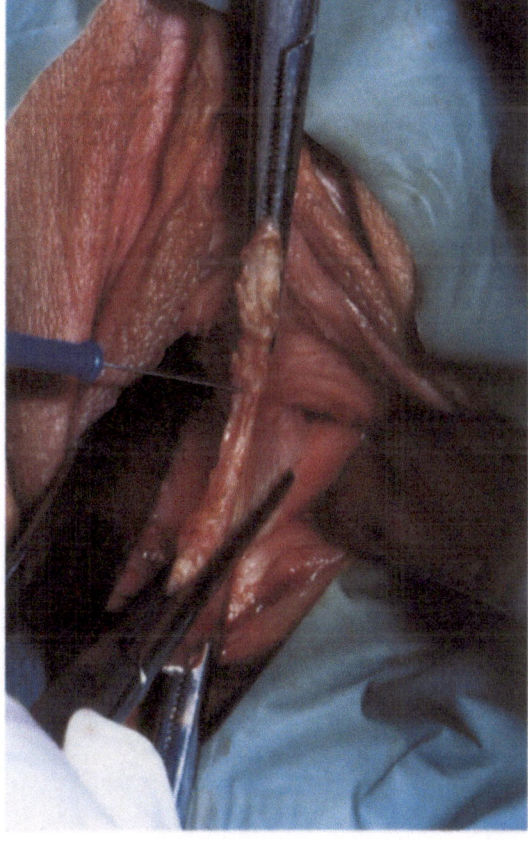

a   b
Figure 33.4 a Vaginal sagittal septum. **b** Resection of the vaginal septum using unipolar coagulation.

normal, single cervical canal 2 months after the first step and a normal uterine cavity 2 months after the second step. Nowadays, all cases of complete uterine septa with or without a vaginal septum are managed in one step.

A double cervix and septate vagina with a normal uterus is an unusual Müllerian anomaly, inconsistent with the current understanding of Müllerian development.[16,17] In such cases, the vaginal septum and the cervical septum can be removed as described previously.

33.2.5 Pre- and Postoperative Management

Following excision of very wide septa, the surgeon's vision may be obscured by pieces of resected tissue and, at times, by uterine bleeding. The Nd:YAG laser produces no debris and carries a reduced risk of bleeding. Several authors have suggested preoperative treatment with danazol or luteinising hormone-releasing hormone agonists;[18] others[9] inject a solution of pitressin into the cervix. Neither pitressin nor hormone administration is required with laser therapy.

Although preoperative hormonal therapy causes atrophy of the endometrium and reduces vascularisation and intraoperative bleeding, it also reduces the depth of the myometrium and therefore increases the risk of perforation and/or myometrial damage. It is suggested that surgery be performed immediately after the end of menstrual bleeding. The literature review by Parazzini et al.[18] pointed out that the only advantage of preoperative use of hormonal therapy was to decrease the operating time.

Postoperatively, a broad-spectrum antibiotic is administered for 3–4 days.

In order to avoid the risk of synechiae, an intrauterine device (IUD; Multiload, Organon, GSS, The Netherlands) is inserted into the uterine cavity. Hormone replacement therapy with oestrogens (100–200 μg ethinyloestradiol) and progestogens (5–15 mg Lynestrenol; Orgametril, Organon, OSS, The Netherlands) is given for 3 months. De Cherney and co-workers,[8] however, use neither hormone replacement therapy nor IUDs. Formerly, Perino and associates[19] administered both oestrogens and medroxyprogesterone and inserted IUDs, but they have recently abandoned these measures and now

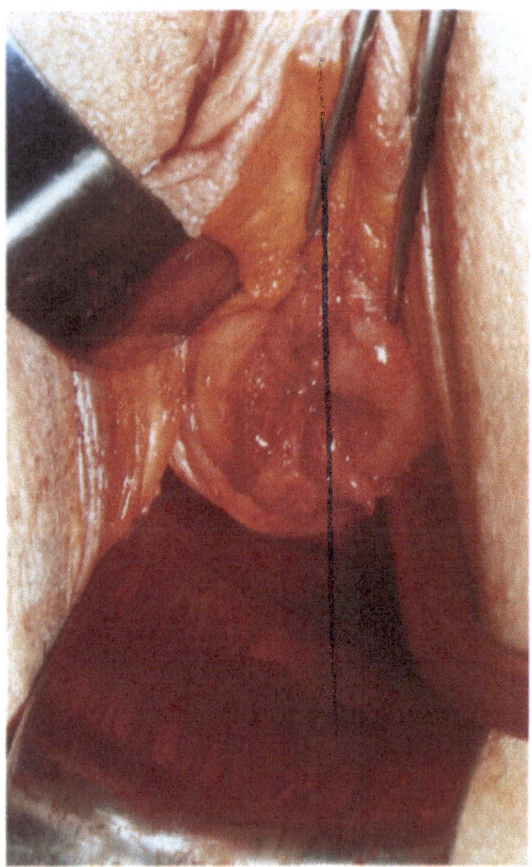
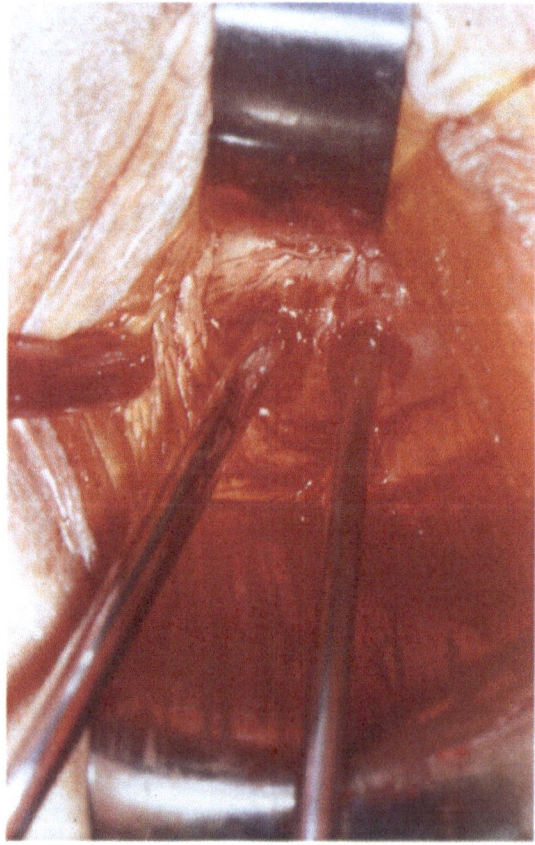

a   b
Figure 33.5 a The external cervical os is completely normal. **b** Dilatation of the cervical canal before the uterine septum resection.

administer no postoperative therapy. Hamou[10] performs a hysteroscopic procedure 1 month after surgery in order to separate synechiae, if necessary.

Almost all authors agree that a follow-up examination should be performed 1–2 months after the operation, irrespective of the postoperative management. Inspection can be made either by means of hysterosalpingography or hysteroscopy. Hamou performs a hysteroscopic inspection 1 month after resection of the septum; in his opinion, this is early enough to prevent the development of synechiae.

In our department, the postoperative morphology of the uterine cavity is systematically evaluated 4 months after the resection. One month after the removal of the IUD, a hysterosalpingography is carried out; the morphology of the uterine cavity almost always resembles that of an arcuate uterus. Indeed, it is preferable not to resect the septum too much, but to leave a sufficient depth of myometrium at the top of the uterus. A hysteroscopy was performed in a first series[12] to confirm that re-epithelialisation of the resected endometrial area had occurred. Nowadays, this procedure is not systematically carried out.

33.2.6 Results and Complications

De Cherney and associates[8] reported the successful use of the urological resectoscope in 72 women, with a term pregnancy rate of 89%. The full-term pregnancy rate reported in various studies ranges from 81 to 89%. Table 33.2 shows the results of hysteroplasty from the literature; the pregnancy rate is 86%. Hysteroscopic resection of an intrauterine septum may benefit patients suffering from infertility or recurrent pregnancy wastage.[20]

Operative hysteroscopy is a safe and effective method of management of uterine septa associated with recurrent pregnancy loss, and makes future vaginal delivery possible. In one of our series of 17 complete uterine septa, 10 out of 17 women became pregnant and no signs of cervical incompetence were observed.[14] The last patient is still being treated with a combination of oestrogens and progestogens. Prophylactic cerclage was never per-

formed after resection of a complete cervical and uterine septum. Following hysteroscopic metroplasty, caesarean section should be performed only for obstetric reasons.

In our series, intraoperative and postoperative complications were encountered in only three cases (1.4%). Classic intraoperative complications such as fluid overload, haemorrhage or perforation could result from the hysteroscopic procedure itself. In our series of 216 patients, no fluid overload or haemorrhage was encountered and perforation was noted in only one case. This was due to the fact that the patient had already undergone a uterine septum resection a few months before, which was considered to be insufficient. The postoperative hysterosalpingography revealed a persistent uterine septum, which needed to be resected a second time. Upon diagnosis of the perforation, laparoscopy enabled us to exclude serious complications such as bowel damage or haemorrhage. Fedele et al.[21] suggested that a remaining uterine septum of less than 1cm in size after hysteroscopic metroplasty does not impair reproductive outcome and therefore does not require a second hysteroscopic surgical procedure.

Two postoperative complications encountered in another hospital were uterine ruptures during delivery. The two cases were twin pregnancies and the labours were very long, taking more than 24 hours. The patients finally delivered by emergency caesarean section. The babies lived and the myometrium was sutured. In both cases, the rupture occurred at the fundus of the uterus. Obviously, in normal conditions, the delivery can be performed vaginally following a uterine septum resection, but in the case of multiple pregnancies, caesarean section should be considered.

33.3 Non-communicating Rudimentary Horns

Pregnancy in a non-communicating rudimentary horn (Figure 33.6a) is uncommon and usually results in miscarriage or uterine rupture. At

Table 33.2. Results of hysteroscopic treatment for uterine septum

Authors	No. of patients treated	No. of pregnancies	No. of pregnancies > 1st trimester		No. of miscarriages	
Corson[9]	18	17	14	(82.3%)	3	(17.6%)
de Cherney[8]	72	72	64	(89%)	8	(11%)
Fayez[25]	19	16	14	(87.5%)	2	(12.5%)
Valle[4]	12	13	11	(84.6%)	2	(15.4%)
March[26]	66	63	55	(87.3%)	8	(12.7%)
Blanc[27]	45	31	25	(81%)	6	(19.3%)
Total	232	212	183	(86%)	29	(13.7%)

hysterography, a hemi-uterus is diagnosed; indeed, the non-communicating rudimentary horn is not opacified (Figure 33.6b). Pregnancies in a non-communicating rudimentary horn are due to transmigration of sperm into the fallopian tube of the affected horn. Most complications occur within the first 20 weeks: the most severe are uterine rupture and maternal death. Raman and colleagues[22] described a 17-week pregnancy occurring in a rudimentary horn, treated by laparotomy and excision. Recently, Dicker and colleagues[23] described the laparoscopic management of a rudimentary horn pregnancy at 8 weeks of amenorrhoea. In order to avoid maternal complications, we systematically perform an excision of the rudimentary horn. A laparoscopic hemihysterectomy can easily be carried out using the same techniques as for laparoscopic hysterectomy.

In rare cases, such non-communicating rudimentary horns can lead to dysmenorrhoea and should then be removed laparoscopically. A Foley catheter is inserted during surgery to empty the bladder. Four laparoscopic puncture sites including the umbilicus are used: 10 mm umbilical, 5 mm right,

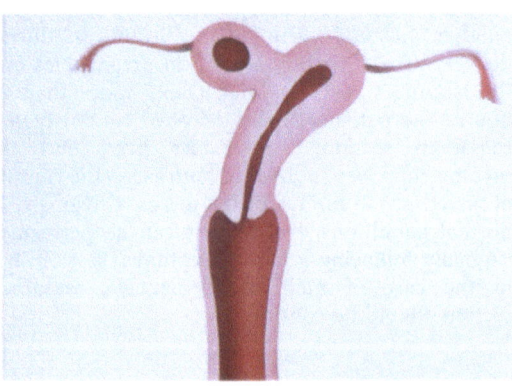

a

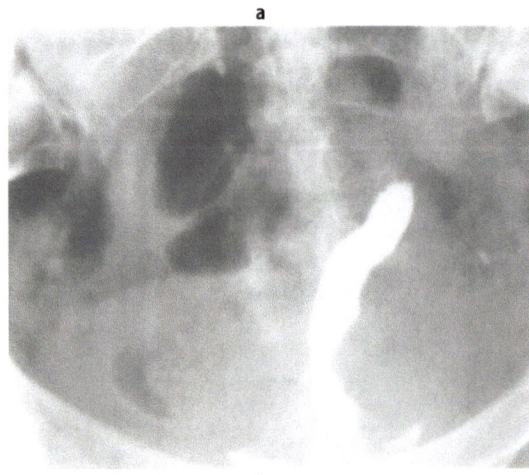

b

Figure 33.6 a Non-communicating rudimentary horn. b Right rudimentary horn. Hysterography: normal left uterine horn.

5 mm medial and 5 mm left lower quadrant sites. These are placed just above the pubic hairline and the lateral incisions are made next to the deep epigastric vessels. A cannula is placed in the single cervix for appropriate uterine mobilisation. A bipolar forceps is used to compress and desiccate the fibrous tissue between the horns. The tissue is then cut with scissors and with a CO_2 laser. Bipolar coagulation is used to coagulate the pedicle. Scissor division is carried out close to the line of desiccation to ensure that a compressed pedicle remains. The mesosalpinx is then cut. If necessary, the peritoneum of the vesico-uterine space is grasped and elevated with forceps, while the scissors dissect the vesico-uterine space. Aquadissection may be used to separate the leaves of the broad ligament, distending the vesico-uterine space and defining the tendinous attachments of the bladder in this area, which are coagulated and cut. The tube of the affected horn is then removed.

The external tubal vessel is identified and exposed by applying traction to the adnexa with an opposite forceps. The dissection of the two horns is performed as follows: if there is true separation of the two horns, the fibrous tissue is coagulated with bipolar coagulation and then cut with scissors or with the CO_2 laser. If there is no external separation of the two horns, the dissection is more difficult; after coagulation, the myometrium must be cut in order to allow the removal of the rudimentary horn. For this purpose, bipolar coagulation and the CO_2 laser or the Nd: YAG laser fibre can be used to achieve coagulation and resection of the myometrium.

In the past, the rudimentary horn was removed either through the trocar of the laparoscope, or through a posterior colpotomy in cases of larger rudimentary horns.

For the past 2 years, the removal of large rudimentary horns has been carried out with the help of a morcellator (Steiner morcellator, Storz, Tuttlingen, Germany) previously described for the removal of the uterus in laparoscopic supracervical hysterectomy.[24]

To date, this procedure has been performed successfully on 20 women in our department. Of the 14 who desired pregnancy, 11 became pregnant and had a normal vaginal delivery (> 36 weeks), except one woman on whom caesarean section was performed for fetal reasons.

33.4 Conclusions

Hysteroscopic resection of an intrauterine septum may benefit patients suffering from infertility or recurrent pregnancy wastage. A partial or complete uterine septum can be easily resected with the help of the Nd:YAG laser. If present, the vaginal septum is also removed during the same procedure. The reproductive outcome of women treated by operative hysteroscopy for an intrauterine septum is reviewed.

To avoid pregnancy in a non-communicating rudimentary horn, the removal of the rudimentary horn and the homolateral tube is performed with the help of bipolar coagulation or the CO_2 laser when the diagnosis is made.

References

1. Edström K, Fernström I (1970) The diagnostic possibilities of a modified hysteroscopic technique. Acta Obstet Gynecol Scand 49:327
2. Donnez J, Nisolle M (1997) Endoscopic laser treatment of uterine malformations. Hum Reprod 12:1381–1387
3. Chervenak FA, Neurwirth RS (1981) Hysteroscopic resection of the uterine septum. Am J Obstet Gynecol 141:351
4. Valle RF, Sciarra JJ (1986) Hysteroscopic resection of the septate uterus. Obstet Gynecol 67:253
5. Gallinat A (1993) Endometrial ablation using the Nd:YAG laser in CO_2 hysteroscopy. In: Leuken RP, Gallinat A (eds) Endoscopic surgery in gynecology. Demeter Verlag GmbH, Berlin, pp 109–116
6. Ashton D, Amin HK, Richart RM et al (1988) The incidence of symptomatic uterine anomalies in women undergoing transcervical tubal sterilization. Obstet Gynecol 72:28–30
7. Nisolle M, Donnez J (1995) Letter to the Editor. Fertil Steril 63:934–935
8. De Cherney AH, Russel LJB, Graebe RA et al (1986) Resectoscopic management of Müllerian defects. Fertil Steril 45:726
9. Corson SL, Batzer FR (1986) CO_2 uterine distension for hysteroscopic septal incision. J Reprod Med 31:710
10. Hamou J (1993) Electroresection of fibroids. In: Sutton C, Diamond M (eds) Endoscopic surgery for gynaecologists. Saunders, London, pp 327–330
11. Daniell JF, Osher S, Miller W (1987) Hysteroscopic resection of uterine septa with visible light laser energy. Colpos Gynecol Laser Surg 3:217
12. Donnez J, Nisolle M (1989) Operative laser hysteroscopy in Müllerian fusion defects and uterine adhesions. In: Donnez J (ed) Laser operative laparoscopy and hysteroscopy. Nauwelaerts Printing, Leuven, pp 249–261
13. Querleu D, Brasme TL, Parmentier D (1990) Ultrasound-guided transcervical metroplasty. Fertil Steril 54:995–998
14. Nisolle M, Donnez J (1996) Endoscopic treatment of Müllerian anomalies. Gynaecol Endosc 5:155–160
15. Rock JA, Murphy AA, Cooper WH (1987) Resectoscopic technique for the lysis of a class V complete uterine septum. Fertil Steril 48:495
16. Candiani M, Busacca M, Natale A et al (1996) Bicervical uterus and septate vagina: report of a previously undescribed Müllerian anomaly. Hum Reprod 11:218–219
17. Goldberg JM, Falcone T (1996) Double cervix and vagina with a normal uterus: an unusual Müllerian anomaly. Hum Reprod 11:1350–1351
18. Parazzini F, Vercellini P, De Giorgi O et al (1998) Efficacy of preoperative medical treatment in facilitating hysteroscopic endometrial resection, myomectomy and metroplasty: literature review. Hum Reprod 13:2592–2597
19. Perino A, Mencaglia L, Hamou J et al (1987) Hysteroscopy for metroplasty of uterine septa: report of 24 cases. Fertil Steril 48:321
20. Goldenberg M, Sivan M, Sharabi Z et al (1995) Reproductive outcome following hysteroscopic management of intrauterine septum and adhesions. Hum Reprod 10:2663–2665
21. Fedele L, Bianchi S, Marchini M et al (1996) Residual uterine septum of less than 1 cm after hysteroscopic metroplasty does not impair reproductive outcome. Hum Reprod 11:727–729
22. Raman S, Tai C, Neom HS (1993) Non-communicating rudimentary horn pregnancy. J Gynecol Surg 9:59–62
23. Dicker D, Nitke S, Shoenfeld A et al (1998) Laparoscopic management of rudimentary horn pregnancy. Hum Reprod 13(2):643–644
24. Donnez J, Nisolle M (1993) Laparoscopic supracervical (subtotal) hysterectomy (LASH). J Gynecol Surg 9:91–94
25. Fayez JA (1986) Comparison between abdominal and hysteroscopic metroplasty. Obstet Gynecol 70:399–406
26. March CM, Israel R (1987) Hysteroscopic management of recurrent abortion caused by septate uterus. Am J Obstet Gynecol 156:834–842
27. Blanc B, d'Ercole C, Gaiato ML et al (1994) Le traitement endoscopique des cloisons utérines. J Gynecol Obstet Biol Reprod 23:596–601

Appendix

Classification of Müllerian Abnormalities

The AFS Classification of Müllerian Anomalies

Patient's Name _____ Date _____ Chart# _____

Age _____ G _____ P _____ Sp Ab _____ VTP _____ Ectopic _____ Infertile Yes _____ No _____

Other Significant History (i.e. surgery, infection, etc.) _____

_____

HSG _____ Sonography _____ Photography _____ Laparoscopy _____ Laparotomy _____

EXAMPLES

I. Hypoplasis/Agenesis
a vaginal   b cervical
c fundal   d tubal   e combined

II. Unicornuate
a communicating   b non-communicating
c no cavity   d no horn

III. Didelphus

IV. Bicornuate
a complete   b partial

V. Septate
a complete**   b partial

VI. Arcuate

VII. DES Drug Related

* Uterus may be normal or take a variety of abnormal forms.
** May have two distinct cervices

Type of Anomaly
Class I _____   Class V _____
Class II _____   Class VI _____
Class III _____   Class VII _____
Class IV _____

Treatment (Surgical Procedures): _____
_____
_____

Prognosis for Conception & Subsequent Viable Infant*

_____ Excellent   (> 75%)

_____ Good   (50 – 75%)

_____ Fair   (25 – 50%)

_____ Poor   (< 25%)
* Based upon physician's judgement.

Recommended Followup Treatment _____
_____
_____

Additional Findings: _____
_____
_____

Vagina: _____
Cervix: _____
Tubes: Right _____ Left _____
Kidneys: Right _____ Left _____

DRAWING

L   R

Part VIII

Early Pregnancy Complications

Contents

Summary

The aetiology of early pregnancy failure is poorly understood. In order to assess early pregnancy failure, knowledge of the normal development of an early pregnancy is essential. Once a diagnosis of miscarriage has been made, management has become increasingly conservative. The rationale behind the expectant management of miscarriage is discussed, as well as the possible role of medical therapy in this context. For many women, no diagnosis can be made at the time of their initial scan; such cases are classified as pregnancies of unknown location. Knowledge of the normal behaviour of human chorionic gonadotrophin (hCG) and progesterone in early pregnancy is needed to manage these cases. The majority of ectopic pregnancies will be visualised by transvaginal ultrasonography. Most laparoscopies now should be for treatment rather than diagnosis. The accurate classification of ectopic pregnancies using ultrasound has opened up the possibility of more conservative management for this condition, whether it be expectant, with methotrexate or surgery. The optimal treatment strategy is not certain. However, systemic methotrexate can be used with success in both single- and multiple-dose regimens, while both laparoscopic salpingotomy and salpingectomy have a role depending on the surgical findings. This section aims to outline a management strategy for early pregnancy complications based on an accurate ultrasound diagnosis and conservative management.

Key points

- The majority of women will choose expectant management for miscarriage
- 84% of women with an incomplete miscarriage, 59% with a missed miscarriage and 52% with an anembryonic pregnancy will resolve their miscarriage within 2 weeks
- Medical treatment with prostaglandins and antiprogesterone agents does not contribute to the management of incomplete miscarriage, but may play a role in missed miscarriage and anembryonic pregnancies
- The use of ultrasonography to follow up women with incomplete miscarriage is not necessary in most cases
- For pregnancies of unknown location, a low serum progesterone value (< 20 nmol/l) is associated with pregnancy failure; a serum hCG rise of over 66% from its baseline value indicates pregnancy viability
- Most ectopic pregnancies should be visualised by ultrasonography
- Local methotrexate therapy under laparoscopic guidance has no role
- Multiple-dose systemic methotrexate therapy regimens are more effective than a single-dose regimen
- Methotrexate is only suitable for haemodynamically stable patients with low initial serum hCG levels (< 3000 IU/l)
- Laparoscopic salpingotomy should be offered to women with tubal pathology suggesting infection. If the contralateral tube is normal, future fertility will be the same whether the affected tube is conserved or not
- The rate of recurrent ectopic pregnancy is approximately 10%
- Serial hCG follow-up essential when the tube is conserved; persistent trophoblast is an indication for systemic methotrexate therapy

Chapter 34

Early Pregnancy Failure

Steven R. Goldstein

34.1 Introduction

Although the blastocyst begins to implant in the endometrium at 3 weeks menstrual age (1 week postconception),[1] the first definitive ultrasound sign of pregnancy is the "gestational sac". Prior to the appearance of the gestational sac, the endometrium is markedly echogenic and the arcuate vessels are somewhat prominent.[2] This, however, is non-diagnostic and can often be seen in the normal late secretory phase. In ultrasound images the gestational sac appears as a thick echogenic ring surrounding a sonolucent centre (Figure 34.1). This sonolucent centre is actually the fluid-filled chorionic sac.[2] This sac already contains the amnion, bilaminar embryonic disc and yolk sac, but these

structures are too small to be imaged, even with the high magnification of our current endovaginal probes. The echogenic ring is the result of a trophoblastic decidual reaction. Early on the entire chorionic sac is surrounded by chorionic villi (Figure 34.2). These villi are symmetrically located. Some villi will bud and branch into secondary and tertiary villi, and become chorion frondosum (the forerunner of the placenta). Other primary villi will regress and become chorion leave. The appearance of the gestational sac predates the fusion of the decidua capsularis and the decidua parietalis. In fact, one can occasionally image a sonolucent endometrial cavity adjacent to the gestational sac.[3] As the gestation progresses, the yolk sac is the first of the structures visualised inside the chorionic sac.[4] This will be followed by the embryonic pole,

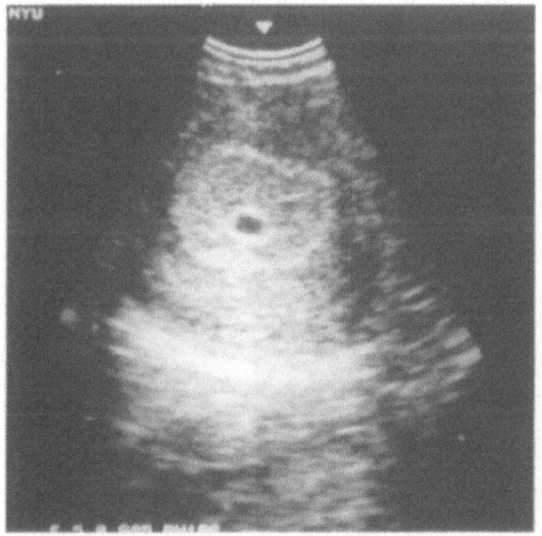

Figure 34.1 The gestational sac is an echogenic ring around a sonolucent centre. In this endovaginal scan at 38 days after the last menstrual period, the sac is seen contained within the decidualised endometrium.

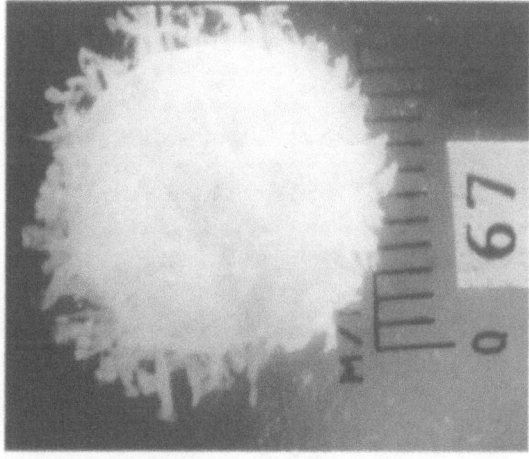

Figure 34.2 Pathologic specimen at 5.5 weeks after the last menstrual period. The chorionic sac grossly appears much like a soft contact lens. Projecting from it are primary trophoblastic villi, which invade maternal decidua and produce the fiercely echogenic ring seen in Figure 38.1.

showing cardiac activity[3] (Figure 34.3). Eventually the amnion surrounding the embryo, but distinctly different from the yolk sac, will be imaged.

Certainly by the time structures are identified within a gestational sac, a definitive diagnosis of intrauterine pregnancy is obvious. The yolk sac when normal is a very regular circular structure up to 6 mm in diameter. It has a very bright echogenic rim around a sonolucent centre. In abnormal pregnancies the yolk sac may be enlarged, irregular or sometimes described as "floating" (see below). The normal embryo will first appear as a thickening along the yolk sac and embryonic cardiac activity will be discernable by m-mode equipment, if available, or by "eyeballing", depending on the type of equipment employed and one's own visual acuity.

The human chorionic gonadotrophin (hCG) produced in ectopic pregnancy can stimulate the uterine endometrium and produce the so-called decidual cast.[5] This can result in a pseudogestational sac, which to some investigators could be confused with a true early intrauterine gestation. Remember this concept predated the development of vaginal ultrasound probes. Such investigators advocated that "the definitive diagnosis of an intrauterine gestation cannot be made until one identifies the embryo within the developing amniotic cavity." However, adherence to such advice merely elongates the window between definitive diagnosis of pregnancy by sensitive radioimmunoassays of hCG (10 days postconception) and the definitive sonographic diagnosis of an intrauterine gestation (as much as 16–20 days later).[6]

Thus, in order to distinguish the true early intrauterine gestation from the pseudogestational sac, investigators described the "double decidual sac".[7,8]

The double decidual sac, with its two concentric rings surrounding a portion of the gestational sac cavity, was thought to represent the decidua parietalis adjacent to decidua capsularis.

Subsequent investigators claim that the early gestational sac is not enveloped by two layers of decidua, as suggested by the double decidual sac concept. They describe an "intradecidual sign" wherin the gestational sac "remains within a thickened decidua on one side of the uterine cavity".[9] There will be cases where this does not appear to be true. One must realise that all our images are two-dimensional. Depending on the scanning plane, the gestational sac may or may not appear centrally or eccentrically located.

Thus, through the high resolution provided by endovaginal probes and reassessment of pathology specimens obtained at curettage, we can better understand the anatomic basis for the sonographic entity known as the gestational sac.

From this it follows that the more normal in appearance a gestational sac is, regardless of being located inside or outside the uterus, the more likely it will be imaged with ultrasound techniques. The natural history of early pregnancies, those that progress and those that fail, has long been of interest to obstetrician–gynaecologists, and more specifically infertility specialists. In the early 1980s, the new-found ability to measure very low hCG levels resulted in numerous studies of the incidence of loss rates in clinically recognised pregnancies as well as clinically unrecognised pregnancies that exhibited small and transitory increases in hCG.[10]

There are wide variations in reported pregnancy loss rates after a normal ultrasound study[11–13] using

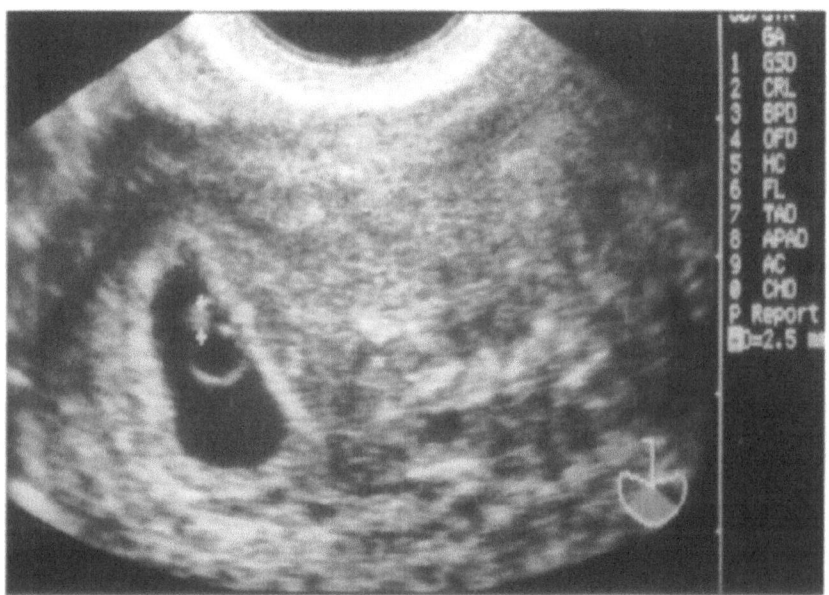

Figure 34.3 Linear embryonic structure (2.5 mm), which shows cardiac activity, seen adjacent to normal–appearing yolk sac at 45 days after the last menstrual period.

improved high-resolution abdominal ultrasound transducers. Times in early pregnancy that a scan was performed and indications for the ultrasound scans varied. In these previous studies, findings were compared with menstrual dating rather than anatomical or embryonic structures. Endovaginal ultrasound probes allow assessment of anatomical and embryological detail not previously appreciated.[14-16]

In one study,[17] 232 women with positive urinary pregnancy tests and no antecedent history of vaginal bleeding had endovaginal sonography performed at the initial visit and at subsequent visits as clinically indicated. Patients were followed until delivery, unless sonographic evidence of non-viability was seen, or spontaneous loss occurred.

Twenty-seven losses occurred during the embryonic period, four losses occurred in the fetal period and there were 201 liveborns. If a gestational sac developed, there was a subsequent loss of viability in the embryonic period of 11.5%; with yolk sac it was 8.5%; an embryo up to 5 mm, 7.2%; an embryo of 6-10 mm, 3.3%; and an embryo larger than 10 mm, 0.5%. No pregnancies lost viability between 8.5 and 14 menstrual weeks. The fetal loss rate after 14 weeks was 2.0%.

Thus, the rate of early pregnancy demise decreases successively with gestational age and is virtually complete by the end of the embryonic period (70 days after onset of the last menstrual period). Subsequent pregnancy losses in the fetal period occur between 14 and 20 weeks. This pattern of early pregnancy demise suggests that there is a period of embryonic loss distinct from a period of fetal loss. The physiological significance of the traditional boundary of the first trimester as an appropriate dividing timeline for early pregnancy may be questioned on the basis of these data.

The successful use of ultrasound requires an understanding of how to apply it in early pregnancy failure. Threatened miscarriage is a clinical term. It is defined as a pregnancy of less than 20 weeks with vaginal bleeding and a closed cervical os. In the past it has been the most common indication for first-trimester ultrasound request. However, all patients with positive pregnancy tests and vaginal bleeding are also at risk of ectopic pregnancy.

Ultrasound findings in the majority of such patients will show a normal-appearing intrauterine gestation (findings will depend on the age of the gestation), with no obvious reason for or source of the clinically apparent vaginal bleeding. If a definitive intrauterine gestation is identified based on the landmarks outlined earlier, sonography may not provide the clinician with the cause for the vaginal bleeding, but the seemingly normal findings may be reassuring to the anxious patient.

Occasionally, on initial ultrasound examination, the uterus shows no gestational sac and an obvious extrauterine pregnancy is diagnosed. This allows one to proceed immediately to therapeutic intervention (Figure 34.4).

If initial ultrasound evaluation of the patient who is pregnant and bleeding fails to reveal a definitive intrauterine gestation, one must resort to following serial beta-subunit determinations until one surpasses a "discriminatory zone" of hCG.[18] A subnormal rate of rise compared to the expected for hCG (66% every 48 hours) indicates either a failing intrauterine gestation or an ectopic gestation.[19,20] At this point, curettage and examination of tissue for the presence of villous material (fetal) compared with "decidua only" (maternal) is an important step in triage.

Once the diagnosis of an intrauterine gestation is firmly established by sonographic criteria, whether or not in combination with serial beta-subunit determination, further questions may arise regarding the normality of that particular gestation.

34.2 Intrauterine Pregnancy Failure

Previously, a blighted ovum was thought of as an anembryonic pregnancy. Sonographically, this was represented by a gestational sac with a mean sac diameter greater than 20 mm without embryo (by transabdominal techniques). This comes from the classic work by Nyberg et al[21] on the major and minor criteria of abnormal gestational sacs. The vaginal probe has further refined these definitions. It would appear that once the mean sac diameter is greater than 8-10 mm (measurement including only the anechoic portion of the chorionic cavity), a yolk sac will become visible.[22] However, the important question is not how early one can see a yolk sac (threshold level), but rather at what point is the lack of such a

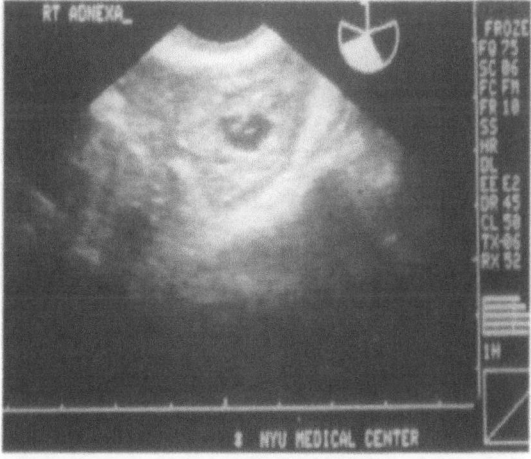

Figure 34.4 Gestational sac containing yolk sac and embryonic pole. This is contained in the right adnexa. The uterus, not pictured in this scanning plane, had no intrauterine gestation.

structure absolutely pathognomonic of non-viable pregnancy, especially allowing for variability in equipment, biology and measuring error (Figure 34.5).

Similarly, a "missed abortion" was previously defined as an embryo of some agreed-upon crown–rump length (usually 15 mm) without cardiac activity but not yet spontaneously passed. Cardiac activity begins 21 days postconception and is actually present before the embryonic structure is large enough to be imaged. This is why with m-mode capability one can often detect a cardiac signal from the lateral edge of the visualised yolk sac. Once again, the question is not how early can cardiac activity be detected, but at what point is its absence absolutely indicative of failed pregnancy (Figure 34.6).

34.3 Embryonic Resorption

The vaginal probe allows us to realise that many so-called "blighted ova" are really cases of intrauterine pregnancy failure with subsequent "embryonic resorption" that previously gave the appearance of an empty sac on transabdominal ultrasound. What we see sonographically will depend on (1) when in development viability is lost and the resorption process begins and (2) when in that resorption process we study the patient. Certainly this explains the process by which the multiple pregnancy is spontaneously reduced to a singleton (previously called the vanishing twin). This is also the process by

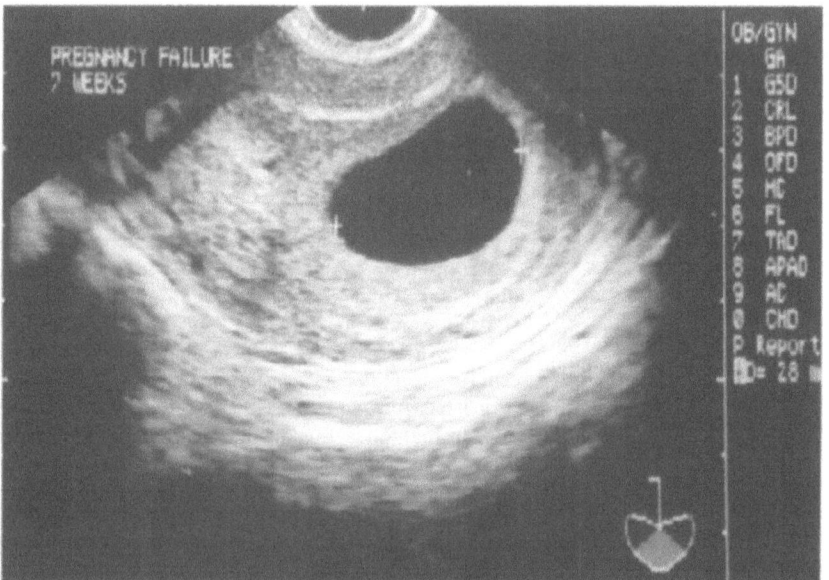

Figure 34.5 Endovaginal scan of a patient at 7 weeks after the last menstrual period. This gestational sac measures 28 mm. It contains no yolk sac or embryonic structure. This is pathognomonic of a failed intrauterine pregnancy.

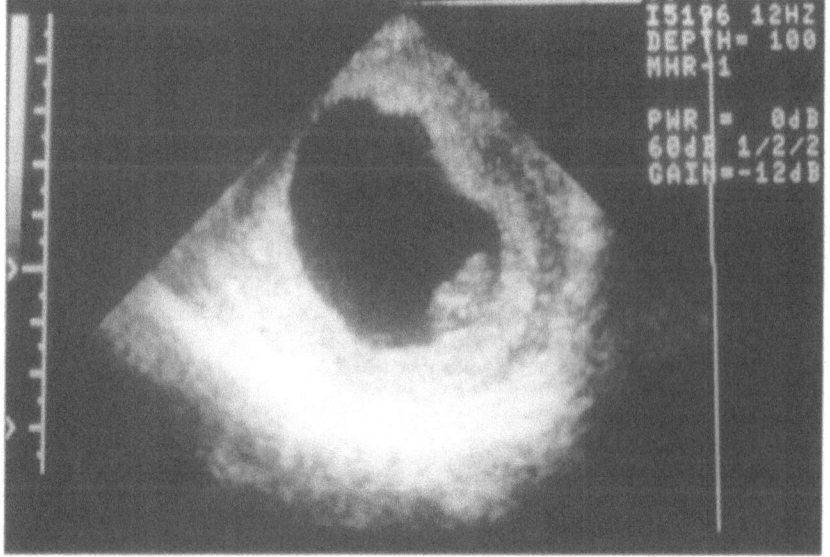

Figure 34.6 Endovaginal ultrasound reveals an 8 mm embryonic structure with a vague morphology. Two weeks previously, there had been a 4 mm normal–appearing embryo with cardiac activity. This is an example of embryonic demise and resorption.

which many singletons become "blighted ova". The vaginal probe has often demonstrated a small embryonic structure at 2, 3 or 4 mm demonstrating cardiac activity, only to have the patient return 2 weeks later and then demonstrate what appears to be a large empty sac, with or without the ability to see the demised embryo.

The incidence of chromosomal abnormalities is generally reported to be increased in such cases of early pregnancy failure. Sonographic abnormalities may be seen in cases prior to embryonic visualisation but after the yolk sac has become apparent. Often such a yolk sac is enlarged, "floating" or poorly formed. Remember the yolk sac, embryonic disc and amnion are present in the earliest gestational sac, but they are too small to be imaged, even with techniques of vaginal probe. The yolk sac portion of this complex is imaged first as the complex enlarges, partially because its sonolucent centre and echogenic rim make it appear very bright and distinct, as opposed to the early ambiguous echogenic thickening of the embryo, which, as already discussed, is best recognised very early by its cardiac pulsations. The endothelial heart tube has folded on itself by 21 days postconception and the cardiovascular system is the first organ system formed in the developing embryo. It, too, is there and beating before it can be imaged with current techniques.

In such pathological pregnancies, whether hCG levels are rising or falling and at what rate will be a function of the condition of trophoblastic tissue and not of the embryonic structures. Sonographically, this is depicted by the echogenic ring (trophoblastic decidual reaction). Many cases of intrauterine pregnancy failure will have high levels of hCG and seemingly normal-appearing villi at the time of curettage. Others will have much lower hCG levels associated with a very poor trophoblastic decidual reaction. This may represent separate aetiologies with mechanisms such as poor implantation, inadequate blood supply or poor flow, or a "fetal factor" such as abnormal chromosomal number or poor embryonic cleavage. However, such cases may also represent the same process merely observed at different points along a naturally occurring "timeline".

34.4 New Considerations for the Failed Pregnancy

Increasingly, pregnancies are being and will be diagnosed as having failed prior to spontaneous passage. There may indeed be a role for cytogenetic analysis as a first step in triage to determine if any further work-up is indicated.

34.4.1 Chromosomal Pregnancy Failure

Various studies show that up to 70% of spontaneous abortions exhibit abnormal chromosomes.[23] Byrne and associates[24] attempted to correlate gross morphology of abortus material with its karyotype and found that various developmental levels could be associated with the various chromosomal anomalies; i.e., conceptuses with karyotypes that occur at term had a greater degree of embryonic development than karyotypes that are never seen among term births. Thus, trisomies 13, 18 and 21 were more often associated with fetuses, and less often with tissue fragments. Focal malformations were multiple and severe in abortuses with triploidy, trisomies 13 and 18, and monosomy X and mild in trisomy 21.

Ohno and colleagues[25] used direct chromosome preparations from chorionic villi instead of traditional tissue culture. This was also carried out in cases of spontaneous abortion. They were the first retrospectively to analyse ultrasound data derived from these pregnancies. All of their 144 patients had at least one ultrasound scan prior to miscarriage. The only detail provided about the ultrasound technique was that it involved a "real-time scanner". The ultrasound findings were merely reported as being "blighted ovum, missed abortion and live abortion" and were based on work of Robinson from 1975.[26] Furthermore, only 32% (47/144) were less than 10 weeks' menstrual age.

A more recent study[27] utilised endovaginal ultrasound transducers of 5–7.5 MHz. It is the first study to use more current concepts of ultrasound landmarks of normal pregnancy and ultrasound indications of definitive pregnancy failure.

The ultrasound appearance of early pregnancy failure in terms of furthest anatomical landmark reached appears not to be significantly different in cases of normal or abnormal karyotypes. It does appear, however, that an abnormal and/or enlarged yolk sac is a non-specific finding of failed pregnancies and does not seem to correlate with karyotypic status. Presumably such an anatomical appearance of the yolk sac is secondary to hydropic change.

It also appears that some karyotypic abnormalities (trisomy 22, mosaics, monosomy X) seem to develop further prior to embryonic demise than others (trisomy 16, multiple trisomies and unusual other variants) (Figures 34.7 and 34.8). Perhaps in the future such information may help to show which chromosomes are involved in the clinical expression of different developmental defects.

The majority of these chromosomal abnormalities are numerical as a result of errors occurring during gametogenesis (chromosomal non-disjunction during meiosis), fertilisation

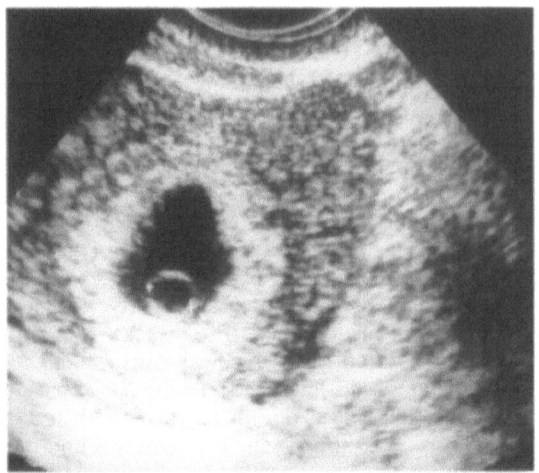

a

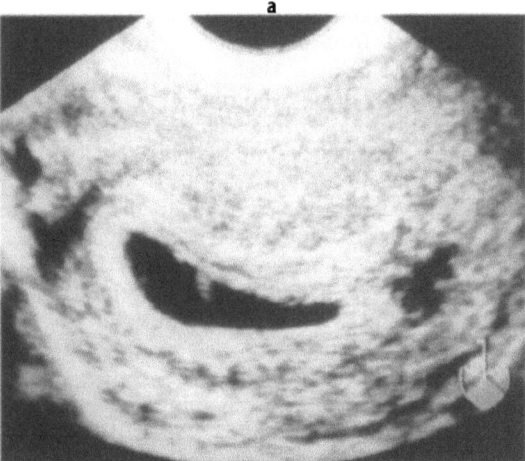

b

(triploidy from dispermy) or the first division of the fertilised ovum (tetraploidy or mosaicism). Of the overall abnormalities, two-thirds will be autosomal trisomies, followed by monosomy X and structural rearrangements. Thus, except for a very small percentage of parental balanced translocations or inversions, the overwhelming majority of these women whose failed pregnancies have abnormal karyotypes would not be expected to show repetitive pregnancy failure.

34.4.2 Non-chromosomal Failure

The reasons for non-chromosomal failure include uterine abnormalities, luteal phase defects, immunological factors, infectious agents, alcohol and smoking, as well as occasional molecular genetic abnormalities lethal to the embryo.

With the first failed pregnancy, cytogenetic analysis of the conceptus will be helpful in subsequent management. If the chromosomes of the conceptus are normal, the couple can undergo evaluation of the various other causes discussed above. If, however, the chromosomes of the conceptus are abnormal, no further work-up or evaluation should be necessary at that time and the likelihood of recurrent loss is very small (unless multiple factors are at play).

Increasingly, failed pregnancies can and should be offered chromosomal analysis. There are two advances that make such an approach possible. First, high-resolution endovaginal ultrasound

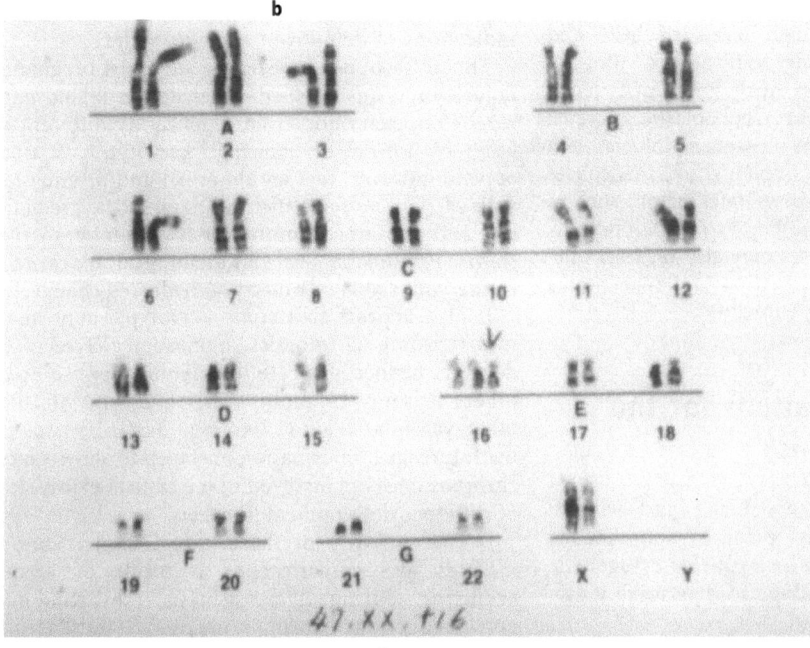

c

Figure 34.7 a Endovaginal scan at 39 days after the last menstrual period. A gestational sac is present. A normal–appearing yolk sac measuring 5 mm (calipers) is seen. **b** Endovaginal scan of the same patient 10 days later. There has been no progressive evolution of normal embryonic structure. The sac is small and flattened with an amorphous echogenic focus seen within it. **c** Karyotype of embryo depicted in **a** and **b**. This represents trisomy 16. No discrete embryonic structure was ever visualised.

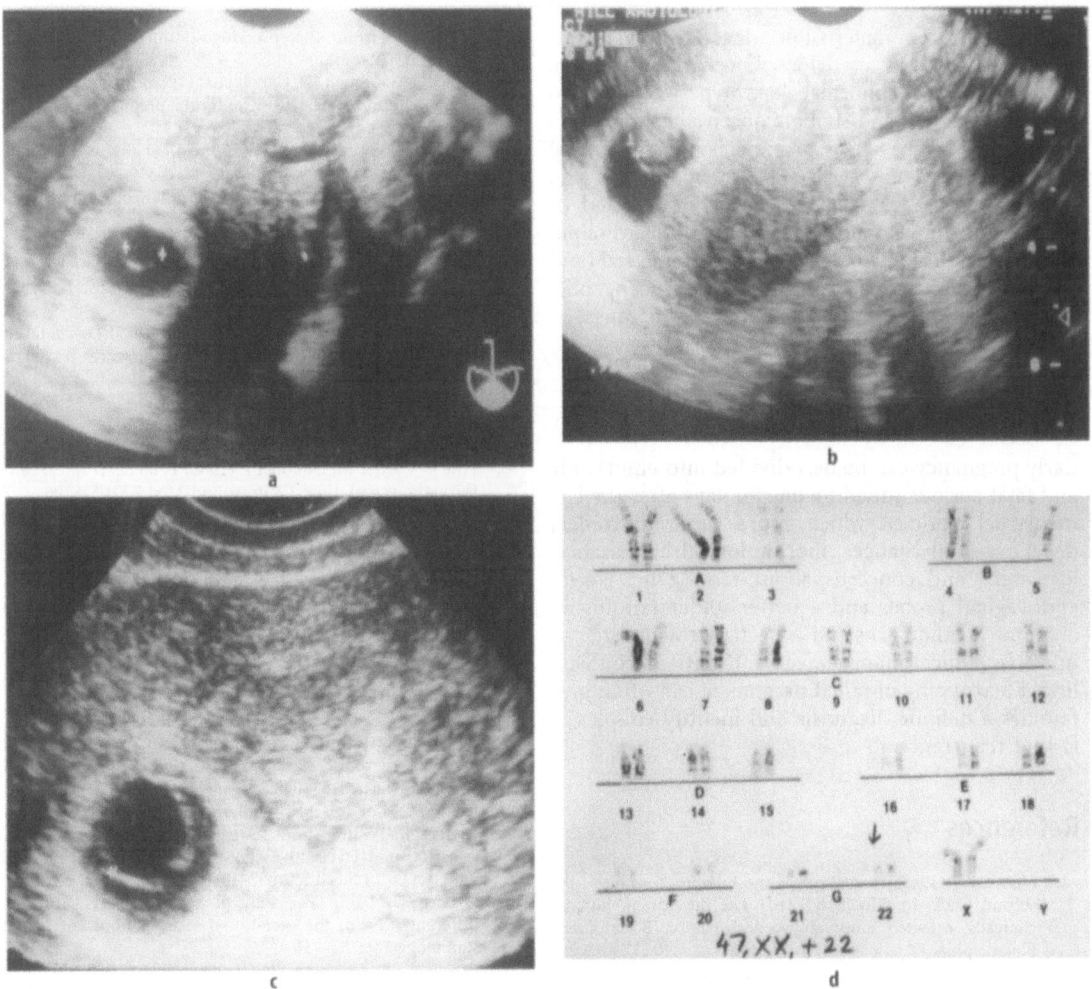

Figure 34.8 a Endovaginal scan of patient at 41 days after the last menstrual period, showing normal–appearing yolk sac measuring 5 mm (calipers). **b** Embryo (7 mm) with cardiac activity noted. This is 10 days after the scan shown in **a** (51 days after the last menstrual period). **c** At 61 days after the last menstrual period (10 days after **b**), the patient complained of vaginal spotting. Endovaginal scan reveals large hydropic yolk sac measuring 11 mm. Discrete embryonic structure is no longer visualised. This is an example of embryonic demise and resorption. **d** Karyotype of embryo shown in **a, b** and **c**, revealing trisomy 22.

transducers have enhanced our understanding of early pregnancy and its normal milestones. This yields an ability to diagnose pregnancy failure consistently prior to spontaneous passage. Ultrasound is employed at the first examination after the missed menses, usually with a positive home monoclonal antibody pregnancy test. The patient is then brought back every 2 weeks until the embryo is greater than 10 mm with cardiac activity. The embryonic loss rate at that point is less than 1%. If intrauterine pregnancy failure is diagnosed sonographically, elective dilatation and curettage is carried out the following day prior to the patient's cramping, bleeding and spontaneous passage. The second advance is the routine examination of tissue from curettage for the presence or absence of chorionic villi or maternal decidua. While initially

done to diagnose unsuspected ectopic pregnancy at the time of elective termination, such examination of tissue in cases of failed intrauterine pregnancy allows a portion of chorion and attached villi to be separated from maternal decidua and submitted for chromosomal study. This avoids the maternal contamination (46XX) that precludes merely submitting "products of conception" for such chromosomal studies. Also, as normal cells will grow better in tissue culture, it seems plausible that some of the spontaneous abortion material karyotyped in old studies may well have represented false-negative cases with contamination of maternal decidua.

Increasingly, pregnancy failure is and will be diagnosed prior to spontaneous passage. Clinicians who have spent 4 months in gynaecological pathology as residents will be able to distinguish chorion and attached villi from maternal decidua. Such embryonic tissue can be easily used for cytogenetic evaluation. The cases with abnormal karyotypes require no further evaluation and should conceive again as soon as possible. The failed pregnancies with normal karyotypes need not await subsequent loss but can immediately be evaluated as clinically suspected or indicated for lupus anticoagulant and anticardiolipin antibodies, luteal phase deficiencies, endometrial (and possible cervical) ureaplasma urealyticum, congential Mullerian abnormalities and submucous myomas.

34.5 Conclusions

Early pregnancy can be best divided into embryonic and fetal periods (dividing line 70 days after the last menstrual period), which more naturally reflect developmental changes, morphological appearance, loss rates and concerns about teratogens. Newer endovaginal probes and a better understanding of anatomical landmarks and expected growth rate can improve clinical management and patient counselling. Karyotyping of failed pregnancy can often give families a definite diagnosis and identify couples at risk of recurrence.

References

1. Moore KL (1988) Formation of the bilaminar embryo: the second week. In: Moore KL (ed) The developing human: clinically oriented embryology, 2nd edn. WB Saunders, Philadelphia, PA
2. Goldstein SR (1991) Pregnancy 1: embryo. In: Goldstein SR (ed) Endovaginal ultrasound, 2nd edn. Wiley-Liss, New York
3. Cadkin AV, McAlpin J (1984) Detection of fetal cardiac activity between 41 and 43 days of gestation. J Ultrasound Med 3:499
4. Sauerbrei E, Cooperberg PL, Poland JB (1980) Ultrasound demonstration of the normal fetal yolk sac. J Clin Ultrasound 8:217
5. Marks WM, Filly RA, Callen PQW et al (1983) The decidual cast of ectopic pregnancy: a confusing ultrasonographic appearance. Radiology 143:223
6. Romero R, Kadar M, Jeanty P et al (1985) Diagnosis of ectopic pregnancy: value of the discriminatory human chorionic gonadotropin zone. Obstet Gynecol 66:357–360
7. Bradley WG, Fiske CE, Filly RA (1982) The double sign of early intrauterine pregnancy: use in exclusion of ectopic pregnancy. Radiology 143:223–226
8. Nyberg DA, Laing FC, Uri-Simmons M et al (1983) Ultrasonic differentiation of the gestational sac of early

9. pregnancy from the pseudogestational sac of ectopic pregnancy. Radiology 146:755–759
10. Yeh HC, Goodman JD, Carr L et al (1986) Intradecidual sign: a US criterion of early intrauterine pregnancy. Radiology 161:463–467
11. Wilcox AJ, Weinberg CR, O'Connor JF et al (1988) Incidence of early pregnancy loss. N Engl J Med 319:189–194
12. Gilmore DH, McNay MB (1985) Spontaneous fetal loss rate in early pregnancy. Lancet i:107–109
13. Wilson RD, Kendrick V, Wittmann BK et al (1986) Spontaneous abortion and pregnancy outcome after normal first trimester ultrasound examination. Obstet Gynecol 67:352–355
14. Simpson JL, Mills JL, Holms LB et al (1987) Low fetal loss rates after ultrasound-proved viability in early pregnancy. JAMA 258:2555–2557
15. Goldstein SR, Snyder JR, Watson C et al (1988) Very early pregnancy detection with endovaginal ultrasound. Obstet Gynecol 72:200–204
16. Fine C, Cartier M, Doubilet P (1988) Fetal heart rates: values throughout gestation. J Ultrasound Med 7:S105–S106
17. Timor-Trisch I, Peisner D, Raju S (1990) Sonoembryology: an organ oriented approach using a high frequency vaginal probe. J Clin Ultrasound 18:286–298
18. Goldstein SR (1994) Embryonic demise in early pregnancy: a new look at the first trimester. Obstet Gynecol 84:294–298
19. Hajenius PJ, Mol BW, Ankum WM et al (1995) Suspected ectopic pregnancy: expectant management in patients with negative sonographic findings and low serum hCG concentrations. Early Pregnancy 1:258–262
20. Kadar N, Bohrer M, Kemmann E et al (1994) The discriminatory human chorionic ganodotropin zone for endovaginal sonography: a prospective, randomized study. Fertil Steril 61:1016–1020
21. Keith SC, London SN, Weitzman GA et al (1993) Serial transvaginal ultrasound scans and beta-human chorionic gonadotropin levels in early singleton and multiple pregnancies. Fertil Steril 59:1007–1010
22. Nyberg D, Laing FC, Filly R et al (1983) Ultrasound differentiation of the gestational sac of ectopic pregnancy. Radiology 146:755–759
23. Rowling SE, Coleman BG, Langer JE et al (1997) First-trimester US parameters of failed pregnancy. Radiology 203:211–217
24. Schmidt-Sarosi C, Schwartz LB, Lublin J et al (1998) Chromosomal analysis of early fetal losses in relation to transvaginal ultrasonographic detection of fetal heart motion after infertility. Fertil Steril 69:274–277
25. Byrne J, Warburton D, Kline J et al (1985) Morphology of early fetal deaths and their chromosomal characteristics. Teratology 32:297–315
26. Ohno M, Maeda T, Matsunobo A (1991) A cytogenetic study of spontaneous abortions with direct analysis of chorionic villi. Obstet Gynecol 77:394–398
27. Robinson HP, Fleming JE (1975) A critical evaluation of sonar "crown rump length" measurements. Br J Obstet Gynaecol 82:702
28. Goldstein SR, Kerenyi T, Scher J et al (1996) Correlation between karyotype and ultrasound findings in patients with failed early pregnancy. Ultrasound Obstet Gynecol 8:314–317

Chapter 35

Ultrasound Diagnosis and Management of Miscarriage

George Condous, Emeka Okaro and Tom Bourne

35.1 Introduction

Miscarriage is known to occur in at least 10–20% of clinical pregnancies.[1] The majority occur before the 13th week. The risk of miscarriage is reduced to 3% if a viable embryo has been seen by ultrasonography. In recent years, early pregnancy units have been introduced in order to improve the efficiency of dealing with women with early pregnancy loss.[2] Management of these women has since changed in many units, with a shift away from a surgical approach to one based on an expectant or "watch and wait" policy.[3] Despite this, in the UK the majority of women with miscarriage are referred to a hospital for assessment and 88% currently undergo surgical evacuation of retained products. The assumption has been that retained products of conception increase the risks of infection and haemorrhage. In fact, less than 10% of women who miscarry experience excessive vaginal bleeding or have infected products of conception within the uterine cavity. In a randomised study, Neilson et al. showed that there was no increased risk of complications for women who underwent expectant management of incomplete miscarriage compared to a surgical approach.[4] The use of non-surgical approaches to the management of miscarriage seems logical.

Knowledge of the normal milestones in early pregnancy that can be seen by ultrasonography is important. The gestational sac becomes visible during week 4, the yolk sac appears during week 5, and the fetal pole with a detectable heartbeat is first seen in week 6.[5] The gestational age of the pregnancy may be uncertain, and in these circumstances early fetal demise can be difficult to diagnose. If the gestation sac diameter is >20 mm without a yolk sac or >25 mm without an embryo, this is classified as an anembryonic pregnancy

(Figure 35.1).[6] If the crown–rump length is at least 6 mm and there is no fetal cardiac activity, or if the crown–rump length is >6 mm with no change at the time of a repeat scan 7 days later, this is classified as a missed miscarriage (early fetal demise).[6] Care must be taken when making this diagnosis, as approximately one-third of embryos with a crown–rump length of less than 5 mm have no demonstrable cardiac activity (Figure 35.2).[7] Whenever there is uncertainty about the viability of a pregnancy, a repeat scan at an interval of 1 week is necessary before a definite diagnosis can be made. Small or irregular gestational sacs, discrepancies between the crown–rump length and gestational age, or an abnormal embryonic heart rate pattern are predictors of a poor pregnancy outcome.[8] An incomplete miscarriage is characterised by a heterogenous appearance and the presence of irregular tissues (Figure 35.3), with or without a gestational sac within the uterine cavity.[6] The endometrial midline echo will usually be distorted. If the endometrial thickness is <15 mm and there is no evidence of retained products of conception, the miscarriage is classified as being complete.[6] Care should be taken in women thought to have a complete miscarriage. As no pregnancy has been seen at any time it is possible that such patients in fact have an ectopic pregnancy. We therefore manage patients with a presumed complete miscarriage in the same way as those where the pregnancy site is uncertain. This is discussed in more detail in chapter 36.

35.2 The Role of Expectant Management

Neilsen et al. have shown expectant management alone to be as effective as surgical evacuation of the

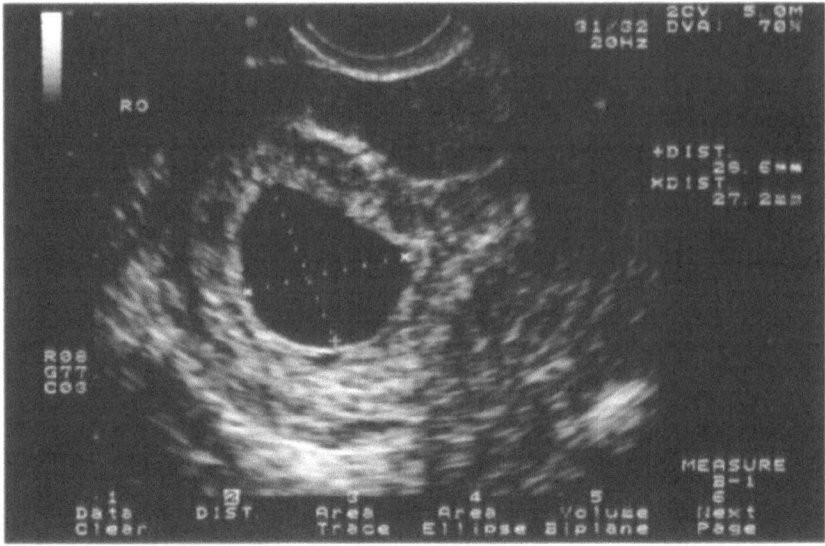

Figure 35.1. An anembryonic pregnancy. The gestation sac measures more than 25 mm and no embryo or yolk sac is seen.

uterus.[4] In a randomised prospective trial, he recruited women with retained products of conception measuring 15–50mm and demonstrated a 71% success rate in the expectant management group. The complication rate (as measured by number of infections or the development of anaemia) was 3% in the expectant group compared to 11% in the surgical group. The duration of bleeding in the expectant group was 1.3 days longer (p<0.02); however, there was no difference in the pain experienced and packed cell volume in each group after 14 days. Poor success rates of between 25 and 43% have been reported.[9,10] This is most likely when the gestation sac is intact and the cervix closed. In such women, resolution may take several weeks and

unless they are counselled appropriately, up to 20% will opt out and request surgical evacuation.[10] The available data suggest there is no difference in psychological morbidity between expectant and surgical management.[11]

Once the diagnosis of miscarriage has been made, the majority of women will choose expectant management. Luise et al. demonstrated that 70% of women with retained products of conception will choose expectant management after appropriate counselling.[6] These data show that women with an incomplete miscarriage can be confidently offered expectant management, as over 80% will complete their miscarriage without surgical intervention within 2 weeks.[12] For other types of miscarriage,

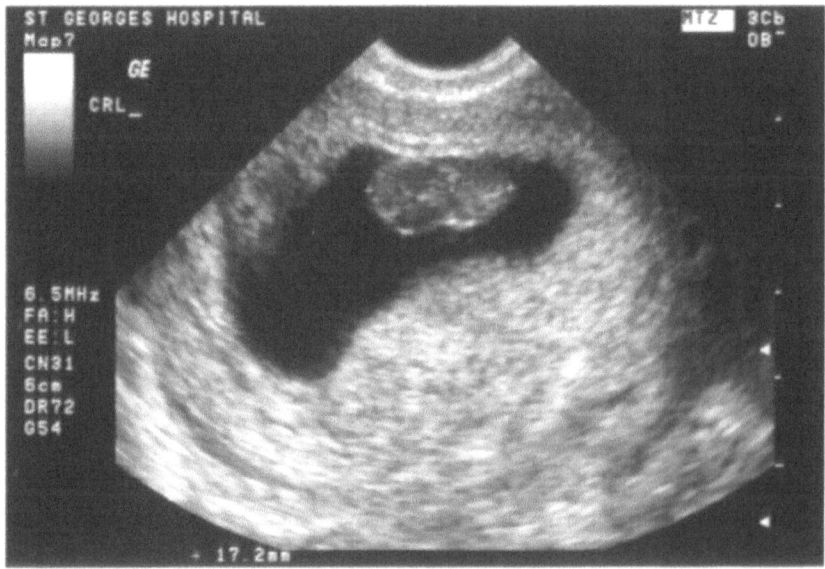

Figure 35.2. A missed miscarriage. Note the crown-rump length of more than 6 mm. The fetal heart is absent.

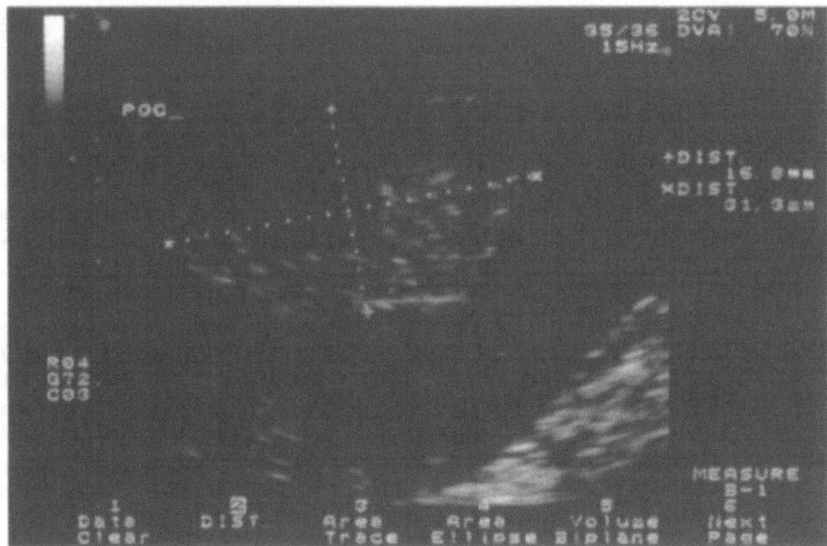

Figure 35.3. An incomplete miscarriage. The cavity appears heterogeneous.

expectant management is less successful. The rate of spontaneous completion of a missed miscarriage may be as high as 84%,[13] while in a more recent study, 76% of missed miscarriages and 66% of anembryonic pregnancies resolved without intervention.[6] Other authors have reported a success rate for expectant management of missed miscarriage of as low as 24.7%.[9] Miscarriage in these two groups is often more painful and less likely to become complete in the same time span as in a patient presenting with an incomplete miscarriage. In the study by Luise et al., only 30% of missed miscarriages and 25% of anembryonic pregnancies had resolved by the end of the first week. By the end of week 2, the number had risen to 59 and 52% respectively[6] (Table 35.1). In this study, some women persisted with expectant management for over a month; as a result, the total number of women achieving their miscarriage increased. However, in practice most women will not choose such an approach. If they have a missed miscarriage or anembryonic pregnancy, women can be told that they have about a 50% chance of resolving their miscarriage without intervention within 2 weeks. After this time, their chances of doing so diminish.

Our anecdotal experience is that while expectant management is valid for women with symptoms attending an early pregnancy unit, the situation is different when the diagnosis is made as a chance finding at the time of a nuchal scan. Our view is that such cases are more likely to experience severe pain or heavy bleeding whether they receive expectant management or medical therapy.

The optimal follow-up for women undergoing expectant management of miscarriage is not standardised. Luise et al. have shown that 91% of women presenting with an incomplete miscarriage resolved their miscarriage: 54% had done so by the end of week 1 and 83% by the end of week 2.[12] After 2 weeks, the odds of a miscarriage becoming complete are significantly reduced. It is therefore a reasonable policy to advise women to give themselves 2 weeks to complete their miscarriage, and that intervention after this time may be reasonable. In this study, neither the presence of a gestational sac within the cavity nor the thickness of the endometrium was clinically useful in determining the outcome of expectant management.[12] Table 35.2 shows the number of days taken to complete a miscarriage related to the ultrasound findings in this study.

Table 35.1. Types of miscarriage and outcomes in patients who chose expectant management. Values are numbers (percentages)

Group classification at diagnosis	Patients	Complete miscarriage		Successful outcome by day 46
		By day 7	By day 14	
Incomplete miscarriage	221 (49)	117 (53)	185 (84)	201 (91)
Missed miscarriage	138 (31)	41 (30)	81 (59)	105 (76)
Anembryonic pregnancy	92 (20)	23 (25)	48 (52)	61 (66)
Total	451 (100)	181 (40)	314 (70)	367 (81)

With permission from Luise et al, (2002) Br Med J 324:873-875[6]

Table 35.2. Presence of a gestational sac (GS) or endometrial thickness (ET) and outcome of expectant management for incomplete, first-trimester miscarriage

Variable	Complete miscarriages No. (% of total)	Days to completion No. (% of group)	Mean (range)
ET (mm)			
<11	30 (13.6)	28 (94.3)	6.8 (2–15)
11–15	54 (24.4)	50 (93.3)	8.8 (2–21)
16–21	41 (18.6)	38 (92.7)	8.9 (1–22)
>21	26 (11.8)	22 (84.6)	10.4 (3–27)
GS (3–28 mm)	70 (31.7)	64 (91.4)	8.7 (2–32)

With permission from Luise et al, (2002) Ultrasound Obstet Gynecol 19: 580–582[12]

Table 35.3 shows the proportion of women completing their miscarriage in relation to time. These data suggest that follow-up for women with incomplete miscarriage need not include ultrasonography. The rate of complications is so low that one follow-up visit after 2 weeks to assess the clinical situation is reasonable. However, women should be able to contact the clinic at any time for advice or support. The emphasis for follow-up should be orientated more towards counselling rather than ultrasound-based assessment of the uterus.

For incomplete miscarriage the high success rate of expectant management means that other interventions are unlikely to alter the outcome. This was confirmed by Neilson et al., who showed no benefit from the use of prostaglandins for the management of incomplete miscarriage.[14] However, for missed miscarriage and anembryonic pregnancies, medical management strategies using both prostaglandins and antiprogesterones may have a role.

35.3 Medical Management of Miscarriage

The use of prostaglandin analogues (misoprostol or gemeprost) with or without antiprogesterone priming (mifepristone) for the medical management of miscarriage is well described.[15–21] Success rates

quoted in the literature vary widely (from 13 to 96%). The outcome depends both on the type of miscarriage treated and the criteria used for follow-up. The total dose of prostaglandin, its duration of use and route of administration also have an effect. Higher success rates (70–96%) are observed when there is an initial diagnosis of incomplete miscarriage;[15,17] however, this is not surprising given the outcome for such miscarriages from expectant management alone. It is unlikely that medical intervention in this group will prove helpful.

The efficacy of medical intervention is not certain. In a randomised clinical trial, Hinshaw et al.[15] demonstrated no statistically significant difference in success rates between surgical and medical management of miscarriage, although patient acceptability for each method was similar. However, this study looked only at incomplete miscarriages. It is of interest that there was a reduction in the number of pelvic infections in the medical management group (p<0.001). However, anecdotally the pain and vaginal bleeding associated with medical management of miscarriage may be a limiting factor influencing its acceptability.[22] A further consideration is that these medical approaches to the management of miscarriage may have economic benefits when compared to surgical evacuation.

In a recent study, Neilsen et al. compared medical management of miscarriage with a combination of antiprogesterone and a prostaglandin E_1 analogue and expectant management alone.[14] There was no improvement in the rate of complete miscarriages achieved in the medical management arm. This may be explained by patient selection, as we know that medical management will not improve the outcome for incomplete miscarriages. A randomised trial examining the impact of medical therapy on the expectant management of missed miscarriage and anembryonic pregnancy is urgently required. Expectant management often results in resorption of retained products of conception with little bleeding; however, bleeding is usual if tissue is passed. In contrast with a medical approach, up to one-third of women will bleed or miscarry during the priming

Table 35.3. Follow-up data from patients undergoing expectant management for an incomplete, first-trimester miscarriage. ERPC, Evacuation of retained products of conception

Time from diagnosis (days)	No. of women	Completed spontaneous miscarriages No. (% in group)	ERPC No. (% in group)	Accumulated spontaneous miscarriages No. (%)
1–7	221	120 (54.3)	8 (3.6)	
8–14	93	64 (68.8)	3 (3.2)	184 (83)
15–21	26	13 (50.0)	5* (19.2)	197 (89)
>22	8	4 (50.0)	4 (50.0)	201 (91)

*Four elective, one emergency
With permission from Luise et al, (2002) Ultrasound Obstet Gynecol 19: 580–582[12]

phase after antiprogesterone alone. Patients must have access to 24-hour emergency facilities in the event of heavy vaginal bleeding.

The infective morbidity of any non-surgical approach, whether it is expectant or medical, has been a cause for concern.[23] However, the available data suggest a reduction in clinical pelvic infection using this approach.[15,24] In relation to long-term complications, it is reassuring that Blohm et al.[25] showed no difference in future fertility rates between those whose miscarriage has been managed expectantly and those who have undergone surgical evacuation.

35.4 Conclusions

In recent years, there has been a trend towards more conservative management for women with first-trimester miscarriage. The majority of women presenting with a miscarriage can be offered expectant management with a reasonable prospect of success and with no increase in the complication rate. Approximately 90% of incomplete miscarriages and 50% of missed miscarriages and anembryonic pregnancies can be expected to miscarry within 2 weeks. The odds of a woman completing her miscarriage with each subsequent week diminish with time. Women can be given an indication of the likelihood of them completing their miscarriage within a 2-week period based on the initial ultrasound diagnosis. Most women will opt for surgical intervention if they have not completed their miscarriage within the 2-week window. The data suggest that the ultrasound appearances of the endometrial cavity contents bear no relation to the outcome of expectant management. The anterior-posterior diameter of the endometrial cavity does not relate to the odds of successful completion. On this basis there seems little sense in repeating ultrasound scans as part of follow-up protocols, as the endometrial cavity contents do not reflect the likelihood of success. Resources for follow-up may be better orientated towards counselling for early pregnancy loss rather than medical intervention. The need for surgery can be based on the presence or absence of pain and bleeding, as well as clinical evidence of infection. The success of expectant management for missed and anembryonic pregnancies is significantly less than for incomplete miscarriage. Medical management is more likely to play a role in these women. A trial comparing medical and expectant management in these pregnancies would be informative at this stage.

Whatever the approach adopted in the management of spontaneous miscarriage, it is the duty of the clinician to ensure the safety of the patient.

Ideally, women should be evaluated in a dedicated early pregnancy unit, the type of miscarriage classified according to an ultrasound scan and the likelihood of successful non-surgical management evaluated. Clinicians should discuss management in the context of a given woman's circumstances. Her clinical and emotional state, her level of understanding and compliance, as well as her access to after-hours emergency facilities are important factors. Expectant management does not suit all women; however, when women express a preference for medical or expectant management, they usually do so because they wish to avoid general anaesthesia and to feel "more in control".[15]

Reassurance and counselling are a significant part of the job for anyone working in an early pregnancy unit. The psychological effects of early pregnancy loss are profound; however, the impact can be ameliorated if couples are handled sensitively. It is helpful for them to know that they can return for reassurance in their next pregnancy. Knowledge of the technical aspects of ultrasonography and serum biochemistry is one of several skills required by people working in this emotionally difficult area.

References

1. Alberman E (1992) Spontaneous abortion: epidemiology. Springer-Verlag, London, pp 9–20
2. Bigrigg MA, Read MD (1991) Management of women referred to early pregnancy assessment unit: care and cost effectiveness. Br Med J 302:577–579
3. Hemminki E (1998) Treatment of miscarriage: current practice and rationale. Obstet Gynecol 91:247–253
4. Neilsen S, Hahlin M (1995) Expectant management of first trimester spontaneous abortion. Lancet 345:84–86
5. Warren WB, Timor-Tritsch IE, Peisner DB et al. (1989) Dating the early pregnancy by sequential appearance of embryonic structures. Am J Obstet Gynecol 161:747–753
6. Luise C, Jermy K, Collins WP et al. (2002) Outcome of expectant management of spontaneous first trimester miscarriage: observational study. Br Med J 324:873–875
7. Levi CS, Lyons EA, Zheng XH et al. (1990) Endovaginal ultrasound: demonstration of cardiac activity in embryos less than 5.0mm in crown-rump length. Radiology 176:71–74
8. Marinez JM, Comas C, Ojuel J et al. (1996) Fetal heart rate patterns in pregnancies with chromosomal disorders or subsequent fetal loss. Obstet Gynecol 87:118–121
9. Jurkovic D, Ross JA, Nicolaides KH (1998) Expectant management of missed miscarriage. Br J Obstet Gynaecol 105:670–671
10. Hurd WW, Whitfield RR, Randolph JF Jr et al. (1997) Expectant management versus elective curettage for the treatment of spontaneous abortion. Fertil Steril 68:601–606
11. Nielsen S, Hahlin M, Möller A et al. (1996) Bereavement, grieving and psychological morbidity after first trimester spontaneous abortion: comparing expectant management with surgical evacuation. Hum Reprod 11:1767–1770
12. Luise C, Jermy K, Collins WP et al. (2002) Expectant management of incomplete, spontaneous first trimester miscarriage: outcome according to initial ultrasound criteria and value of follow-up visits. *Ultrasound Obstet Gynecol*, 19:580–582

13. Schwarzler P, Holden D, Nielsen S et al. (1999) The conservative management of first trimester miscarriages and the use of colour Doppler sonography for patient selection. Hum Reprod 14:1341–1345

14. Neilsen S, Hahlin M, Platz-Christensen J (1999) Randomised trial comparing expectant with medical management for first trimester miscarriages. Br J Obstet Gynaecol 106:804–807

15. Hinshaw HKS (1997) Medical management of miscarriage. Problems in early pregnancy: advances in diagnosis and management. RCOG Press, London, pp 284–295

16. el-Refaey H, Hinshaw K, Henshaw R et al. (1992) Medical management of missed abortion and anembryonic pregnancy. Br Med J 305:1399

17. Henshaw RC, Cooper K, el-Refaey H et al. (1993) Medical management of miscarriage: non-surgical uterine evacuation of incomplete and inevitable spontaneous abortion. Br Med J 306:894–895

18. Chung TK, Cheung LP, Lau WC et al. (1994) Spontaneous abortion: a medical approach to management. Aust NZ J Obstet Gynaecol 34:432–436

19. de Jonge ET, Makin JD, Manefeldt E et al. (1995) Randomised clinical trial of medical evacuation and surgical curettage for incomplete miscarriage. Br Med J 311:662

20. Chung TK, Cheung LP, Leung TY et al. (1995) Misoprostol in the management of spontaneous abortion. Br J Obstet Gynaecol 102:832–835

21. Nielsen S, Hahlin M, Platz-Christensen J (1997) Unsuccessful treatment of missed abortion with a combination of an antiprogesterone and a prostaglandin E1 analogue. Br J Obstet Gynaecol 104:1094–1096

22. Johnson N, Priestnall M, Marsay T et al. (1997) A randomised trial evaluating pain and bleeding after a first trimester miscarriage treated surgically or medically. Eur J Obstet Gynecol Reprod Biol 72:213–215

23. Jurkovic D (1998) Editorial: Modern management of miscarriage: is there a place for non-surgical treatment? Ultrasound Obstet Gynecol 11:161–163

24. Chipchase J, James D (1997) Randomised trial of expectant versus surgical management of spontaneous miscarriage. Br J Obstet Gynaecol 104:840–841

25. Blohm F, Hahlin M, Nielsen S et al. (1997) Fertility after a randomised trial of spontaneous abortion managed by surgical evacuation or expectant treatment. Lancet 349:995

Chapter 36

Ultrasound Diagnosis and Management of Pregnancy of Unknown Location and Ectopic Pregnancy

George Condous, Emeka Okaro and Tom Bourne

36.1 Introduction

The introduction of the vaginal ultrasound probe and the wider availability of facilities to measure serum levels of human beta-chorionic gonadotrophin (βhCG) and progesterone have revolutionised the management of early pregnancy complications. In the past, the mainstay of the assessment of a patient with a possible ectopic pregnancy was the negative predictive value of demonstrating an intrauterine pregnancy. Any women with a positive pregnancy test and an empty uterus at the time of her scan required further investigation, usually in the form of a laparoscopy. However, using transvaginal ultrasonography (TVS) it is possible to detect an intrauterine gestation sac at 5 weeks gestation, regardless of patient obesity or bladder fullness.[1] Hence an intrauterine pregnancy can be seen in more women presenting with early pregnancy problems. However, despite these advances, ectopic pregnancy remains a major diagnostic challenge. The incidence of ectopic pregnancy is rising (1.1% of pregnancies in the UK), and although the associated mortality is falling (0.4 per 100 ectopic pregnancies), it is still the fourth most common cause of direct maternal death reported in the UK.[2]

While the increased resolution obtained by TVS represents a significant advance, it creates its own problems. The earlier patients present to the early pregnancy unit, the more women will have an inconclusive ultrasound scan, where no ultrasound features of either an extra- or intrauterine pregnancy can be seen. It is the role of the early pregnancy team to follow through such patients until a diagnosis is established, on the basis of either ultrasound findings or serum βhCG and progesterone values.

36.2 Pregnancy of Unknown Location

36.2.1 Definition

Of women presenting to an early pregnancy unit, in 8–31%[3,4] a pregnancy will not be visualised by ultrasound and so no diagnosis can be made. They are given the label "pregnancy of unknown location" (PUL). This is defined by TVS as there being no signs of either an intra- or extrauterine pregnancy or retained products of conception in a woman with a positive pregnancy test (i.e. serum βhCG > 5 IU/l). This management approach should also apply to women where it is thought there has been a complete miscarriage. Women with a PUL should be managed expectantly on the basis of measurements of serum levels of βhCG and progesterone. This can be on an outpatient basis. Expectant management has been shown to be safe, to reduce the need for unnecessary surgical intervention and is not associated with any serious adverse outcomes. Nevertheless, 9–29%[3,5] of these women will require surgical intervention due to a worsening clinical condition or non-declining serum βhCG (Figure 36.1).

36.2.2 The Discriminatory Zone and Serial Monitoring of Biochemical Markers

When the location of pregnancy cannot be confirmed on the basis of an ultrasound scan, the use of biochemical markers and their interpretation is the cornerstone of management. An understanding of the discriminatory zone, the doubling time of serum βhCG in early normal pregnancy and the correlation between low serum progesterone and

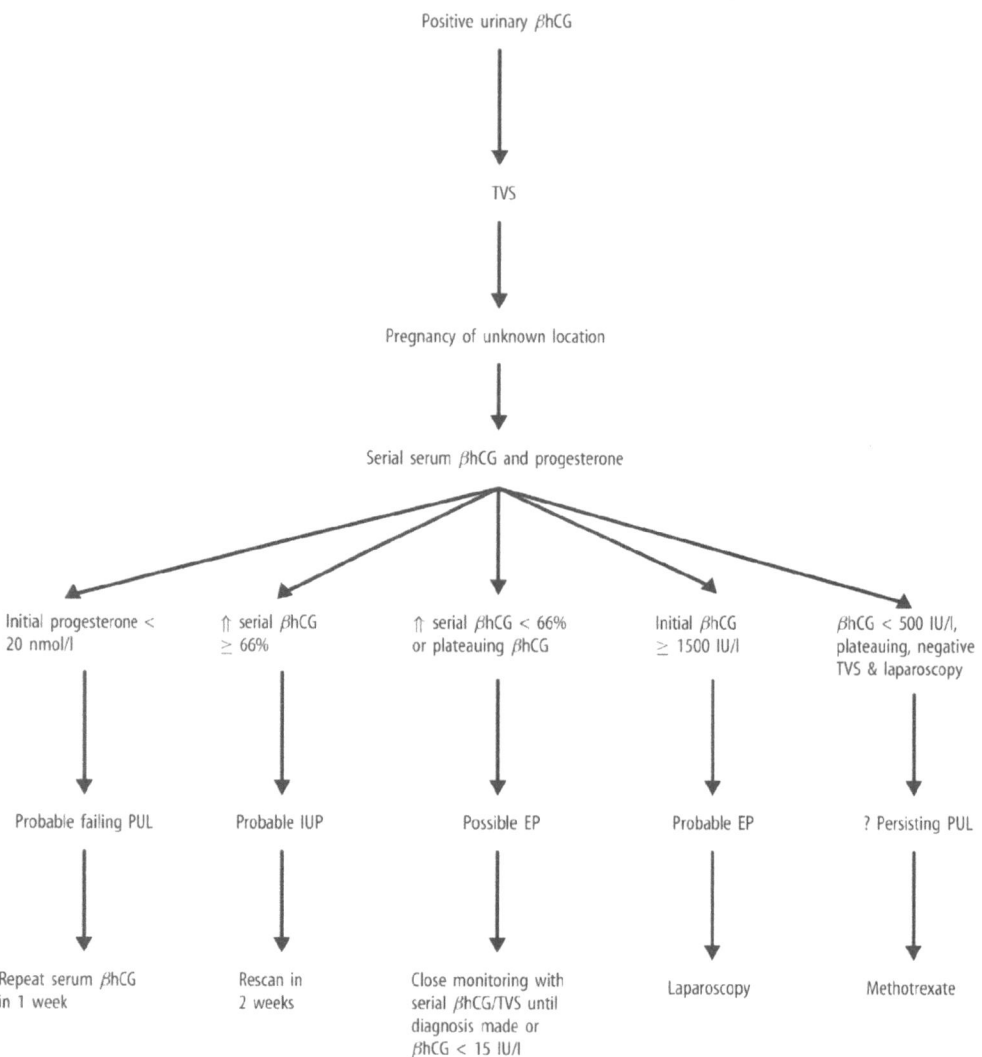

Figure 36.1 Flow chart for the management of pregnancies of unknown location. PUL, Pregnancy of unknown location; βhCG, human beta-chorionic gonadotrophin; TVS, transvaginal ultrasound scan; IUP, intrauterine pregnancy; EP, ectopic pregnancy

spontaneous resolution of pregnancy are all important biophysiological concepts in the management of pregnancies of unknown location.

The concept of combining ultrasound with measurements of serum βhCG using a discriminatory zone is well described.[6–8] By correlating the serum βhCG values to the size of an intrauterine gestational sac, a value can be chosen that corresponds to the threshold above which an intrauterine gestation sac should be seen. If a sac cannot be seen above the threshold value, steps must be taken to determine whether the pregnancy is abnormal or ectopic.

Barnhart et al.[8] showed that above a discriminatory level of 1500 IU/l, an intrauterine gestation sac was seen in 91.5% of cases, compared with 28.6% when levels were below 1500 IU/l. However, it should be noted that the discriminatory zone might vary among institutions due to different types of equipment, the frequency of the probe used and assay techniques. It is also dependent on operator experience. Higher serum βhCG titres are seen in early multiple pregnancies and may lead to unnecessary concern about the location of the pregnancy.

In practice, a single measurement of βhCG will not be diagnostic in the majority of cases. In most cases when the serum βhCG is above the discriminatory zone and an ectopic pregnancy is present, it will be large enough to be visualised by ultrasonography. The problem arises at lower serum βhCG levels or in the smaller number of cases when an ultrasound diagnosis cannot be made. In these cases it is not possible to distinguish between a PUL that will develop into a normal intrauterine pregnancy and one that subsequently becomes an ectopic pregnancy, on the basis of the rate of serum βhCG increase. This can be expressed as the slope of the log βhCG time curve or as the percentage increase in serum βhCG over a given sampling interval. For practical purposes, the rate is most easily determined from two samples drawn 48 hours apart. The difference between the two serum βhCG values obtained is represented as a percentage of the initial value. In normal intrauterine pregnancies, there should be a 66% rise over the baseline value over 48 hours.[9] Using this well-known algorithm is not without its pitfalls, as approximately 15% of normal intrauterine pregnancies screened in this way will appear abnormal, and 13% of ectopic pregnancies will give contradictory results and delay the diagnosis beyond 48 hours. It is possible to have either a "sick" intrauterine or a "flourishing" ectopic pregnancy, and both can give conflicting results.

Pregnancies of unknown location should be stratified into those with either a low or high risk of ectopic pregnancy. The vast majority of these will be at low risk and in turn are made up of failing PUL and viable intrauterine pregnancies. A failing PUL may be intrauterine or extrauterine and generally will resolve spontaneously. A failing PUL is not necessarily a failing intrauterine pregnancy. These pregnancies are never seen on TVS, their baseline serum progesterone at presentation will be < 20 nmol/l and serial serum βhCG levels fall. A baseline serum progesterone level of < 20 nmol/l will identify a failing PUL with a positive predictive value of $\geq$ 95%.[5] This compares favourably with complex multiparameter diagnostic models.[5] In contrast, viable intrauterine pregnancies usually demonstrate a > 66% increase in serial serum βhCG levels taken at 48-hour intervals. However, not all will be ongoing viable pregnancies.

In our unpublished series of 209 consecutive PUL, 87.4% were at low risk of ectopic pregnancy and made up of either intrauterine pregnancies or failing PUL. Approximately 10% of PUL are at high risk and are subsequently revealed to be ectopic pregnancies. In our series, 10.5% were ectopic pregnancies. While the use of serum biochemistry has a high predictive value for either an intrauterine pregnancy or a failing PUL, this is not the case with ectopic pregnancy. Serum biochemistry may pick out a patient who is at risk of ectopic pregnancy, but it is rarely diagnostic. The serial serum βhCG and progesterone levels do not follow a set formula in these women and so serial ultrasound scans need to be performed every 48-72 hours until the diagnosis declares itself. One cannot overemphasise that biochemical results should not be taken in isolation and the clinical assessment and subsequent ultrasound findings are essential to the ongoing management. When the diagnosis of ectopic pregnancy has been established (and this should be possible by TVS in the majority of cases), appropriate medical or surgical management should be initiated. The overall rate of intervention for PUL managed expectantly in our series is 12.1%, which is consistent with the figure of 9% published by other groups.[5]

36.2.3 Persisting Pregnancies of Unknown Location

To date there are no published data in the literature relating to persisting PUL. This small subset of women are defined as those in whom the serum βhCG levels fail to decline, where there is no evidence of trophoblast disease, and the location of the pregnancy cannot be identified by ultrasound or laparoscopy. In general, the serum hCG levels are low (< 500 IU/l) and have reached a plateau. We have successfully treated four such women with methotrexate 50 mg/m^2 and their serum βhCG levels subsequently resolved.

In our view, great care should be taken before giving medical treatment for a PUL when the site of the pregnancy has not been identified. A positive serum βhCG does not always indicate pregnancy. Germ cell tumours may secrete βhCG and should be considered, especially if a women is adamant that she cannot be pregnant. In our series we have seen one placental site tumour and one posterior fossa germ cell tumour present in this way.

36.3 Ectopic Pregnancy

36.3.1 Tubal Ectopic Pregnancies

The ratio of intrauterine to ectopic pregnancies in the UK may be as high as 50:1. The consequences

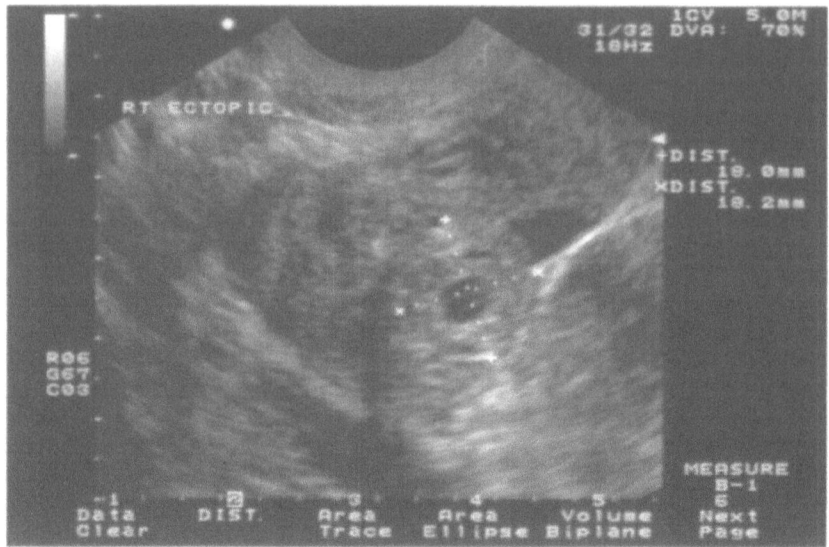

Figure 36.2. Classic appearance of an ectopic pregnancy. Note the "bagel" like ring.

of misdiagnosis are potentially severe and include maternal death. Unfortunately, clinical history and examination may not be helpful. The introduction of transvaginal ultrasound has meant that while the finding of an intrauterine pregnancy is of value, attempts can be made to try to identify the ectopic gestation sac itself. The presence of an ectopic pregnancy is virtually ruled out by the identification of an intrauterine pregnancy by ultrasonography. The frequency of heterotopic pregnancy in spontaneous conceptions is estimated between 1:10,000 and 1:50,000, but as high as 1:100 in assisted conceptions.[10] In general, confirmation of an intrauterine pregnancy is considered sufficient to rule out an ectopic pregnancy unless symptoms persist.

Those women with a high risk of ectopic pregnancy should be advised that they should present to an early pregnancy unit as soon as they know they are pregnant. Those with a previous history of an ectopic pregnancy fall into this category and they should undergo TVS to check the location of the pregnancy. Although the exact aetiology is unknown, there are numerous other risk factors, including: pelvic inflammatory disease, sexually transmitted infections, tubal surgery/sterilisation, peritubal adhesions, use of intrauterine devices (although this is contentious), use of the progesterone-only pill, and use of post-coital contraception. Women with such risk factors may also be encouraged to have an early scan to confirm pregnancy location. Unfortunately, it is still possible

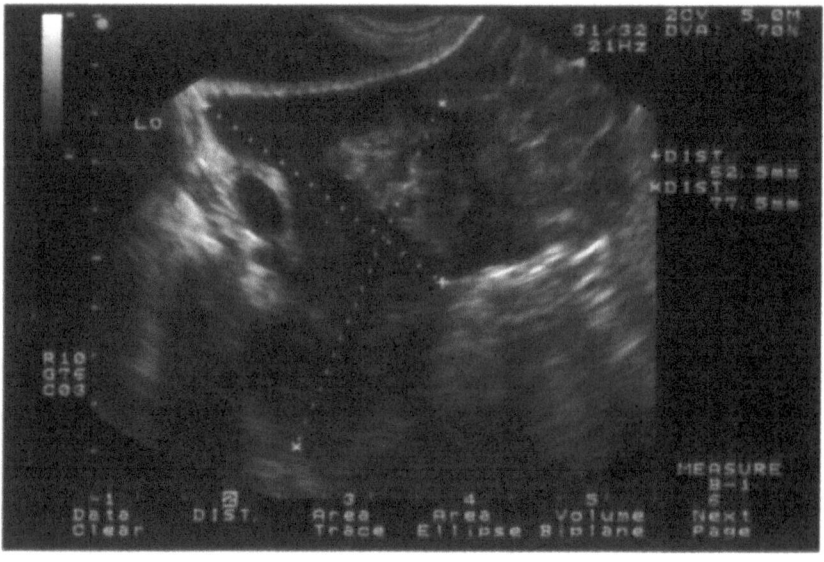

Figure 36.3. Blood in the pouch of Douglas. Blood gives a particulate "ground glass" appearance in comparison to serous fluid, which is anechoic.

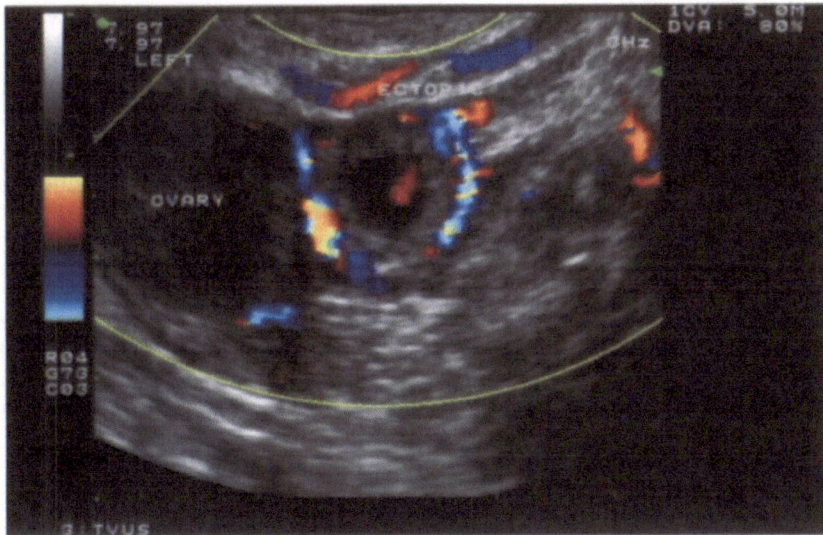

Figure 36.4. A viable tubal ectopic pregnancy.

to see ultrasound reports that read "empty uterus, ectopic pregnancy cannot be excluded". This is not helpful and will invariably lead to the patient undergoing an unnecessary laparoscopy. Transvaginal ultrasonography together with the use of quantitative serum βhCG levels should avoid this. If an ectopic pregnancy is present, TVS should detect it in 80–90% of cases. Misdiagnosis should be a rare event and the standard of care in any early pregnancy unit should be determined by its false-positive and negative rates for the diagnosis of ectopic pregnancy.

Discrete point tenderness in the adnexal region is an important clinical finding. Such a finding may worry some operators, but the use of a vaginal probe during a scan is less traumatic than a bimanual pelvic examination and provides more information.

In our experience, we have had no problems with ectopic rupture during a scanning procedure, though clearly a suspected ectopic pregnancy should be assessed in an environment where resuscitation is available.

The appearances of an ectopic pregnancy on TVS may be highly variable. Classically they are described as the "bagel sign" with a hyperechoic ring around the gestation sac in the adnexal region (Figure 36.2), but more often are seen as a small homogenous mass next to the ovary.[11] The dimensions of the ectopic pregnancy should be described, as should the presence of an embryo with or without a heartbeat. Haematoceles have a characteristic appearance, and the amount of bleeding that has occurred commented upon by looking for fluid or blood in the pouch of Douglas (Figure 36.3). The

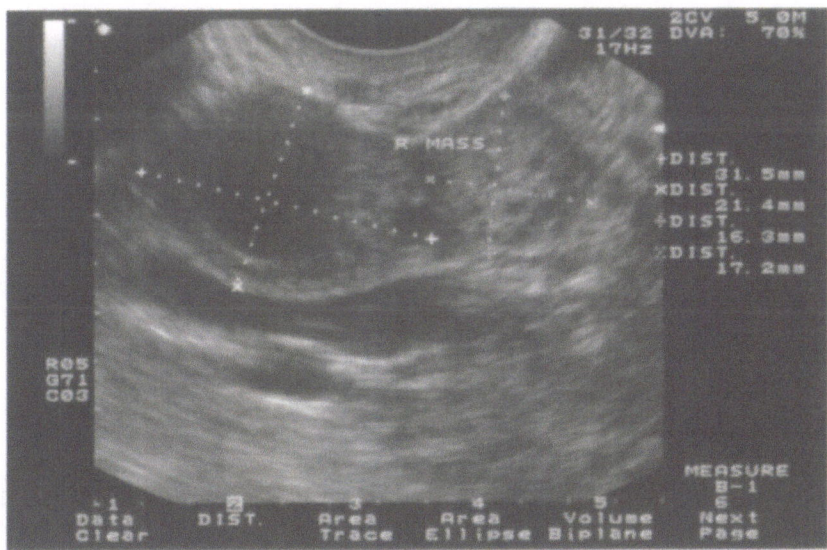

Figure 36.5. A homogenous mass in the tube consistent with a small ectopic pregnancy.

appearances of blood and clot as opposed to serous fluid are quite different and should not be confused. This information is of importance to the clinician, as the management options for ectopic pregnancy are rapidly changing, and depend very much on the ultrasound appearances and the level of serum βhCG. For example, Ylöstalo et al.[12] managed 15% of their ectopic pregnancies conservatively and observed spontaneous resolution in 64.6%. Follow-up for these women involved ultrasound scans and measurements of serial serum βhCG titres until they dropped to < 15 IU/l. Inclusion criteria stipulated that the patient had to be stable, compliant, and with no evidence of haemoperitoneum on TVS, or other signs of tubal rupture.

Brown et al.[13] pooled data from published studies and concluded that the most appropriate TVS criterion on which to diagnose ectopic pregnancy is any non-cystic adnexal mass. This leads to a positive predictive value of 96.3%, a negative predictive value of 94.8%, specificity of 98.9% and sensitivity of 84.4%. This performed better than the visualisation of an embryo with a heartbeat in the adnexa, an adnexal cystic mass, or an adnexal mass with an echogenic or "tubal" ring (Figure 36.4). This will not surprise experienced operators who will have seen many ectopic pregnancies that appear as an homogenous small mass next to the ovary with no evidence of a sac or embryo (Figure 36.5).

The corpus luteum is a useful guide when looking for an ectopic pregnancy, as it will be on the ipsilateral side in over 85% of cases.[14] The issue of the so-called "pseudosac" is controversial. This is a misnomer and probably represents a fluid collection or debris in the cavity. It is possible to confuse this with an early gestational sac; however, this sign is largely based on historical data and relates to the use of transabdom-inal ultrasonography. Using high-resolution vaginal probes, misinterpretation is less likely.

The early detection and classification of an unruptured ectopic pregnancy may allow minimally invasive procedures to be performed under TVS control. Injection of methotrexate and 50% dextrose have been used to avoid major surgical intervention.[15] Similarly, intratubal injection of potassium chloride and/or systemic methotrexate has been used in unruptured interstitial pregnancies, with complete resolution in 86.6%.[16] Detailed reviews of treatment strategies for ectopic pregnancy are described elsewhere in this book. However, all rely on the accurate characterisation of the tubal pregnancy by ultrasonography and serum biochemistry.

36.3.2 Non-tubal Ectopic Pregnancies

Ectopic pregnancies are classified according to their site of implantation. At least 95% of ectopic pregnancies will be tubal and the vast majority of these will be ampullary. Other sites account for only 5% of ectopic pregnancies, but they contribute a disproportionate number of serious complications. They may be difficult to diagnose, and are associated with significant haemorrhage leading to a higher morbidity and mortality than tubal ectopic pregnancy.

Cornual or interstitial pregnancies account for about 2% of ectopic pregnancies.[17] The sonographic image of the cornual/interstitial pregnancy is that of a bulge in the cornual area of the uterus where an extremely thin myometrial mantle surrounds the hyperechoic ring of the gestational sac (Figures 36.6 and 36.7).[18] The gestation sac should be located more than 1 cm from the endometrial echo. Colour

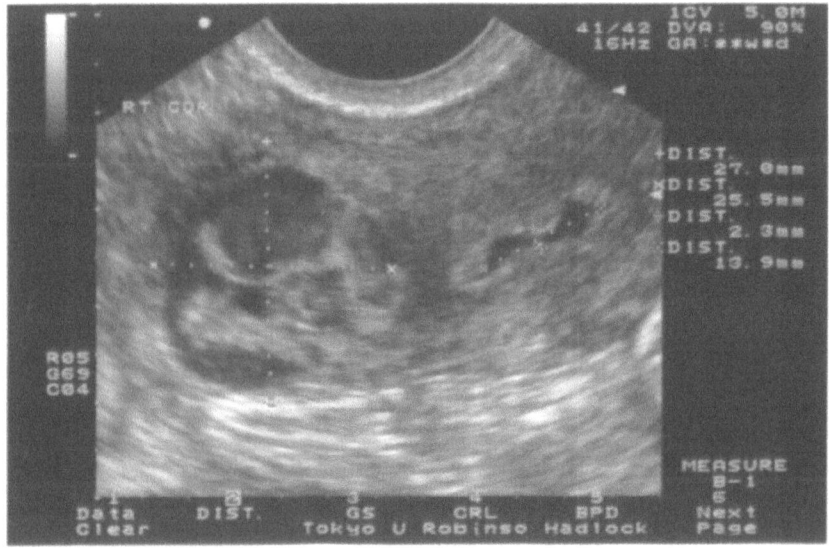

Figure 36.6. A cornual ectopic pregnancy without colour Doppler.

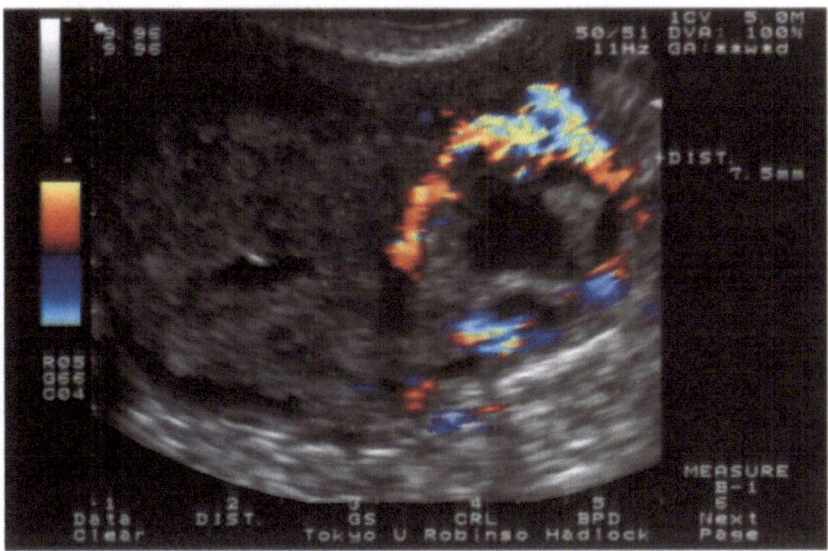

Figure 36.7. A cornual ectopic pregnancy with colour Doppler.

flow Doppler studies may help to localise the pregnancy. Hypoechogenic lesions situated in the cornual region may persist for 1 year or more following treatment, despite resumption of normal menstruation.

Cervical ectopic pregnancies are rare (Figure 36.8). The cervix is classically barrel shaped. It is important to differentiate this from an intact gestational sac passing through the cervix, which usually causes intense pain, whereas true cervical pregnancies are often relatively asymptomatic. Colour Doppler studies may assist in the diagnosis. The uterine artery is a useful anatomical marker and the presence of blood flow around the gestation sac is more suggestive of an implanted sac rather than one passing though the cervix. Ovarian pregnancy is also rare and has an incidence of 1:7000 deliveries and 1:34 ectopic pregnancies.[19] Diagnosis can be difficult, but the finding of an hyperechoic chorionic ring, which moves with the ovary, is suggestive.

All non-tubal ectopic pregnancies represent a treatment problem. However, in general a surgical approach is more hazardous and the mainstay of treatment is either systemic or local administration of methotrexate. In our unit we rely on a single-dose methotrexate regimen for the treatment of ectopic and cornual pregnancies and have rarely had problems with this approach. Although the choice of medical and surgical management for the management of tubal ectopic pregnancy is debated, our view is that medical therapy should be the first-line treatment for non-tubal ectopic gestations. A detailed description of medical management strategies is given in Chapter 37.

Abdominal pregnancies are rare and tend to be diagnosed later in pregnancy. The ultrasound features are well described and include the finding of an empty uterus separate from the fetus, no uterine mantle around the pregnancy or fetus, placenta in an unusual location and extreme oligohydramnios resulting in crowding of the fetal structures.[20,21]

Fortunately, heterotopic pregnancies are unusual; however, with the advent of reproductive technologies, their number is steadily increasing. This has already been touched on earlier, but a high index of suspicion should be present when a patient has become pregnant with the help of an assisted conception unit.

36.4 Conclusions

The introduction of TVS, facilities for rapid measurement of serum levels of βhCG and progesterone, alongside the development of dedicated early pregnancy units have changed the management of early pregnancy complications. The diagnosis of ectopic pregnancy is now based on the positive visualisation of a pregnancy outside the uterus and the emphasis for management moved towards less invasive treatment. In general, ectopic pregnancies are now diagnosed at an earlier stage in their natural history and so the classic presentation of acute abdominal pain secondary to tubal rupture is fortunately rare. Most ectopic pregnancies are now detected at a relatively asymptomatic stage and so options for treatment have widened. However, the increased sensitivity of ultrasound comes with a price. The number of women presenting with inconclusive scans increases, as women are encouraged to present earlier. The psychological morbidity engendered by the uncertainty of these scans is largely unknown, but may be significant.

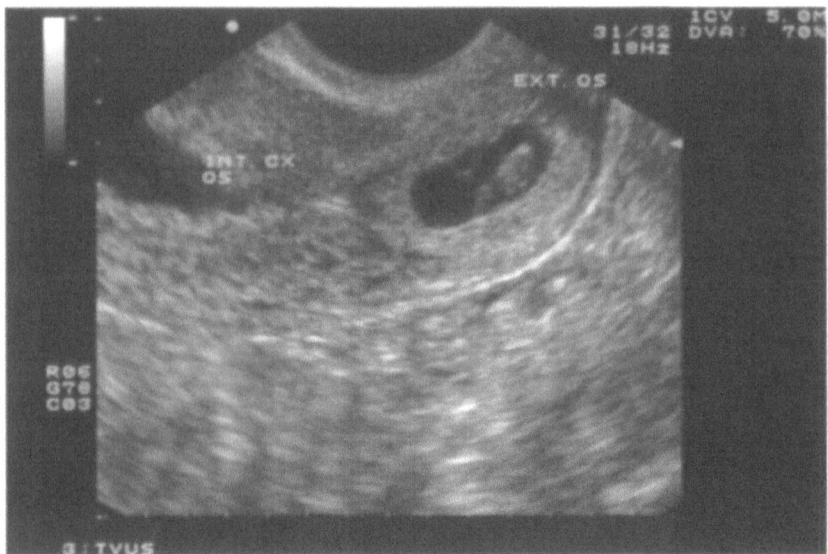

Figure 36.8 A cervical ectopic pregnancy.

An understanding of normal and abnormal serum βhCG and progesterone behaviour is vital for those involved in the management of pregnancies of unknown location. Strict follow-up criteria must be enforced for these women and patient compliance is essential. A proportion of biochemical changes in early pregnancy will be idiosyncratic and the clinical picture of the patient must never be obscured by obsessive concentration on either ultrasound findings or serum measurement of βhCG or progesterone.

There is a great scope to expand our knowledge of PUL and in doing so create better algorithms to predict which PUL will become a viable or failing intrauterine pregnancy, but more importantly predict which PUL will become an ectopic pregnancy. If we can identify those women with greatest risk of ectopic pregnancy either at the time of presentation or with fewer visits, we can direct our resources, both clinically and ultimately financially.

Most ectopic pregnancies should now be positively identified by an ultrasound scan and the remainder should be identified at follow-up. Where the pregnancy site is uncertain, serum progesterone measurements will identify the majority of cases where the pregnancy will fail and serial βhCG measurements will predict viability in others. Only 10% will have an ectopic pregnancy. Careful outpatient evaluation is important to avoid unnecessary intervention. In most cases an ectopic pregnancy is no longer an emergency, but will be diagnosed and managed in the outpatient department or scheduled for day surgery. The application of less invasive approaches to treatment is reliant on accurate characterisation of an ectopic pregnancy, so the availability of transvaginal ultrasound and laboratory services at the point of first contact with the patient is essential. This chapter has focussed on the technical aspects of the diagnosis and management of possible ectopic pregnancy; however, the psychological morbidity for women must be kept in mind at all times. The rapid processing of patients through early pregnancy units and on to medical therapy or surgery may be an efficient approach to management, but for many women the experience can be extremely traumatic and they need time to absorb the information given to them. As we overcome the technical difficulties associated with the management of potential ectopic pregnancy, we must not forget a patient's emotional needs.

References

1. Warren WB, Timor-Tritsch IE, Peisner DB et al. (1989) Dating the early pregnancy bysequential appearance of embryonic structures. Am J Obstet Gynecol 161:747–753
2. "Why Mothers Die", Triennial Report (1997–1999) Confidential Enquiry into Maternal Deaths, United Kingdom
3. Hahlin M, Thorburn J, Bryman I (1995) The expectant management of early pregnancies of uncertain site. Hum Reprod 10:1223–1227
4. Banerjee S, Aslam N, Zosmer N et al. (1999) The expectant management of women with pregnancies of unknown location. Ultrasound Obstet Gynecol 14:231–236
5. Banerjee S, Aslam N, Woelfler B et al. (2001) Expectant management of early pregnancies of unknown location: a prospective evaluation of methods to predict spontaneous resolution of pregnancy. Br J Obstet Gynaecol 108:158–163
6. Barnhart KT, Simhan H, Kamelle SA (1999) Diagnostic accuracy of ultrasound above and below the beta-hCG discriminatory zone. Obstet Gynecol 94:583–587

7. Kadar N, DeVore G, Romero R (1981) Discriminatory hCG zone: its use in the sonographic evaluation for ectopic pregnancy. Obstet Gynecol 58:156–161

8. Peisner DB, Timor-Tritsch IE (1990) The discriminatory zone of beta-hCG for vaginal probes. J Clin Ultrasound 18:280–285

9. Kadar N, Caldwell BV, Romero R (1981) A method of screening for ectopic pregnancy and its indications. Obstet Gynecol 58:162–166

10. Ludwig M, Kaisi M, Bauer O et al. (1999) Heterotopic pregnancy in a spontaneous cycle: do not forget about it! Eur J Obstet Gynecol Reprod Biol 87:91–93

11. Lerner JP, Monteagudo A (1995) Vaginal sonographic puncture procedures. In: Goldstein SR, Timor-Tritsch IE (eds) Ultrasound in Gynecology, Churchill-Livingstone, New York, Ch 15, p 228

12. Ylöstalo P, Cacciatore B, Koskimies A et al. (1991) Conservative treatment of ectopic pregnancy. Ann NY Acad Sci 626:516–523

13. Brown DL, Doubilet PM (1994) Transvaginal sonography for diagnosing ectopic pregnancy: positivity criteria and performance characteristics. J Ultrasound Med 13:259–266

14. Jurkovic D, Bourne TH, Campbell S et al. (1992) The diagnosis of ectopic pregnancy using transvaginal color flow imaging. Fertil Steril 57:68–73

15. Feichtinger W, Kemeter P (1987) Conservative treatment of ectopic pregnancy by transvaginal aspiration under sonographic control and methotrexate injection. Lancet 14 (1):381–382

16. Benifla JL, Fernandez H, Sebban E et al. (1996) Alternative to surgery for treatment of unruptured interstitial pregnancy: 15 cases of medical treatment. Eur J Obstet Gynecol Reprod Biol 70:151–156

17. Kallchman GG, Meltzer RM (1966) Interstitial pregnancy following homolateral salpingectomy: report of 2 cases and review of the literature. Am J Obstet Gynecol 96:1139–1141

18. Jafrie SZ, Loginsky SJ, Bouffard JA et al. (1987) Sonographic detection of interstitial pregnancy. J Clin Ultrasound 15:253–257

19. Rimes HG, Nosal RA, Gallagher JC (1983) Ovarian pregnancy: a series of 24 cases. Obstet Gynecol 61:174

20. Hertz RH, Timor-Tritsch IE, Sokol RJ et al. (1977) Diagnostic studies and fetal assessment in advanced extrauterine pregnancy. Obstet Gynecol 50:63–65

21. Stanley JH, Horger EO III, Fagan CJ et al. (1986) Sonographic findings in abdominal pregnancy. Am J Radiology 147:1043–1046

Chapter 37

Systemic and Local Therapy of Ectopic Pregnancy

Petra J. Hajenius, Ben-Willem J. Mol, Wim M. Ankum and Fulco Van der Veen

37.1 Introduction

The diagnosis of ectopic pregnancy can be made by non-invasive methods as a result of sensitive pregnancy tests in urine and serum and high-resolution transvaginal ultrasonography. These have been integrated in reliable diagnostic algorithms.[1-4] These algorithms, in combination with the increased awareness and knowledge of risk factors among both clinicians and patients, enable an early and accurate diagnosis of ectopic pregnancy. As a consequence, the clinical presentation of ectopic pregnancy has changed from a life-threatening disease –necessitating emergency surgery – to a more benign condition in sometimes even asymptomatic patients. This in turn has resulted in major changes in the options available for therapeutic management.

As laparoscopy is no longer needed for the diagnosis of ectopic pregnancy, medical treatment has increasingly become of interest. Systemic or local administration of drugs into the gestational sac has been introduced in selected patients with an unruptured ectopic pregnancy without active bleeding. Important selection criteria are ectopic pregnancy size, maximum serum human chorionic gonadotrophin (hCG) concentrations and absence of fetal cardiac activity.

The drug of interest in the medical treatment of ectopic pregnancy is methotrexate. Methotrexate is a folic acid antagonist and inhibits de novo synthesis of purines and pyrimidines, thus interfering with DNA synthesis and cell proliferation. The drug has been widely used in the treatment of gestational trophoblastic disease since 1956.[5] Secondary to its effect on highly proliferative tissues, methotrexate has a strong dose-related potential for toxicity. Side-effects include stomatitis, conjunctivitis, gastritis-enteritis, impaired liver function, bone marrow depression and photosensitivity. The administration of folinic acid decreases side-effects of the drug. In 40 years of clinical experience with methotrexate, this drug has been shown to be safe. In women treated with methotrexate for gestational trophoblastic disease, no adverse effects on reproductive outcome have been reported.[6,7]

Initially, ectopic pregnancy was treated with methotrexate administered systemically in a multiple-dose regimen in combination with folinic acid, similar to the treatment of gestational trophoblastic disease.[8,9] More recently, a single-dose regimen has been advocated to minimise side-effects and to improve patients' compliance.[10] Further efforts to attain maximal efficacy while minimising or eliminating side-effects have resulted in various protocols with locally administered methotrexate into the gestational sac, under either sonographic[11] or laparoscopic guidance.[12]

In this chapter, a systematic review is given of the uncontrolled studies updated to 1997 and the few randomised controlled trials available so far in the treatment of tubal pregnancy with methotrexate. In this review, treatment success, tubal patency and future fertility are analysed. Treatment success is defined as an uneventful decline of serum human hCG to undetectable levels by primary treatment. Additional surgical or medical interventions for tubal rupture, clinical symptoms or persistent trophoblast are therefore regarded as treatment failures. Persistent trophoblast is defined as rising or plateauing serum hCG concentrations after primary conservative treatment, for which additional treatment (surgical or medical) is necessary. Tubal patency is defined as the passage of dye at hysterosalpingography or at second-look laparoscopy in the homolateral tube. Future fertility is defined as a spontaneous subsequent intrauterine pregnancy or repeat ectopic pregnancy in patients desiring future pregnancy. Based on the available evidence, consequences for clinical practice are outlined and recommendations for future studies are discussed.

37.2 Uncontrolled Studies

37.2.1 Systemic Methotrexate

In 1985, Chotiner was the first to describe a patient with tubal pregnancy treated successfully with systemic methotrexate in a multiple-dose regimen,[8] according to an earlier report by Tanaka et al in 1982, who had treated a patient with interstitial ectopic pregnancy with a similar regimen.[9] The patient had ovarian hyperstimulation syndrome, and surgery was therefore contraindicated. The results of uncontrolled studies on systemic methotrexate in a multiple-dose regimen are summarised in Tables 37.1 and 37.2.[13-21] Haemodynamically stable patients with a laparoscopically confirmed small unruptured tubal pregnancy and no active bleeding, and serum hCG concentrations varying between 40 and 59 000 IU/l, were included in these studies. The mean primary success rate was 92%, the mean tubal patency rate 78%, the mean intrauterine pregnancy rate 59%, and the mean repeat ectopic pregnancy rate 8%.

In 1989, Stovall et al individualised the methotrexate dosage, which ultimately led to a single-dose regimen to improve patient compliance, to minimise side-effects and to reduce overall costs.[10] The results of uncontrolled studies reporting on systemic methotrexate in a single-dose regimen are summarised in Tables 37.3 and 37.4.[22-30] Haemodynamically stable patients with a small unruptured tubal pregnancy, without fetal cardiac activity and no signs of active bleeding on transvaginal sonography, and serum hCG concentrations varying between 45 and 49 473 IU/l were included in these studies. No confirmative laparoscopy was performed in these patients. The mean primary success rate was 75%, the mean tubal patency rate 84%, the mean intrauterine pregnancy rate 58%, and the mean repeat ectopic pregnancy rate 8%.

The 75% success rate of the single-dose regimen is low compared to the 92% success rate of the multiple-dose regimen. This is the result of additional interventions after the initial treatment for clinical symptoms and/or persistent trophoblast. Whether side-effects in the single-dose regimen are reduced compared to the multiple-dose regimen is questionable. Although Stovall et al reported no significant side-effects of the single-dose regimen,[10] more recent studies reported side-effects in up to 41% of patients.[24-27]

37.2.2 Local Methotrexate

In 1987, Feichtinger was the first to use the transvaginal puncture technique – originally developed for oocyte retrieval in in-vitro fertilisation (IVF) procedures – to treat a patient with tubal pregnancy with low-dose local methotrexate.[11] The results of uncontrolled studies on local methotrexate injected transvaginally under ultrasound guidance are summarised in Tables 37.5 and 37.6.[31-39] Haemodynamically stable patients with a visible tubal pregnancy on transvaginal sonography, and serum hCG concentrations varying between 60 and 105 000 IU/l were included in these studies. The mean primary success rate was 62%, the mean tubal patency rate 88%, the mean intrauterine pregnancy rate 32%, and the mean repeat ectopic pregnancy rate 7%.

In 1989, Pansky was the first to describe the treatment of tubal pregnancy with local methotrexate administered laparoscopically.[12] The results of uncontrolled studies on local methotrexate under laparoscopic guidance are summarised in Tables 37.7 and 37.8.[40-49] Haemodynamically stable patients with a small unruptured ectopic pregnancy, no active bleeding, and serum hCG concentrations varying between 77 and 57 880 IU/l were included in these studies. The mean primary success rate was 77%, the mean tubal patency rate 87%, the mean intrauterine pregnancy rate 47%, and the mean repeat ectopic pregnancy rate 8%.

Side-effects of local methotrexate have been reported to be none to minimal. Moreover, reported side-effects were the result of additional systemic methotrexate treatment for persistent trophoblast.

37.3 Summary of Uncontrolled Studies

Treatment of tubal pregnancy with methotrexate has been limited to haemodynamically stable patients with a small unruptured tubal pregnancy (< 4 cm) and no signs of active bleeding.

In most studies reporting on systemic methotrexate, no additional criteria were used, as these early studies were descriptive case series. Only recently, prospective studies have used upper limits for serum hCG concentrations, with a maximum of 10 000 IU/l.

In nearly all studies reporting on systemic methotrexate in a single-dose regimen, patients with fetal cardiac activity were excluded, as this feature was supposed to have an adverse effect on clinical outcome. Although no upper limit for the serum hCG concentration was reported, mean serum hCG concentrations exceeded the level of 4000 IU/l in only a few studies.

Table 37.1. Inclusion criteria and short-term outcome of systemic methotrexate in a multiple-dose regimen. n, Number of patients; TVS, transvaginal sonography; MTX, methotrexate; im, intramuscular; CF, folinic acid; Ø, diameter; u, urinary human chorionic gonadotrophin (hCG)

Author	Year	n	Serum hCG (IU/l)	Inclusion criteria TVS	Laparoscopy	Serum hCG Range (IU/l)	Dose MTX (im)	CF (im)	Failure Surgery n	Additional MTX n	Success n	%
Ory	86	6			Ø < 4 cm Unruptured No fluid	103–25 410	1 mg/kg (days 0,2,4,6)	0.1 mg/kg (days 1,3,5,7)	1		5	83
Kooi	87	10			Unruptured No fluid	40–17 000	50 mg (days 0,2,4,6)	15 mg oral (days 1,3,5,7)		1	9	90
Ichinoe	87	23				80–16 000 (u)	0.4 mg/kg (days 0–4)		1		22	96
Sauer	87	21			Ø < 3 cm Unruptured No bleeding	65–59 000	1 mg/kg (days 0,2,4,6)	0.1 mg/kg (days 1,3,5,7)	1	2	18	86
Stovall	91	96		Ø < 3 cm No fluid	Ø < 3.5 cm Unruptured No bleeding		1 mg/kg (days 0,2,4,6)	0.1 mg/kg (days 1,3,5,7)	4		92	96
Brynsen	91	9			Unruptured No bleeding		0.4 mg/kg (days 0–4)		2		7	78
Isaacs	92	4				224–2360	1 mg/kg (days 0,2,4)	0.1 mg/kg (days 1,3,5)			4	100
Prapas	92	20	< 10 000	No cardiac activity No fluid	Unruptured	2500–9500	1 mg/kg	0.1 mg/kg	1		19	95
Chryssikopulos	96	3	< 2000		No bleeding Ø < 5 cm Unruptured No fluid		(days 0,2,4,6) 0.3 mg/kg oral (days 0–4)	(days 1,3,5,7)	3		0	0
All		192							13	3	176	92

Table 37.2. Long-term outcome of systemic methotrexate in a multiple-dose regimen

Author	Year	n	Tubal patency n/n	%	Intrauterine pregnancy n/n	%	Ectopic pregnancy n/n	%
Ory	86	6	1/2	50				
Kooi	87	10			2/4	50	1/4	25
Ichinoe	87	23	10/19	53				
Sauer	87	21	15/20	75				
Stovall	91	96	49/58	85	33/56	59	4/56	7
Bryalsen	91	9	5/5	100				
Prapas	92	20	14/17					
Chryssikopulos	96	3	3/3	100	2/3	67	0/3	0
All		187	97/124	78	37/63	59	5/63	8

Table 37.3. Inclusion criteria and short-term outcome of systemic methotrexate in a single-dose regimen. SD, Standard deviation; DC, diagnostic curettage; TVS, transvaginal sonography; MTX, methotrexate; Ø, diameter; hCG, human chorionic gonadotrophin

Author	Year	n	Inclusion criteria Serum hCG (IU/l)	TVS	Serum hCG Mean ± SD or range (IU/l)	MTX dose (im)	Failure Surgery n	Additional MTX n	Success n	%
Stovall	93	120	↑After DC	Ø < 3 cm	3950 ± 1193	50 mg/m²	7	4	109	91
Henry	94	61	↑After DC	Ø < 3.5 cm No cardiac activity No bleeding		50 mg/m²	9	16	36	59
Glock	94	35	↑After DC	Ø < 3.5 cm No cardiac activity No bleeding	1388 ± 464	50 mg/m²	5		30	86
Ransom	94	21		Ø < 3.5 cm No cardiac activity	1575 ± 1350	50 mg/m²	6	1	14	66
Wolf	94	12	≤ 6000	Ø < 4 cm	1907 ± 1422	75 mg		1	11	92
Gross	95	17	< 15000	Ø < 3 cm No cardiac activity Unruptured	3320 (158–12420)	50 mg/m²	1		16	94
Corsan	95	44		Ø < 3.5 cm No cardiac activity	2517 ± 3144	50 mg/m²	11	10	23	52
Stika	96	50		Ø < 3.5 cm Unruptured	1896 ± 2399	50 mg/m²	11	7	32	64
Yao	96	21		Unruptured	1581 ± 471		Not reported	Not reported	14	67
Thoen	97	47		Ø < 3.5 cm No cardiac activity	803 (45–49473)	50 mg/m²	4	7	36	77
All		428							321	75

Table 37.4. Long-term outcome of systemic methotrexate in a single-dose regimen

Author	Year	n	Tubal patency n/n	%	Intrauterine pregnancy n/n	%	Ectopic pregnancy n/n	%
Stovall	93	120	51/62	82	34/49	69	5/49	10
Glock	94	35	10/13	77	3/15	20	0/15	0
Corsan	95	44	21/23	91				
All		199	82/98	84	37/64	58	5/64	8

Studies reporting on local treatment with methotrexate have included more advanced ectopic pregnancies with fetal cardiac activity and high serum hCG concentrations. It is not inconceivable that additional aspiration of the tubal content before injecting methotrexate might positively influence the effectiveness of methotrexate and thus the short-term outcome.

Overall, systemic methotrexate in a multiple-dose regimen seems to be the most effective treatment; in the single-dose regimen and the local administration routes, additional methotrexate or surgical interventions for clinical symptoms and/or persistent trophoblast are more often necessary. Tubal patency and fertility outcome seem to be comparable between the different routes of administration, taking into account the fact that only few studies reported on these outcome measures, with variable follow-up periods.

Table 37.5. Inclusion criteria and short-term outcome of methotrexate injected transvaginally under sonographic guidance. SD, Standard deviation; TVS, transvaginal sonography; MTX, methotrexate; Ø, diameter; hCG, human chorionic gonadotrophin; EP, ectopic pregnancy

| Author | Year | Inclusion criteria | | Serum hCG | MTX dose | | Failure | Success | |
		Serum hCG n (IU/l)	TVS	Mean ± SD or range (IU/l)		Surgery n	Additional MTX n	n	%
Feichtinger	87	9 ↑	EP visible		10–50 mg	2	1	6	67
Leeton	88	2	Vital EP	4900/15 000	50 mg			2	100
Menard	90	17	Ø < 6 cm No fluid	58–19 400	50 mg	4		13	76
Schiff	92	7	EP visible	2103 (649–5690)	50 mg			7	100
Atri	92	25 15% ↑ in 24 hours	EP visible	5798 (60–21 000)	1 mg/kg	6	6	13	52
Tulandi	92	40 15% ↑ in 24 hours	EP visible	3884–6563	1 mg/kg	11	9	20	50
Fernandez	93	100 Score ≤ 12		4930 (65–46 740)	1 mg/kg	17	28	55	55
Darai	96	100	No signs of rupture No cardiac activity	11 614 (192–105 000)	1 mg/kg	22	12	66	66
Merz	96	30	EP visible	4551 (210–21 420)	1 mg	5	7	18	60
Yao	96	19	EP visible	3366 ± 862	1 mg/kg	Not reported	Not reported	15	79
All		349						215	62

Table 37.6. Long-term outcome of methotrexate injected transvaginally under sonographic guidance

Author	Year	n	Tubal patency n/n	%	Intrauterine pregnancy n/n	%	Ectopic pregnancy n/n	%
Feichtinger	89	9	2/2	100				
Tulandi	92	40	9/11	82	2/11	18	2/11	18
Atri	92	25	10/13	77	2/13	15	1/13	8
Fernandez	93	100	72/80	90	31/58	53	3/58	5
Darai	96	100			15/75	20	6/75	8
Merz	96	30	12/14	86	4/14	29	0/14	0
All		304	105/120	88	54/171	32	12/171	7

37.4 Randomised Controlled Trials

So far, 18 randomised controlled trials have been published in the treatment of tubal pregnancy with methotrexate, describing 12 different comparisons. Table 30.9 summarises the number of patients included and the rate ratios (RR) of short-term and long-term outcomes, with the corresponding 95% confidence intervals (CI).

37.4.1 Systemic Methotrexate

Treatment with systemic methotrexate is described in the following studies:

- systemic methotrexate in a multiple-dose intramuscular regimen versus laparoscopic salpingostomy;[50–53]
- systemic methotrexate in a single-dose intramuscular regimen versus laparoscopic salpingostomy;[54–57]

- methotrexate 25 mg/m^2 versus 50 mg/m^2 both in a single-dose intramuscular regimen;[58]
- systemic methotrexate in a single-dose intramuscular regimen versus the same regimen in combination with oral mifepristone;[59]
- systemic methotrexate in an oral regimen versus prostaglandins and hyperosmolar glucose under laparoscopic guidance;[60]
- systemic methotrexate in a low-dose oral regimen versus expectant management.[61]

37.4.2 Local Methotrexate

The following studies are on local methotrexate treatment:

- methotrexate transvaginally under sonographic guidance versus laparoscopic salpingostomy;[54,62]
- methotrexate under laparoscopic guidance versus laparoscopic salpingostomy;[63–66]

Table 37.7. Inclusion criteria and short-term outcome of intratubal methotrexate under laparoscopic guidance. TVS, transvaginal sonography; MTX, methotrexate; , diameter; hCG, human chorionic gonadotrophin

Author	Year	n	Inclusion criteria Serum hCG (IU/l)	Inclusion criteria TVS	Laparoscopy	Serum hCG Mean and/or range (IU/l)	MTX dose	Surgery n	Failure Additional MTX n	Success n	%
Kool	90	25		No cardiac activity	Unruptured No bleeding	130–19 000	100 mg	1	7	17	68
Mardesic	90	4			⌀ < 3 cm	97–3018	20 mg			4	100
Kojima	90	9			⌀ < 5 cm Unruptured No bleeding	160–16 000	525 mg		1	8	89
Thompson	91	18			⌀ < 4 cm Unruptured	7000 (77–57 880)	20 mg	1		17	94
Wolf	91	9			⌀ < 4 cm Unruptured No bleeding	34–17100	15 mg	1		8	89
Pansky	92	59			⌀ < 3 cm Unruptured No bleeding	626 (25–3200)	12.5 mg		12	47	80
Groutz	93	10	↑ /=	No cardiac activity	⌀ < 4 cm	225–10660	50 mg	1		9	90
Shalev	95	44	> 1500 and ↑		⌀ < 4 cm Unruptured	3729 (156–37 000)	50 mg	17		27	61
All		178						21	20	137	77

Table 37.8. Long-term outcome of intratubal methotrexate under laparoscopic guidance

Author	Year	n	Tubal patency N/n	%	Intrauterine pregnancy n/n	%	Ectopic pregnancy n/n	%
Pansky	89	59	19/21	90				
Kooi	90	25			9/14	64	0/14	0
Mardesic	90	4	3/3	100				
Kojima	90	9	9/9	100				
Thompson	91	8	8/8	100				
Pansky	93	51			21/31	68	4/31	13
Shalev	95	44	13/19	68	12/44	27	3/44	7
All		210	52/60	87	42/89	47	7/89	8

- methotrexate transvaginally under sonographic guidance versus methotrexate under laparoscopic guidance;[67]
- methotrexate transvaginally under sonographic guidance versus systemic methotrexate in a single-dose intramuscular regimen;[54,68,69]
- methotrexate under laparoscopic guidance versus the same regimen in combination with systemic methotrexate;[70]
- methotrexate versus prostaglandins both transvaginally under sonographic guidance combined with the systemic administration of the drug.[71]

37.4.3 Systemic Methotrexate in a Multiple-dose Intramuscular Regimen versus Laparoscopic Salpingostomy

In a multicentre study[50] involving 100 haemodynamically stable women with a laparoscopically confirmed unruptured tubal pregnancy without fetal cardiac activity and no signs of active bleeding, no significant differences were found in primary treatment success (RR 1.2, 95% CI 0.93, 1.4) and tubal preservation (RR 0.98, 95% CI 0.87, 1.1), thus ruling out large differences in short-term treatment effect.

Tubal patency rate, assessed in 81 women, was not higher after systemic methotrexate (RR 0.93, 95% CI 0.64, 1.4). Eighteen months after completion of the trial, fertility outcome was assessed in 74 patients trying to conceive.[51] Out of 34 women in the systemic methotrexate group, 12 had a spontaneous intrauterine pregnancy, two had an intrauterine pregnancy through IVF–embryo transfer (ET), whereas three had a spontaneous ectopic pregnancy. Out of 40 women in the laparoscopic salpingostomy group, 16 had a spontaneous intrauterine pregnancy, two had an intrauterine pregnancy through IVF–ET, whereas four had a spontaneous ectopic pregnancy. Cox proportional hazard estimates of the RR were 0.89 (95% CI 0.42, 1.9) for spontaneous intrauterine pregnancy, and 0.77 (95% CI 0.17, 3.4) for repeat ectopic pregnancies.

Other outcome measures analysed were serum hCG clearance time, complications, health-related quality of life, and costs. Mean serum hCG clearance time was not significantly different (19 versus 14 days). Sixty-one per cent of the women undergoing systemic methotrexate therapy experienced complications and/or side-effects compared to only 12% in the salpingostomy group. In the salpingostomy group, virtually all complications comprised the side-effects of systemic methotrexate in women treated for persistent trophoblast.

Health-related quality of life was more severely impaired after systemic methotrexate than after laparoscopic salpingostomy.[52] Medically treated women showed more limitations in physical role and social functioning, had worse health perceptions, less energy, more pain, more physical symptoms, a worse overall quality of life, and were more depressed than surgically treated women (p < 0.05).

Treatment with systemic methotrexate after a confirmatory laparoscopy was significantly more expensive than laparoscopic salpingostomy.[53] Mean total costs per patient were $5721 for systemic methotrexate and $4066 for laparoscopic salpingostomy, with a mean difference of $1655 (95% CI $906, $2414). Re-interventions, only required in women with initial serum hCG concentrations > 1500 IU/l, generated considerable additional costs due to prolonged hospital stay (4.5 versus 2.5 days). Furthermore, costs due to loss of productivity were higher in the systemic methotrexate group (lost labour days 38 versus 28). Subgroup analysis indicated that only in patients with an initial serum hCG concentration < 1500 IU/l, the difference in total costs between systemic methotrexate ($4399) and laparoscopic salpingostomy ($4185) was less; however, this was not significant ($214, 95% CI $283, $676).

In a scenario analysis, it was calculated that systemic methotrexate was less costly compared to laparoscopic salpingostomy, only if administered as part of a totally non-invasive treatment strategy and in patients with an initial serum hCG concentration < 1500 IU/l (total costs $2991). In such a scenario without a confirmatory laparoscopy, total costs were equal to laparoscopic salpingostomy in patients with an initial serum hCG concentration varying between 1500 and 3000 IU/l

Table 37.9. Randomised trials with methotrexate (MTX). Values are rate ratios and 95% confidence intervals

Author	Year	Comparison	n	Treatment success	Persistent trophoblast	Tubal patency	Intrauterine pregnancy	Ectopic pregnancy
Hajenius	97	Systemic MTX in a multiple-dose im regimen	100	1.2 (0.93–1.4)	0.29 (0.08–0.99)	0.93 (0.64–1.4)	0.89 (0.42–1.9)	0.77 (0.17–3.4)
Dias Pereira	00	versus laparoscopic salpingostomy						
Fernandez	98	Systemic MTX in a single-dose im regimen versus	207	0.83 (0.71–0.97)	3.6 (1.7–8)	1.1 (0.74–1.5)	0.99 (0.55–1.8)	0.27 (0.02–4.5)
Saraj	98	laparoscopic salpingostomy						
Sowter	01							
Yalcinkaya	96	25mg/m² MTX versus 50mg/m² MTX both in a	40	1.3 (0.75–2.1)	0.75 (0.27–2.0)			
		single-dose im regimen						
Gazvani	98	Systemic MTX in a single-dose im regimen v	50	0.82 (0.62–1.1)	4.0 (0.48–33)	0.85 (0.60–1.2)		
		ersus the same regimen in combination with oral						
		mifepristone						
Landstrom	98	Systemic MTX in an oral regimen versus	31	1.1 (0.84–1.3)				
		prostaglandins and hyperosmolar glucose under						
		laparoscopic guidance						
Korhonen	96	Systemic MTX in a low-dose oral regimen versus	60	1.0 (0.76–1.3)				
		expectant management						
Fernandez	98	MTX transvaginally under sonographic guidance	78	0.83 (0.68–1.0)	4.2 (0.88–20)	0.99 (0.78–1.3)	1.6 (1.1–2.3)	0.26 (0.03–2.1)
		versus laparoscopic salpingostomy						
Mottla	92	MTX under laparoscopic guidance versus	127	0.92 (0.81–1.0)	1.6 (0.62–4.2)	1.1 (0.78–1.6)	0.98 (0.71–1.3)	0.37 (0.02–8.6)
O-Shea	94	laparoscopic salpingostomy						
Zilber	96							
Porpora	96							
Tzafettas	94	MTX transvaginally under sonographic guidance	36	1.6 (1.0–2.5)	0.32 (0.07–1.4)			
		versus MTX under laparoscopic guidance						
Fernandez	98	MTX transvaginally under sonographic guidance	95	1.2 (0.95–1.5)			1.2 (0.70–1.9)	1.3 (0.06–29)
Cohen	96	versus systemic MTX in a single-dose im regimen						
Shulman	92	MTX under laparoscopic guidance versus the same	15	0.86 (0.63–1.2)				
		regimen in combination with systemic MTX						
Fernandez	91	MTX versus prostaglandins both transvaginally	21	1.0 (0.54–1.8)	Not specified	0.88 (0.67–1.1)		
		under sonographic guidance combined with the						
		systemic administration of the drug						

($3885), whereas in patients with an initial serum hCG concentration > 3000 IU/l, systemic methotrexate would still be more costly ($4975).

37.4.4 Systemic Methotrexate in a Single-dose Intramuscular Regimen versus Laparoscopic Salpingostomy

The combined results of three studies[54-56] involving 207 haemodynamically stable women with a small unruptured tubal pregnancy showed that systemic methotrexate in a single-dose intramuscular regimen was significantly less successful than laparoscopic salpingostomy in the elimination of tubal pregnancy (RR 0.83, 95% CI 0.71, 0.97). This was mainly a result of the significantly higher persistent trophoblast rate (RR 3.6, 95% CI 1.7, 8), necessitating additional methotrexate injections, which were successful, as is reflected by a comparable tubal preservation rate (RR 1.1, 95% CI 0.95, 1.2).

In 77 patients, tubal patency could be assessed and showed no significant differences between the two treatment groups (RR 1.1, 95% CI 0.74, 1.5). The number of subsequent intrauterine pregnancies was similar (RR 0.99, 95% CI 0.55, 1.8), whereas the number of repeat ectopic pregnancies was lower (RR 0.27, 95% CI 0.02, 4.5), although these findings were not significantly different.

Other outcome measures analysed were serum hCG, serum progesterone clearance time, hospital stay, quality of life and costs. Mean time for serum hCG to decrease to undetectable levels was significantly less after laparoscopic salpingotomy (8–20 days after surgery versus 18–28 days after methotrexate). Serum progesterone clearance time was significantly less after laparoscopic salpingotomy (20 versus 27 days). Mean hospital stay was shorter in the methotrexate group because women were hospitalised for at least 2 days after laparoscopic salpingostomy, whereas methotrexate was given on an outpatient basis (1 versus 2 days).

Women treated with methotrexate had significantly better physical functioning than after laparoscopic surgery (p < 0.01). No differences were found in psychological functioning.[56]

Single-dose methotrexate resulted in a 52% saving in direct costs compared to laparoscopic surgery.[57] Mean direct costs per patient were $ NZ 1470 and $ NZ 3083, respectively. This significant difference of $ NZ 1613 (95% CI $ NZ 1166, $ NZ 2061) was the result of savings due to reduced theatre usage and hospital stay. Furthermore, single-dose methotrexate resulted in a 40% saving in indirect costs: mean indirect costs per patient were $ NZ 1141 and $ NZ 1899, respectively, with a mean difference of $ NZ 758 (95% CI $ NZ 277, $ NZ 1240).

In a scenario analysis, it was calculated that the cost savings of single-dose methotrexate remained under a wide range of alternative assumptions about unit costs. Subgroup analysis indicated that in patients with an initial serum hCG concentration > 1500 IU/l, the difference in indirect costs is lost due to the prolonged follow-up and a higher rate of surgical re-intervention.

37.4.5 Methotrexate 25 mg/m^2 versus 50 mg/m^2 both in a Single-dose Intramuscular Regimen

In a small double-blinded study[58] involving 40 haemodynamically stable women with an unruptured tubal pregnancy, a lower dose of methotrexate was as effective as a higher dose of methotrexate in the elimination of ectopic pregnancy (RR 1.3, 95% CI 0.75, 2.1). Persistent trophoblast did not occur more frequently (RR 0.75, 95% CI 0.27, 2.0). No data were available on tubal patency and future fertility.

Other outcome measures analysed were serum hCG clearance time and side-effects. Mean serum hCG clearance time was comparable (27 days), whereas the one woman who developed side-effects was found in the higher dose treatment group.

37.4.6 Systemic Methotrexate in a Single-dose Intramuscular Regimen versus the same Regimen in Combination with Oral Mifepristone

In a small study[59] involving 50 haemodynamically stable women with a small laparoscopically confirmed unruptured tubal pregnancy, systemic methotrexate alone was less successful than in combination with mifepristone in the elimination of the tubal pregnancy (RR 0.82, 95% CI 0.62, 1.1). This was mainly the result of the higher persistent trophoblast rate (RR 4.0, 95% CI 0.48, 33), necessitating a second injection, although mean serum hCG concentrations were low in both treatment groups, i.e. 346 IU/l (range 52–12 700) and 497 IU/l (range 30–4200), respectively. Both findings, however, were not significantly different.

No differences were found in tubal preservation (RR 0.92, 95% CI 0.78, 1.1) nor in overall tubal patency rate (RR 0.85, 95% CI 0.60, 1.2), which could be assessed for 24 women. No data were available on future fertility.

Other outcome measures analysed were serum hCG clearance time and side-effects. Mean serum hCG clearance time did not differ significantly (21 versus 14 days), whereas two women in each treatment group developed side-effects.

37.4.7 Systemic Methotrexate in an Oral Regimen versus Prostaglandins and Hyperosmolar Glucose under Laparoscopic Guidance

In a multicentre study[60] involving 31 haemodynamically stable women with a laparoscopically confirmed unruptured tubal pregnancy and a serum hCG concentration < 3000 IU/l, no significant differences were found in primary treatment success (RR 1.1, 95% CI 0.84, 1.3) between non-invasive oral management and local injection therapy. Mean serum hCG concentrations, however, were low, i.e. 810 IU/l (range 104–3085) and 932 IU/l (range 54–4446), respectively. No data were available on tubal patency or future fertility.

37.4.8 Systemic Methotrexate in a Low-dose Oral Regimen versus Expectant Management

In a double-blinded placebo-controlled randomised trial[61] involving 60 haemodynamically stable women with a small tubal pregnancy without fetal cardiac activity and a serum hCG concentration < 5000 IU/l, no significant differences were found in primary treatment success (RR 1.0, 95% CI 0.76, 1.3) and serum hCG clearance time (27 versus 24 days). However, mean serum hCG concentrations were low, i.e. 395 IU/l (range 61–4279) in the methotrexate group and 211 IU/l (range 20–1343) in the expectant group. In this placebo-controlled trial, 23% of the patients in both treatment groups needed surgical intervention. The authors did not mention which patients failed, why they failed and how they were managed subsequently. No data were available on tubal patency or future fertility.

37.4.9 Methotrexate Transvaginally under Sonographic Guidance versus Laparoscopic Salpingostomy

The results of an updated study[54] involving 78 women with an ectopic pregnancy with a pretherapeutic score < 13 showed that methotrexate transvaginally under sonographic guidance was significantly less successful than laparoscopic salpingostomy in the elimination of the tubal pregnancy (RR 0.83, 95% CI 0.68, 1.0). This was mainly the result of the higher persistent trophoblast rate (RR 4.2, 95% CI 0.88, 20), for which additional systemic methotrexate injections were necessary. In all patients, additional interventions were conserva-

tive and successful, which is reflected in a 100% tubal preservation rate.

In the original study,[62] in which 40 women were randomised, homolateral tubal patency was assessed in 35 women and no difference was found (RR 0.99, 95% CI 0.78, 1.3). The number of subsequent intrauterine pregnancies was significantly higher (RR 1.6, 95% CI 1.1, 2.3) and the number of repeat ectopic pregnancies lower (RR 0.26, 95% CI 0.03, 2.1), although this finding was not significantly different.

Other medical outcome measures analysed were serum hCG clearance time and hospital stay. Mean serum hCG clearance time was significantly longer after methotrexate treatment (29 versus 14 days), which could be explained by the higher initial serum hCG concentration in this treatment group (3805 versus 2591 IU/l). Mean hospital stay was shorter because women were hospitalised for at least 2 days after laparoscopic salpingostomy, whereas methotrexate was given on an outpatient basis (1 versus 2 days).

37.4.10 Methotrexate under Laparoscopic Guidance versus Laparoscopic Salpingostomy

The combined results of four studies[63–66] involving 127 haemodynamically stable women with a small unruptured tubal pregnancy without signs of active bleeding showed that methotrexate under laparoscopic guidance was significantly less successful than laparoscopic salpingostomy in the elimination of the tubal pregnancy (RR 0.92, 95% CI 0.81, 1.0). This was the result of the high surgical intervention rate for persistent trophoblast in the methotrexate group (RR 1.6, 95% CI 0.62, 4.2). Especially in the study by Mottla et al,[63] the initial rise in serum hCG was wrongly interpreted as treatment failure by the authors, because they were unfamiliar with the serum hCG clearance patterns after methotrexate. However, these additional surgical interventions had no impact on tubal preservation (RR 0.95, 95% CI 0.88, 1.0).

Two studies reported on tubal patency in 36 women.[64,65] In one, an overall tubal patency could be calculated.[64] No significant differences were found (RR 1.1, 95% CI 0.78, 1.6). Only one study reported on future fertility in 34 women.[66] The number of subsequent intrauterine pregnancies was comparable (RR 0.98, 95% CI 0.71, 1.3), whereas the number of repeat ectopic pregnancies was lower (RR 0.37, 95% CI 0.02, 8.6), although these findings were not significantly different.

Other outcome measures analysed were operation time, serum hCG clearance time, hospital stay and complications. Apart from a shorter operation time (varying between 32 and 53 versus 67 and 86 minutes) and a longer hospital stay (3 versus 2 days) in the methotrexate group, no significant differences were found between the two treatment groups.

37.4.11 Methotrexate Transvaginally under Sonographic Guidance versus Methotrexate under Laparoscopic Guidance

The results of a small study[67] involving 36 haemodynamically stable women with a small unruptured ectopic pregnancy showed that treatment success of methotrexate administered transvaginally under ultrasound guidance was significantly better than the "blind" intratubal injection under laparoscopic guidance (RR 1.6, 95% CI 1.0, 2.5). In addition, mean serum hCG clearance time was significantly shorter in women treated by this administration route (17 versus 29 days). No data were available on tubal patency and future fertility.

37.4.12 Methotrexate Transvaginally under Sonographic Guidance versus Systemic Methotrexate in a Single-dose Intramuscular Regimen

The combined results of three studies[54,68,69] involving 95 women with a small unruptured ectopic pregnancy showed no significant difference in primary treatment success between the two treatments (RR 1.2, 95% CI 0.95, 1.5). In the local methotrexate group, the tubal content was aspirated. Only one woman in the systemic methotrexate group developed mild side-effects.

No significant differences were found in the number of subsequent intrauterine pregnancies (RR 1.2, 95% CI 0.70, 1.9) and repeat ectopic pregnancies (RR 1.3, 95% CI 0.06, 29).

37.4.13 Methotrexate under Laparoscopic Guidance versus the same Regimen in Combination with Systemic Methotrexate

In a small study[70] involving only 15 haemodynamically stable women with a small unruptured tubal pregnancy, local methotrexate alone was less successful than this regimen in combination with systemic methotrexate in the elimination of the tubal pregnancy (RR 0.86, 95% CI 0.63, 1.2). No data were available on tubal patency and future fertility.

Other outcome measures analysed were serum hCG clearance time, complications and side-effects. Mean serum hCG clearance time did not differ significantly (20 versus 21 days), whereas no complications or side-effects were seen in both treatment groups.

37.4.14 Methotrexate versus Prostaglandins both Transvaginally under Sonographic Guidance Combined with the Systemic Administration of the Drug

In a small study[71] involving 21 haemodynamically stable women, no significant difference was found in primary treatment success (RR 1.0, 95% CI 0.54, 1.8). The authors did not mention the number of additional surgical interventions done per treatment group. Tubal patency was lower in the methotrexate group, although this finding was not significantly different (RR 0.88, 95% CI 0.67, 1.1). No data were available on pregnancy outcome in women with desire for future fertility.

Other outcome measures analysed were serum hCG clearance time, hospital stay and side-effects. Mean serum hCG clearance time was longer in the methotrexate group (28 versus 18 days). Hospital stay was 3 days in both groups, whereas only one woman in each treatment group developed side-effects.

37.5 Summary of Randomised Controlled Trials

In the evaluation of the different administration routes, systemic methotrexate seems to be the most effective route. It seems clear that there is no place for local methotrexate under laparoscopic guidance. This mode of administration is less effective than laparoscopic salpingostomy in the elimination of tubal pregnancy. Moreover, with local methotrexate under laparoscopic guidance, the risks of anaesthesia and trocar insertion are still present, whereas if laparoscopy is still needed for diagnostic purposes, laparoscopic surgery is the obvious choice of treatment. Although the transvaginal administration of methotrexate under sonographic guidance is less invasive and more effective than the laparoscopically "blind" intratubal injection, this technique requires visualisation of an ectopic gestational sac and specific skills and expertise of the clinician. However, compared to laparoscopic salpingostomy, local methotrexate transvaginally under sonographic guidance is less effective in the elimination of tubal pregnancy. Compared to the local routes of administration, systemic methotrexate is more practical, easier to administer, and less dependent on clinical skills. Furthermore, in combination with non-invasive diagnostic tools, systemic methotrexate offers the option of a totally non-invasive outpatient management.

Based on the available evidence, methotrexate in a single-dose intramuscular regimen is not effective enough to advocate its routine use. Additional injections for inadequately declining serum hCG concentrations are frequently necessary.

The single randomised trial comparing systemic methotrexate in a multiple-dose intramuscular regimen versus laparoscopic salpingostomy showed no significant differences in short- and long-term medical outcome measures. Health-related quality of life was more severely impaired after systemic methotrexate. However, in a case-control study, women indicated that they were willing to trade off the increased treatment burden of systemic methotrexate for the benefit of a totally non-invasive management of tubal pregnancy.[72] In such a treatment scenario, it was calculated that systemic methotrexate would become less expensive only in women with an initial serum hCG concentration < 1500 IU/l, whereas costs would be similar to laparoscopic salpingostomy in women with an initial serum hCG concentration between 1500 and 3000 IU/l, and higher in patients with an initial serum hCG concentration > 3000 IU/l.

The single randomised trial comparing systemic methotrexate versus expectant management in tubal pregnancy is clinically not informative. The oral route of administration and the low dosage of methotrexate are uncommon and likely to fail, virtually resulting in a comparison between two placebo treatments, as is demonstrated by the 23% failure rate in both treatment groups.

In view of the possible side-effects of methotrexate as a chemotherapeutic agent, this drug has been compared with prostaglandins. However, prostaglandin therapy may induce side-effects such as cardiac arrhythmia, cardiopulmonary oedema and gastrointestinal complaints. The two randomised controlled trials comparing these two medical treatments show no significant differences in treatment success, nor in side-effects.

37.6 Conclusions

Laparoscopic surgery has been advocated by many specialists in the field as the cornerstone for the treatment of ectopic pregnancy.[73-76] This technique has proven to be safe and feasible in virtually all patients. So far, no consensus has been reached as to whether laparoscopic surgery should be performed conservatively or radically.[77-79] The inherent drawbacks of salpingostomy, i.e. the risk of persistent trophoblast and repeat tubal pregnancy generating additional costs, are only justified if this approach results in a higher spontaneous intrauterine pregnancy rate, thereby saving the treatment burden and costs of subsequent infertility treatment after salpingectomy. A review of cohort studies comparing fertility outcome after salpingostomy and salpingectomy for tubal pregnancy showed no beneficial effect of conservative surgery on the intrauterine pregnancy rate, whereas the risk of repeat ectopic pregnancy was increased, although not significantly.[80] A retrospective comparative study performing life table analysis showed a beneficial effect of salpingostomy as compared to salpingectomy for tubal pregnancy towards fertility outcome in women with contralateral tubal pathology.[81] Whether salpingostomy is beneficial in women without tubal pathology is still unknown. Therefore, a randomised controlled trial comparing salpingostomy versus salpingectomy in these patients should be carried out urgently.

If the diagnosis of tubal pregnancy is established non-invasively, medical treatment with systemic methotrexate in a multiple-dose intramuscular regimen is an alternative treatment option, thereby offering a complete non-invasive outpatient management. However, this treatment option can only be recommended for haemodynamically stable women with an unruptured tubal pregnancy and no signs of active bleeding presenting with low initial serum hCG concentrations (< 3000 IU/l), after properly informing them about the risks and benefits of the available treatment options.

References

1. Ankum WM, Van der Veen F, Hamerlynck JVThH et al (1993) Laparoscopy: a dispensable tool in the diagnosis of ectopic pregnancy? Hum Reprod 8:1301–1306
2. Ankum WM, Van der Veen F, Hamerlynck JVThH et al (1993) Transvaginal sonography and human chorionic gonadotropin measurements in suspected ectopic pregnancy: a detailed analysis of a diagnostic approach. Hum Reprod 8:1307–1311
3. Mol BWJ, Hajenius PJ, Engelsbel S et al (1998) Serum human chorionic gonadotropin measurement in the diagnosis of ectopic pregnancy when transvaginal sonography is inconclusive. Fertil Steril 70:972–981
4. Mol BWJ, Hajenius PJ, Engelsbel S et al (1999) Can noninvasive diagnostic tools predict tubal rupture or active bleeding in patients with tubal pregnancy? Fertil Steril 71:167–173
5. Li MC, Hertz R, Spencer DB (1956) Effect of MTX therapy on choriocarcinoma and chorioadenoma. Proc Soc Exp Biol Med 93:361–364
6. Thiel DH, Ross GT, Lipsett MB (1970) Pregnancies after chemotherapy of trophoblastic neoplasms. Science 169:1326–1327

7. Walden PAM, Bagshaw KD (1976) Reproductive performance of women successfully treated for gestational trophoblastic tumors. Am J Obstet Gynecol 125:1108–1114

8. Chotiner HC (1985) Nonsurgical management of ectopic pregnancy associated with severe hyperstimulation syndrome. Obstet Gynecol 66:740–743

9. Tanaka T, Haydshi H, Kutsuzawa T et al (1982) Treatment of interstitial ectopic pregnancy with methotrexate: report of a successful case. Fertil Steril 37:851–852

10. Stovall TG, Ling FW, Buster JE (1989) Outpatient chemotherapy of unruptured ectopic pregnancy. Fertil Steril 51:435–438

11. Feichtinger W, Kemeter P (1987) Conservative treatment of ectopic pregnancy by transvaginal aspiration under sonographic control and methotrexate injection. Lancet 14 Feb i:381–382

12. Pansky M, Bukowski I, Golan A et al (1989) Local methotrexate injection: a nonsurgical treatment of ectopic pregnancy. Am J Obstet Gynecol 161:393–396

13. Ory SJ, Alelei L, Villanueva AL et al (1986) Conservative treatment of ectopic pregnancy with methotrexate. Am J Obstet Gynecol 154:1299–1306

14. Kooi GS, Kock HCLV (1987) De behandeling met methotrexaat wegens tubaire graviditeit. Ned Tijdschr Geneesk 131:2359–2364

15. Ichinoe K, Wake N, Shinkai N et al (1987) Nonsurgical therapy to preserve oviduct function in patients with tubal pregnancies. Am J Obstet Gynecol 156:484–487

16. Sauer MV, Gorill MJ, Rodi IA et al (1987). Nonsurgical management of unruptured pregnancy: an extended trial. Fertil Steril 48:752–755

17. Stovall TG, Ling FW, Gray LA et al (1991) Methotrexate treatment of unruptured ectopic pregnancy: a report of 100 cases. Obstet Gynecol 77:749–753

18. Byrjalsen C, Toft B (1991) Medical treatment of ectopic pregnancy. Acta Europ Fertil 22:99–101

19. Isaacs J, Meeks GR, Hampton HL et al (1992) Treatment of unruptured ectopic pregnancy with methotrexate. J Miss State Med Assoc 33:81–85

20. Prapas J, Prapas N, Prapa S et al (1992) Conservative treatment of ectopic pregnancy with intramuscular administration of methotrexate. Acta Europaea Fertilitatis 23:25–28

21. Chryssikopulos A, Grigoriu O, Vitoratos N (1989) Treatment of ectopic pregnancy by methotrexate. Geburtsh u Fraenheilk 49:753–754

22. Stovall TG, Ling FW (1993) Single-dose methotrexate: an expanded clinical trial. Am J Obstet Gynecol 168:1759–1765

23. Henry MA, Gentry WL (1994) Single injection of methotrexate for treatment of ectopic pregnancies. Am J Obstet Gynecol 171:1584–1587

24. Glock JL, Johnson JV, Brumsted JR (1994) Efficacy and safety of single-dose systemic methotrexate in the treatment of ectopic pregnancy. Fertil Steril 62:716–721

25. Ransom MX, Garcia AJ, Bohrer M et al (1994) Serum progesterone as a predictor of methotrexate success in the treatment of ectopic pregnancy. Obstet Gynecol 83:1033–1037

26. Wolf GC, Nickisch SA, George K et al (1994) Completely nonsurgical management of ectopic pregnancies. Gynecol Obstet 37:332–335

27. Gross Z, Rodriguez JJ, Stalnaker BL (1995) Ectopic pregnancy. Nonsurgical, outpatient evaluation and single-dose methotrexate treatment. J Reprod Med 40:371–374

28. Corsan GH, Karacan M, Qasim S et al (1995) Identification of hormonal parameters for successful systemic single-dose methotrexate therapy in ectopic pregnancy. Hum Reprod 10:2719–2722

29. Stika CS, Anderson L, Frederiksen MC (1996) Single-dose methotrexate for the treatment of ectopic pregnancy: Northwestern Memorial Hospital three-year experience. Am J Obstet Gynecol 174:1840–1848

30. Thoen LD, Creinin MD (1997) Medical treatment of ectopic pregnancy with methotrexate. Fertil Steril 68:727–730

31. Leeton J, Davison G (1988) Nonsurgical management of unruptured tubal pregnancy with intra-amniotic methotrexate: preliminary report of two cases. Fertil Steril 50:167–169

32. Ménard A, Créquat J, Mandelbrot L et al (1990) Treatment of unruptured tubal pregnancy by local injection of methotrexate under transvaginal sonographic control. Fertil Steril 54:47–50

33. Schiff E, Shalev E, Bustan M et al (1992) Pharmacokinetics of methotrexate after local tubal injection for conservative treatment of ectopic pregnancy. Fertil Steril 57:688–690

34. Atri M, Bret PM, Tulandi T et al (1992) Ectopic pregnancy: evolution after treatment with transvaginal methotrexate. Radiology 185:749–753

35. Tulandi T, Atri M, Bret P et al (1992) Transvaginal intratubal methotrexate treatment of ectopic pregnancy. Fertil Steril 58:98–100

36. Fernandez H, Baton C, Beniflan JL et al (1993) Methotrexate treatment of ectopic pregnancy: 100 cases treated by primary transvaginal injection under sonographic control. Fertil Steril 59:773–777

37. Darai E, Benifla JL, Naouri M et al (1996) Transvaginal intratubal methotrexate treatment of ectopic pregnancy. Report of 100 cases. Hum Reprod 11:420–424

38. Merz E, Bahlmann F, Weber G et al (1996) Unruptured tubal pregnancy: local low-dose therapy with methotrexate under transvaginal ultrasonographic guidance. Gynecol Obstet Invest 41:76–81

39. Yao M, Tulandi T, Falcone T (1996) Treatment of ectopic pregnancy by systemic methotrexate, transvaginal methotrexate, and operative laparoscopy. Int J Fertil Menopausal Stud 41:470–475

40. Kooi S, Kock HC (1990) Treatment of tubal pregnancy by local injection of methotrexate after adrenaline injection into the mesosalpinx: a report of 25 patients. Fertil Steril 54:580–584

41. Mardesic T, Cepicky P, Vido I et al (1990) Conservative nonsurgical treatment of early detected tubal pregnancies with intra-amniotic methotrexate. Zentralbl Gynakol 112:497–499

42. Kojima E, Abe Y, Morita M et al (1990) The treatment of unruptured tubal pregnancy with intratubal methotrexate injection under laparoscopic control. Obstet Gynecol 75:723–725

43. Thompson GR, O'Shea RT, Seman E (1991) Methotrexate injection of tubal ectopic pregnancy. A logical evolution? Med J Aust 154:469–471

44. Wolf GC, Witt BR (1991) Outpatient laparoscopic management of ectopic pregnancy with a local methotrexate injection. J Reprod Med 36:489–491

45. Pansky M, Bukoversusky I, Golan A et al (1992) Methotrexate local injection for unruptured tubal pregnancy: an alternative to laparotomy? Int J Gynaecol Obstet 37:265–270

46. Groutz A, Luxman D, Cohen JR et al (1993) Rising beta-hCG titres following laparoscopic injection of methotrexate into unruptured, viable tubal pregnancies. Br J Obstet Gynaecol 100:287–288

47. Shalev E, Peleg D, Bustan M et al (1995) Limited role for intratubal methotrexate treatment of ectopic pregnancy. Fertil Steril 63:20–24

48. Pansky M, Langer R, Bukoversusky J et al (1993) Reproductive outcome after local methotrexate injection for tubal pregnancy. Fertil Steril 60:85–87

49. Porpora MG, Oliva MM, De Cristofaro A et al (1996) Comparison of local injection of methotrexate and linear salpingostomy in the conservative laparoscopic treatment of ectopic pregnancy. J Am Assoc Gynecol Laparosc 3:271–276

50. Hajenius PJ, Engelsbel S, Mol BWJ et al (1997) Randomised trial of systemic methotrexate versus laparoscopic salpingostomy in tubal pregnancy. Lancet 350:774–779

51. Dias de Pereira G, Hajenius PJ, Mol BWJ et al (1999) Fertility outcome after systemic methotrexate and laparoscopic salpingostomy for tubal pregnancy. Lancet 353:724–725

52. Nieuwkerk PT, Hajenius PJ, Van der Veen F et al (1998) Systemic methotrexate versus laparoscopic salpingostomy in tubal pregnancy: the impact on patients' health related quality of life. Fertil Steril 70:511–517

53. Mol BWJ, Hajenius PJ, Engelsbel S et al (1999) Treatment of tubal pregnancy in The Netherlands: an economic comparison of systemic methotrexate administration and laparoscopic salpingostomy. Am J Obstet Gynecol 181:945–951

54. Fernandez H, Capella-Allouc Y, Vincent S et al (1998) Randomised trial of conservative laparoscopic treatment and methotrexate administration in ectopic pregnancy and subsequent fertility. Hum Reprod 13:3239–3243

55. Saraj AJ, Wilcox JG, Najmabadi S et al (1998) Resolution of hormonal markers of ectopic gestation: a randomised trial comparing single dose intramuscular methotrexate with salpingostomy. Obstet Gynecol 92:989–994

56. Sowter MC, Farquhar CM, Petrie KJ et al (2001) A randomised trial comparing single dose systemic methotrexate and laparoscopic surgery for the treatment of unruptured ectopic pregnancy. Br J Obstet Gynaecol 180:192–203

57. Sowter MC, Farquhar CM, Gudex G (2001) An economic evaluation of single dose systemic methotrexate and laparoscopic surgery for the treatment of unruptured ectopic pregnancy. Br J Obstet Gynaecol 180:204–212

58. Yalcinkaya TM, Brown SE, Thomas DW et al (1996) A comparison of 25 mg/m^2 and 50 mg/m^2 dose of methotrexate for the treatment of ectopic pregnancy. Abstract of the Scientific Oral and Poster Sessions of the American Society for Reproductive Medicine. November, O-027, Boston, USA

59. Gazvani MR, Baruah DN, Alfirevic Z et al (1998) Mifepristone in combination with methotrexate for the medical management of tubal pregnancy: a randomized controlled trial. Hum Reprod 13:1987–1990

60. Landstrom G, Bryman I, Ekstrom P et al (1998) Ectopic pregnancy: local medical treatment versus oral methotrexate therapy – a multicentre pilot study. Abstracts of the 14th Annual Meeting of the ESHRE, O-073, Goteborg

61. Korhonen J, Stenman UH, Ylostalo P (1996) Low-dose oral methotrexate with expectant management of ectopic pregnancy. Obstet Gynecol 88:775–778

62. Fernandez H, Pauthier S, Doumerc S et al (1995) Ultrasound-guided injection of methotrexate versus laparoscopic salpingotomy in ectopic pregnancy. Fertil Steril 63:25–29

63. Mottla GL, Rulin MC, Guzick DS (1992) Lack of resolution of ectopic pregnancy by intratubal injection of methotrexate. Fertil Steril 57:685–687

64. O-Shea RT, Thompson GR, Harding A (1994) Intra-amniotic methotrexate versus CO2 laser laparoscopic salpingotomy in the management of tubal ectopic pregnancy – a prospective randomized trial. Fertil Steril 62:876–878

65. Porpora MG, Oliva MM, De Cristofaro A et al (1996) Comparison of local methotrexate and linear salpingostomy in the conservative laparoscopic treatment of ectopic pregnancy. J Am Assoc Gynecol Laparosc 3:271–276

66. Zilber U, Pansky M, Bukoversusky I et al (1996) Laparoscopic salpingostomy versus laparoscopic local methotrexate injection in the management of unruptured ectopic gestation. Am J Obstet Gynecol 175:600–602

67. Tzafettas J, Anapliotis S, Zournatzi V et al (1994) Transvaginal intra-amniotic injection of methotrexate in early ectopic pregnancy. Advantages over the laparoscopic approach. Early Hum Dev 39:101–107

68. Fernandez H, Bourget P, Ville Y et al (1994) Treatment of unruptured tubal pregnancy with methotrexate: pharmacokinetic analysis of local versus intramuscular administration. Fertil Steril 62:943–947

69. Cohen DR, Falcone T, Khalife S et al (1996) Methotrexate: local versus intramuscular. Fertil Steril 65:206–207

70. Shulman A, Maymon R, Zmira N et al (1992) Conservative treatment of ectopic pregnancy and its effect on corpus luteum activity. Gynecol Obstet Invest 33:161–164

71. Fernandez H, Baton C, Lelaidier C et al (1991) Conservative management of ectopic pregnancy: prospective randomized clinical trial of methotrexate versus prostaglandin sulprostone by combined transvaginal and systemic administration. Fertil Steril 55:746–750

72. Nieuwkerk PT, Hajenius PJ, Van der Veen F et al (1998) Systemic methotrexate versus laparoscopic salpingostomy in tubal pregnancy: patient preference for systemic methotrexate. Fertil Steril 70:518–522

73. Gomel V (1995) For tubal pregnancy, surgical treatment is usually best. Clin Obstet Gynecol 38:353–361

74. Grainger DA, Seifer DB (1995) Laparoscopic management of ectopic pregnancy. Curr Op Obstet Gynecol 7:277–282

75. Clasen K, Camus M, Tournaye H et al (1997) Ectopic pregnancy: let's cut! Strict laparoscopic approach to 194 consecutive cases and review of the literature on alternatives. Hum Reprod 12:596–601

76. Yao M, Tulandi T (1997) Current status of surgical and nonsurgical management of ectopic pregnancy. Fertil Steril 67:421–433

77. Dubuisson JB, Morice P, Chapron C et al (1997) Salpingectomy – the laparoscopic surgical choice for ectopic pregnancy. Hum Reprod 11:1199–1203

78. Dela Cruz A, Cumming DC (1997) Factors determining fertility after conservative or radical surgical treatment for ectopic pregnancy. Fertil Steril 68:871–874

79. Korell M, Albrich W, Hepp H (1997) Fertility after organ-preserving surgery for ectopic pregnancy: results of a multicenter study. Fertil Steril 68:220–223

80. Mol BWJ, Hajenius PJ, Ankum WM et al (1996) Conservative versus radical surgery for tubal pregnancy. Letter to the editor. Acta Obst Gynecol Scand 75:866–867

81. Mol BWJ, Matthijsse HM, Tinga DJ et al (1998) Fertility after conservative and radical surgery for tubal pregnancy. Hum Reprod 13:1804–1809

Chapter 38

The Laparoscopic Approach of Ectopic Pregnancy

Hervé Fernandez

38.1 Introduction

Over the past two decades, the frequency of ectopic pregnancies has increased markedly, reaching roughly 2% of all births in the industrialised countries.[1] This rate seems to be stabilising in France and the USA, and has even declined slightly in Scandinavia since the beginning of the 1990s. Improved sensitivity of the plasma human chorionic gonadotrophin (hCG) immunoassay, use of progesterone assays to determine the activity of ectopic pregnancies, and improvement in the quality of transvaginal ultrasonography allow early diagnoses. Either decision-making algorithms[2] or scoring systems[3] can then be used to determine whether medical or surgical treatment is indicated. In specialised centres, these decision-aiding methods have led to successful medical treatment of 30–40% of ectopic pregnancies, but no study has shown their efficacy in more widespread application. In 1992, however, an exhaustive registry of ectopic pregnancies was established in the French region of Auvergne, from which we can calculate, on a regional scale, the percentage of ectopic pregnancies treated with each of the available approaches. Thus, overall, from 1992 through 1996, 10% of patients were treated by laparotomy, 10% medically and 80% laparoscopically (Table 38.1). Within this "laparoscopic" group, radical (salpingectomy) and conservative (salpingotomy) approaches were evenly distributed.

38.2 Laparoscopic Approach

38.2.1 Laparotomy versus Laparoscopy

Three treatment trials have conclusively answered the question: is laparoscopy better than laparotomy? (Table 38.2).[4-6]

The laparoscopic approach results in equal efficacy, less haemorrhaging and less pain, at the same time as it shortens hospitalisation and recovery time. Moreover, it is less costly.

Nonetheless, two of the three studies[4,6] found a higher rate of persistent ectopic pregnancy among the women with laparoscopic surgery. This observation is probably related more to the learning curve for laparoscopic surgery than to any objective aspect of this procedure.

38.2.2 The Role of Laparoscopy in the Diagnosis of Ectopic Pregnancy

The various clinical presentations of ectopic pregnancies can be summed up in three main categories:

- haemoperitoneum, which indicates an emergency situation;
- suspected ectopic pregnancy, which requires an hCG assay and an ultrasound examination;

Table 38.1. Treatment of ectopic pregnancy (1993–1996) as part of French regional registry

	1993 (n = 205)	1994 (n = 213)	1995 (n = 205)	1996 (n=170)
Laparotomy	25 (122)	19 (8.9)	26 (12.7)	13 (7.7)
Laparoscopy	171 (83.4)	182 (85.5)	166 (81)	138 (82.1)
Radical	46.3%	45.5%	46.3%	48.8%
Conservative	53.7%	54.5%	53.7%	51.2%
Success	91.8%	94%	93.6%	96.5%
Methotrexate	4.4%	5.6%	5.9%	10.1%
Success	66.7%	58.3%	58.3%	70.6%

Table 38.2. Summary of three prospective, randomised trials comparing laparoscopy surgery with laparotomy for the treatment of ectopic pregnancy. NA, Not applicable or not available. Values in parentheses are percentages

	Murphy et al[4]		Vermesh et al[5]		Lindorff et al[6]	
	Laparoscopy	Laparotomy	Laparoscopy	Laparotomy	Laparoscopy	Laparotomy
Total no. of patients	26	36	30	30	52	57
Estimated blood loss (ml)	$60\pm61^*$	115 ± 115	$79\pm18^*$	195 ± 24	NA	NA
Analgesia (mg of morphine)	26 ± 43	58 ± 37	NA	NA	NA	NA
Hospital stay (days)	1.1 ± 0.8	2.7 ± 0.7	$1.4\pm0.1^*$	3.3 ± 0.2	$2.2\pm0.1^*$	5.4 ± 0.2
Time to normal activity (days)	17.9 ± 9	62 ± 49	NA	NA	$10.9\pm0.9^*$	24.1 ± 0.9
Complications						
Converted to laparotomy	0	NA	2	NA	2	NA
Persistent ectopic pregnancy	3/17 (18)	0	1/30 (3.3)	1/30 (3.3)	8/52 (15.4)	1/57 (1.8)
Blood transfusion	1	2	0	0	0	0
Febrile morbidity	0	3	1	1	0	0
Subsequent laparotomy	0	0	0	0	5^a	2^b
Subsequent repeat laparoscopy	0	0	0	0	2^a	1^a
Oral methotrexate	0	0	0	0	1^a	0
Subsequent fertility	8	10	19	21	42	45
No. desiring conception	8	10	19	21	42	45
No. of intrauterine pregnancies	7 (88)	5 (50)	13 (68)	15 (71)	22 (52)	20 (44)
No. of recurrent ectopic pregnancies	0	2 (20)	1 (5)	4 (19)	4 (10)	5 (11)

$^*p < 0.01$; ^{a}for persistent ectopic pregnancy; ^{b}one subfascial haematoma and one haematosalpinx with ovarian torsion.

- atypical cases that are often difficult to differentiate from an early spontaneous miscarriage.

Ectopic pregnancy associated with haemoperitoneum always suggests the threat of a tubal rupture. In the literature, the incidence of haemoperitoneum ranges from 18 to 34% of ectopic pregnancies.[7-9] In this situation, the clinical picture, confirmed by a urine sample positive for hCG, requires laparoscopy both for diagnosis and treatment. In the 1992–96 listings of the Auvergne registry, 153 patients underwent surgery for tubal rupture; for 70% of them, this emergency surgery was laparoscopic. It therefore appears that the experience of gynaecological surgeons and the skills of anaesthetists in case of haemodynamic instability now permit the treatment of acute haemoperitoneum by laparoscopy. In this population, radical treatment was practised in 80% of cases.

The most common diagnostic situations fall into the second group, suspected ectopic pregnancy, where decision-aiding algorithms and scoring systems help decide whether medical or surgical treatment is most appropriate. Centres with expertise in treating ectopic pregnancies obtain a diagnostic sensitivity of 95–100% for ultrasound examinations performed and interpreted according to laboratory test results.[10] In this case, diagnostic laparoscopy is generally unnecessary, and laparoscopy will be used only for therapeutic ends, once it

is decided that medical management is not appropriate. On the other hand, the Auvergne data show that diagnostic laparoscopy is still performed almost half the time, thereby revealing the still limited application of the use of ultrasound for the diagnosis of ectopic pregnancies. There is thus a substantial disparity by centre and by region in the methods for diagnosing ectopic pregnancies. If laparoscopy is used for diagnosis, it will, of course, be used immediately thereafter for treatment as well.

Atypical cases are essentially characterised by doubt as to whether miscarriage or ectopic pregnancy is present. In this group, curettage or hysteroscopy may be used to look for chorionic villi in order to ascertain the diagnosis. In these situations, associated with relatively inactive ectopic pregnancies, laparoscopy should be avoided, so that strategies of expectant or medical management can be used.

38.2.3 The Role of Laparoscopy in the Treatment of Ectopic Pregnancy

Since 1973, laparoscopy has allowed conservative treatment and diagnosis during the same procedure.[11] Laparoscopic salpingectomy was first proposed in 1981.[12] This advance re-ignited the debate between proponents of conservative and of radical treatment. Because no randomised treatment trials

Table 38.3. Rate of persistent ectopic pregnancy after conservative surgery by salpingectomy

	Year	Total no.	Laparoscopy No. of persistent ectopic pregnancies	%
Hajenius	1997	49	14	29
Hoppe	1994	101	13	12.9
Seifer	1993	103	16	15.5
Murphy	1992	26	3	11.5
Lundorff	1991	52	8	15.4
Keckstein	1990	22	1	4.5
Henderson	1989	15	3	20
Vermesh	1989	30	1	3.3
Brumsted	1988	25	1	4
Silva	1988	8	1	12.5
Pouly	1986	317	11	3.5

have been performed, there is still no consensus about which treatment for ectopic pregnancy best preserves fertility. Nonetheless, we can sum up current data by the following points:

- there is practically no failure after radical treatment (< 0.5%), while the failure rate reported after conservative treatment ranges from 3 to 29% (Table 38.3);[13]
- there is no difference between the two treatments in the rate of repeat ectopic pregnancies;[14]
- subsequent fertility is the same for both treatments among young (< 30 years) women with no other risk factor for infertility. For women with a previous history of infertility, however, the best results have been obtained with conservative treatment.[15]

38.2.4 When Is Conservative Treatment Most Appropriate?

Four principal criteria help to determine the appropriateness of conservative treatment: operability, risk of failure, desire to conserve fertility and prognosis for fertility, that is, the probability of an intrauterine pregnancy and of another ectopic pregnancy.

38.2.4.1 Operability

Experienced surgeons can treat 95% of tubal pregnancies conservatively, by a technique that includes aspiration and lavage to remove the haemoperitoneum, clean the pelvis, and evaluate the main

prognostic features before deciding on radical or conservative treatment (Figure 38.2). It is easier to use three suprapubic trocars, because the tube can be exposed more easily and a 10mm salpingotomy incision made at the interface of the inner one-third and outer two-thirds of the haematosalpinx, on the side opposite the mesosalpinx (Figure 38.3). The trophoblast is aspirated, carefully to avoid fragmentation, through the salpingotomy (Figure 38.4). The surgery is completed by lavage of the peritoneal cavity, which removes clots and trophoblastic material. The salpingotomy is not sutured.

Three elements related to operability contra-indicate conservative treatment: location, haemostasis and tubal condition.

In tubal pregnancies, interstitial location makes conservative treatment risky, because a cornual tubal incision can cause haemorrhage that is difficult to control with laparoscopy. In these situations, medical treatment by methotrexate, with laparoscopically guided puncture – or better still, during the diagnostic ultrasound examination – may be effective.

Although tubal rupture is not in itself a contra-indication to conservative treatment, the ensuing tubal damage makes conservation essentially illusory, and thus explains why a salpingectomy is performed in 80% of ruptures. Once the salpingotomy has been performed, haemostasis may be difficult to achieve. If heavy bleeding continues, despite lavage with warm water and tubal compression by haemostatic forceps for 10 minutes, a salpingectomy may be performed.

38.2.4.2 Risk of Failure

Failure is of course the most common complication of conservative treatment, and at a rate that varies highly between reports.[13] An early assessment of the risk of failure is possible by comparing the patient's rate of hCG decrease to a reference diagram (Figure 38.1).[16] Should this rate reach the alert zone, a methotrexate injection may be proposed. The failure rate appears higher when the tubal pregnancy is greater than 4cm, when tubal accessibility is hindered by adhesions, and when the hCG concentration is greater than 20 000 mIU/ml. Hagstrom et al[17] noticed a higher failure rate for active ectopic pregnancies, defined by an hCG level > 5000 mIU/ml and a progesterone level > 10 ng/ml (or 30 nmol/ml). In these circumstances, they propose that a single intramuscular dose of 1.5 mg/kg of methotrexate be administered simultaneously with the conservative treatment. Early diagnosis of failures reduces the rate of secondary surgery to between 1 and 3%.

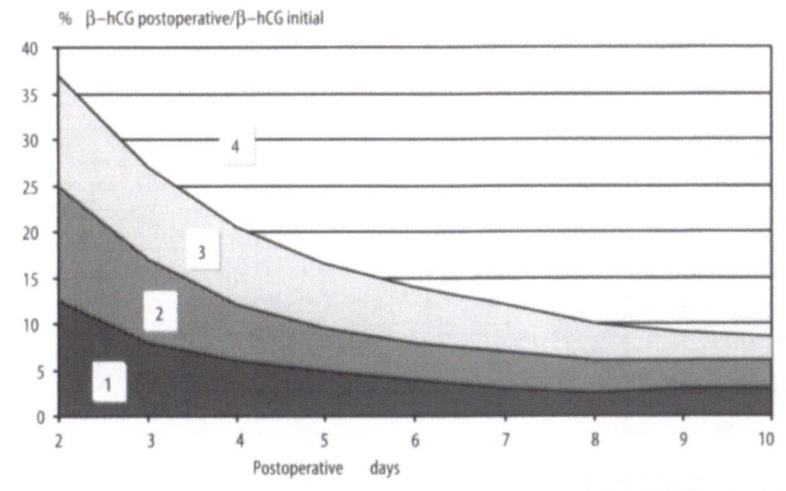

Figure 38.1. Treatment success according to postoperative β-human chorionic gonadotrophin (β-hCG) level.[16]

38.2.4.3 Desire for Pregnancy

It is often difficult at the moment of surgery to determine whether the patient desires future pregnancies. This criterion should not be considered in deciding whether conservative or radical surgery is indicated.

38.2.5 Radical Treatment by Laparoscopy

All available evidence indicates that radical treatment can be used in all ectopic pregnancies.

Three suprapubic entries are used for this treatment, which begins by grasping the tube with a grip clamp placed at the isthmus. This traction allows the tubal isthmus and the mesosalpinx to be exposed. Using bipolar coagulation, the salpingectomy proceeds in a retrograde manner, from the uterine horn up to the ovarian fimbria. The electrocautery dissection will take place at the level of the fimbria of the uterine tube to avoid injury to the lumbo-ovarian ligament (Figure 38.5).

Extraction of the tube can be accomplished in an endoscopic removal bag introduced in a 12mm trocar for voluminous ectopic pregnancies or in a standard trocar, for salpingectomies of smaller volume (Figure 38.6). Abdominal-pelvic lavage is necessary to avoid the risk, albeit small, of recurrent ectopic pregnancy.

Salpingectomy is indicated principally for patients who do not desire further pregnancies, in situations of broken or very altered tubes for which any conservative treatment appears impossible, for patients with a previous ectopic pregnancy or tubal surgery in the same tube as the pregnancy, when uncontrollable haemorrhaging occurs initially or subsequently after

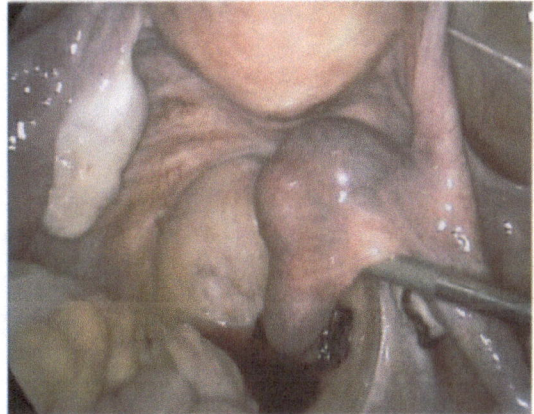

Figure 38.2. Laparoscopic evaluation of operability

conservative surgery has been tried, or when a haematosalpinx of 6cm or more is present.

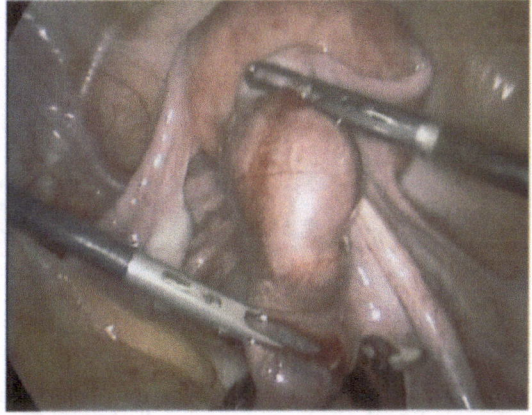

Figure 38.3. Laparoscopic evaluation of operability using multiple trocars

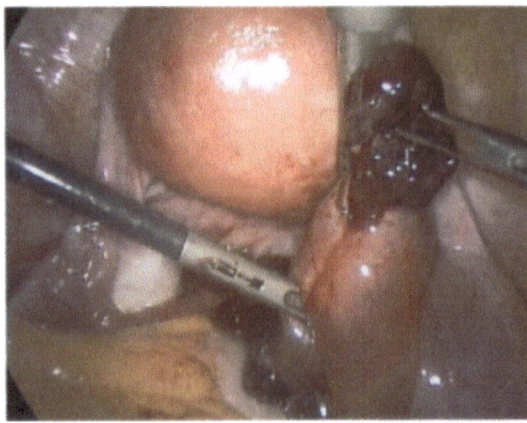

Figure 38.4. Conservative Treatment by Laparoscopy

Table 38.4. Fertility after conservative laparoscopic surgery

	Year	n	% Intrauterine pregnancies	% Ectopic pregnancies
De Cherney	1987	69	52	16
Donnez	1990	138	51	10
Pouly	1991	223	67	12
Paulsen	1992	48	54	31
Lundorff	1992	42	52	7
Total		520	58	12

Table 38.5. Fertility after salpingectomy by laparoscopy

	Year	n	Intrauterine pregnancies n	Intrauterine pregnancies %	Ectopic pregnancies n	Ectopic pregnancies %
Isner	1994	32	20	64	2	6
Dubuisson	1996	145	73	50.3	22	15.2
Fernandez	1998	184	104	56.3	19	10.3

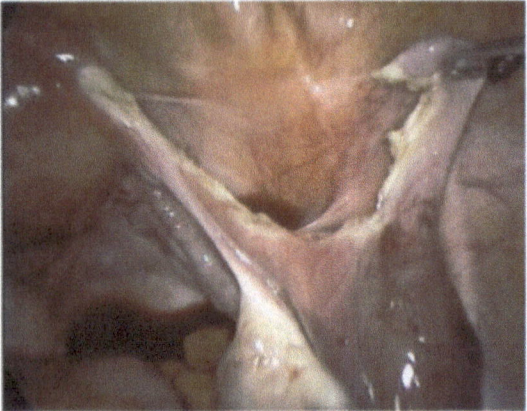

Figure 38.5. Radical Treatment by Laparoscopy

38.3 Prognosis for Fertility

This prognosis can be assessed by balancing the probability of an intrauterine pregnancy and the risk of a repeated ectopic pregnancy (Tables 38.4 and 38.5).

Conservative treatment should be favoured when tubal and ovarian anomalies suggest previous tubal infection, because it offers the best chance for future fertility. In contrast, when the true pelvis is normal, fertility will be identical regardless of the choice of surgery, especially among patients whose ectopic pregnancy occurred while using an intrauterine device for contraception.

Salpingectomy is preferable in case of major tubular anomalies: in-vitro fertilisation methods can be suggested to the patient. In Dubuisson's[20] and our series of 145 and 184 patients respectively, treated by laparoscopic salpingectomy, the fertility rate was over 80%, similar to that observed after conservative treatment among women with no risk factors.[16] The rate of recurrent ectopic pregnancies was close to 10% and it thus seems clear that salpingectomy does not protect against recurrent ectopic pregnancy and that this rate of recurrence is equivalent to that observed after conservative laparoscopic treatment.

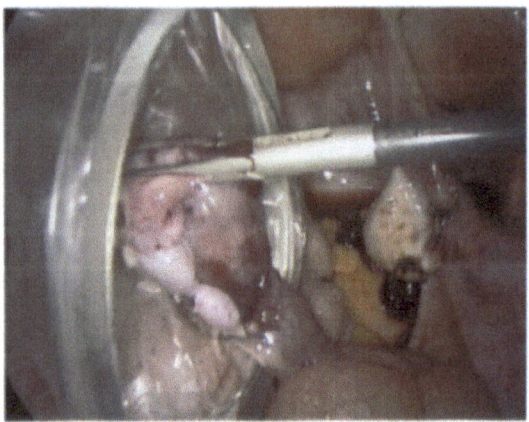

Figure 38.6. Radical Treatment by Laparoscopy

As we have seen, patients with a healthy pelvis have identical fertility rates, whether or not the tube is conserved. In these circumstances, radical treatment is preferable because it avoids any risk of trophoblastic retention.

Finally, if the patient is young and the other tube healthy, salpingectomy does not change her chances for subsequent fertility. The salpingectomy presents other advantages, including its simplicity, the lack of special equipment required, and the low rate of persistent trophoblast (< 1% compared with 29% after conservative treatment). It is probably only in cases with a history of infertility and damaged tubes that conservative treatment may remain indicated, with a slightly higher rate of intrauterine pregnancy.

38.4 Conclusions

Conservative laparoscopic treatment remains the reference treatment for ectopic pregnancy. Nonetheless, analysis of the fertility of the subgroups of women with no risk factors for infertility shows that fertility does not depend on the type of treatment. Recent treatment trials comparing conservative and medical treatment have found identical success rates and identical subsequent fertility.[18,19] In contrast, in situations where the tubal condition appears irremediable, a bilateral salpingectomy can be performed and the patient referred, if she so desires, to an in-vitro fertilisation programme.

The lack of any differential effect on subsequent fertility means that treatment should be selected according to criteria favouring the least trauma, the easiest application, and, probably, even if so far it has not been well evaluated, the least expensive.

In the future, the analysis of new strategies may, at one extreme or another, determine that laparoscopy alone should be used for radical treatment, and medical treatment reserved for situations in which conservation is possible. Nonetheless, only treatment trials will definitively answer this question.

References

1. Coste J, Job-Spira N, Aublet-Cuvelier B et al (1994) Incidence of ectopic pregnancy, first results of a population based register in France. Hum Reprod 9:742–745
2. Carson SA, Buster JE (1993) Ectopic pregnancy. New Engl J Med 329:1174–1180
3. Fernandez H, Lelaidier C, Thouvenez V et al (1991) The use of a pretherapeutic, predictive score to determine inclusion criteria for the non-surgical treatment of ectopic pregnancy. Hum Reprod 6:995–998
4. Murphy AA, Nager CW, Wujek JJ et al (1992) Operative laparoscopy versus laparotomy for the management of ectopic pregnancy: a prospective trial. Fertil Steril 57:1180–1185
5. Verrnesh M, Silva PD, Rosen GF et al (1989) Management of unruptured ectopic gestation by linear salpingostomy: a prospective, randomized clinical trial of laparoscopy versus laparotomy. Obstet Gynecol 73:400–407
6. Lundorff P, Thorbum J, Hahlin M et al (1991) Laparoscopic surgery in ectopic pregnancy: a randomized trial versus laparotomy. Acta Obstet Gynecol Scand 70:343–348
7. Saxon D, Falcone T, Mascha EJ et al (1997) A study of ruptured tubal ectopic pregnancy. Obstet Gynecol 90:46–49
8. Bogdanskiene G, Dirsaite J, Telyceniene O et al (1997) Fertility after ectopic pregnancy: preliminary analysis of a population-based register in Lithuania. 12, Abstract book 1, 340
9. DiMarchi JM, Kosasa TS, Hale RW (1989) What is the significance of the human chorionic gonadotrophin value in ectopic pregnancy? Obstet Gynecol 74:851–855
10. Cacciatore B, Korhonen J, Stemman UH et al (1995) Transvaginal sonography and serum hCG in monitoring of presumed ectopic pregnancies selected for expectant management. Ultrasound Obstet Gynecol 5:297–300
11. Bruhat MA, Manhes H, Mage G et al (1980) Treatment of ectopic pregnancy by means of laparoscopy. Fertil Steril 33:411–414
12. Dubuisson JB, Aubriot FX, Foulot H et al (1990) Reproductive outcome after laparoscopic salpingectomy for tubal pregnancy. Fertil Steril 53:1004-1007
13. Seiler DB (1997) Persistent ectopic pregnancy: an argument for heightened vigilance and patient compliance. Fertil Steril 68(3):402–404
14. Yao M, Tulandi T (1997) Current status of surgical and nonsurgical management of ectopic pregnancy. Fertil Steril 67(3):421–433
15. Job-Spira N, Bouyer J, Pouly JL et al (1996) Fertility after ectopic pregnancy: first results of a population based cohort study in France. Hum Reprod 11:99–104
16. Pouly JL, Chapron C, Manhes H et al (1991) Multifactorial analysis of fertility after conservative laparoscopic treatment of ectopic pregnancy in a series of 223 patients. Fertil Steril 56:453–460
17. Hagstrom HG, Hahlin M, Betinegarg-Eden B et al (1994) Prediction of persistent ectopic pregnancy after laparoscopic salpingostomy. Obstet Gynecol 84:798–802
18. Hajenius PJ, Engelsbel S, Mol BWJ et al (1997) Randomised trial of systemic methotrexate versus laparoscopic salpingostomy in tubal pregnancy. Lancet 350:774–779
19. Fernandez H, Pauthier S, Doumerc S et al (1995) Ultrasound-guided injection of methotrexate versus laparoscopic salpingotomy in ectopic pregnancy. Fertil Steril 63:25–29
20. Dubuisson JB, Morice P, Chapron C et al (1996) Salpingectomy – the laparoscopic surgical choice for ectopic pregnancy. Hum Reprod 11:1199–1203

Part IX

Early Prenatal Diagnosis and Obstetric Endoscopy

Contents

Summary

In the context of this book, we decided to limit our discussion of pregnancy to the first trimester, hence the absence of a discussion about mid-trimester amniocentesis from this section. Historically, invasive procedures such as amniocentesis were offered only on the basis of maternal age. The relatively recent introduction of nuchal translucency screening and biochemical testing has allowed an estimate of risk to be given for younger women as well. Hence couples can now make a more informed choice about whether to have an invasive diagnostic procedure. The arguments for nuchal translucency screening are discussed in depth. The introduction of high-resolution ultrasonography has meant that some serious congenital abnormalities are being diagnosed at earlier gestations; these are described.

A review of invasive procedures in early pregnancy is given. For invasive procedures, early amniocentesis is associated with a unacceptable fetal loss rate and is not used in clinical practice. Coelocentesis is a useful research tool that offers the chance to study materno-embryonic transfer and may give a route for the introduction of transduced cells in the context of fetal somatic gene therapy. Chorionic villus biopsy (CVS) remains the technique of choice for obtaining a fetal karyotype in the first trimester. Whether this should be performed transcervically or transabdominally is open to debate. The appropriate route may depend on operator experience or on factors such as placental location. The relative merits of CVS and mid-trimester amniocentesis are disputed, but many feel that in experienced hands the miscarriage rate of both procedures is similar.

Currently, endoscopy has a limited role, but as the technique evolves technically, it seems likely that the range of procedures that can be performed in utero will widen. Furthermore, as with many new procedures, they are often tried initially on extreme cases where the prognosis is grim, which may give rise to misleading results. For the moment, endoscopy is generally limited to the management of feto-fetal transfusion syndrome and to occlude the cord when there are complications of monochorionic twins. How far this type of surgery can develop remains to be seen.

Key points

- The sensitivity of nuchal translucency for aneuploidy is approximately 80% for a 5% false-positive rate

- Training in nuchal translucency measurement and regular audit of the screening programme is mandatory

- The sensitivity of screening is improved by the addition of serum biochemical testing. Using a combined approach, there is a 85–90% detection rate of Down's syndrome with a 5% false-positive rate. Nasal bone hypoplasia may also lead to an improvement in test performance

- Even if the karyotype is normal, an increased nuchal translucency measurement is associated with an increased risk of a congenital abnormality and the prognosis worsens with increasing nuchal translucency

- Increased nuchal translucency (> 3.5 mm/> 99th centile) is a better indication for screening for congenital heart defects with fetal echocardiography than maternal/obstetric history

- With appropriate training, 50–60% of other fetal anatomical defects can be detected at the same time as the nuchal translucency scan at 11–14 weeks

- Early amniocentesis before 13 full weeks of gestation has an unacceptably high miscarriage rate. Coelocentesis is a useful research tool but is not currently clinically useful

- CVS may be performed transabdominally or transcervically, with similar outcomes

- In experienced hands, the miscarriage rate associated with CVS may be the same as for mid-trimester amniocentesis

- Fetal endoscopic surgery may be used for treatment of feto–fetal transfusion syndrome, occlusion of the umbilical cord in monochorionic twins and division of amniotic bands

Chapter 39

Nuchal Translucency and Early Diagnosis of Congenital Anomalies

Federico Prefumo, Amar Bhide and Basky Thilaganathan

39.1 Introduction

It has been known for a long time that Turner syndrome is associated with septate cystic hygromata in the second trimester of pregnancy. In contrast, the abnormal thickening of nuchal soft tissues in the first trimester of pregnancy has been termed "nuchal translucency" (NT). This term has later been used generally to indicate the measurement of the maximum thickness of the subcutaneous translucency between the skin and the soft tissue overlying the cervical spine of the fetus. Abnormally increased NT measurements, with or without fetal hydrops, have been demonstrated to be associated with a number of aneuploidies (including trisomy 21, 18, 13 and sex chromosome abnormalities), genetic syndromes and structural fetal abnormalities.

39.2 Pathophysiology

The pathophysiology of NT is not yet well understood. It has been suggested that fluid collects in the nuchal region of the fetus much like it does in dependent oedema in later life. This occurs partly because of the fetal tendency to lie on the back and partly because of the laxity of the skin of the neck. The accumulation of fluid can represent the end point of several pathological processes. For example, chromosome 21 contains the gene that codes for type VI collagen. In trisomy 21 one subunit of this collagen can be over-expressed, resulting in connective tissue that has a more elastic composition. Further to this, many aneuploidies are associated with congenital heart defects (CHD). The latter, independent from their aetiology, may cause heart failure and the subsequent accumulation of extra-

vascular fluid. The failure of fetal movements, as a result of neuromuscular abnormalities, may also cause increased NT. Finally, intrathoracic tumours or an abnormally narrow rib cage can obstruct venous and lymphatic return from the upper half of the body, leading to fluid accumulation and oedema.

39.3 Natural History

Nuchal translucency is a transient finding, and most of the fetuses with abnormally increased measurements experience resolution over time.[1,2] There is therefore a narrow window of opportunity, between 10 and 14 weeks of gestation, to detect abnormal fluid collections. The immaturity of the fetal lymphatic system and the high peripheral resistance of the placenta are thought to contribute to the appearance of nuchal fluid. After 14 weeks, the lymphatic system has developed sufficiently to drain away any excess fluid, and changes to the placental circulation will result in a drop in peripheral resistance, making the fluid much less likely to accumulate. Furthermore, increased NT between 10 and 14 weeks generally resolves with advancing gestation, regardless of whether fetal pathology is present or the type of fetal pathology.

39.4 Measurement Technique

Consistency in the measurement technique is of the utmost importance in order to obtain reproducible results with an NT screening programme. The method for NT measurement has been standardised by the Fetal Medicine Foundation, and can be carried out transabdominally in the majority of cases. A sagittal section of the fetus must be obtained for measurement of the maximum thickness of the subcutaneous translucency between the skin and the soft tissue overlying the cervical spine. Since the measurement is a few millimetres in magnitude, and because even fractions of a millimetre can make a difference in risk calculations, the image must be magnified, with the fetus occupying at least three-quarters of the screen (Figure 39.1). The ultrasound machine should allow measurements with a precision of at least 0.1 mm. Calipers must be placed in an out-to-out position (Figure 39.2).

Care should be taken to distinguish between fetal skin and amnion, because at this gestation both structures appear as thin membranes. This can be achieved by waiting for spontaneous fetal movement away from the amniotic membrane; alternatively, the fetus can moved off the amnion by having the mother cough and/or tapping the maternal abdomen. Other pitfalls in NT measurements include the presence of an encephalocele, a nuchal cord or an amniotic band. Reference values for NT are dependent on crown–rump length, and are shown in Figure 39.3.

As with any ultrasound-based measurement, NT remains highly operator-dependent. Published studies have demonstrated satisfactory inter- and intra-observer variability, with most of the measurement error being produced as a consequence of poor calliper placement. The importance of adequate training, coupled with careful follow-up and audit of the results in an NT screening programme, cannot be overstated.

39.5 Screening for Chromosomal Abnormalities

Early reports showing an association between increased first-trimester NT and chromosomal abnormalities used a thickness of 3–5 mm as a marker of increased fetal aneuploidy risk. Unlike the second trimester, in which cystic hygromata were most often associated with Turner syndrome, first-trimester NT is frequently associated with Down's syndrome, the most common aneuploidy at this gestation.

In the early 1990s, an algorithm was developed to provide individualised risk assessment based on NT measurement at 10–14 weeks of pregnancy for patients requesting screening for Down's syndrome.[3] A background risk was established by accounting for maternal age, gestational age and previous pregnancies affected by Down's syndrome. The background risk was used to calculate a test or adjusted risk using the likelihood ratios for NT, which are based on multiples of the median NT measurement for a particular gestational age (Figure 39.4).

Several authors criticised NT screening on the basis that the test was difficult to implement and that the risk algorithm was based on data from a high-risk population. More recent studies, however, have shown that NT can be successfully measured in nearly all cases and that, after appropriate sonographic training, the test is also effective when applied to low-risk populations. The data from six studies, which reported on the implementation of NT screening during the period 1998–1999, are shown in Table 39.1.[4–9] These series show that between 43 and 100% of fetuses affected by Down's syndrome can be detected, depending on the combination of fetal NT and maternal age used to identify a high-risk group.

Nuchal translucency measurement also seems to be an effective screening test for chromosomal abnormalities other than trisomy 21. In the largest published series from a general population,[7] the detection rates of an NT measurement > 95th percentile for trisomy 18, 13, Turner syndrome and

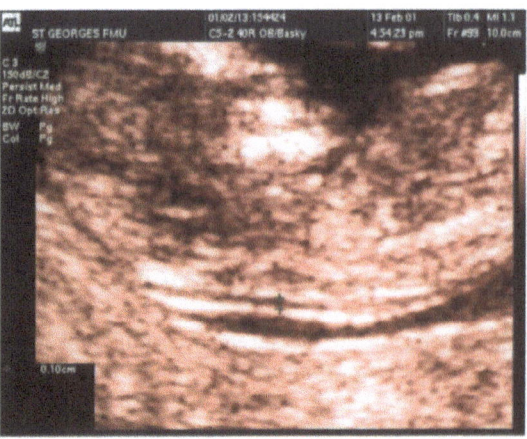

Figure 39.1. Ideal ultrasound image for nuchal translucency measurement. Note the size of the image, the location of focal point and the placement of callipers.

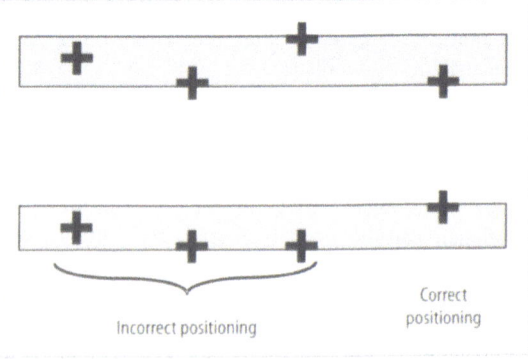

Figure 39.2. Correct and incorrect calliper placement for nuchal translucency measurement.

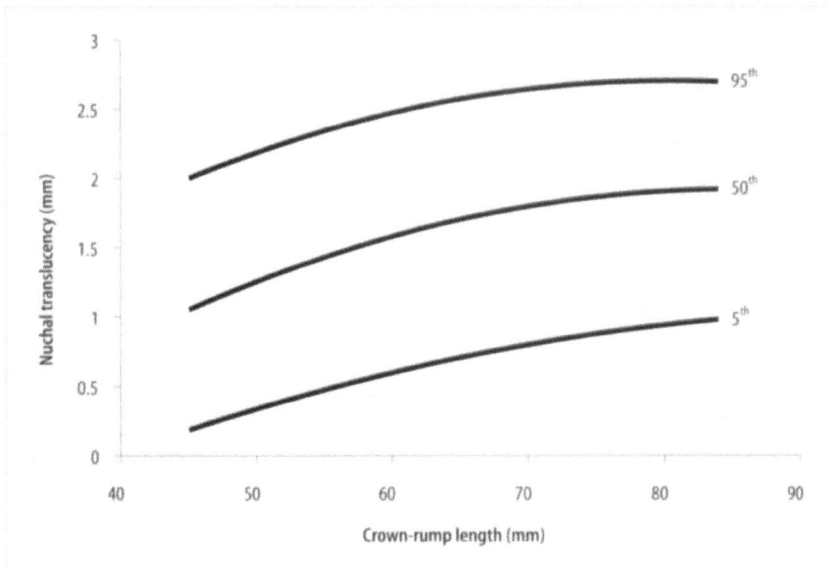

Figure 39.3. Reference range for nuchal translucency measurement.

triploidy were 75%, 72%, 87% and 59%, respectively. Increased NT also seems to be a clinically useful marker for unbalanced translocations.[10] The bigger the increase in NT, the higher the prevalence of chromosomal abnormalities: this has been reported to be 0.33%, 21%, 33%, 50% and 64% for NT measurements $\leq$ 3.5 mm, 3.5–4.4 mm, 4.5–5.4 mm, 5.5–6.4 mm and $\geq$ 6.5 mm, respectively.[11]

In order to improve the performance of the test, there have been various attempts to combine NT screening with first-trimester maternal biochemistry or other ultrasound findings. At the moment, the most successful approach seems to be the combination of NT measurement with maternal serum free human beta-chorionic gonadotrophin and pregnancy-associated plasma protein-A levels. According to several published series, combining first-trimester maternal biochemistry improves the sensitivity for Down's syndrome up to 90%, while maintaining the same false-positive rate. A detailed financial analysis also shows that nuchal screening alone or in combination with maternal serum biochemistry, are the most cost-efficient tests for the detection of Down's syndrome.[12]

Alternative strategies to improve screening efficiency have been developed to reduce the false-positive rate by subjecting pregnancies that are found to be at high risk to a second tier of screening. The latter tests are usually more complex and expensive, making them unsuitable for use with a low-risk population. Data are available for the isolation of fetal cells from the maternal circulation, ultrasound assessment of fetal nasal bone ossification[13] and ductus venosus blood flow (Figures 39.5 and 39.6). However, further evidence must be obtained before these methods can be recommended for clinical use. We refer to a recent review for a more complete discussion of these issues.[14]

Table 39.1. Studies examining the implementation of fetal nuchal translucency (NT) screening in an unselected population. MA, Maternal age

Reference	Gestation (weeks)	Number	Screening cut-off	False-positive rate (%)	Detection rate trisomy 21
Hafner et al, (1998)[4]	10^{+0}–13^{+6}	4233	NT > 2.5 mm	1.7	3 of 7 (43%)
Theodoropoulos et al, (1998)[5]	10^{+4}–13^{+6}	3550	NT > 95th centile	2.9	10 of 11 (91%)
	10^{+4}–13^{+6}	3550	NT + MA: risk > 1 in 300	4.9	10 of 11 (91%)
Pajkrt et al, (1998)[6]	10^{+0}–14^{+6}	1473	NT > 3.0 mm	2.2	6 of 9 (67%)
			NT + MA: risk > 1 in 100	8.1	7 of 9 (78%)
			NT + MA: risk > 1 in 300	19.8	9 of 9 (100%)
Snijders et al, (1998)[7]	10^{+4}–13^{+6}	96 127	NT > 95th centile	4.4	234 of 326 (72%)
			NT + MA: risk > 1 in 300	8.3	268 of 326 (82%)
Whitlow et al, (1999)[8]	11^{+0}–14^{+6}	6634	NT > 99th centile	1.0	13 of 23 (57%)
Schwarzler et al, (1999)[9]	10^{+1}–13^{+6}	4523	NT > 2.5 mm	3.1	8 of 12 (67%)
	10^{+1}–13^{+6}	4523	NT + MA: risk > 1 in 270	4.7	10 of 12 (83%)

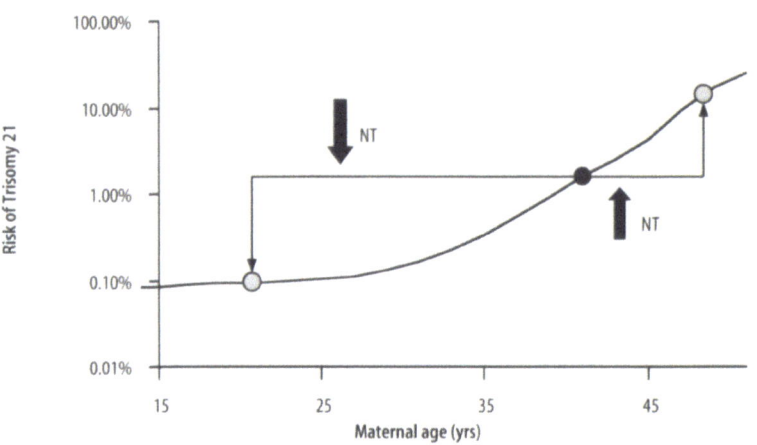

Figure 39.4. Down syndrome risk with respect to maternal age. The effects of increased and decreased nuchal measurement are shown starting from the a-priori risk (•).

39.6 Increased NT and Normal Karyotype

Despite the association between NT and aneuploidies, a substantial proportion of fetuses with increased NT have a normal karyotype. As the collection of fluid is supposed to be the result of fetal abnormalities, it is not surprising that chromosomally normal fetuses with an increased NT have a worse prognosis when compared to fetuses with a normal NT. Table 39.2 shows data from published studies regarding the outcome of pregnancies with an increased NT.[11,15–22] In the largest series from an unselected population,[21] fetuses with an NT over the 99th centile had an adverse pregnancy outcome (miscarriage, intrauterine death, or termination for fetal abnormality) in 17.8% of cases (relative risk 12.2, 95% CI 7.2–20.8) versus 1.5% for those with a normal measurement. The corresponding figure was 6.8% for NT measurements above the 95th centile (relative risk 4.7, 95% CI 2.8–7.9). A high association was observed in all studies between increased NT and early spontaneous pregnancy loss.

The incidence of major structural abnormalities and genetic syndromes is also increased in fetuses with an abnormal NT, and an increasing number of conditions are being reported in association with increased first-trimester NT (Table 39.3).[11] Although in some cases the defect may be purely coincidental, in other cases there may be a true association operating through one or more of the mechanisms previously suggested to be responsible for NT increase: cardiac dysfunction in association with abnormalities of the heart and great arteries; venous congestion in the head and neck in association with the constriction of the fetal body in amnion rupture sequence or superior mediastinal compression found in diaphragmatic hernia or the narrow chest in skeletal dysplasia; failure of lymphatic drainage due to abnormal or delayed development of the lymphatic system or impaired fetal movements in various neuromuscular disorders; altered composition of the subcutaneous connective tissue and fetal anaemia or hypoproteinaemia.

It is important to emphasise that the likelihood of any adverse outcome and the strength of the association with any structural abnormality vary with the extent at which NT is increased. In the series by Souka et al.,[11] the chance of the livebirth of a neonate with no structural defects was 85.9% for NT measurements between 3.5 and 4.4 mm, but dropped to 31.2% for measurements ≥ 6.5 mm. Studies with a long-term follow-up have also raised the possibility of an association between increased NT and later neurodevelopmental delay in the absence of structural abnormalities.[18,20,22] However, further studies are necessary to clarify these findings.

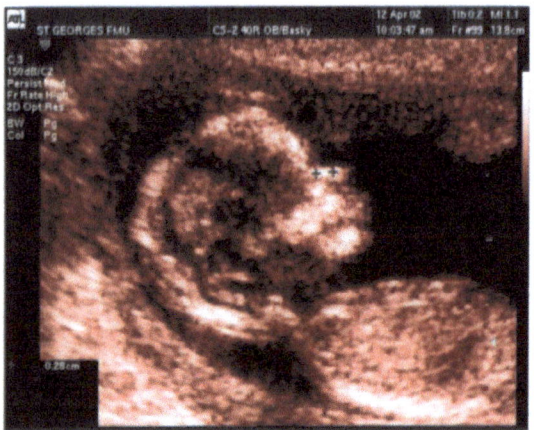

Figure 39.5. Fetal profile demonstrating the nasal bone.

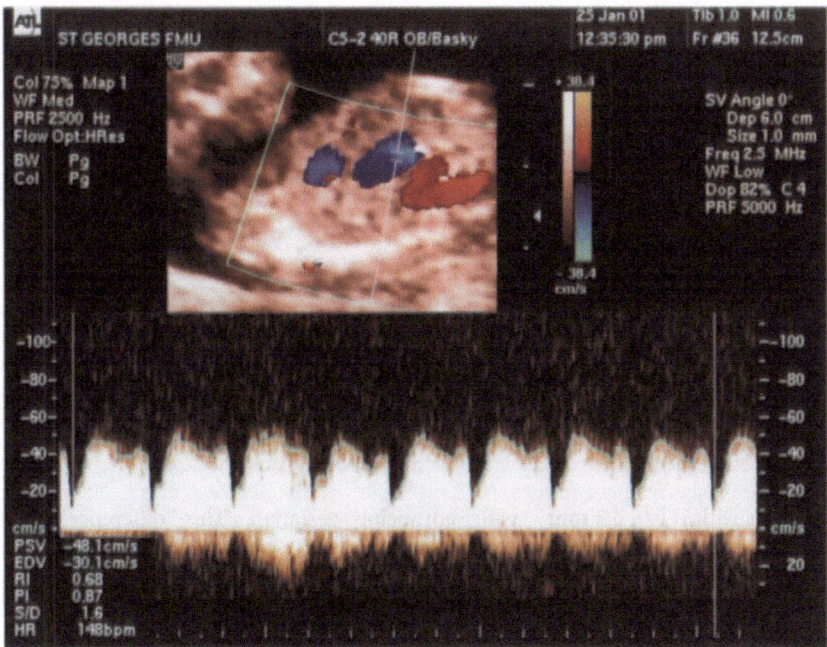

Figure 39.6. Biphasic fetal ductus venosus waveform obtained using pulsed wave Doppler in the first trimester.

39.7 Nuchal Translucency and Congenital Heart Defects

One of the associations most consistently reported by all the studies is the one between increased NT and structural cardiac abnormalities. A study of 29,154 singleton pregnancies[23] showed that NT was above the 95th centile in 56% of cases with a major cardiac defect. This sonographic marker could, therefore, also be used to identify a subgroup of pregnancies at high risk for CHD that would benefit from specialist fetal echocardiography at a tertiary referral centre. However, data from unselected populations have shown that NT alone is not a reliable screening test for congenital cardiac abnormalities, with sensitivities of around 15% for CHD.[21,24]

Although the sensitivity of NT screening for major CHD is much lower than previously suggested, the data clearly demonstrate an increased likelihood of CHD with increasing NT measurements. Hence, fetuses with first-trimester NT measurements ≥ 3.5 mm have a major CHD prevalence of 50/1000 pregnancies, or 5%. The risk of major CHD in fetuses with NT ≥ 3.5 mm is therefore significantly greater than with established risk factors currently in use. The risk of both minor and major CHD combined in pregnancies complicated by maternal diabetes, family history of CHD or previous pregnancy affected by CHD is around 1–3%. Thus, by identifying a high-risk group with increased NT, fetal echocardiography can be carried out earlier in pregnancy, as the majority of complex CHDs can be identified from as early as 12 weeks. Despite the relatively low sensitivity, the policy of targeted early

Table 39.2. Studies examining the outcome of pregnancies with an increased first-trimester nuchal translucency (NT)

Reference	NT	Population screened	No. of women scanned	Increased NT (%)	Increased NT (number)	Aneuploidy	Poor outcome (%)	Developmental delay
Pandya et al, (1995)[15]	> 3 mm	Selected	Not stated		1015	19%	8	No follow-up
Chaban et al, (1996)[16]	> 3 mm	Selected	Not stated		54	48%	39	No follow-up
Fukada et al, (1997)[17]	> 5 mm	Selected	996	1.2	12	75%	100	No follow-up
Van Vugt et al, (1998)[18]	> 3 mm	Not stated	Not stated		63	Excluded	21	3.2%
Bilardo et al, (1998)[19]	> 3 mm	Selected	1911	4.4	74	34%	32	No follow-up
Adekunle et al, (1999)[20]	$\geq$ 4 mm	Unselected	4975	0.8	53	28%	37	5%
Michailidis and Economides (2001)[21]	$\geq$ 9th centile / $\geq$ 99th centile	Unselected	6650	3.7 / 1.3	251 / 86	Excluded	13 / 18	No follow-up
Souka et al, (2001)[11]	$\geq$ 3.5 mm	Selected	Not stated		1320	Excluded	23	No follow-up
Hiippala et al, (2001)[22]	> 3 mm	Unselected	10,507	0.5[a]	50[a]	Excluded		6%

[a] This figure only includes children with a normal karyotype still available for clinical follow-up at 2–7 years of age.

Table 39.3. Most common abnormalities associated with increased nuchal translucency

Cardiac

Structural
Congenital diaphragmatic hernia
Exomphalos
Body stalk anomaly

Musculoskeletal
Achondrogenesis
Osteogenesis imperfecta
Jeune's thoracic dystrophy
Campomelic dysplasia
Fetal akinesia deformation sequence

Genetic syndromes
Noonan
Beckwith–Wiedemann
Fryn
Smith–Lemli–Opitz

fetal echocardiography in fetuses with NT ≥ 3.5 mm is likely to be more rewarding for the detection of CHDs, than current policies based on the maternal or obstetric history.

39.8 Detection of Structural Abnormalities in the First Trimester

There are now many case reports and series that have reported the detection of fetal anomalies at 10–14 weeks of gestation. Few studies, however, have examined the sensitivity of first-trimester ultrasound in the detection of structural abnormalities. Since a recent comprehensive review of the literature,[25] little other than case reports have been published. It is important to remember that, although some abnormalities are the same at 12 and 20 weeks of gestation, the features of other congenital anomalies may change with advancing gestation. This difference occurs because of the earlier stage of embryological development and because secondary pathological mechanisms have not yet altered the appearance of certain conditions. For example, the diagnosis of exomphalos cannot be confirmed before 12 weeks, when the physiological hernia of the midgut would be expected to resolve (Figure 39.7). Similarly, the prenatal diagnosis of anencephaly at 20 weeks of gestation relies on the demonstration of an absent cranial vault and cerebral hemispheres, whereas at 10–14 weeks of gestation, acrania and exencephaly are seen (Figure 39.8). With advancing gestation, there is progressive deterioration of the exposed neural tissue, resulting in the finding of anencephaly in the second trimester.

In a series of 6443 pregnancies from an unselected population screened for anatomical defects at 10–14 weeks of pregnancy,[26] 59% of the structural anomalies were detected at this early stage of pregnancy. Anomalies of the central nervous system, neck and gastrointestinal tract were most readily

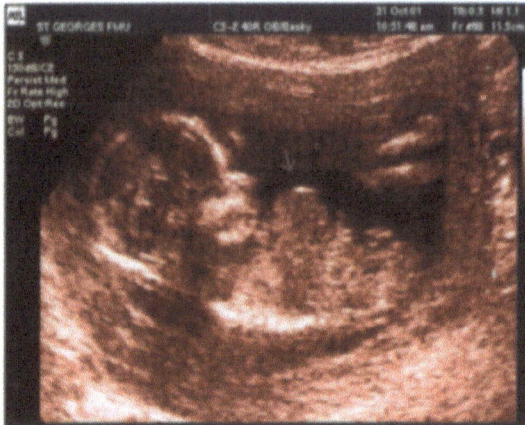

Figure 39.7. Fetal exomphalos diagnosed during the nuchal translucency scan.

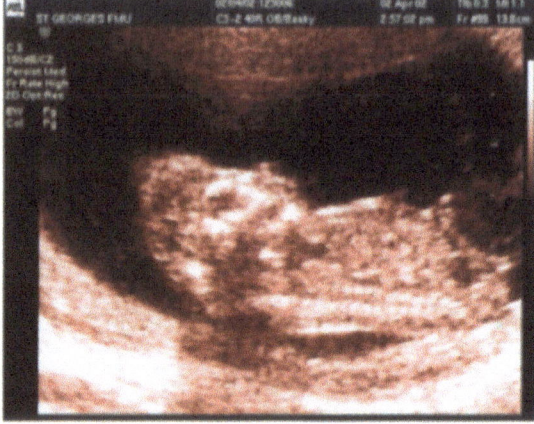

Figure 39.8. Fetal exencephaly, noted by the absence of an echogenic skull vault. The brain matter is seen floating in the amniotic fluid at this stage.

identified, whereas abnormalities of the heart were harder to determine. Skeletal and facial abnormalities were often missed. The study confirmed that, although a significant proportion of defects can be detected at this early gestation, ultrasound is not capable of screening for some major anomalies, and a 20-week scan should still be performed. In this series, the combination of a first- and second-trimester anomaly scan detected 81% of structural congenital abnormalities.

39.9 Multiple Pregnancies

Twins account for about 1% of all pregnancies, with two-thirds being dizygotic and one-third monozygotic (identical). In dizygotic pregnancies, each zygote develops its own amnion (diamniotic) and placenta (dichorionic). Monozygotic pregnancies may also be dichorionic, or there may be sharing of the same placenta (monochorionic), amniotic sac (monoamniotic) and even fetal organs (conjoined or Siamese). Chorionicity and amnionicity depend on how soon, after fertilisation, the single embryonic mass splits into two. The perinatal mortality rate in twins is around six times higher than in singletons. This increased mortality is about 3–4 times higher in monochorionic than dichorionic twin pregnancies, with the highest rate of mortality before 24 weeks of gestation. Any effort to reduce this excess loss can only be achieved through early identification of monochorionic pregnancies by ultrasound examination in early pregnancy and the development of appropriate methods of surveillance and intervention during the second trimester.

Chorionicity is best determined by ultrasound examination at 6–9 weeks of gestation, when in dichorionic twins there is a thick septum between the chorionic sacs. After 9 weeks, this septum becomes progressively thinner to form the chorionic component of the inter-twin membrane, but it remains thick and easy to identify at the base of the membrane as a triangular tissue projection. This, when visible, is known as the λ-sign. In monochorionic twins the triangular tissue projection is absent, resulting in the T-sign. With the introduction of first-trimester scanning between 11 and 14 weeks, sonographic examination of the base of the inter-twin membrane for the presence of the lambda and T-signs provides reliable distinction between dichorionic and monochorionic pregnancies (Figures 39.9 and 39.10).

The finding of increased NT in twin pregnancies must be interpreted with caution. The sensitivity of this finding for fetal aneuploidy is unchanged in twin pregnancies. However, the false-positive rate of increased NT is doubled to approximately 10%,

mainly due to the effect/inclusion of monochorionic twins. The finding of increased NT in one or both monochorionic twins increases the risk of the development of twin-to-twin transfusion syndrome fourfold to about 40%. Hence, with this finding in monochorionic twins, serial ultrasound surveillance as well as prenatal diagnosis should be considered.

39.10 Three-dimensional Ultrasound

The availability of ultrasound systems capable of three-dimensional (3D) imaging has produced much enthusiasm and expectations in the world of obstetric ultrasound. However, the continuous improvement in the technical capabilities of these systems, together with the lack of properly designed studies, does not yet allow critical evaluation of the impact of 3D ultrasound on first-trimester scanning. This technique has the potential of improving our knowledge of normal and abnormal embryonic development,[27] as well as

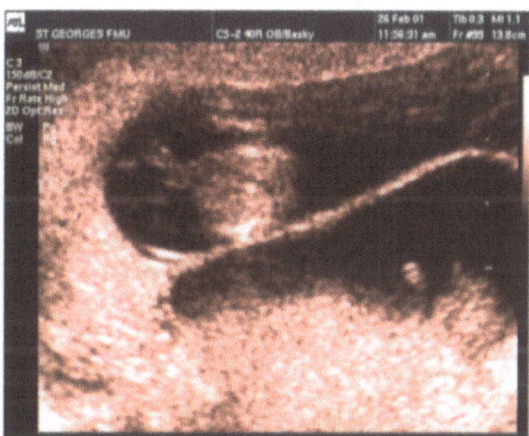

Figure 39.9. Dichorionic twin pregnancy with a λ-sign.

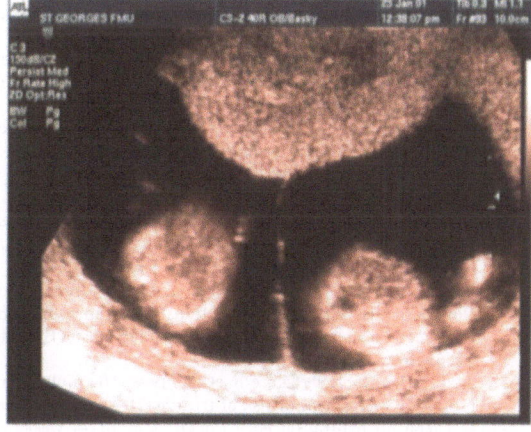

Figure 39.10. Monochorionic twin pregnancy with a T-sign.

helping in the assessment of fetal anatomy.[28] Single case reports have suggested a role for early 3D ultrasound in the diagnosis of specific fetal abnormalities. However, in a routine setting, 2D scanning still proves superior to 3D ultrasound for the assessment of fetal morphology.[29]

For what specifically concerns NT measurement, a few reports compared 2D and 3D transvaginal ultrasound assessment of NT.[30,31] They found that measurement using a 3D technique was significantly quicker, providing an almost ideal mid-sagittal view of the fetus even when fetal lie was suboptimal in terms of a 2D scan. They also showed reduced intraoperative variability between measurements made in three dimensions. These results were not confirmed in subsequent studies.[29]

39.11 Conclusions

The sensitivity of NT for aneuploidy is about 80% for a 5% false-positive rate. In fetuses with normal karyotype, prognosis worsens as NT increases. An NT above 3.5 mm or above the 99th centile mandates further screening of the fetal heart, and has a higher sensitivity for cardiac defects than a screening programme based on maternal or obstetrical history.

With appropriate training, 50%–60% of other fetal anatomical defects can be detected at the same time as the NT scan at 11–14 weeks. Training in NT measurement and regular audit of the screening programme and policy is mandatory.

References

1. Pandya PP, Kondylios A, Hilbert L et al. (1995) Chromosomal defects and outcome in 1015 fetuses with increased nuchal translucency. Ultrasound Obstet Gynecol 5:15–19
2. Pajkrt EGI, Mol BW, van Lith JM et al. (1998) Weekly nuchal translucency measurements in normal fetuses. Obstet Gynecol 91:208–211
3. Pandya PP, Snijders RJ, Johnson SP et al. (1995) Screening for fetal trisomies at 10 to 14 weeks of gestation. Br J Obstet Gynaecol 102:957–962
4. Hafner E, Schuchter K, Liebhart E et al. (1998) Results of routine fetal nuchal translucency measurement at weeks 10–13 in 4233 unselected pregnant women. Prenat Diagn 18:29–34
5. Theodoropoulos P, Lolis D, Papageorgiou C et al. (1998) Evaluation of first-trimester screening by fetal nuchal translucency and maternal age. Prenat Diagn 18:133–137
6. Pajkrt E, van Lith JMM, Mol BWJ et al. (1998) Screening for Down's syndrome by fetal nuchal translucency measurement in a general obstetric population. Ultrasound Obstet Gynecol 12:163–169
7. Snijders RJ, Noble P, Sebire N et al. (1998) UK multicentre project on assessment of risk of trisomy 21 by maternal age and fetal nuchal-translucency thickness at 10–14 weeks of gestation. Lancet 352:343–346
8. Whitlow BJ, Chatzipapas IK, Lazanakis ML et al. (1999) The value of sonography in early pregnancy for the detection of fetal abnormalities in an unselected population. Br J Obstet Gynaecol 106:929–936
9. Schwarzler P, Carvalho JS, Senat MV et al. (1999) Screening for fetal aneuploidies and fetal cardiac abnormalities by nuchal translucency thickness measurement at 10–14 weeks of gestation as part of routine antenatal care in an unselected population. Br J Obstet Gynaecol 106:1029–1034
10. Sepulveda W, Be C, Youlton R et al. (2001) Nuchal translucency thickness and outcome in chromosome translocation diagnosed in the first trimester. Prenat Diagn 21:726–728
11. Souka AP, Krampl E, Bakalis S et al. (2001) Outcome of pregnancy in chromosomally normal fetuses with increased nuchal translucency in the first trimester. Ultrasound Obstet Gynecol 18:9–17
12. Gilbert RE, Augood C, Gupta R et al. (2001) Screening for Down's syndrome: effects, safety, and cost effectiveness of first and second trimester strategies. Br Med J 323:1–6
13. Cicero S, Curcio P, Papageorghiou A et al. (2001) Absence of the nasal bone in fetuses with trisomy 21 at 11–14 weeks of gestation: an observational study. Lancet 358:1665–1667
14. Hyett J, Thilaganathan B (1999) First trimester screening for fetal abnormalities. Curr Opin Obstet Gynecol 11:563–569
15. Pandya PP, Snijders RJM, Johnson S et al. (1995) Natural history of trisomy 21 fetuses with increased nuchal translucency thickness. Ultrasound Obstet Gynecol 5:381–383
16. Chaban FK, Van Splunder P, Los FJ et al. (1996) Fetal outcome in nuchal translucency with emphasis on normal karyotype. Prenat Diagn 16:537–541
17. Fukada Y, Yasumizu T, Takizawa M et al. (1997) The prognosis of fetuses with transient nuchal translucency in the first and early second trimester. Acta Obstet Gynecol Scand 76:913–916
18. Van Vugt JMG, Tinnemans BWS, Van Zalen-Sprock RM (1998) Outcome and early childhood follow-up of chromosomally normal fetuses with enlarged nuchal translucency at 10–14 weeks' gestation. Ultrasound Obstet Gynecol 11:407–409
19. Bilardo CM, Pajkrt E, de Graaf I et al. (1998) Outcome of fetuses with enlarged nuchal translucency and normal karyotype. Ultrasound Obstet Gynecol 11:401–406
20. Adekunle O, Gopee A, El-Sayed M et al. (1999) Increased first trimester nuchal translucency: pregnancy and infant outcomes after routine screening for Down's syndrome in an unselected antenatal population. Br J Radiol 72:457–460
21. Michailidis GD, Economides DL (2001) Nuchal translucency and pregnancy outcome in karyotypically normal fetuses. Ultrasound Obstet Gynecol 17:102–105
22. Hiippala A, Eronen M, Taipale P et al. (2001) Fetal nuchal translucency and normal chromosomes: a long-term follow-up study. Ultrasound Obstet Gynecol 18:18–22
23. Hyett JA, Perdu M, Sharland GK et al. (1999) Screening for congenital heart disease with fetal nuchal translucency at 10–14 weeks of gestation. Br Med J 318:81–85
24. Mavrides E, Cobian-Sanchez F, Tekay A et al. (2001) Limitations of using first-trimester nuchal translucency measurement in routine screening for major congenital heart defects. Ultrasound Obstet Gynecol 17:106–110
25. Souka AP, Snijders RJ, Novakov A et al. (1998) Defects and syndromes in chromosomally normal fetuses with increased nuchal translucency thickness at 10–14 weeks of gestation. Ultrasound Obstet Gynecol 11:391–400
26. Whitlow BJ, Chatzipapas IK, Economides DL (1998) The effect of fetal neck position on nuchal translucency measurement. Br J Obstet Gynaecol 105:872–876
27. Blaas HG, Eik-Nes SH, Berg S et al. (1998) In-vivo three-dimensional ultrasound reconstructions of embryos and early fetuses. Lancet 352:1182–1186

28. Hull AD, James G, Salerno CC et al. (2001) Three-dimensional ultrasonography and assessment of the first-trimester fetus. J Ultrasound Med 20:287–293

29. Michailidis GD, Papageorgiou P, Economides DL (2002) Assessment of fetal anatomy in the first trimester using two- and three-dimensional ultrasound. Br J Radiol 75:215–219

30. Kurjak A, Kupesic S, Ivancic-Kosuta M (1999) Three-dimensional transvaginal ultrasound improves measurement of nuchal translucency. J Perinat Med 27:97–102

31. Eppel W, Worda C, Frigo P et al. (2001) Three- versus two-dimensional ultrasound for nuchal translucency thickness measurements: comparison of feasibility and levels of agreement. Prenat Diagn 21:596–601

Chapter 40

Early Amniocentesis

Karin Sundberg

40.1 Introduction

It is generally accepted that pregnant women who are considered at increased risk for abnormal outcome because of chromosome abnormalities are offered prenatal karyotyping. Advanced maternal age or ultrasound-detected fetal malformations are among the indications where abnormal fetal karyotypes are frequently found.

During the 1970s, ultrasound-guided amniocentesis in the 16th week of pregnancy became the standard technique for fetal karyotyping. Neural tube defects are also detected by amniocentesis by measuring the level of alpha-fetoprotein in the amniotic fluid. In the mid-1980s, standard amniocentesis (SAC) carried out at 16 weeks was shown to be associated with an increased risk of postprocedure fetal loss of 1% (0.3–1.5%).[1]

First-trimester chorion villus sampling (CVS) was introduced during the late 1980s as an alternative method for fetal karyotyping, to attempt to avoid late terminations of affected pregnancies after midtrimester amniocentesis. Although fetal safety after CVS has been shown to be similar to that after SAC,[2] there are certain disadvantages associated with CVS. The sampling procedure is technically more complicated to perform, and neural tube defects cannot be detected from chorionic tissue. However, the most severe difficulty associated with CVS is the cytogenetic inconsistency of the chorionic tissue, which causes diagnostic errors in more than 1% of the samples, because of false-positive results that need follow-up.

As a natural consequence, early amniocentesis (EAC), defined as amniocentesis carried out before 14 weeks of pregnancy, has been evaluated in several cohort studies to evaluate the possibilities and potential advantages of advancing amniocentesis into the earlier weeks of pregnancy.[3,4] Most of these cohort studies from the late 1980s and early 1990s included amniocentesis at 13–14 weeks, but results from three randomised studies of the safety and feasibility of EAC at 11 and 12 weeks are now available and constitute the key references of this chapter.[5–7]

40.2 Sampling Techniques

Like SAC, EAC is carried out transabdominally under real-time ultrasound-guided insertion of a needle with stiletto. The needle gauges are between 20 and 22. It has been claimed that the thinnest 22-gauge needle should reduce the procedure-related risk of fetal loss, but convincing data have not been published.

Some centres use guided needle insertion, by means of a dotted line on the screen showing the route of the needle during insertion. Others use the freehand technique. As the amniotic membrane is mostly separated from the chorionic membrane in these early weeks, special care has to be taken not to tear the thin and loosely bound amniotic membrane during needle insertion. In addition, the amniotic membrane may cause problems during aspiration. It is easily drawn towards the needle tip, which can be difficult to visualise using the transabdominal route. Increasing the gain during sampling and placing the needle tip in front of the fetal abdomen, where the largest pool of amniotic fluid is located, is therefore recommended.

Regarding the volume aspirated, most centres use the same volume in ml as the number of gestational weeks of the pregnancy, i.e. 10 ml for 10 weeks of pregnancy, 14 ml for 14 weeks, although no evidence for this widely used policy is available.

The transvaginal route has also been evaluated as an option for EAC because of the better visualisation of the membranes during aspiration. However, this method was abandoned as a result of increased risk of infection in the samples.[8]

40.2.1 The Filter Technique

Two problems are associated with EAC compared to SAC. First, the very low concentration of vital cells in these early weeks results in significantly higher culture failure rates of around 2% compared to SAC, where culture failures are rare events (0.2%).[7] Second, there is a limited volume available for aspiration. The total volume in these early weeks is usually less than 100 ml. Both problems are overcome when EAC is carried out with the filter technique (EAF).

The filter technique was developed for sampling amniotic fluid at 12 weeks, with the main purpose of increasing the cell yield in the sample.[6] At the same time, only a limited amount of fluid is removed. The fluid is circulated during sampling in a closed, sterile system of disposable utensils with a cell filter inserted. This filter catches all cellular components in the fluid when it is reinjected into the amniotic cavity. Volumes of 12–15 ml of amniotic fluid are circulated two to three times during sampling, increasing the cell yield significantly. Also the volume reduction of the intra-amniotic fluid is limited. A filter system for sampling early amniotic fluid is shown in Figure 40.1.

40.3 Diagnostic Safety

Increased culture failure rates after EAC were found in most of the early cohort studies. This was expected, as the cell concentration is much lower in the first trimester.[9] In two early series, the culture failure rates were shown to be directly correlated to the gestational week at sampling.[8,10] Thus, EAC as a clinical diagnostic test has only rarely been applied before 11 full weeks of gestation.

It was suspected too, that EAC could turn out to be a technically more difficult test to carry out, due to the membrane separation and the limited volume. However, conflicting data on the sampling success of EAC have been published. The Canadian randomised multicentre study found a significant increase in sampling failures in the EAC group compared to SAC, but the two smaller single-centre randomised studies that compared EAC with CVS both found very low sampling failure rates (Table 40.1). This finding might be explained by a larger degree of variety in experience among the individuals performing the sampling in a multicentre trial.

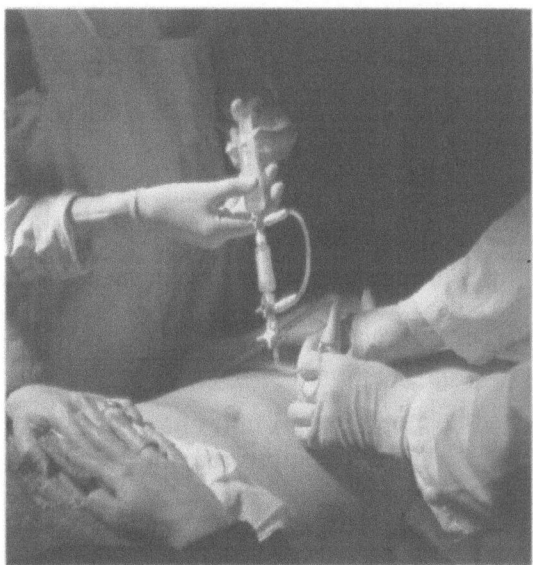

Figure 40.1. A filter system for early amniocentesis. This system was used to obtain the results of the Copenhagen trial. It is a disposable system of sterile utensils with a cell filter (Duropore, pore size 0.65 microns from Millipore A/S) inserted. At sampling, the system is attached to a standard amniocentesis needle of 20 gauge immediately after insertion. The amniotic fluid is aspirated through the tubing beside the filter and reinjected through the cell filter. The direction of the fluid is operated by use of the three-way valves. The system shown removes approximately 5ml of amniotic fluid in total.

40.3.1 Cytogenetic Aspects

Confined placental mosaicism causes diagnostic problems after CVS.[11] It was initially feared that similar problems could occur after EAC, as a larger proportion of the amniotic cells is derived from the membranes in these weeks.[3] Nevertheless, no studies so far have been able to demonstrate that false-positive diagnoses occur more frequently after EAC. The Canadian randomised trial found only one diagnostic error among all 4374 amniocenteses. It was in the EAC group, but was probably due to maternal contamination. Maternal contamination might be more frequent among EAC due to more difficult sampling conditions, but the problem is of limited importance because of its rare occurrence.

Table 40.1. Culture and sampling failure rates after early amniocentesis in three randomised studies. CVS, Chorion villus sampling; SAC, standard amniocentesis

Trial	Culture failure rate (%)	Sampling failure rate (%)
London[5]	2.3 vs 0.5 (CVS)	0.2 vs 0.8 (CVS)
Copenhagen[6]	0.2[a] vs 0.9[b] (CVS)	0.2[a] vs 0.7 (CVS)
Canada[7]	1.7 vs 0.2 (SAC)	3.1 vs 0.4[b] (SAC)

[a] The filter technique was used for sampling early amniotic fluid (see Figure 40.1); [b] significant difference.

Banding quality by means of number of bands on the chromosomes has also been evaluated for both EAC and EAF.[12,13] High band counts are obtained after EAC and EAF and the band numbers are similar to SAC and higher than after CVS.

Only very few publications are available concerning mosaicism on EAC. One demonstrated a case of true trisomy 15 mosaicism diagnosed at 12 weeks by EAF.[14] Further, EAF has also been shown to be a successful method for follow-up on mosaicism after CVS, indicating that EAF and EAC have the same cytogenetic consistency as SAC.[15]

40.3.2 Alpha-fetoprotein and Acetylcholinesterase in Amniotic Fluid

One of the major benefits of EAC is the option of early detection of neural tube defects and abdominal wall defects, by measuring alpha-fetoprotein and acetylcholinesterase in the amniotic fluid. A reliable test method, with no increased risk of false-positive diagnoses, and the normal ranges for amnion alpha-fetoprotein and acetylcholinesterase for late first-trimester has been published.[16] However, only few cases of neural tube defects and abdominal wall defects detected by EAC have been reported so far.

40.3.3 Fluorescence In Situ Hybridisation

Fluorescence in situ hybridisation is a numerical test for chromosomal aneuploidy that can be applied to uncultured cells, with overnight diagnosis of the number of specific chromosomes. It has been shown to be a useful test when applied to trophoblastic cells from CVS and amniotic cells from SAC, and EAF has also been evaluated as a method that can successfully obtain enough cells for both fluorescence in situ hybridisation and karyotyping of the same sample.[17] The purpose is to reduce the reporting time of an abnormal result after EAC/EAF, and thus avoid prostaglandin-induced abortions. The culture time of amniotic fluid cells is often several weeks, pushing many pregnancies sampled late in the first trimester well into the second trimester before a termination can be undertaken.

40.4 Safety of Early Amniocentesis

The general attitude towards EAC was very positive and the results promising in the first series published during the early 1990s, including more than 5000 sampled pregnancies.[3] Only very few suggested safety problems associated with EAC, because of a correla-

tion between leakage after sampling and subsequent increased fetal loss rates or orthopaedic postural deformities among the infants.[18]

40.4.1 Randomised Studies

Results from three randomised studies concerning the risks associated with EAC are now available: two single-centre studies both ended prematurely,[5,6] and one well-powered multicentre study was completed.[7] Details on the design of the studies, gestational ages, control groups and sampling techniques used are given in Tables 40.2 and 40.3.

40.4.1.1 The London Study

The first published study, from King's College, London,[5] was only partly randomised, as the participants were allowed to choose between EAC and CVS and randomisation. The background data were comparable between the group that was allowed to choose and the randomised group, so the study could be accepted as a randomised study. The trial stopped early due to collapse of recruitment, after publicity in the early 1990s that CVS caused limb reduction defects.[19]

40.4.1.2 The Copenhagen Study

The Copenhagen study from 1997[6] randomised between EAF at 12 weeks and CVS at 11 weeks.

Table 40.2. Study design of the three randomised studies of early amniocentesis (EAC). Values are mean gestational age at sampling in full weeks. SAC, Standard amniocentesis; CVS, chorion villus sampling

Trial	No.	SAC	EAC	CVS
London[5]	1201		11 weeks (10–13)	11 weeks (10–13)
Copenhagen[6]	1160		12 weeks[a] (11–13)	11 weeks (10–12)
Canada[7]	4374	15 weeks (11–17)	12 weeks (10–17)	

[a] EAC in the Copenhagen study was obtained with the filter technique (see Figure 34.1).

Table 40.3. Sampling techniques used in the three randomised trials. EAC, Early amniocentesis

Trial	Needle size for EAC	Transplacental sampling	Mean volume
London[5]	20 gauge	No	11 ml
Copenhagen[6]	20 gauge	Yes	Filter (5 ml)
Canada[7]	22 gauge	Yes	11 ml

Total fetal loss was compared after randomisation at 10 weeks. This trial also ended prematurely primarily due to the suspicion that EAF caused talipes equino varus (TEV), which was verified after data evaluation.

40.4.1.3 The Canadian Study

The Canadian Early and Mid-trimester Amniocentesis Trial, from 1998, compared EAC with SAC. More than 4000 women were included and the study reached the expected number of participants, which allowed more solid conclusions to be made.

40.4.2 Fetal Loss After Early Amniocentesis

Fetal loss was found to be significantly increased after EAC in the London and the Canadian study, with an increased loss rate of 3.0% and 1.7% respectively (Table 40.4). Both studies used a similar standard sampling technique, but different needle sizes. The gestational age at sampling differed too, indicating that sampling at earlier gestational ages further increases the risk of fetal loss. Also the different approach to transplacental sampling might have influenced the high loss rate after EAC found in the London study.

The Copenhagen study of 12-week EAF could not demonstrate the increased loss rate found in the two other studies, indicating that the filter technique might lower the risk of fetal loss, but the low power of the study allows no final conclusions to be drawn concerning this topic.

40.4.3 Increased Risk of Talipes Equino Varus After Early Amniocentesis

A surprisingly high percentage of 1.6% of the infants were born with TEV after EAC in the London study. Although the difference was not significant, it was much higher than in the CVS group and higher than the expected background incidence of $1:800$.

The same high frequency of TEV was found in the Copenhagen study and here the difference was

highly significant ($p < 0.01$). These results were verified in the Canadian study with an even higher level of significance ($p < 0.0001$) (Table 40.5) Although the mechanism or aetiology of TEV after EAC is not understood, the fact that leakage increases the risk indicates that damage of the amniotic membrane is in some way involved.

40.4.4 Procedure-Related Leakage of Amniotic Fluid

Temporary leakage of amniotic fluid associated with amniocentesis is a well-known iatrogenic complication that occurs in 1.7% of cases after SAC.[1] In the literature on EAC, most cohort studies and the Canadian randomised study are in agreement that EAC is associated with higher leakage rates compared to SAC. The Canadian study found that 1.7% had leakage of amniotic fluid after SAC and 3.5% leaked after EAC. The Copenhagen study of EAC found 4.4% leakage of amniotic fluid after EAF. Thus the leakage of amniotic fluid after EAC seems to be associated with twice the leakage rate of SAC.

Leakage after EAC also increases the risk of subsequent fetal loss up to 40%, which is twice the risk of fetal loss after leaking subsequent to SAC, where the risk has been shown to be 18%.[20]

The Canadian and Copenhagen studies both found that leakage increased the risk of the infant being born with TEV. In the Canadian study, as many as 15% of the children born after leakage of amniotic fluid had TEV.

40.4.5 Lung Function After Early Amniocentesis

That amniocentesis was associated with respiratory distress syndrome and pneumonia among the newborn was shown in the classical trial of risks of SAC by Ann Tabor.[1] A significant difference ($p < 0.05$) between the amniocentesis group and the control group, which had no invasive testing, could not be explained by prematurity. The mechanism is un-

Table 40.4. Randomised studies of procedure-related fetal loss after early amniocentesis (EAC). Values are total fetal loss rates. SAC, Standard amniocentesis; CVS, chorion villus sampling

Trial	No.	SAC (%)	EAC (%)	CVS (%)	Significance
London[5]	1201		5.3	2.3	S
Copenhagen[6]	1160		5.4	4.8	NS
Canada[7]	4374	5.9	7.6		S

Table 40.5. Frequency of talipes equino varus (TEV) among children exposed to early amniocentesis (EAC), standard amniocentesis (SAC) or chorion villus sampling (CVS) during pregnancy in the three randomised studies

Trial	EAC (no./% TEV)	SAC (no./% TEV)	CVS (no./% TEV)
London[5]	675/1.6%		536/0.56%
Copenhagen[6]	527/1.7%		531/none
Canada[7]	2022/1.4%	2050/0.1%	
Total	3224/1.5%	2050/0.1%	1067/0.28%

known. An animal study of lung function after fetal exposure to amniocentesis indicated that it was the needle insertion itself, not the amount of fluid aspirated, that was associated with impaired lung function.[21] Only few and small studies are available on this topic, and none are conclusive concerning the effect of EAC on lung function. A recent follow-up study on 1-year-old children exposed to CVS or EAC found a significant correlation between first-trimester sampling CVS or EAC and increased respiratory morbidity compared to a control group.[22] Concerning lung function after EAC and EAF, none of the randomised studies found any trend towards impaired lung function after EAC, but the respiratory status of the children was only clinically evaluated after birth, and no lung function tests were applied. Further follow-up studies of the effects of EAC and SAC on fetal lung development are needed.

40.4.6 Transplacental Needle Passage may be an Important Risk Factor

Although the study of Tabor et al[1] showed a significant ($p < 0.05$) increased loss rate when transplacental needle passage was used for SAC, later studies have not been able to confirm this trend, and a significant reduction of the leakage rate is observed after transplacental needle passage.[23] Transplacental needle passage seems not to increase the risk of subsequent fetal loss after EAC or EAF either. Among the EAF obtained in the Copenhagen study, 19% had transplacental sampling and none of these had postprocedural leakage or gave birth to children with TEV. This strongly suggests that transplacental sampling might be a safer sampling technique for EAC too. No data are available yet from larger studies concerning this topic.

40.5 Conclusions

It has been demonstrated that amniocentesis can be performed successfully early in pregnancy, and that cultured cells from first-trimester amniotic fluid is cytogenetically reliable. It has also been shown that by use of the filter technique, it is possible to reduce the culture failure rate significantly to the level of SAC.

However, concerning fetal safety, it has now clearly been shown in two independent randomised trials that EAC is associated with a significantly increased risk of postprocedure fetal loss. Another severe side-effect of EAC and EAF has also been demonstrated – a highly significant correlation between the occurrence of TEV after EAC or EAF. The fact that large cohort studies have not been able

to disclose the risk of affecting children with talipes by EAC is thought-provoking. It clearly emphasises the importance of conducting randomised trials before introducing new diagnostic methods into the routine, however promising they may seem.

Given our present knowledge, EAC before 13 full weeks of gestation must be abandoned because of associated fetal risks. Further, it must be emphasised that no results of randomised trials on the safety of amniocentesis between 13 and 15 weeks are available. Thus, amniocentesis between 13 and 15 weeks must still be considered an experimental approach and should not take place outside controlled trials. Results from randomised multicentre trials are necessary before amniocentesis at 13 and 14 weeks can be considered as safe as that at 16 weeks.

References

1. Tabor A, Philip J, Madsen M et al (1986) Randomised controlled trial of genetic amniocentesis in 4606 low-risk women. Lancet June 7:1287–1292
2. Smidt-Jensen S, Permin M, Philip J et al (1992) Randomised comparison of transabdominal and transcervical chorionic villus sampling and amniocentesis. Lancet 340:1237–1244
3. Wilson RD (1995) Early amniocentesis: a clinical review. Prenat Diagn 15:1259–1273
4. Sundberg K, Jørgensen FS, Tabor A et al (1995) Experience with early amniocentesis. J Perinat Med 23:149–158
5. Nicolaides K, Brizot ML, Patel F et al (1994) Comparison of chorionic villus sampling and amniocentesis for fetal karyotyping at 10–13 weeks' gestation. Lancet 344:435–439
6. Sundberg K, Bang J, Smidt-Jensen S et al (1997) Randomised study of risk of fetal loss related to early amniocentesis versus chorionic villus sampling. Lancet 350:697–703
7. Wilson RD, Johnson J, Windrim R et al (1998) The Canadian Early and Mid-trimester Amniocentesis Trial (CEMAT) group: randomized trial to assess safety and fetal outcome of early and mid-trimester amniocentesis. Lancet 351:242–247
8. Jørgensen FS, Bang J, Lind A-M et al (1992) Genetic amniocentesis at 7–14 weeks of gestation. Prenat Diagn 12:277–283
9. Elejalde BR, de Elejalde MM, Acuna JM et al (1990) Prospective study of amniocentesis performed between weeks 9 and 16 of gestation: its feasibility, risks, complications and use in early genetic prenatal diagnosis. Am J Med Genet 35:188–196
10. Rooney DE, Maclachlan N, Smith J et al (1989) Early amniocentesis: a cytogenetic evaluation. Br Med J 299:25
11. Hahnemann JM, Vejerslev LO (1997) Accuracy of cytogenetic findings on CVS - diagnostic consequences of CVS mosaicism and non-mosaic discrepancy in centres contributing to EUCROMIC 1986–1992. Prenat Diagn 17:801–820
12. Lundsteen C, Maahr J, Gerdes T (1994) Metaphase quality can be monitored by automatic counting of bands. Clin Genet 45:62–66
13. Kerber S, Held KR (1993) Early genetic amniocentesis – 4 years' experience. Prenat Diagn 13:21–27
14. Sundberg K, Brocks V, Jacobsen JR et al (1994) True trisomy 15 mosaicism, detected by amniocentesis at 12 weeks of gestation and fetal echocardiography. Prenat Diagn 14:559–563
15. Sundberg K, Lundsteen C, Philip J (1996) Early amniocentesis for further investigation of mosaicism diagnosed by chorion villus sampling. Prenat Diagn 16:1121–1127

16. Jørgensen FS, Sundberg K, Loft AGR et al (1995) Alpha-fetoprotein and acetylcholinesterase in first and early second trimester amniotic fluid. Prenat Diagn 15:621

17. Bryndorf T, Sundberg K, Christensen B et al (1994) Early and rapid exclusion of Down's syndrome. Lancet 343:802

18. Penso CA, Sandstrom MM, Garber MF et al (1990) Early amniocentesis: report of 407 cases with neonatal follow-up. Obstet Gynecol 76:1032-1036

19. Firth HV, Boyd PA, Chamberlain P et al (1991) Severe limb abnormalities after chorion villus sampling at 56-66 days' gestation. Lancet 337:762-763

20. Tabor A (1988) Thesis: Genetic amniocentesis. Indications and risks. Danish Medical Bulletin

21. Hislop A, Fairweather DV (1982) Amniocentesis and lung growth: an animal experiment with clinical implications. Lancet 2:1271-1272

22. Greenough A, Yuksel B, Naik S et al (1998) First trimester invasive procedures: effects on symptom status and lung volume in very young children. Pedriatric Pulmonology 24(6):415-422

23. Giorlandino C, Morbili L, Bilancioni E et al (1994) Transplacental amniocentesis: is it really a higher-risk procedure? Prenat Diagn 14:803-806

Chapter 41

Coelocentesis

Eric Jauniaux, Davor Jurkovic and Beatrice Gulbis

41.1 Introduction

With the development of amniocentesis for genetic investigation,[1] the amniotic fluid became the first fluid available to study the fetal environment in utero. Analyses of amniotic fluid have been performed from the third month of gestation onwards and have demonstrated important variations in gas tension, acid–base status and biochemical composition with gestational age and differences compared with maternal blood.

During the 1970s, amniotic fluid biochemistry was occasionally investigated in the first trimester. Because of technical difficulties in recognising accurately the different anatomical structures of the early gestational sac in utero, it is likely that most of the few samples obtained in these studies, before 12 weeks of gestation, were a mixture of coelomic fluid and amniotic fluid. In fact, the original anatomical finding that the extraembryonic coelom is a fluid cavity, which surrounds the embryo and fetus during most of the first trimester,[2] was completely ignored by most authors of the 1960s and 1970s. Furthermore, some authors believed that it was a thin virtual space containing a gelatinous substance that could not be aspirated.

The advent of high-resolution transvaginal ultrasound transducers at the end of the 1980s has enabled a more detailed morphological assessment of the early gestational sac in utero. In particular, the membrane separating the exocoelomic and amniotic cavities can now be clearly identified and coelomic fluid can be selectively aspirated from 5 weeks of gestation. In 1991, two independent teams, based respectively at King's College Hospital Medical School[3] and St Bartholomew's Hospital Medical College,[4] reported what they believed were the first data on the biochemistry of the extraem-

bryonic coelom. However, in 1958, McKay et al[5] had already published a paper on the protein content of the coelomic and amniotic fluids of five first-trimester normal pregnancies, obtained during hysterectomy. Although the number of samples studied was extremely small, the total protein concentration found by these authors in coelomic or chorionic fluid was very similar to that found in our studies, more than three decades later.[3] This chapter presents a summary of a decade of investigation of the coelomic fluid in research and clinical practice.

41.2 Embryology of Human Adnexae

The formation of the placenta begins between 13 and 15 days after ovulation, corresponding to stage 6 of embryonic development and to the end of the fourth week after the last menstrual period.[2] The primary villi are composed of a central mass of cytotrophoblast surrounded by a thick layer of syncytiotrophoblast. During the following week of gestation, they acquire a central mesenchymal core from the extraembryonic mesoderm and become branched, forming the secondary villi. The appearance of embryonic blood vessels within the mesenchymal core transforms the secondary villi into tertiary villi. At the end of the fifth gestational week, all three primitive types of placental villi can be found but tertiary villi progressively predominate. Up to weeks 9–10 postmenstruation, which corresponds to the last week of the embryonic period (stages 19–23), villi cover the entire surface of the chorionic sac. As the gestational sac grows during fetal life, the villi associated with the decidua capsularis, surrounding the amniotic sac, degenerate forming the chorion laeve, whereas the villi associated with the decidua basalis proliferate forming the chorion frondosum or definitive placenta.[2]

The extraembryonic coelom or exocoelomic cavity develops during the fourth week after the last menstrual period.[2] It surrounds the blastocyst, which is composed of two cavities separated by the bilaminar embryonic disk, i.e. the amniotic cavity and the primary yolk sac (Figure 41.1). At the end of the fourth week of gestation, the developing exocoelomic cavity splits the extraembryonic mesoderm into two layers, the somatic mesoderm, lining the trophoblast and the splanchnic mesoderm, covering the secondary yolk sac and the embryo (Figure 41.1). There is no anatomical barrier between the mesenchyme of the placental fetal plate and the exocoelomic or chorionic cavity.[2] At approximately 31 days menstrual age, the gestational sac is 2–3 mm in diameter and can be detected by means of transvaginal ultrasound imaging.

The amniotic cavity develops during the third week of pregnancy from the inner cell mass of the implanted blastocyst and grows inside the extraembryonic coelom, fusing with the placental chorionic plate at the end of the first trimester. The amniotic cavity is smaller than the exocoelomic cavity up to 9 weeks of gestation. Thus, during the second and third months of pregnancy the embryo and subsequently the fetus is surrounded by the amniotic cavity, which is surrounded by the exocoelomic cavity and the secondary yolk sac.

The secondary yolk sac is an independent organ floating inside the exocoelomic cavity (Figure 41.1). It forms at the beginning of the fifth week postmenstruation and develops rapidly so that by the 37th menstrual day it is larger than the amniotic cavity. From the sixth week of gestation it appears as a spherical and cystic structure covered by numerous superficial small vessels merging at the basis of the vitelline duct. This connects the yolk sac to the ventral part of the embryo, the gut and main blood circulation. An external mesothelial layer facing the extraembryonic coelom, a vascular mesenchyme and an endodermal layer facing the yolk sac cavity form the wall of the secondary yolk sac. The extraembryonic human circulation is first established within the vitelline duct artery via the dorsal aorta. During the tenth week of gestation, the yolk sac starts to degenerate and rapidly ceases to function.[2]

41.3 Technique of Sampling

Coelomic fluid as well as amniotic fluid can be retrieved by transvaginal puncture. Fluid aspiration is always performed under ultrasonographic guidance using a 5 MHz curvilinear transvaginal probe (Aloka SSD-680; Aloka Co., Japan) through an 18-gauge needle guide attached to the shaft of the probe.[1,6] When the two compartments are clearly visualised, coelomic fluid is first aspirated using a 20-gauge needle (Figure 41.2). Subsequently, a second 20-gauge needle is reintroduced through the guide and the needle advanced into the amniotic cavity to aspirate amniotic fluid.

The exocoelomic cavity can be visualised from 5 to 12 weeks' gestation and coelomic fluid is

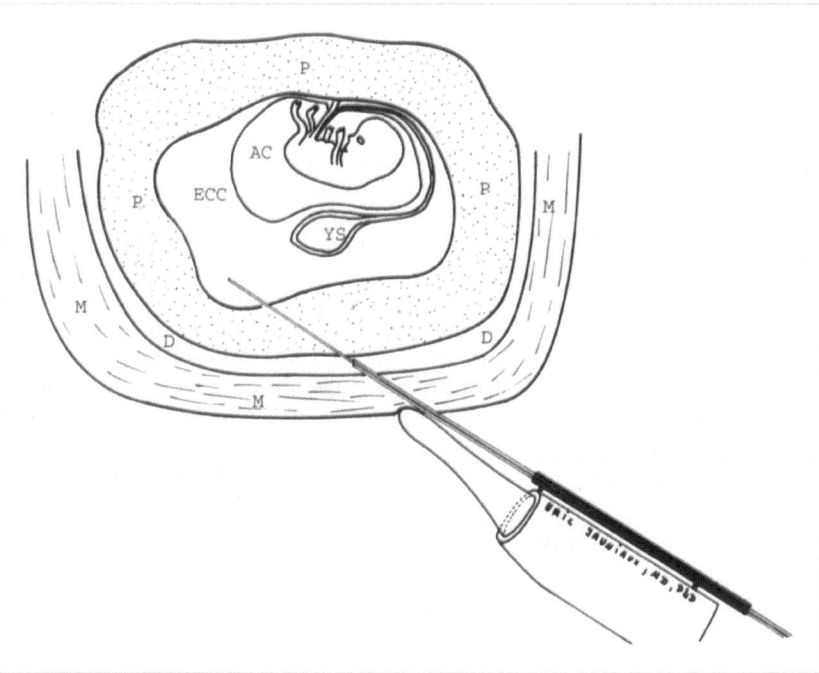

Figure 41.1. Schematic representation of a human pregnancy at 8 weeks, showing the exocoelomic cavity (ECC) puncture under transvaginal ultrasound guidance. The 18 gauge needle guide attached to the shaft of the probe is introduced inside the uterine wall. Exocoelomic fluid is first aspirated through a 20 gauge needle and subsequently another 20 gauge needle is introduced inside the amniotic cavity (AC). M, Myometrium; D, decidua; P, placenta; YS, yolk sac; E, embryo. (Modified from Jauniaux et al.[16])

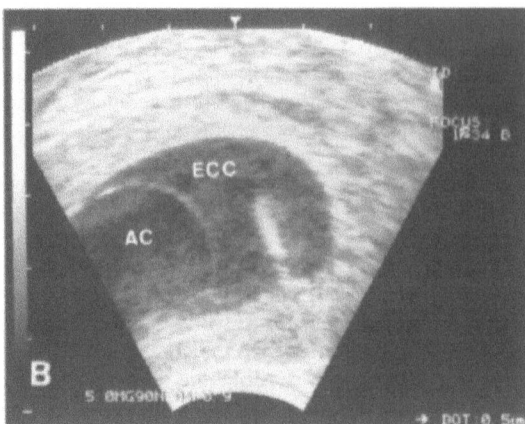

Figure 41.2. Coelocentesis at 7 weeks' gestation. *ECC*, Exocoelomic cavity; *AC*, amniotic cavity.

aspirated with a high success rate close to 100% in pregnancies between 6 and 10 weeks.[6] The amniotic cavity can be clearly identified only from the beginning of the seventh week of gestation and amniotic fluid can be obtained in all cases from 8 weeks onwards. The volume of fluid obtained from the exocoelomic cavity varies between 2 and 8 ml at 6 and 10 weeks, respectively, whereas amniotic fluid volume samples increase exponentially from 3 to 30 ml between 7 and 12 weeks. In all cases, exocoelomic fluid is yellow-coloured and more viscous than amniotic fluid, which is always clear.

41.4 Coelocentesis for Prenatal Diagnosis

Coelocentesis has a success rate of more than 95% between 7 and 10 weeks of gestation and, in theory, is the ideal alternative for early amniocentesis and chorion villus sampling (CVS) because the risk of directly injuring the growing embryo or damaging its placenta is almost non-existent. Furthermore, the procedure is easy to learn, induces only minimal discomfort to the mother and is associated with a very low rate of contamination of the sample by maternal cells.[6-12]

The high failure rate of cell growth from coelomic samples limits the applications of coelocentesis to DNA analysis.[6,7,10,11] Jurkovic et al[7] have amplified the β-globin DNA in 58 series of matched samples of coelomic fluid, placental tissue and maternal blood. In 53 cases, a normal maternal β-globin genotype was detected. In three of the five cases, where maternal haemoglobin phenotype was HbAS, heterozygosity for the sickle mutation was found on analysis of coelomic fluid and placental tissue. Three further coelomic fluid and placental samples were found to be heterozygous for transmission of the sickle gene, whereas the corresponding maternal haemoglobin phenotype was normal, thus indicating paternal transmission. These original results were confirmed by Findlay et al[10] and Makrydimas et al,[11] who studied DNA fingerprinting in 23 series of samples and the β-globin gene in known carriers of β-thalassaemia, respectively.

Using various culture systems, we successfully obtained a karyotype in about 70% of 250 coelomic fluid samples (unpublished data). Cruger et al,[9] using a mixed medium of fresh Amniomax medium in plastic flaskettes, were able to culture and performed successful cytogenetic analysis in nine out of ten coelomic fluid samples. However, in our experimental series of 250 samples, we found wide variations in the number of cells obtained per ml of coelomic fluid and that more than 50% of these cells were apoptotic after 9 weeks of gestation. Finally, cytogenetic results from coelocentesis may be obscured by contamination of the sample by mosaicism and pseudomosaicism at a rate similar (1–2%) to that observed in CVS.

Theoretically, the incidence of fetal loss after coelocentesis should be similar to that associated with early amniocentesis (2-4%). There are still no data about the relative long-term risks of coelocentesis. Ross et al[12] performed coelocentesis in 20 singleton first-trimester pregnancies, 2–13 days before planned termination for psychosocial reasons. During the follow-up period, there were five miscarriages (25%). All cases had a specific appearance on ultrasound scan, i.e. the gestational sac was filled with echogenic material and the fetus was no longer discernible. These results suggest that aspiration of less than 2 ml out of 6–10 ml of coelomic fluid may induce permanent changes in the delicate balance of pressure between the fluid cavities of the early gestational sac and/or that bleeding occurs inside the exocoelomic cavity. This phenomenon will inevitably lead to a major haemorrhage with secondary collapse of the yolk sac and amniotic cavity. Although coelocentesis is not associated with immediate feto-maternal haemorrhage,[13] the higher rate of culture failure of coelomic samples and immediate postprocedure pregnancy loss after coelocentesis compared to CVS or early amniocentesis, has made this technique unsuitable for routine prenatal diagnosis at the moment.

41.5 Coelocentesis to Study the Composition of the Extraembryonic Coelom

The coelomic fluid composition has been studied in various species of marine invertebrates.[14] In humans, the coelomic and amniotic fluids differ in their relative biochemical composition.[3,15-20] In particular, their protein pattern varies widely (Figure 41.3), suggesting that they have a different origin. Overall these studies indicate that the coelomic fluid contains numerous specific trophoblastic proteins (Table 41.1) and that the exocoelomic cavity is to be considered as the physiological liquid extension of the placental villous mesenchyme.

Almost all individual proteins are at higher concentrations in the exocoelomic than in the amniotic cavity, suggesting that the thin membrane

Table 41.1. Comparison of coelomic versus amniotic fluid protein composition. AFP, Alpha-fetoprotein; hCG, human chorionic gonadotrophin; ND, not detectable

Protein	Coelomic fluid	Amniotic fluid
Total protein (g/l)	3.5 ± 0.7	0.2 ± 0.2
AFP (kIU/l)	$21\,816 \pm 12\,667$	$27\,096 \pm 11\,822$
Albumin (g/l)	1.7 ± 0.5	ND
Pre-albumin (g/l)	0.04 ± 0.02	ND
IgG (mg/dl)	32 ± 21	ND
HcG (mIU/ml)	$165\,607 \pm 78\,543$	1752 ± 1451

separating these two compartments, which later becomes the amniotic epithelium, is not permeable to molecules with a high molecular weight (Figure 41.4a). The total protein concentration in matched samples decreases significantly from maternal serum to the coelomic cavity and from the latter to the amniotic cavity.[3,15-19]

Between 6 and 12 weeks of gestation, the mean level of total protein is 18 times lower in the coelomic fluid than in maternal serum and 54 times higher in the coelomic cavity than in the amniotic cavity.[16,17] Total protein concentrations in the coelomic fluid are not influenced by changes in maternal serum protein levels during the first trimester. The total protein concentration in the exocoelomic cavity increases with advancing gestation, while it decreases in the maternal serum. Furthermore, no correlation is found between alpha-fetoprotein (AFP), albumin and pre-albumin levels in coelomic fluid and those of maternal serum, indicating that the placental transfer rate of these specific proteins is probably independent of their respective concentrations on each side of the placental barrier.[17]

Alpha-fetoprotein is the only large protein in similar concentration in the exocoelomic and amniotic cavity during the first trimester (Figure 41.4b). It is produced by the secondary yolk sac up to 10 weeks of gestation and by the embryonic liver from 6 weeks until delivery. Analysis of Concanavalin A affinity molecular variants of AFP have demonstrated that both exocoelomic fluid and amniotic fluid AFP molecules were mainly from yolk sac origin, while maternal serum AFP molecules were mainly from fetal liver origin.[16,17] These results suggest that the human secondary yolk sac also has an excretory function and secretes AFP towards embryonic and extraembryonic compartments. In humans, molecules of AFP are also synthesised by the vitelline duct, which has the same cellular constitution as the yolk sac, and excreted in the amniotic fluid at the level where the duct fuses with the primitive umbilical cord. Yolk sac AFP could also shift in the amniotic fluid via the vitelline duct and the embryonic gut when the anal membranes break down at around 10 weeks postmenstruation. By contrast, most AFP molecules

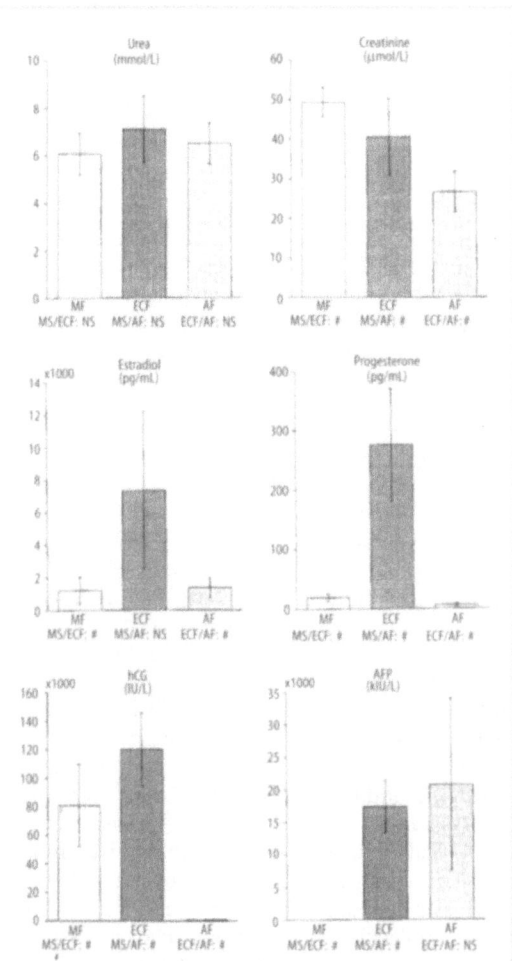

Figure 41.3. Concentrations of urea, creatinine and hormones in the maternal serum (*MS*), coelomic fluid (*ECF*) and amniotic fluid (*AF*). *NS*, No statistical difference in concentration; #p < 0.05.

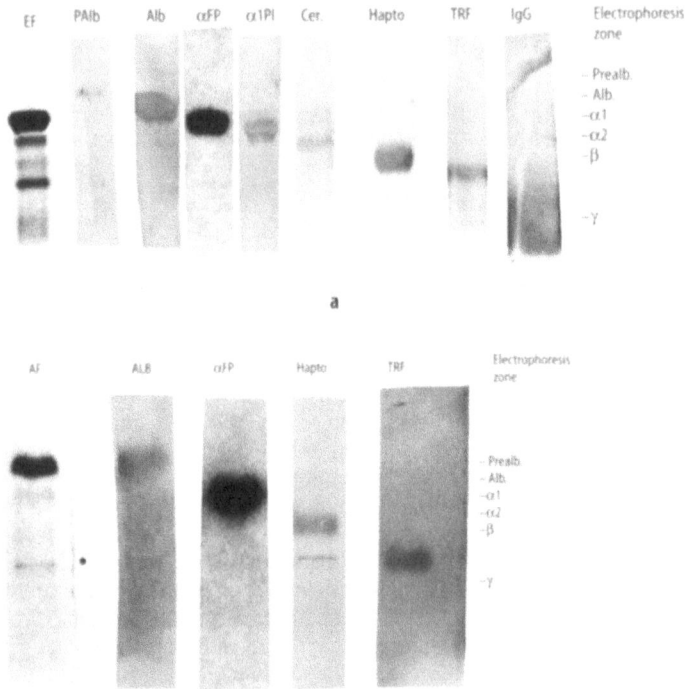

a

b

Figure 41.4. Electrophoresis of proteins in (**a**) coelomic fluid and (**b**) amniotic fluid. Note that the coelomic fluid contains many more proteins.

from fetal liver origin are probably transferred from the embryonic circulation to the maternal circulation, mainly across the placental villous membrane.

We have so far always used mechanical cervical dilatation by means of hygroscopic dilators before coelocentesis. Hypan dilators expand to apply radial force to the cervical canal walls and are mainly used to dilate the cervix prior to surgical termination of pregnancy. By contrast, prostaglandin analogues are uterotonic agents, which produce a rise in intracellular calcium concentration, leading to contraction of the myometrial cells, and also cause cervical ripening through other mechanisms. Prostaglandin analogues, when used for cervical ripening, provoke a breakdown of the placental barrier, resulting in an increase of transfer of AFP molecules from the fetal fluid compartments into the maternal circulation. This suggests that these drugs also increase the placental permeability to sodium, with secondary accumulation of this ion in the coelomic fluid. Thus, these drugs should be avoided in experiments designed to study the composition of embryonic fluids.

Following these initial descriptive studies of the composition of the embryonic fluid, we have investigated the influence of the placenta and the secondary yolk sac on the composition of the coelomic fluid.[18,19] Indeed, the turnover of the coelomic fluid is slow and any protein synthesised by the trophoblast and/or any molecule crossing the placental barrier from the maternal circulation is

likely to accumulate inside the exocoelomic cavity (Figure 41.5). The study of series of matched samples of coelomic fluid and placental tissue or yolk sac samples offers a unique opportunity to study the metabolic functions of these organs in vivo.

Within the context of a better understanding of the fetal nutritional pathways, we have also studied the transfer of molecules from the exocoelomic fluid to the fetal circulation and digestive system through the wall of the secondary yolk sac.[20] After electrophoresis and immunoblotting with specific antibodies, the β-subunit of human chorionic gonadotrophin (hCG) was detected in all placental homogenates and culture media but was not revealed in any of the corresponding yolk sac tissue samples. Reverse transcription–polymerase chain reaction showed that all placental samples express β-hCG mRNA, whereas all yolk sac and liver samples express AFP mRNA. The distribution of the placental-specific protein hCG in yolk sac and coelomic fluid and the absence of hCG mRNA expression in yolk sac tissue provide the first biological evidence of its absorptive function. Similarities in the composition of the yolk sac and coelomic fluid suggest that there is a free transfer for most molecules between the two corresponding compartments through the layers of its wall. Conversely, an important concentration gradient exists for most proteins between the extraembryonic coelomic cavity and the amniotic cavity, indicating

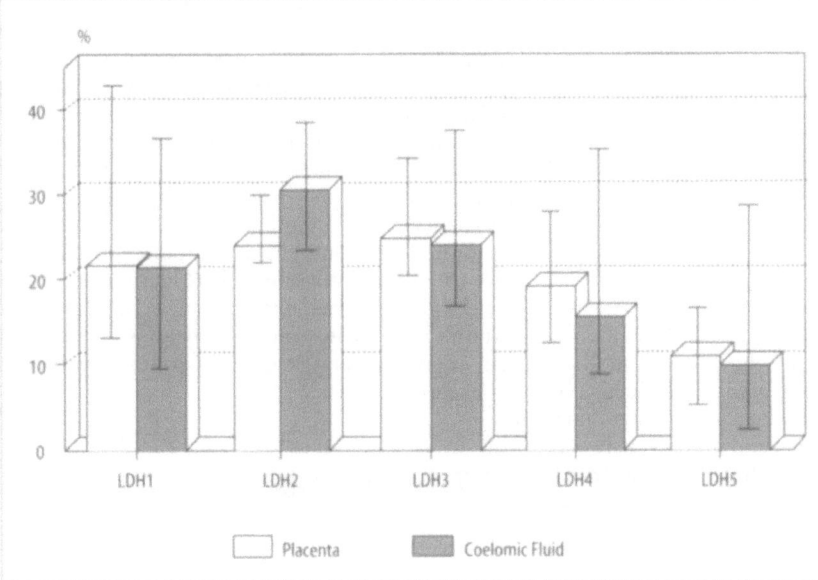

Figure 41.5. Pattern of lactate dehydrogenase (*LDH*) isoenzymes in matched samples of placenta tissue and coelomic fluid samples, providing evidence that coelomic fluid composition is mainly influenced by the placental metabolism.

that molecule transfer is limited at the level of the amniotic membrane, which separates the corresponding fluids. The yolk sac lumen contains digestive enzymes, which are not found inside the extraembryonic coelomic cavity but are present in increasing concentrations in the amniotic cavity as pregnancy advances. These findings suggest that the yolk sac membrane is an important zone of transfer between the extraembryonic and embryonic compartments and that the main flux of molecules occurs from outside the yolk sac, i.e. from the extraembryonic coelomic cavity to its lumen and subsequently to the embryonic gut and circulation.

41.6 Coelocentesis: A New Model to Study Drug Transfer in Early Pregnancy

Biological substances present in the maternal circulation early in pregnancy must cross the villous barrier to reach the embryonic compartments. When the definitive placenta forms at the end of the first trimester, materno-fetal transfers may also occur at the level of the free amniotic membranes. Maternal or placental proteins filtered in the extraembryonic coelomic cavity are probably absorbed by the secondary yolk sac, which is in direct continuity with the primitive digestive system throughout embryonic development.[19]

Placental transfers have been mainly studied in experimental animals such as guinea pigs and monkeys because they have haemochorial placentas similar to those of humans. In lower vertebrates, the yolk sac serves as the principal membrane for placental exchanges. In particular, rodents have a subsidiary yolk sac placenta, which completely envelops the fetus through the whole gestation and serves as the principal site for acquisition of protein by the fetus. Due to the complexity of the experimental situation in the intact animal and the considerable embryological differences between human and some animal species, the precise mechanism of transfer of many substances across the human placenta has not been elucidated. Transfer of protein across the human placenta has been studied in vivo by the injection of radiolabelled albumin or immunoglobin in the maternal circulation before delivery. This type of investigation was subsequently abandoned because of the damage that radioactive substances can cause to the developing fetal organs. Materno-fetal transfers in humans have been more satisfactorily investigated in vitro by using isolated, dually perfused placenta. Thus, available data concerning the mechanisms of transfer of most drugs and their interference with embryonic development in the human fetus is of limited value.

Diazepam is a lipophilic and undissociated drug with a low molecular weight of about 280 Daltons and a terminal half-life of 43 hours. Diazepam and its metabolites bind 95% to albumin and easily cross biological membranes via water-filled extracellular channels or directly through the cells, as is the case for the trophoblastic barrier (Table 41.2).[21] Our data suggested that diazepam enters the amniotic cavity mainly via the fetal circulation and subsequently through the fetal skin, which remains poorly

Table 41.2. Mean concentrations of various drugs in maternal serum and embryonic fluids 525 min after a single intravenous bolus (diazepam 0.1 mg/kg, fentanyl 1.5 g/kg, propofol 3 mg/kg, inulin 5 mg/kg) or after chronic intake (cotinine).[20,24] ND, Not detectable

Drugs	Maternal serum	Coelomic fluid	Amniotic fluid
Diazepam (ng/ml)	189	6.9	7.4
Fentanyl (ng/ml)	1.3	ND	1.1
Propofol (g/ml)	1.96	ND	ND
Inulin (mg/ml)	6.9	5.1	3.0
Cotinine (ng/ml)	72	99	108

keratinised until the end of the fourth month of pregnancy.[22] The rare and variable presence of diazepam inside the coelomic cavity may reflect chronic accumulation in benzodiazepine users. In contrast, inulin is a hydrophilic non-electrolyte molecule of 5200 Daltons, for which there is no specific transport system, and which is cleared from the circulation by glomerular filtration.[22] Inulin was detected in all fetal and maternal samples. A trend towards increasing inulin concentration was noted in the exocoelomic cavity with advancing time. Coelomic and maternal serum inulin concentrations were similar within 20 minutes after injection.

Amniotic inulin concentrations were always lower than coelomic concentration irrespective of gestational age or advancing time after injection. These results suggest that the study of drug transfer in the first trimester of human pregnancy is feasible using samples obtained from the exocoelomic cavity.

Propofol is a short-acting intravenous general anaesthetic agent with a rapid onset of action, which is extensively used in various surgical procedures and in particular, in surgical termination of pregnancy before 24 weeks of gestation. Propofol is detectable in all maternal and fetal serum samples, whereas no propofol is found in coelomic or amniotic fluid samples at any stage of gestation.[23] The pharmacodynamics of propofol found in pregnant women at 12–18 weeks of gestation are similar to those described at term. This indicates that our data can be extrapolated to the period of gestation between 24 and 37 weeks and that our model can be used to study the placental transfer of other analgesic drugs in early pregnancy. Although propofol has no known teratogenic effect in humans, our results also indicate that in continuing pregnancies the fluid cavities surrounding the developing embryo will not act as a reservoir for this drug.

The rapid changes in the gestational sac anatomy during the first trimester and, in particular, the degeneration of two-thirds of the original placenta tissue during formation of placental membranes (chorion laeve) induce inherent technical limitations of quantifying the volume of the remaining func-

tional tissue. Thus the permeability of the placenta during the first trimester to inulin or other substances cannot be determined accurately during that period of gestation. In-vitro studies will require the development of different models based on specific anatomical differences existing before and after 12 weeks of gestation. These studies have demonstrated that the permeability of the placenta is greater in early pregnancy than at term, but also because of the slow turnover of coelomic fluid, substances to which the mother is chronically exposed are likely to accumulate inside the exocoelomic cavity.[19] This prolonged exposure to toxins such as tobacco carcinogens[24] has important teratological implications and should be explored further.

41.7 Conclusions

The exocoelomic cavity was probably the last remaining physiological body fluid cavity to be explored in the human embryo. Its unique anatomical position has enabled us to study the protein metabolism of the early placenta and secondary yolk sac and to explore materno-embryonic transfer pathways. The exocoelomic cavity, which forms inside the extraembryonic mesoderm alongside the placental chorionic plate, is now believed to be an important transfer interface and a reservoir of nutrients for the embryo. Maternal or placental proteins filtered in the extraembryonic coelomic cavity are probably absorbed by the secondary yolk sac, which is in direct continuity with the primitive digestive system throughout embryonic development. Coelocentesis is a possible technique for the prenatal diagnosis of genetic disorders and in particular congenital haemoglobinopathies. However, the only study, so far, evaluating the safety of coelomic fluid aspiration in ongoing pregnancies, has shown that the risk of miscarriage after coelocentesis is around 25%.[12] This finding and the high failure rate of cell growth from coelomic fluid currently limits the applications of coelocentesis to explore the biology of materno-embryonic exchanges at a time of gestation when fetal blood cannot be obtained. Our findings will help to develop therapeutic protocols making use of fetal somatic gene therapy by injecting transduced cells into the exocoelomic cavity. The selective sampling of fluid from the exocoelomic cavity has also offered a novel approach to the study of transfer of drugs and toxins across the early human placenta and a unique tool to explore fetal physiology in vivo.

References

1. Steele MW, Breg WR (1966) Chromosome analysis of human amniotic fluid cells. Lancet i:383–385
2. Jones CPJ, Jauniaux E (1995) Ultrastructure of the materno-embryonic interface in the first trimester of pregnancy. Micron 2:145–173
3. Jauniaux E, Jurkovic D, Gulbis B et al (1991) Biochemical composition of exocoelomic fluid in early human pregnancy. Obstet Gynecol 78:1124–1128
4. Wathen NC, Cass PL, Kitau MJ et al (1991) Human chorionic gonadotrophin and alpha-fetoprotein levels in matched samples of amniotic fluid, extraembryonic exocoelomic fluid, and maternal serum in the first trimester of pregnancy. Prenat Diagn 11:145–151
5. McKay DG, Richardson MV, Hertig AT (1958) Studies of the function of early human trophoblast. III. A study of the protein structure of mole fluid, chorionic and amniotic fluids by paper electrophoresis. Am J Obstet Gynecol 75:699–707
6. Jurkovic D, Jauniaux E, Campbell S et al (1993) Coelocentesis: a new technique for early prenatal diagnosis. Lancet 341:1623–1624
7. Jurkovic D, Jauniaux E, Campbell S et al (1995) Detection of sickle gene by coelocentesis in early pregnancy: a new approach to prenatal diagnosis of single gene disorders. Hum Reprod 10:1287–1289
8. Gavril P, Jauniaux E, Gulbis B et al (1995) Changes in the coelomic fluid composition following two different methods of cervical ripening. Hum Reprod 10:2453–2455
9. Cruger DG, Bruun-Petersen G, Kolvraa S (1996) Early prenatal diagnosis: standard cytogenetic analysis of coelomic cells obtained by coelocentesis. Prenat Diagn 16:945–949
10. Findlay I, Atkinson G, Chambers M et al (1996) Rapid genetic diagnosis at 7–9 weeks gestation: diagnosis of sex, single gene defects and DNA fingerprint from coelomic samples. Hum Reprod 11:2548–2553
11. Makrydimas G, Georgiou I, Kranas V et al (1997) Prenatal diagnosis of b-thalassaemia by coelocentesis. Molec Hum Reprod 3:729–731
12. Ross JA, Jurkovic D, Nicolaides K (1997) Coelocentesis: a study of short term safety. Prenat Diagn 17:913–917
13. Makrydimas G, Lolis D, Georgiou I et al (1997) Feto-maternal bleeding following coelocentesis. Hum Reprod 12:845–846
14. Snowden AM, Vasta GR (1994) A dimeric lectin from coelomic fluid of the starfish Oreaster reticulatus cross-reacts with the sea urchin embryonic substrate adhesion protein, echinonectin. Ann NY Acad Sci 712:327–329
15. Gulbis B, Jauniaux E, Jurkovic D et al (1992) Determination of protein pattern in embryonic cavities of early human pregnancies: a model to understand materno-embryonic exchanges. Hum Reprod 7:886–889
16. Jauniaux E, Gulbis B, Jurkovic D et al (1993) Protein and steroid levels in embryonic cavities of early human pregnancy. Hum Reprod 8:782–787
17. Jauniaux E, Gulbis B, Jurkovic D et al (1994) Relationship between protein concentrations in embryological fluids and maternal serum and yolk sac size during human early pregnancy. Hum Reprod 9:161–166
18. Jauniaux E, Gulbis B (1997) Embryonal physiology. In: Jauniaux E, Barea R, Edwards R (eds) Embryonic medicine and therapy. Oxford University Press, Oxford, pp 223–243
19. Jauniaux E, Gulbis B (2000) Fluid compartments of the embryonic environment. Hum Reprod Update 6:268–278
20. Gulbis B, Jauniaux E, Cotton F et al (1998) Protein and enzyme patterns in the fluid cavities of the first trimester gestational sac: relevance to the absorptive role of secondary yolk sac. Molec Hum Reprod 9:857–862
21. Jauniaux E, Jurkovic D, Lees C et al (1996) In vivo study of diazepam transfer across the first trimester human placenta. Hum Reprod 11:889–892
22. Jauniaux E, Lees C, Jurkovic D et al (1997) Transfer of inulin across the first trimester human placenta. Am J Obstet Gynecol 176:33–36
23. Jauniaux E, Gulbis B, Shannon C et al (1998) Placental propofol transfer and fetal sedation during maternal general anaesthesia in early pregnancy. Lancet 352:290–291
24. Jauniaux E, Gulbis B, Acharya G et al (1999) Maternal tobacco exposure and cotinine levels in fetal fluids in the first half of pregnancy. Obstet Gynecol 93:25–29

Chapter 42

Chorion Villus Sampling in the First Trimester

The-Hung Bui and David T.Y. Liu

42.1 Introduction

The main objectives of invasive prenatal diagnosis are to offer prospective parents, who choose to undergo such a procedure, the assurance of having unaffected children when the risk of having a child with a specific genetic disorder is deemed unacceptably high, and to permit optimal management or treatment of affected pregnancies or fetuses. Prenatal diagnosis does not address all possible birth defects or genetic diseases. It only allows one to convert a risk figure for a specific genetic disease or structural defect to a certainty; this is not equivalent to the assurance of having a normal child.

In the 30 years since fetal diagnosis was introduced, our ability to diagnose genetic disorders and structural abnormalities prenatally has both expanded and has been enhanced by the remarkable advances made in laboratory sciences, the availability of increasingly sophisticated ultrasonographic modalities and the rapid evolution of invasive sampling techniques. Both mid-trimester amniocentesis and first-trimester chorion villus sampling (CVS) are now well-established techniques for conditions that require the analysis of a fetal sample.[1] The major advantage of CVS is that results are obtained at an earlier gestational age than with mid-trimester amniocentesis, allowing the option of earlier term-ination in the event of an abnormal result. Also, the ability to achieve early diagnosis by CVS is a significant step towards the potential for fetal therapy of some genetic disorders because it can be offered before irreversible damage has occurred.[2]

The decision as to whether or not to undergo an invasive diagnostic procedure must be made by the woman herself or by the concerned couple after all risks, options and possible outcomes have been thoroughly discussed as part of the genetic counselling process that should take place prior to any prenatal genetic test.

This chapter focuses on the current techniques used for CVS in the first trimester, when the procedure is optimally performed, its appropriateness for a given indication, as well as its safety and diagnostic accuracy.

42.2 Anatomy of First-trimester Gestation

A practical understanding of the anatomy of first-trimester gestation, as well as some knowledge of the morphology and histology of first-trimester villi will facilitate adequate sampling by the operator.

At this early stage, the inner amnion and outer chorion are not yet fused and the space between these membranes defines the coelomic cavity or extraembryonic coelom (Figure 42.1a). Degenerating villi cover most of the chorionic membrane, forming the chorion laeve, whereas fast-growing villi that anchor loosely into the underlying decidua basalis make the chorion frondosum, a tissue that will subsequently become the placenta (Figure 42.1c). The chorion frondosum is therefore the preferred sampling site due to the rich mitotic activity of its villi.

Histologically, a first-trimester villus has a mesenchymal core that is surrounded by an inner layer of cytotrophoblasts and an outer layer of syncytiotrophoblasts (Figure 42.1b). There is a dense cytotrophoblastic cell column at its end. Mitotic activity is observed in both the mesenchymal core and the cytotrophoblasts, but not in the syncytiotrophoblasts.

42.3 Indications for Chorion Villus Sampling and Turnaround Time

A detailed account of the many genetic, multifactorial and acquired disorders amenable to prenatal diagnosis by laboratory investigations is

324

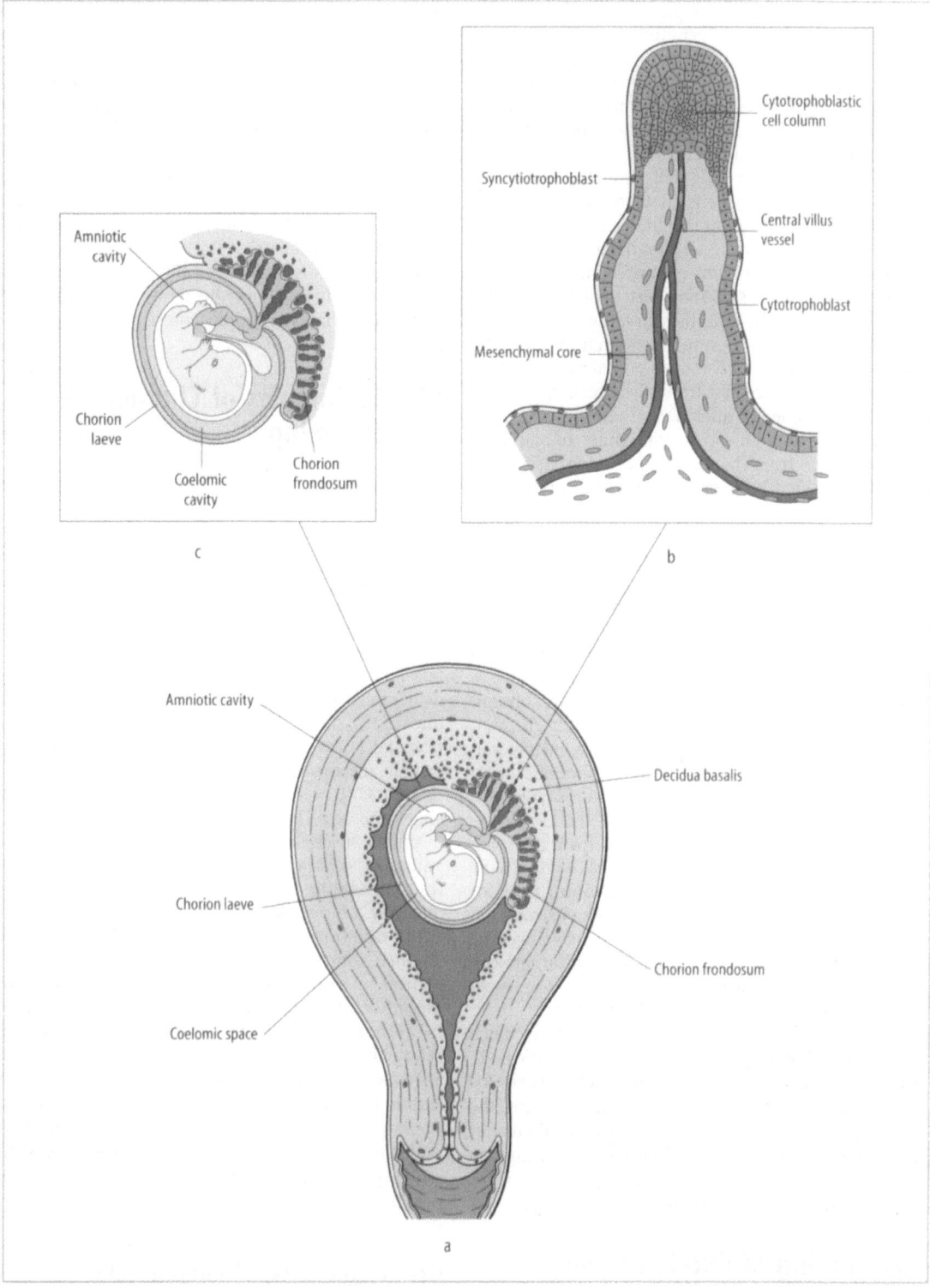

Figure 42.1. a, c Intrauterine gestation in the first trimester (9–13 weeks). The coelomic cavity is defined by the amniotic and chorionic membranes, which are not yet fused. **b** A single chorion villus. The outer syncytiotrophoblasts and inner cytotrophoblasts surround the mesenchymal core. High mitotic activity is found in the cytotrophoblastic cell column.

outside the scope of this chapter and can be found in textbooks on medical genetics. As the field is advancing rapidly, contact should be made with a medical genetics unit or other specialised laboratory to inquire into the current possibility of prenatal diagnosis whenever there are any doubts about a potentially diagnosable disorder.

The indications for CVS fall generally into three broad categories: cytogenetic, metabolic and molecular disorders. The most common indication for invasive first- and second-trimester prenatal diagnosis is chromosome analysis for advanced maternal age. However, a positive screening test – nuchal translucency thickness of the fetus measured by ultrasound or biochemical maternal serum test – may become the major indication for chromosome analysis on villous tissue in places where first-trimester screening tests for Down's syndrome are offered.[3,4]

After sampling, chorionic villi must be carefully dissected away from the maternal decidual tissue and can be examined by a variety of laboratory techniques. The two methods currently used for chromosome preparations involve two different types of cells. Direct villi processing or overnight culture relies on the actively dividing cells from cytotrophoblasts (about one in 400 cells is undergoing mitotic division) and may provide a karyotype within hours or 1 day after CVS. These cells are mostly to be found in the cytotrophoblastic cell column and have a limited life span in tissue culture. Therefore, obtaining intact villi at CVS will facilitate direct chromosome preparations in the laboratory. However, because of problems with mosaicism and the lower chromosome banding quality of such karyotypes, it is common practice also to make use of the fibroblasts grown in long-term tissue cultures from the mesenchymal core for a more reliable cytogenetic analysis.[5] Thus, the traditional turnaround time for karyotyping after CVS is 7–14 days because of differences in cell culture and villi processing. The advent of fluorescence in-situ hybridisation can contribute to an earlier diagnosis for the most common numerical chromosome aberrations.

The yield of cells and DNA from a CVS is much greater than that obtained from 20ml of amniotic fluid. Hence, biochemical or DNA analysis can usually be carried out directly on chorionic villi, obviating the need for and delay of a cell culture, as is required after mid-trimester amniocentesis. Chorion villus sampling is therefore generally preferred over amniocentesis for the two latter categories of investigations.

42.4 Timing of Chorion Villus Sampling

First-trimester CVS is optimally performed between 10 and 13 weeks of gestation to avoid the high background spontaneous miscarriage rate occurring in earlier gestation, but still allowing results to be available within the first trimester. Additionally, by this gestational age, the chorion frondosum is easily identified as a hyperechoic homogenous area on ultrasound scan. Earlier sampling has been suspected to increase the risk of fetal abnormalities caused by disruptive damage[6] and is associated with a higher fetal loss rate. The obvious advantage of CVS is that results are obtained at an earlier gestational age than after an amniocentesis. Termination of pregnancy, should it be chosen, is medically safer and emotionally less traumatic than the termination that might follow mid-trimester amniocentesis.

42.5 Techniques of Chorion Villus Sampling

Chorion villus sampling aided by transcervical endoscopy was first reported in the late 1960s but was soon abandoned because of a high frequency of complications and unreliable results. Chinese investigators performed blind transcervical CVS for fetal sex determination with a relatively high rate of success in the mid-1970s. However, it was the development of real-time ultrasound that made it possible to introduce fine sampling devices into the developing placenta accurately and safely in the mid-1980s, thus allowing successful and dependable prenatal chromosome, biochemical and DNA analysis in the first trimester.

The CVS techniques can be used for both singleton and twin pregnancies.[7] Chorion villus sampling uses continuous abdominal ultrasound guidance and can be performed by either the transcervical or the transabdominal route. The vast majority of pregnant women can be sampled by either technique. Patient or physician preference will dictate which approach is used. Occasionally, clinical findings will support one approach over the other. Operators need therefore to be proficient in both sampling methods to improve procedure safety and provide increased patient choice. At least 5–10 mg of chorionic villous tissue (wet weight) should be retrieved, depending on the indication for prenatal diagnosis (cytogenetic, biochemical or molecular). The use of antibiotic prophylaxis without any maternal risk factors is controversial. Rh-prophylaxis is given as indicated.

42.5.1 Transcervical Chorion Villus Sampling

In the first trimester (10–13 weeks) and occasionally within the early second trimester, the transcervical route for CVS offers a welcome approach. Clinicians find ready access to the sampling site, particularly if placentation is posterior. Women, too, find passage of sampling implements through the cervix readily acceptable and any discomfort felt compares favourably with mid-trimester amniocentesis.[8] On a scale of 1 to 10, the latter indicating the most discomfort, women undergoing transcervical CVS scored the procedure as between 2 and 3.[8]

The lithotomy position allows introduction of a speculum for access to the cervix. The cervix and vaginal walls are cleaned with an antiseptic solution before insertion of the catheter or biopsy forceps. Scanning with a 3.5–5 MHz curvilinear or similar probe defines the best placental site for sampling. Continued scanning is maintained to guide the chosen implement to the desired sampling area. An anterior placenta is approached by pulling the speculum downward while the tip of the implement is directed upward. When the placenta is posterior, the tip of the implement is rotated 180 downward after passing the internal os of the cervix as the speculum is lifted to aid the manoeuvre. Aspiration is the most widely used technique for collection of chorionic villi. This process is facilitated by moving the implement gently back and forth to enhance capture of the villus sample.

Occasionally, two consecutive attempts may be needed to obtain adequate villous material. This is particularly likely when a sizeable amount of villi is needed for metabolic studies. Two consecutive samplings have not been shown to increase fetal loss rate in over 2000 procedures (D.T.Y. Liu et al., unpublished observations). If more than two attempts are required, it is advisable to delay further sampling after an interval of a week. If miscarriage does not follow sampling within 3 weeks, the subsequent course of pregnancy is similar to that of the general population.

Varying concentrations of venous lakes or lacunae are found in many early placentas.[9] Their presence can be classified from grade I to grade IV, the latter indicating an area where most of the placenta is replaced by lacunae. These areas are best avoided, as entry into them can result in blood-stained samples or contribute to spotting after diagnosis.

There are two fundamental types of instruments, which depend upon aspiration to collect villi: the Liu sampler and disposable plastic catheters.

42.5.1.1 The Liu Sampler

The Liu sampler is a cannula about 14 gauge and 2 mm in diameter with a calculated curve to facilitate intrauterine manoeuvre. A rounded and closed end enhances safety. The upper aspect of the cannula tip is flattened to reflect sound and assist tip localisation.

The collection portal (1.5 × 2.0 mm) is placed at either the left or right side to ensure that aspiration will not exert suction pressure against the delicate amniotic sac. The portal is also bevelled, with the cutting point away from the tip. When suction is applied, villi will be cut to assist collection and reduce trauma. The cannula can be reused to reduce cost.

42.5.1.2 Disposable Plastic Catheters

There are various designs of these cannulas, all employing the principle of a flexible polyethylene tube, which relies on a malleable metal trocar to provide rigidity and shape. The stainless metal trocar is also echogenic and assists ultrasound-guided placement. Removal of the trocar prior to aspiration, however, will cause distortion to the shape of the plastic tube. This will cause trauma and interfere with the placement. Furthermore, localisation is more difficult once the metal trocar is removed because plastic is less echogenic than metal.

42.5.1.3 Biopsy Forceps

Rigid straight or curved biopsy forceps have also been used with both routes.[10] The end of these metal forceps can be fashioned to provide a suitable curve for transcervical sampling. The forceps are guided to the sampling site by ultrasound scanning. Chorion villi are collected by opening and closing a small set of jaws. Villi are avulsed when the forceps are withdrawn. As the forceps is sizeable compared to a cannula or needle, more trauma and placental disruption is inevitable.

42.5.2 Transabdominal Chorion Villus Sampling

For the transabdominal approach, the skin is prepared using iodine or alcohol solution. Care should be taken to avoid the bowel and urinary bladder. Either a needle guide attached to the ultrasound probe or a freehand technique is utilised to insert a 19- or 20-gauge spinal needle under ultrasound guidance. Transabdominal double-needle CVS techniques have been described with a larger outer sheath (17–18 gauge) and a smaller aspirating needle (19–20 gauge).[11] Negative pressure is applied to a 20 or 30 ml syringe attached to the end of the needle to aspirate the villous tissue into the syringe.

Initially, CVS was only done transcervically. Presently, the transabdominal approach is often chosen for fundal and anterior placental locations and transcervical CVS for posterior placentation. If only the transcervical approach is used, manipulation of the uterus by cervical tenaculum or speculum may sometimes be necessary for fundal or anterior placental position.

42.6 Safety and Accuracy of Chorion Villus Sampling

Amniocentesis performed at 15–18 weeks of gestation has been the gold standard approach for prenatal cytogenetic diagnosis with a high accuracy (99.4–99.8%) and an estimated procedure-related loss rate of 0.5–1%.[1] The advantage of an early diagnosis must be weighed against any increased risk of fetal loss that CVS may present. In common with all invasive diagnostic procedures, there is a small but unavoidable risk of miscarriage after CVS.

Selection acting on karyotypically abnormal fetuses occurs throughout the course of pregnancy. Spontaneous miscarriage rates vary with maternal age and decrease with advancing pregnancy.[12] The rate of spontaneous miscarriage decreases rapidly in the first trimester and by 10 weeks' gestation the incidence levels off to below 2%.[12] Appreciation of this change will advise that sampling should be conducted after the ninth week of gestation. In Nottingham, UK, around 11% of referrals for first-trimester transcervical CVS either miscarried or misaborted before the diagnostic test. In women less than 35 years of age, the spontaneous miscarriage rate is less than 4% for established pregnancies. It is 4–4.5% between 35 and 40 years of age. In women over 40 years, a miscarriage rate of 13–15% can be expected. Women intending to undergo villus sampling should appreciate that this natural fetal loss rate is in excess of that associated with the diagnostic procedure.

This background spontaneous miscarriage rate can make it difficult to identify the true procedure-related fetal loss rate. Studies trying to differentiate the risk between early and later invasive prenatal procedures compare total fetal loss rate (spontaneous loss, procedure-related loss, termination of pregnancy due to diagnosis) from a predetermined gestational age rather than postprocedural loss because the background fetal loss is higher in earlier gestation. This approach eliminates any bias that may occur when comparing procedures performed at significantly different gestational ages and also takes into account karyotypically abnormal embryos that miscarry before an amniocentesis or an elective termination following CVS. Just comparing postprocedural fetal loss rates would be otherwise confounding.

42.6.1 Chorion Villus Sampling versus Mid-trimester Amniocentesis

Chorion villus sampling compared to mid-trimester amniocentesis has received extensive evaluation in three randomised trials and one large case-control study.[11,13–16] No significant increased risk of total pregnancy losses was found in the CVS group compared to the amniocentesis group in three of these studies.[11,14,15] In the early Canadian and US studies, CVS was performed transcervically and both studies were undertaken when many operators were still gaining experience with the procedure.[13–15] The MRC–European multicentre randomised CVS trial was associated with a significant excess loss rate of 4.6% in the CVS group compared to the amniocentesis group.[16] In this study, CVS was performed by several different methods. A possible explanation for the different results found in the MRC–European trial is that loss rate may be higher in less experienced centres.[17] Many centres in that study contributed very few patients, which may reflect less experience in CVS when the study was performed. Also of interest is that the largest contributing centre showed no excess loss rate in the CVS group compared with the amniocentesis group.[16] As with all surgical procedures, the experience of the operators is a major determinant of risk.

42.6.2 Transabdominal versus Transcervical Chorion Villus Sampling

Comparison of transabdominal and transcervical CVS has shown both procedures to be equally safe and accurate in their prediction (diagnostic accuracy of 97.5–99.6%).[5,14,17–19] The randomised, prospective study conducted in the USA found no difference in the postprocedural pregnancy losses between the two approaches.[19] Of interest is that the overall postprocedural fetal loss rate of 2.5% was 0.8% lower[19] than that found in the initial USA study, which compared CVS to second-trimester amniocentesis.[15] As the difference in fetal loss rate between amniocentesis and CVS was just 0.8% in the first USA study,[15] this suggests that when centres are becoming equivalently experienced, amniocentesis and CVS may have the same risk of pregnancy loss.[19]

Some studies have indicated a decreased procedural risk for fetal loss with transabdominal CVS.[11,20] In a randomised study, transcervical CVS – the procedure for which the conducting centre had less experience – had a relative fetal loss risk of 1.7 compared with either transabdominal CVS or mid-trimester amniocentesis, whereas no difference was found between the two latter procedures.[11]

However, other investigators found that fetal loss following transcervical CVS compared favourably with the transabdominal approach.[17] There is a learning curve for each technique of CVS and, once achieved, expertise will require constant practice to maintain the desired standard.[17]

In experienced operators' hands, it is estimated that the fetal loss rate is about 1% by transcervical intervention. This is similar to that for first-trimester transabdominal villus sampling and late amniocentesis, but better than that for early (less than 13 weeks) amniocentesis, which no longer can be viewed as an alternative to first-trimester CVS.[21]

42.6.3 Spotting and Infections

A difference between the two techniques is that the transcervical technique results in a greater risk of postprocedural spotting and minimal bleeding, while the transabdominal technique increases uterine discomfort with cramps. Spotting of blood after cervical instrumentation is observed in 12.1% of cases (D.T.Y. Liu et al., unpublished observations). This spotting, often of cervical origin, can last for a few days, but we have not found an association with increased obstetric complications. It makes good sense not to provoke the situation by excessive exercise, nor to engage in coital activity while bleeding is still evident. Vaginal infection is understandably an issue of concern when a transcervical route is chosen. Experience from several centres and our own 1000 consecutive bacteriological examinations of cervical swabs indicated that the risk of introducing infection is not significant. The cervix, however, should be cleansed with an antiseptic lotion prior to sampling. Following this simple precautionary step, neither maternal infection nor fetal loss due to infection exerts a major influence on the outcome of over 2000 of our procedures. Understandably, when vaginal infection is suspected or evident, bacteriological examination with cervical swabs and prescription of antibiotics are advised. These steps are pertinent both for transabdominal and transcervical sampling. Infection also compromises cytocultures; therefore, where this is likely, the cytogeneticists must be informed. Maternal evaluation for infection indicates that a low rate of bacteraemia can follow CVS, so antibiotic prophylaxis is recommended for women with abnormal cardiac valves.

42.6.4 Prenatal Diagnosis in Twin Gestations

Prenatal diagnosis in twin gestations and higher-order multiple gestations poses particular difficulties in terms of safety and technique of invasive procedures, interpretation of laboratory results, and the dilemmas produced by the finding of discordant abnormality. Prenatal diagnosis by both CVS and amniocentesis can be safely performed in multiple pregnancy with a similar accuracy.[7] Although total fetal loss after amniocentesis in a twin pregnancy is at least double that for a singleton, much of this additional risk is probably secondary to the inherent hazards of twins and not procedure-related. In experienced centres, CVS is equally safe and efficacious, and allows an earlier diagnosis, which may be beneficial when discordant results are found, because selective fetal reduction is safer and technically easier in the first trimester.

42.6.5 Confined Placental Mosaicism and Uniparental Disomy

Evaluation of the safety and accuracy of CVS subsequently shifted focus. Questions concerning the clinical significance of maternal cell contamination, confined placental mosaicism, uniparental disomy, and possible associations between vascular disruptive limb abnormalities and CVS when the procedure is performed at gestational ages prior to 9 weeks have been raised.

Confined placental or chorionic mosaicism is defined as a discrepancy between the karyotype in the chorionic and fetal tissues. It was first described in 1983 and has been shown in about 1% of CVS.[5] Confined chorionic mosaicism originates generally from the cytotrophoblasts that cover the chorionic villus. These cells are dividing rapidly and may have chromosomal or molecular errors that are not representative of the fetal status. Confined chorionic mosaicism can be confirmed only when a normal karyotype from the amniocytes is found after an additional amniocentesis.[5] Cordocentesis may be necessary in certain specific chromosomal situations to clarify the discrepancy. More reliable in the prediction of the fetal karyotype is cytogenetic analysis of fibroblasts grown in long-term cultures from the mesenchymal core of the chorionic villus.[5,22]

Chorion villus sampling mosaicism usually represents an abnormal cell line confined to the placenta, which often involves chromosomal trisomy.[5,23] Such mosaicism may occur when there is complete dichotomy between a trisomic karyotype in the placenta and a normal diploid fetus or when both diploid and trisomic components are present within the placenta. Gestations with pure or significant trisomy in placental lineages associated with a diploid fetal karyotype probably result from a trisomic zygote that has lost one copy of the trisomic chromosome in the embryonic progenitor cell during cleavage, a phenomenon that has been called trisomic rescue.[23,24] Uniparental disomy would be expected to occur in one-third of such cases. Uniparental disomy – both copies of one chromosome pair inherited from the same parent instead of the usual one chromosome from each parent – in the fetus may be associated with confined placental mosaicism for certain chromosomes.[24] Trisomy of chromosomes 7, 9, 15 and 16 are the most common among gestations with these dichotomic confined placental mosaicisms.[5,23] Pregnancies with trisomy 16 confined to the placenta are associated with intrauterine growth restriction, low birth weight or fetal death, and are correlated with high levels of trisomic cells in the term placenta.[23] For these reasons, careful follow-up with medical and ultrasound examination for fetal growth is strongly recommended when confined placental mosaicism is identified.

Contamination by maternal decidual tissue is always a potential problem, but it can be minimised with very careful attention to cleaning the chorionic villi of any maternal decidual cells under the dissecting microscope prior to tissue culturing.[5,22] Long-term tissue culturing increases the contamination risk if villi are not appropriately cleaned. This has not posed a significant problem in most cytogenetic laboratories with experience in CVS, but may be a problem in smaller centres with a reduced patient load.[22]

42.6.6 Teratogenicity of Chorion Villus Sampling

A cluster of vascular disruptive anomalies (oromandibular-limb hypogenesis syndrome and limb reduction defects) was reported in 1991 in pregnancies exposed to CVS at 55–66 days' gestation or earlier. This was further supported in different countries by both cohort and case-control studies in which a gestation-specific gradient of risk was found.[6] To evaluate the risk for limb or other defects, an international registry of CVS was established by the World Health Organisation committee on CVS in 1992. The consensus of data based on 138 000 infants born after CVS does not support any increased risk or specific pattern of limb defects if CVS is performed after the ninth week of gestation.[17] However, the potential teratogenicity of CVS after 10 weeks' gestation is still controversial and continues to be debated.[6] The existing evidence suggests a continuum of risk for transverse limb deficiency following CVS; the risk diminishing with advancing gestation from values perhaps 10–20 fold above background before 9 weeks, to levels approaching background at 10–11

weeks and beyond. Thus, it appears that anxiety about fetal limb defects is unfounded when sampling is conducted after the stage of major organogenesis (after 9–10 weeks). However, women should be made aware that there is a natural limb defect rate of 6–7 per 10 000 births in the general population.[6,17]

42.7 Conclusions

Over the past decade, large collaborative studies on CVS performed in the first trimester have shown that it has a similar safety and accuracy to mid-trimester amniocentesis, and compares favourably to early amniocentesis. There remain some controversies regarding its usefulness in multiple gestations, the clinical significance of confined placental mosaicism, and possible teratogenicity of CVS. However, first-trimester CVS is now an established alternative to mid-trimester amniocentesis for prenatal diagnosis.

References

1. Stranc LC, Evans JA, Hamerton JL (1997) Chorionic villus sampling and amniocentesis for prenatal diagnosis. Lancet 349:711–714
2. Bui T-H, Jones DRE (1998) Stem cell transplantation into the fetal recipient: challenges and prospects. Curr Opin Obstet Gynaecol 10:105–108
3. Snijders RJ, Noble P, Sebire N et al. (1998) UK multicentre project on assessment of risk of trisomy 21 by maternal age and fetal nuchal-translucency thickness at 10–14 weeks of gestation. Fetal Medicine Foundation First Trimester Screening Group. Lancet 352:343–346
4. Haddow JE, Polamaki GE, Knight GJ et al. (1998) Screening of maternal serum for fetal Down's syndrome in the first trimester. N Engl J Med 338:955–961
5. Hahnemann JM, Vejerslev LO (1997) Accuracy of cytogenetic findings on CVS - diagnostic consequences of CVS mosaicism and non-mosaic discrepancy in centres contributing to EUCROMIC 1986–1992. Prenat Diagn 17:801–820
6. Firth H (1997) Chorion villus sampling and limb deficiency - cause or coincidence? Prenat Diagn 17:1313–1330
7. Wapner RJ (1995) Genetic diagnosis in multiple pregnancies. Semin Perinatol 19:351–362
8. Liu DTY, Jeavons B, Pearson D et al. (1988) Patient experience of transcervical chorion villus sampling as an out-patient procedure. J Psychosomat Obstet Gynaecol 8:113–118
9. Liu DTY, Agbaje R, Preston C et al. (1991) Intraplacental sonolucent spaces: incidences and relevance to chorionic villus sampling. Prenat Diagn 11:805–808
10. Fortuny A, Borrell A, Soler A et al. (1995) Chorionic villus sampling by biopsy forceps. Results of 1580 procedures from a single centre. Prenat Diagn 15:541–550
11. Smidt-Jensen S, Permin M, Philip J et al. (1992) Randomized comparison of amniocentesis and transabdominal and transcervical chorionic villus sampling. Lancet 340:1237–1244
12. Liu DTY, Jeavons B, Preston C et al. (1987) A prospective study of spontaneous miscarriage in ultrasonically normal pregnancies and relevance to chorion villus sampling. Prenat Diagn 7:223–227

13. Canadian Collaborative CVS-Amniocentesis Clinical Trial Group (1989) Multicenter randomized clinical trial of chorion villus sampling and amniocentesis: first report. Lancet i:1–7

14. Lippman A, Tomkins DT, Shine J et al. and the Canadian Collaborative CVS-Amniocentesis Clinical Trial Group (1992) Canadian multicentre randomised clinical trial of chorion villus sampling and amniocentesis: final report. Prenat Diagn 12:385–467

15. Rhoads GG, Jackson LG, Schlesselman SE et al. (1989) The safety and efficacy of chorionic villus sampling for early pregnancy diagnosis of cytogenetic abnormalities. N Engl J Med 320:609–663

16. Medical Research Council Working Party on the Evaluation of Chorion Villus Sampling (1991) Medical Research Council European trial of chorion villus sampling. Lancet 337:1491–1499

17. Kuliev A, Jackson L, Froster U et al. (1996) Chorionic villus safety. Am J Obstet Gynecol 174:807–811

18. Brambati B, Terzian E, Tognoni G (1991) Randomized clinical trial of transabdominal versus transcervical chorionic villus sampling methods. Prenat Diagn 11:285–293

19. Jackson LG, Zachary JM, Fowler SE et al. and the US National Institute of Child Health and Human Development Chorionic-Villus Sampling and Amniocentesis Study Group (1992) A randomized comparison of transcervical and transabdominal chorionic-villus sampling. N Engl J Med 327:594–598

20. Chueh JT, Goldberg JD, Wohlferd MM et al. (1995) Comparison of transcervical and transabdominal chorionic villus sampling loss rates in nine thousand cases from a single center. Am J Obstet Gynecol 173:1277–1282

21. The Canadian Early and Mid-trimester Amniocentesis Trial (CEMAT) group: randomized trial to assess safety and fetal outcome of early and mid-trimester amniocentesis. Lancet 351:242–247

22. Ledbetter DH, Zachary JM, Simpson JL et al. (1992) Cytogenetic results from the US Collaborative Study on CVS. Prenat Diagn 12:317–345

23. Robinson WP, Barrett IJ, Bernard L et al. (1997) Meiotic origin of trisomy in confined placental mosaicism is correlated with presence of fetal uniparental disomy, high levels of trisomy in trophoblast, and increased risk of fetal intrauterine growth restriction. Am J Hum Genet 60:917–927

24. Ledbetter DH, Engel E (1995) Uniparental disomy in humans: development of an imprinting map and its implications for prenatal diagnosis. Hum Mol Genet 4:1757–1764

Chapter 43
Obstetric Endoscopy

Eduard Gratacós, Yves Ville and Jan Deprest

43.1 Introduction

Fetoscopy was introduced in fetal medicine in the 1970s as an invasive technique for the diagnosis of fetal malformations or to guide invasive procedures. Advances in high-resolution ultrasound imaging made the use of fetoscopy unnecessary for these indications and the technique was abandoned during the 1980s. Several changes have contributed to the reintroduction of fetoscopy in fetal medicine. Endoscopy has evolved technically and become less invasive with the development of new instruments and smaller endoscopes, and its surgical possibilities have increased substantially as a result of video-endoscopic technology. In addition, knowledge about the pathophysiology and natural history of fetal diseases has made it possible to identify conditions in which surgical intervention on the fetus or its adnexae could prevent fetal death or irreversible neonatal damage. Fetoscopy may allow these operations to be performed by minimally invasive access, overcoming important complications associated with open fetal surgery. However, fetoscopy also has limitations and there is still much scope for research. Over the past years, a few indications for fetoscopy have gained acceptance in fetal medicine. Most operative fetoscopies involve operations on the placenta, cord or membranes, which is regarded as "obstetric" endoscopy, but a few fetoscopic surgical procedures on the fetus have already been performed.

In this chapter we will focus on obstetric endoscopy, its indications and associated complications. Preliminary experience and potential future applications of endoscopic fetal surgery are also discussed.

43.2 Technical Aspects of Fetoscopy

43.2.1 Endoscopes

Fetoscopes combine a small diameter to minimise the access diameter with a sufficient length to bridge the maternal abdominal wall and span the whole distance of the amniotic cavity. Over the past years the quality and resolution of the endoscopes have improved, and endoscopes with up to 50 000 pixels are already being marketed. Fibre-endoscopes with diameters from 1.2 to 2.3 mm and a working length of 25 cm or more and a 0 angle of view are now used (Figure 43.1). Fibre-optics are normally preferred over rod-lenses for image and light transmission, because they allow smaller diameters and the scopes can be bent to a certain degree. A curved fetoscope may improve the angle of vision over the placenta and membranes when the insertion is not perpendicular to the area of interest (Figure 43.1).

43.2.2 Uterine Access: Insertion and Fixation of the Cannula and Intruments

Fetoscopy can be performed percutaneously or through a maternal laparotomy of variable size. Single-port procedures are usually done through a percutaneous access, where a sheath loaded with a sharp trocar is introduced under ultrasound guidance. In certain situations or when more than one port is needed, displacement of the uterus with respect to a cannula fixed in the abdominal wall could produce wall lacerations and bleeding. A mini- or formal laparotomy is then preferred by some surgeons to avoid this risk. Thus, in cases of anterior placenta, for laser coagulation of placental vessels, Deprest et al[1] have suggested performing a mini-laparotomy to access the uterus through the uterine fundus or lateral wall, although Ville et al[2] overcome this difficulty by a very lateral insertion of the endoscope under Doppler visualisation of uterine vessels. For more complex fetoscopic operations involving multiple uterine ports, the need for laparotomy seems more indisputable and in the few

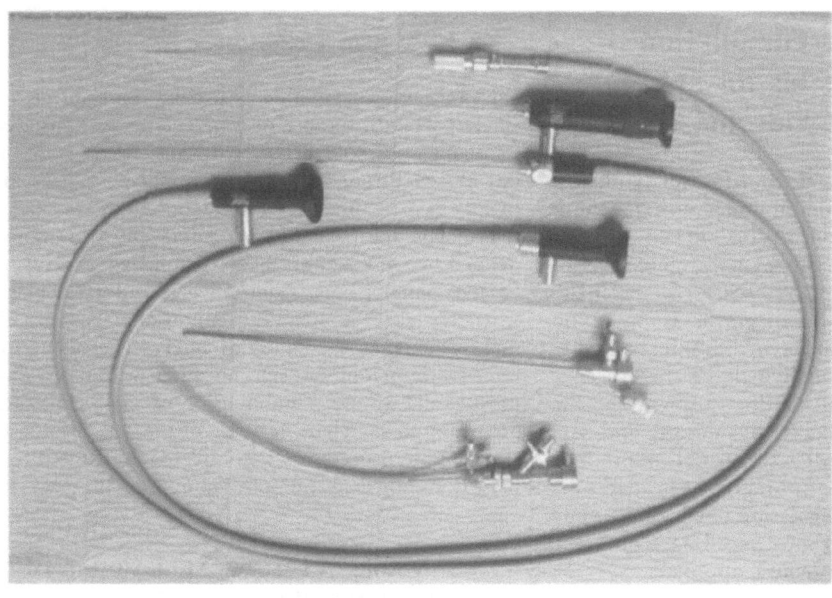

Figure 43.1. Overview of our fibre-optic endoscopes: 1.0 and 2.0 mm 0 fibre scopes with deported eyepieces, 1.2 mm endoscope with conventional eyepiece. Straight and curved sheaths are shown at the bottom of the image.

cases reported to date,[3,4] a midline laparotomy has been performed.

In single-port procedures the sheath accommodating the endoscope can be inserted directly into the amniotic cavity. The use of an external cannula offers substantial advantages, as it avoids friction with the uterine wall and allows the use of different instruments through the same insertion. The use of external cannulas varies between groups. Some use them systematically, while others do so only in complex procedures due to an anterior placenta or when the use of different scopes or instruments in the same procedure is expected. We use vascular access cannulas as external cannulas; these are available in any diameter between 5 and 15 Fr (1.6–5 mm). Initially, uterine insertion was performed with the Seldinger technique, resulting in gradual expansion of the myometrial and membrane stab wound. More recently, purpose-designed uterine trocars in various diameters to fit the cannulas have been developed within the Eurofoetus programme[5] and are now available. These trocars simplify substantially the insertion procedure and are rapidly gaining acceptance. The diameter of the external cannula is chosen according to the largest instrument to be used during the procedure. The cannulas offer a leakproof seal and a plastic side channel for infusion or removal of fluid. They offer the additional advantage of being flexible, which allows the insertion of curved instrumentation.

43.2.3 Image Display and Distension Media

The fetoscope is connected to a good-quality light source and a video camera. Endoscopic vision is normally limited to a few centimetres depth and therefore in many cases ultrasound guidance to complement the procedure becomes essential. The fetoscopic images can be combined on the same screen with real-time ultrasound images via a so-called Twin-video system (Karl Storz, Brussels, Belgium).

In most clinical applications, physiological saline solution at body temperature is used when amniotic fluid needs to be replaced in order to improve vision, or to create the necessary working space. A fluid environment is satisfactory for endoscopic procedures on fetal adnexae, but it limits surgical performance for more complex operations on the fetus. Working with gas as a distension medium facilitates endoscopic surgery significantly, but there are some concerns regarding fetal safety. Using gas for uterine distension is a tempting solution to reduce operating time and improve surgical performance in fetal surgery. Carbon dioxide amniodistension has been reported in the first four attempts of in-utero fetoscopic covering of myelomeningocele.[4] However, use of this gas in fetoscopic surgery may raise safety concerns. Amniodistension with CO_2 rapidly induces fetal acidosis and hypercarbia in fetal sheep,[6] even in the presence of compensatory maternal hypocarbia induced by aggressive maternal hyperventilation.[7] Alternative gases to CO_2, such as helium and N_2O, have been used in human endoscopy, and they might be good candidates for amniodistension. We recently demonstrated that, in fetal sheep, N_2O amniodistension did not induce any demonstrable metabolic fetal effects, but resulted in a 60% reduction in operation length and bleeding episodes compared to fluid amniodistension.[8]

43.3 Nd:YAG Laser Coagulation of Placental Vessels for Feto-fetal Transfusion Syndrome

Pre-viable severe feto-fetal transfusion syndrome (FFTS) is the most common indication for fetoscopy. This complication occurs in 10–15% of monochorionic multiple pregnancies, and is associated with an almost 100% risk of perinatal mortality.[9] The ultrasound diagnosis is based on monochorionicity and the polyhydramnios–oligohydramnios sequence. It usually includes the presence of a distended fetal bladder in the recipient and the absence of bladder filling in the donor, and less frequently discordant fetal sizes. Serial amniodrainage has been the mainstay of therapy for FFTS over the past decade. Laser coagulation of chorionic plate vessels has recently been introduced as a probably more cause-oriented therapeutic approach.

43.3.1 The Rationale for Laser Coagulation

Placental vascular communications, and therefore bilateral blood transfer, exist in virtually all monochorionic pregnancies, but only about 15% of these women present with FFTS. The development of the syndrome is likely to be associated with a particular vascular pattern favouring a unidirectional imbalance in net blood flow between the fetuses. Anatomical placental studies suggest that FFTS is characterised by the presence of one (or a few) arterio-venous anastomosis in combination with a paucity of arterio-arterious or veno-venous anastomoses.[10] These arterio-arterious and veno-venous communications are normally found in uncomplicated monochorionic pregnancies where they allow flow in either direction and can therefore compensate any blood transfer imbalance due to unidirectional arterio-venous communications.

Indeed, an arterio-venous anastomosis is not a real anatomical anastomosis but a cotyledon that is fed by an artery from one fetus and drained by a vein from the other. The afferent and efferent branches of this shared cotyledon run over the placental surface and plunge into the chorionic plate almost at the same point (Figure 43.2a). Interruption of these vessels should eliminate the abnormal communication and therefore the pathological inter-twin blood transfer. Our group has recently demonstrated in an experimental animal model that laser coagulation of vessels feeding the cotyledon at the place where they overrun the chorionic plate leads to its functional elimination.[11] Recent data from perfusion studies in FFTS cases treated by laser confirm effective separation of twin circulations.[12]

43.3.2 Surgical Techniques

Nd:YAG laser coagulation is usually done through a single port with the use of a percutaneously inserted fetoscope. A 400–600 m Nd:YAG laser fibre is introduced through the operative sheath. There are mainly two methods for coagulation. Vessels can be selected on the basis of their fetoscopic appearance, defined by De Lia et al[12] as fetoscopic laser occlusion of chorioangiopagus. Alternatively, and particularly when the view or operating conditions are suboptimal, systematic coagulation of all vessels crossing the inter-twin membrane can be carried out.[2] Today, most units use a combination of both methods according to the characteristics of the case. The laser coagulation procedure is completed by amniodrainage until normalisation of the amniotic fluid occurs.

43.3.3 Results of Laser Coagulation in Feto-fetal Transfusion Syndrome

Fetal survival following laser coagulation has been consistently reported to be around 55–68% with a risk of about 5% for neurological injury in survivors.[2,12–15] These results appear to compare favourably with those reported for amniodrainage. Both a retrospective compilation of amniodrainage series published until 1997,[16] as well as a recently reported prospective multicentre study,[17] yielded a 60% survival rate with about 19% risk for neurological impairment. In the best available comparison to date, the results of laser (n = 73) at one institution were prospectively compared with those of amniodrainage (n = 43) at another.[13] The inclusion criteria for both groups were the same, all cases being severe pre-viable FFTS of comparable gestational age at diagnosis. The survival rate and neurological morbidity for the laser group were 61 and 6% respectively, and those of amniodrainage 51 and 19%. Recently, a randomised multicentre trial comparing laser with amniodrainage in the management of FFTS (http://www.eurofoetus.org) has been set up in the context of the Eurofoetus programme, a research project supported by the European Commission.[5]

43.4 Fetoscopy for Cord Occlusion in Complicated Monochorionic Twins

43.4.1 The Rationale and Different Techniques for Cord Occlusion

Selective feticide may be indicated in monochorionic twins for several reasons. Probably the most

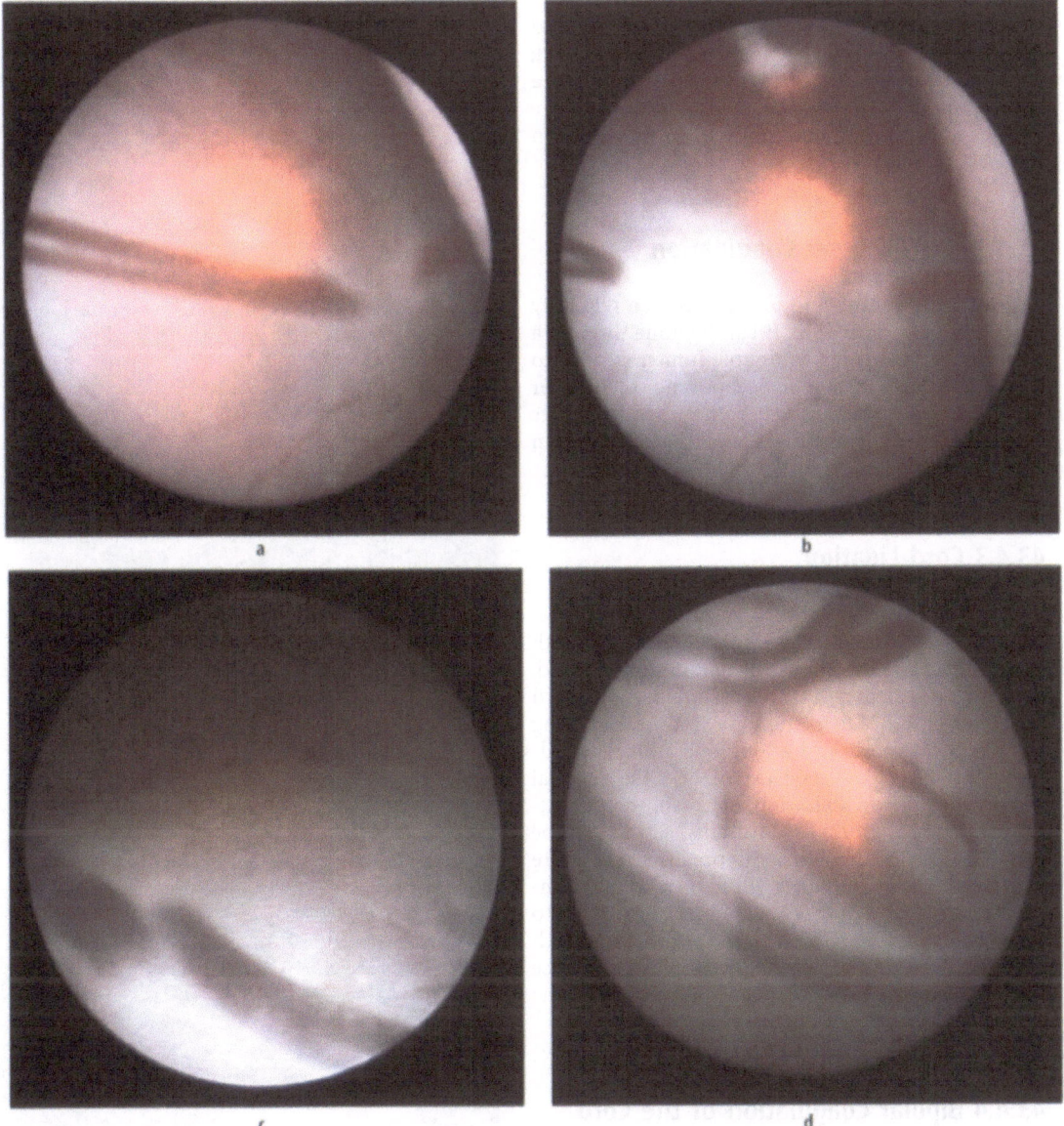

Figure 43.2. Fetoscopic appearance of anastomosing vessels on a monochorionic placenta. Artery-to-vein anastomosis prior to (a) and after (b) coagulation. c Artery-to-artery anastomosis. d Superficial chorionic plate vessels crossing the intertwin membrane.

common and clear-cut indication is the so-called "twin reversed arterial perfusion" sequence, where a normal twin acts as a pump for an acardiac co-twin through an arterio-arterial anastomosis. In severe cases, the situation carries a substantial risk for fetal death or neurological damage in the normal fetus. Monochorionic pregnancies where one fetus presents with a major anomaly are another indication for selective feticide, because of the high risk of acute feto-fetal transfusion in case of fetal death of the affected twin. Finally, FFTS cases refractory to therapy and/or with impending fetal demise may

also benefit from selective feticide. The risk of embolisation to the co-twin makes it impossible to use conventional feticide techniques with intracardiac injection of potassium chloride in monochorionic pregnancies. An additional reason is the already mentioned risk of acute transfusion after death of one fetus. The vascular communication between both fetuses must therefore be interrupted completely and permanently, and occlusion of the umbilical cord or major fetal vessels seems the most logical approach. Ultrasound-guided sclerosation or embolisation of major fetal vessels with different substances has been reported, but the efficacy and safety of this method has not been demonstrated; the largest series reported by Denbow et al[18] had a 70% failure rate. Umbilical cord occlusion therefore appears to be the best option for selective feticide in monochorionic twins.

43.4.2 Nd:YAG Laser Coagulation

Nd:YAG laser coagulation of the cord is a relatively quick and easy procedure. It can be done through a single insertion, using a double-lumen needle to accommodate a 1.0 mm fetoscope and 400m laser fibre. It has been performed from 16 weeks but its efficacy is limited above 20–22 weeks' gestation or in extremely hydropic cords,[19] where it tends to fail.

43.4.3 Cord Ligation

Ligation of the umbilical cord results in immediate, complete and permanent interruption of both arterial and venous flow in the umbilical cord, whatever its diameter. However, fetoscopic cord ligation is usually a demanding procedure, involving the use of two ports and a long operation. According to available published experience, the survival rate in the co-twin following successful cord ligation is 71% (n = 15/21).[20] Mortality can largely be explained by the high risk of preterm premature rupture of the membranes (PPROM), which complicates up to 47% of cases, with about 30% prior to 32 weeks' gestation. Given these results, the search for other techniques that could simplify or reduce the invasiveness of cord ligation while achieving the same efficacy has continued.

43.4.4 Bipolar Coagulation of the Cord

Bipolar coagulation is not necessarily an endoscopic procedure, as it can be performed entirely under ultrasound guidance through a single port. We prefer to combine the ultrasound view with endoscopic assessment prior to, during and after the procedure (Figure 43.3). This is done through the same port, which avoids the need for a second port insertion. However, in cases of difficult performance under ultrasonographic control alone, a second port may be added for fetoscopy, to help guide the procedure. The cord can be grasped through the membranes, avoiding the surgical creation of monoamniotic twins. In a recently reported series with ten cases,[21] including twin reversed arterial perfusion sequences and discordant monochorionic twin gestations up to 26 weeks' gestation, the procedure

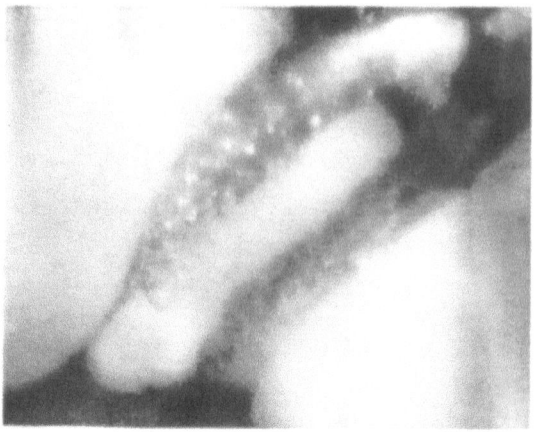

a

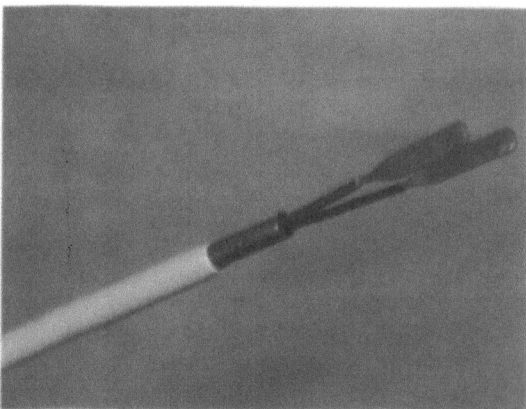

b

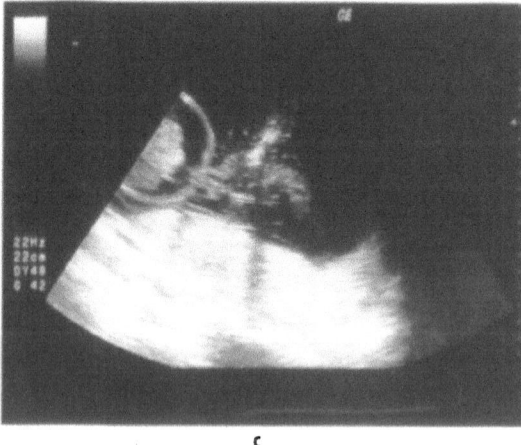

c

Figure 43.3. a Technique of fetoscopic cord coagulation, using a 3 mm bipolar forceps. **b** Smaller instruments are now available, like this 7.0 Fr (2.3mm) bipolar forceps, which can be manipulated under ultrasound control. **c** Ultrasound image: local heat production is visible as turbulence and steam bubbles.

was successful in all cases and operating time was usually limited to 15 minutes. Preterm premature rupture of the membranes with fetal or neonatal death occurred in two cases (20%), with the remaining eight cases delivering at a mean of 35 weeks' gestation. Survival rate after this preliminary experience is apparently similar to cord ligation. However, in our opinion, the simpler nature of this procedure makes it preferable to cord ligation, even if two ports must be used. It is expected that fewer associated complications and better survival rates will be observed after the learning curve. We have demonstrated the safety and performance of bipolar forceps as small as 2.4 mm in animal experiments.[22] In our clinical experience, the diameter of the forceps used has decreased over time, and now forceps with diameters ranging from 2.4 to 2.7 mm are being used.

43.4.5 Clinical Algorithm for Cord Occlusion

Our current algorithm for cord occlusion is as follows.[23] In cases eligible for cord occlusion before 21 weeks' gestation, micro-endoscopy-guided Nd: YAG laser coagulation is attempted initially. If the laser is not effective or at later gestational ages, bipolar cord coagulation is performed, first under sonographic guidance only and if necessary under endoscopic control. Sono-endoscopic cord ligation is kept as a second option if the former fails.

43.5 Lysis of Amniotic Bands

Amniotic band syndrome is a sporadic condition that occurs in 1 : 1200–1 : 15 000 live births, carrying a high risk for deformities of the fetus, mainly consisting of limb amputation at variable levels. Experimental work in sheep has shown that release of the constriction can restore anatomy and function of the limb.[24] The diagnosis of amniotic bands can be made by ultrasound, and in selected cases where other anomalies are ruled out, fetoscopic liberation of amniotic bands could be performed early enough to prevent irreversible limb damage. Quintero has reported treatment of two cases using endoscopic techniques.[25] Lysis of bands at 22 and 23 weeks respectively, restored adequate blood flow distal to the obstruction, and only mild or minimal limb dysfunction was present at birth.

43.6 Complications of Fetoscopic Procedures

43.6.1 Iatrogenic Preterm Premature Rupture of Membranes

The most common complication of any fetoscopic procedure is iatrogenic PPROM. There are no formal studies evaluating the risk factors for iatrogenic PPROM, but on the basis of current clinical experience its incidence appears to increase with the duration, complexity and number of ports used in the procedure. Thus, laser coagulation for FFTS is associated with a 10% incidence that has not decreased after the learning curve.[2,13] As previously stated, cord ligation was complicated with iatrogenic PPROM in up to 47% of cases in the largest series reported to date.[20] Finally, the incidence of PPROM in the first eight published cases of tracheal occlusion for congenital diaphragmatic hernia, a procedure involving the use of four ports, was 62% (5/8).[3] The influence of other factors such as the use of and volume of amnioinfusion, previous invasive procedures, haemorrhage, underlying conditions or pre-existing contractions may also be relevant, but it is more difficult to estimate from available published clinical experience. The above figures illustrate the importance of iatrogenic PPROM in fetoscopy and the need to prevent or minimise this complication to allow further implementation of fetoscopy for more complex operations.

The most intuitive way to approach this problem would be to seal the entry site at the time of the intervention. The material used for sealing should ideally promote wound repair mechanisms. Several techniques have been proposed or used, trying to seal the traumatic membrane defect and reduce the incidence of iatrogenic PPROM, but only a few of them have been studied in animal or in-vitro experiments. Quintero has reported preliminary experience with the use of amnioinfused cryoprecipitate and platelets in seven cases of PPROM after fetoscopy or amniocentesis.[26] Cessation of amniorrhoea was observed in three cases, but two unexplained fetal deaths occurred shortly after treatment.

Our group has demonstrated the feasibility of using collagen plugs to seal the fetoscopic access site in primates[27] and the efficacy of this method to seal single membrane defects and prevent oligohydramnios-related pulmonary hypoplasia in a fetal rabbit model.[28] However, the technique has not been tested formally for long periods of time or in humans.

Recent results might even question the theoretical basis for the use of plugs in fetal membranes. While it is uncertain whether the fetal membranes can indeed heal, recent experiments conducted by our group suggest that a potential mechanism to avoid leakage after uterine trauma could be the ability of amnion and chorion to glide over each other.[29] This could facilitate a relative displacement of the respective hole at each membrane, which would reduce or even eliminate the resulting membrane defect. If this was true, the use of plugs could be harmful by fixing amnion and chorion attached to the uterine wall. It is expected that future clinical experience and research will help clarify this matter.

In any case, regardless of the potential development of solutions that could minimise the risk, PPROM will probably remain a significant complication when several ports are inserted in the amniotic cavity. This emphasises the need for surgical approaches that minimise the size and number of trocar insertions.

43.6.2 Other Complications and the Launch of a Collaborative Registry

Possibly, the most common complication of fetoscopy after iatrogenic PPROM is uterine wall bleeding.[30] Haemorrhage is normally mild and self-limited, although in some cases intra-amniotic bleeding can hamper the endoscopic view and render fetoscopic surgery impossible. Serious intra-abdominal bleeding after a percutaneous procedure is very uncommon, but has been reported,[2] requiring laparotomy and blood transfusion. This complication is obviously very unlikely if the procedure is carried out through a mini- or formal laparotomy, as it can be identified early and controlled.

Chorioamnionitis appears to be an uncommon complication.[2] Amniotic fluid embolism is another theoretical complication of operative fetoscopy, but has not been reported yet. Other maternal complications can be related in particular to the surgical procedure on the fetus or placenta and cord. For instance, in our experience, a maternal mirror syndrome consisting of generalised oedema and oliguria has occurred following a laser procedure for FFTS. This illustrates the possibility of uncommon but serious complications associated with operative fetoscopy in general or with a particular fetoscopic operation. Patients should be counselled likewise and monitored closely for any of these complications. The implementation of new fetoscopic operations involving exchange of large amounts of fluid or uterine distension with gas might result in new complications, but further experience is required. The small number of procedures carried out in a single centre will considerably limit estimates on rare complications. A database has recently been set up for the prospective and multicollaborative collection of data, with support from the European Commission, making "fetoscopy" registry possible.[5] Data can be entered via the internet and the registry is open to all centres worldwide (http://www.eurofoetus.org).

43.7 Embryofetoscopy and Fetoscopy in the First Trimester of Pregnancy

There are a few indications for diagnostic fetoscopy in the first trimester of pregnancy. At these gesta-tional ages, technical features of endoscopes, indications and associated complications probably differ from fetoscopy in the second trimester. Embryoscopes have a smaller diameter than fetoscopes used in the second trimester. Today, fibre-optics of 0.5–1.0 mm are available. These optics are semi-flexible, contain 10 000 pixels or more, and have a 70 field of vision. Because of the limited field of view, the endoscope must be directed to the area of interest under ultrasound. Introduction is done through a single 18-gauge needle or a double needle to allow aspiration or the use of other instrumentation.

The term embryofetoscopy is probably more appropriate before 12 weeks of gestation, while fetoscopy can be used for procedures at later gestational ages.[23] However, a more relevant differentiation relates to the embryonic space accessed. Early in gestation, before the chorion and amnion leaves fuse, the exocoelomic space allows for insertion of a microendoscope and observation of the embryo without entering the amniotic cavity. This technique can be done transcervically or transabdominally, although the first approach has almost been abandoned. The exocoelomic approach should reduce the incidence of complications related to membrane disruption, as the amnion is not wounded, although no figures are yet available in the literature. Later than 10 weeks' gestation, the amniotic cavity must be accessed through a transabdominal puncture. The rate and type of complications in the latter case should be similar to those of early amniocentesis, but further experience is required to estimate risks.

Extracoelomic embryofetoscopy can be offered to a very small number of selected families at high risk for genetic conditions. On the other hand, early sonographic suspicion of fetal anomalies at 11–14 weeks' gestation can be confirmed or ruled out by intra-amniotic fetoscopy. At this time the procedure can be combined with an amniocentesis. First-trimester fetoscopy is being used for early diagnosis in a limited but increasing number of congenital malformations.[31]

43.8 Endoscopic Fetal Surgery

Fetoscopy has the theoretical advantage of minimally invasive access, which should reduce the likelihood of preterm delivery and other complications associated with the need for a hysterotomy in open fetal surgery. Probably the most relevant experience with operative fetoscopy to date is tracheal clipping for the in-utero treatment of congenital diagphragmatic hernia, which has been reported in 16 cases.[32] There were six survivors, and the fetoscopic modification of the procedure improved survival and reduced associated preterm labour compared with previous cases managed by open surgery. Before tracheal occlusion, the most experience with fetoscopy had been achieved in fetuses with fetal lower urinary tract obstruction. Laser for posterior urethral valves or placement of vesico-amniotic shunts have been performed,[33] but associated anomalies or irreversible damage prior to the therapy have limited the survival rates for this approach. Methods to identify those cases that would benefit from in-utero correction are now under evaluation. Nd:YAG laser coagulation has been used to achieve flow reduction within a sacrococcygeal teratoma of a mid-trimester fetus.[34] Neither procedure mimics the open surgical intervention, i.e. resection of the tumour, but they can alleviate the in-utero effects of the disease and prevent irreversible damage. Finally, in-utero fetoscopic covering of a myelomeningocele by glueing maternal split-thickness skin graft has been reported in four cases, with long-term infant survival in two cases.[4]

43.9 Conclusions

The experiences described above illustrate the feasibility of endoscopic fetal surgery. However, there is still much scope for research, and in the meantime some surgical procedures may be better performed through open surgery. Aside from its complications, fetoscopy poses the surgical challenge of performing complex operations on a delicate patient and in a very unfriendly environment. Reduced working space, suboptimal positioning of the surgical patient, and lack of specific instruments and surgical skills are limiting factors for operative fetoscopy. Fetoscopic operations must be carefully designed and extensive training is required. How far endoscopic fetal surgery can develop is still to be seen, but on a theoretical basis a standardised fetoscopic operation should reduce substantially the aggressiveness of open surgery. The use of surgery on the fetus might become more acceptable in the future, and new indications for fetal operations or invasive monitoring could be developed.

References

1. Deprest J, Van Schoubroeck D, Van Ballaer P et al (1998) Alternative access for fetoscopic Nd:YAG laser in TTS with anterior placenta. Ultrasound Obstet Gynecol 12:347–352
2. Ville Y, Hecher K, Gagnon A et al (1998) Endoscopic laser coagulation in the management of severe twin transfusion syndrome. Br J Obstet Gynaecol 105:446–453
3. Harrison MR, Mychaliska GB, Albanese CT et al (1998) Correction of congenital diaphragmatic hernia in utero. IX: Fetuses with poor prognosis (liver herniation and low lung-to-head ratio) can be saved by fetoscopic temporary tracheal occlusion. J Pediatr Surg 33:1017–1023
4. Bruner JP, Richards WO, Tulipan NB et al (1999) Endoscopic coverage of fetal myelomeningocele in utero. Am J Obstet Gynecol 180:153–158
5. Gratacós E, Deprest J (2000) Current experience with fetoscopy and the Eurofoetus registry for fetoscopic procedures. Eur J Obstet Gynecol Reprod Biol 92:151–159
6. Luks FI, Deprest JA, Marcus M et al (1994) Carbon dioxide pneumamnios causes acidosis in the fetal lamb. Fetal Diagn Ther 9:101–104
7. Gratacós E, Wu J, Devlieger R et al (2001) Effects of amniodistention with carbon dioxide on fetal acid-base status during fetoscopic surgery in a sheep model. Surg Endosc 15:368–372
8. Gratacós E, Wu J, Devlieger R et al (2002) Nitrous oxide amniodistention reduces operation time as compared to fluid amniodistention while inducing no changes in fetal acid-base status in a sheep model for endoscopic fetal surgery. Am J Obstet Gynecol 186:538–543
9. Blickstein I (1990) The twin–twin transfusion syndrome. Obstet Gynecol 76:14–22
10. Machin GA, Keith LG (1998) Can twin-to-twin transfusion syndrome be explained, and how is it treated? Clin Obstet Gynecol 41:104–113
11. Branisteanu-Dumitrascu I, Deprest J, Evrard V et al (1999) Time-related cotyledonary effects of laser coagulation of superficial chorionic vessels in an ovine model. Prenat Diagn 19:205–210
12. De Lia JE, Kuhlmann RS, Lopez KP (1999) Treating previable twin–twin transfusion syndrome with fetoscopic laser surgery: outcomes following the learning curve. J Perinat Med 27:61–67
13. Hecher K, Plath H, Bregenzer T et al (1999) Endoscopic laser surgery compared to serial amniocentesis in the treatment of severe twin–twin transfusion syndrome. Am J Obstet Gynecol 180:717–724
14. Gratacós E, Van Schoubroeck D, Carreras E et al Transient hydropic signs in the donor fetus after fetoscopic laser coagulation in severe twin–twin transfusion syndrome: incidence and clinical relevance. Ultrasound Obstet Gynecol, submitted
15. Quintero RA, Morales WJ, Allen MH et al (1999) Staging of twin–twin transfusion syndrome. J Perinatol 19:550–555
16. Ville Y (1997) Monochorionic twins: "les liasons dangereuses." Ultrasound Obstet Gynecol 10:82–85
17. Mari G (1998) Amnioreduction in twin–twin transfusion syndrome – a multicenter registry, evaluation of 579 procedures. Am J Obstet Gynecol 177:S28(Abstract)
18. Denbow ML, Overton TG, Duncan KR et al (1999) High failure rate of umbilical vessel occlusion by ultrasound guided injection of absolute alcohol or enbucrilate gel. Prenat Diagn 19:527–532
19. Hecher K, Hackeloër BJ, Ville Y (1997) Umbilical cord coagulation by operative microendoscopy at 16 weeks gestation in an acardiac twin. Ultrasound Obstet Gynecol 10:130–132
20. Deprest JA, Evrard VA, Van Ballaer PP et al (1998) Fetoscopic cord ligation. Eur J Obstet Gynecol Reprod Biol 81:157–164
21. Deprest J, Audibert F, Van Schoubroeck D et al (1999) Bipolar cord coagulation of the umbilical cord in complicated monochorionic twin pregnancy. Am J Obstet Gynecol 1(Suppl)
22. Yesildaglar N, Zikulnig L, Gratacós E et al (2000) Bipolar-coagulation with small diameter forceps in animal models for in utero cord obliteration. Hum Reprod 15:865–868
23. Challis D, Gratacós E, Deprest J (1999) Selective termination in monochorionic twins. J Perinat Med 27:327–338
24. Crombleholme TM, Dirkes K, Withney TM et al (1995) Amniotic band syndrome in fetal lambs. I. Fetoscopic release and morphometric outcome. J Pediatr Surg 30:974–978
25. Quintero RA, Morales WJ, Phillips J et al (1997) In utero lysis of amniotic bands. Ultrasound Obstet Gynecol 10:316–320

26. Quintero RA, Morales WJ, Allen M et al (1999) Treatment of iatrogenic previable premature rupture of membranes with intra-amniotic injection of platelets and cryoprecipitate (amniopatch): preliminary experience. Am J Obstet Gynecol 181:744–749

27. Luks FI, Deprest JA, Peers KH et al (1999) Gelatin sponge plug to seal fetoscopy port sites: technique in ovine and primate models. Am J Obstet Gynecol 181:995–996

28. Gratacós E, Wu J, Yesildaglar N et al (2000) Successful sealing of fetoscopic access sites with collagen plugs in the rabbit model. Am J Obstet Gynecol 182:142–146

29. Gratacós E, Devlieger R, Decaluwe H et al (2000) Is the angle of needle insertion influencing the created defect in human fetal membranes? Evaluation of the agreement between specialists' opinions and ex vivo observations. Am J Obstet Gynecol 182:646–649

30. Deprest J, Gratacos E (1999) Obstetrical endoscopy. Curr Opin Obstet Gynecol 11:195–203

31. Ville Y (1997) Diagnostic embryoscopy and fetoscopy in the first trimester of pregnancy. Prenat Diagn 17:1237–1246

32. Albanese C, Chiba T, Paek B et al (2000) Fetal tracheal occlusion for severe left congenital diaphragmatic hernia. Am J Obstet Gynecol 182:S182(Abstract)

33. Quintero RA, Johnson MP, Romero R et al (1995) In utero percutaneous cystoscopy in the management of fetal lower obstructive uropathy. Lancet 346:537–540

34. Hecher K, Hackelöer B-J (1996) Intra-uterine endoscopic laser surgery for fetal sacrococcygeal teratoma. Lancet 347:470

Index